Life stage group	Potassium (g/d)	Chloride (g/d)	Calcium (mg/d)	Phosphorus (mg/d)	Magnesium (mg/d)	Iron (mg/d)	Zinc (mg/d)	Selenium (µg/d)	Iodine (µg/d)	Copper (µg/d)	Manganese (mg/d)	Fluoride (mg/d)	Chromium (µg/d)	Molybdenum (µg/d)	Water (L/d)[8]
Infants															
0-6 mo	0.4*	0.18*	200*	100*	30*	0.27*	2*	15*	110*	200*	0.003*	0.01*	0.2*	2*	0.7*
6-12 mo	0.7*	0.57*	260*	275*	75*	11	3*	20*	130*	220*	0.6*	0.5*	5.5*	3*	0.8*
Children															
1-3 y	3.0*	1.5*	700	460	80	7	3	20	90	340	1.2*	0.7*	11*	17	1.3*
4-8 y	3.8*	1.9*	1,000	500	130	10	5	30	90	440	1.5*	1*	15*	22	1.7*
Males															
9-13 y	4.5*	2.3*	1,300	1,250	240	8	8	40	120	700	1.9*	2*	25*	34	2.4*
14-18 y	4.7*	2.3*	1,300	1,250	410	11	11	55	150	890	2.2*	3*	35*	43	3.3*
19-30 y	4.7*	2.3*	1,000	700	400	8	11	55	150	900	2.3*	4*	35*	45	3.7*
31-50 y	4.7*	2.3*	1,000	700	420	8	11	55	150	900	2.3*	4*	35*	45	3.7*
51-70 y	4.7*	2.0*	1,000	700	420	8	11	55	150	900	2.3*	4*	30*	45	3.7*
>70 y	4.7*	1.8*	1,200	700	420	8	11	55	150	900	2.3*	4*	30*	45	3.7*
Females															
9-13 y	4.5*	2.3*	1,300	1,250	240	8	8	40	120	700	1.6*	2*	21*	34	2.1*
14-18 y	4.7*	2.3*	1,300	1,250	360	15	9	55	150	890	1.6*	3*	24*	43	2.3*
19-30 y	4.7*	2.3*	1,000	700	310	18	8	55	150	900	1.8*	3*	25*	45	2.7*
31-50 y	4.7*	2.3*	1,000	700	320	18	8	55	150	900	1.8*	3*	25*	45	2.7*
51-70 y	4.7*	2.0*	1,200	700	320	8	8	55	150	900	1.8*	3*	20*	45	2.7*
>70 y	4.7*	1.8*	1,200	700	320	8	8	55	150	900	1.8*	3*	20*	45	2.7*
Pregnancy															
≤18 y	4.7*	2.3*	1,300	1,250	400	27	12	60	220	1,000	2.0*	3*	29*	50	3.0*
19-30 y	4.7*	2.3*	1,000	700	350	27	11	60	220	1,000	2.0*	3*	30*	50	3.0*
31-50 y	4.7*	2.3*	1,000	700	360	27	11	60	220	1,000	2.0*	3*	30*	50	3.0*
Lactation															
≤18 y	5.1*	2.3	1,300	1,250	360	10	13	70	290	1,300	2.6*	3*	44*	50	3.8*
19-30 y	5.1*	2.3	1,000	700	310	9	12	70	290	1,300	2.6*	3*	45*	50	3.8*
31-50 y	5.1*	2.3	1,000	700	320	9	12	70	290	1,300	2.6*	3*	45*	50	3.8*

Sources: Data compiled from *Dietary Reference Intakes for Calcium, Phosphorus, Magnesium, Vitamin D, and Fluoride.* Washington, DC: National Academies Press; 1997. *Dietary Reference Intakes for Thiamin, Riboflavin, Niacin, Vitamin B₆, Folate, Vitamin B₁₂, Pantothenic Acid, Biotin, and Choline.* Washington, DC: National Academies Press; 1998. *Dietary Reference Intakes for Vitamin C, Vitamin E, Selenium, and Carotenoids.* Washington, DC: National Academies Press; 2000. *Dietary Reference Intakes for Vitamin A, Vitamin K, Arsenic, Boron, Chromium, Copper, Iron, Manganese, Molybdenum, Nickel, Silicon, Vanadium, and Zinc.* Washington, DC: National Academies Press; 2000. *Dietary Reference Intakes for Water, Potassium, Sodium, Chloride, and Sulfate.* Food and Nutrition Board. Washington, DC: National Academies Press; 2005. *Dietary Reference Intakes for Calcium and Vitamin D.* Washington, DC: National Academies Press; 2011. These reports may be accessed via http://nap.edu.

HUMAN NUTRITION
Healthy Options for Life

John J.B. Anderson, PhD

Professor Emeritus
Schools of Public Health and Medicine
University of North Carolina at Chapel Hill
Chapel Hill, North Carolina

Martin M. Root, PhD

Assistant Professor
Appalachian State University
Boone, North Carolina

Sanford C. Garner, PhD

Project Manager/Senior Scientist
Integrated Laboratory Systems, Inc.
Durham, North Carolina

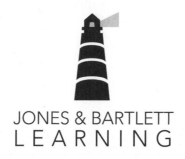

JONES & BARTLETT
LEARNING

World Headquarters
Jones & Bartlett Learning
5 Wall Street
Burlington, MA 01803
978-443-5000
info@jblearning.com
www.jblearning.com

Jones & Bartlett Learning books and products are available through most bookstores and online booksellers. To contact Jones & Bartlett Learning directly, call 800-832-0034, fax 978-443-8000, or visit our website, www.jblearning.com.

Production Credits

Chief Executive Officer: Ty Field
President: James Homer
Chief Product Officer: Eduardo Moura
Executive Publisher: William Brottmiller
Executive Editor: Rhonda Dearborn
Editorial Assistant: Sean Fabery
Associate Director of Production: Julie C. Bolduc
Production Editors: Jessica Steele Newfell, Louis C. Bruno, Jr.
Senior Marketing Manager: Andrea DeFronzo
Art Development Editor: Joanna Lundeen
Illustrations: Troy Liston
VP, Manufacturing and Inventory Control: Therese Connell
Composition: Cenveo Publisher Services
Cover Design: Kristin E. Parker
Photo Research and Permissions Coordinator: Lauren Miller
Cover Image: © iStockphoto/Thinkstock
Printing and Binding: Courier Companies
Cover Printing: Courier Companies

To order this product, use ISBN: 978-1-4496-9874-4

Library of Congress Cataloging-in-Publication Data
Anderson, John J. B. (John Joseph Baxter), 1934– author.
  Human nutrition : healthy options for life / by John J. B. Anderson, Martin M. Root, Sanford C. Garner.
    p. ; cm.
  Includes bibliographical references and index.
  ISBN 978-1-4496-4741-4 (pbk. : alk. paper)
  I. Root, Martin Menzo, 1951– author. II. Garner, Sanford C., author. III. Title.
  [DNLM: 1. Nutritional Physiological Phenomena. 2. Food. QU 145]
  RA784
  613.2—dc23
                                        2013035512

6048

Printed in the United States of America
18 17 16 15 14   10 9 8 7 6 5 4 3 2 1

We dedicate this book to our greatest supporters:
Betsey Anderson, Connie Root, and Donna Garner.

Brief Contents

Contents

Preface

The selection of foods is much more important than most of us realize, as the variety of foods we eat provide us with the nutrients and nonnutrients that allow us to grow from childhood into adulthood. Beyond foods, the size of our servings or plates requires lifetime monitoring; typically by adulthood, far too many of us consume excessive amounts of foods that contribute to common adult chronic diseases of affluence, which are detailed in this text. Healthy consumption of reasonable amounts of foods helps promote health, especially when other healthy behaviors are practiced. We can achieve this task every day of our lives through wise and judicious food selection. Although the approach followed in this text is science based, much of the material can be followed with only a rudimentary knowledge of biology and chemistry. Our emphasis has been to find the best and most reliable science and to present these findings on health and nutrition in an understandable way that not only informs but encourages lifelong healthy diets and lifestyle.

Healthy food choices begin with plant sources. Animal sources need not be excluded from one's diet, but serving sizes must be closely monitored to minimize the consumption of fat, cholesterol, fried foods, and packaged meats. By making careful food selections, individuals can reduce their intakes of salt, sugar, highly refined grain products, and many processed foods while choosing vegetables, fruits, whole grains, nuts, and seeds as the major sources of nutrients. Plant foods contain natural chemicals or molecules that act in diverse ways to provide health benefits. Focusing more on plant foods in this text and less on animal products is more in line with recent research that promotes health and reduces the risks of chronic diseases. This novel preventive approach relating to adult diseases follows logically from the role of healthy eating in the promotion of lifelong health.

This text is designed as a starting point for students to gain knowledge and understanding of nutrition and how healthy food choices support the proper functioning of the human body. Emphasis has been placed on diet and linkages or associations with health and disease. In today's world, major concerns revolve increasingly around the so-called chronic diseases, including obesity, type 2 diabetes mellitus, cardiovascular diseases, diet-related cancers, and osteoporosis. We now know more than ever about the significance of poor diets—that is, low intakes of micronutrients in the face of excessive caloric intakes—to the development of chronic diseases. These diseases are a major factor in early deaths for the unhealthy, while at the same time healthy individuals with good health behaviors, including diet, are living on average into their 80s or even later.

This book provides special emphasis on several topics, among them food processing and food safety, type 2 diabetes mellitus, and cardiovascular disease. Additionally, a full chapter is devoted to diet-related cancers and other diet-related chronic diseases. These topics are rarely covered in an introductory nutrition text to the extent they are covered here. We advocate strongly that these diet-related diseases and lifestyle risk factors need fuller coverage at this time in our history, and exploding scientific information about these topics seems to support this view.

A major goal of this text is to enable students to become more sophisticated in their own rationales for the selection of healthy foods in appropriate serving sizes that promote health and prevent diet-related diseases. Several activities in each chapter offer ways in which greater understanding of nutritional concepts may be advanced. Nutrition explanations are based on biology, chemistry, and the social sciences. The chemical elements are briefly noted, and the use of organic molecules is limited to a few illustrative structures. Biochemical pathways are provided, mostly with word descriptions but occasionally with chemical structures as needed. The use of figures, flow charts, tables, and other visuals helps the student understand basic concepts of nutrition. Many photos are included to demonstrate both the healthy outcomes of good nutrition and the unhealthy developments that follow long-term adverse eating habits. Healthy eating patterns, based on modern behavioral approaches, are emphasized as the pathways to health across the lifecycle. Several components of this book enhance student learning. Important features of each chapter include chapter outlines and summaries, in-text keyword definitions, in-text highlights of key points, activities, selected references, and student activities. References at the end of each chapter, though limited, are intended to enable students to go beyond our explanations and to explore other aspects of the topics presented.

The lengthy glossary includes key definitions designed to help students master the terminology of nutrition. Many of the terms are likely to be new to students, and a major effort has been made to make the definitions clear.

Acknowledgments

We are indebted to a number of colleagues and interested individuals who have contributed to the improvement of this text in various ways. Included in this group are Boyd R. Switzer, Linda Kastleman, and Philip J. Klemmer. In addition, Liza Cahoon, Mellanye Lackey, and other librarians at UNC Health Sciences Library have helped greatly in finding references used by us in this offering. We no doubt have not included others who have contributed, and we apologize for our oversight.

We also appreciate the many helpful contributions of the staff of Jones & Bartlett Learning who have transformed our written material into a highly readable textbook that enhances student learning.

We are grateful for the interest the following reviewers showed in reviewing this book's manuscript:

Michelle B. Alexander, MPH, CHES, Thomas Nelson Community College, Williamsburg, VA

Dr. Cherylann Dozier, Eastern New Mexico University, Portales, NM

Roberta T. Feehan, RN, PhD, Kean University, Union, NJ

Dr. Shahla Khan, University of North Florida, Jacksonville, FL

Dr. Yevgeniya Lapik, Harold Washington College, Chicago, IL

Lorinda Lindemulder, RN, MSN., Trinity Christian College, Palos Heights, IL

Kylie Paranto, MS, RD, Metropolitan State University of Denver, Denver, CO

Nancy Munoz, DCN, MHA, RD, LDN, Genesis HealthCare, LLC, University of Massachusetts, Amherst, Amherst, MA

Liz Quintana, EdD, RD, LD, CDE, West Virginia University School of Medicine, Morgantown, WV

Rizwana Rahim, PhD, Roosevelt University, East-West University, Chicago, IL

Dr. Stephen Wuerz, Highland Community College, Highland, KS

How to Use This Book

Pedagogy

This text has many learning objects that clarify key topics and enhance student learning.

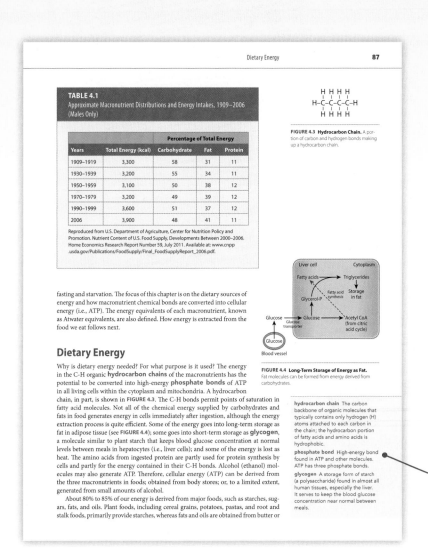

TABLE 4.1
Approximate Macronutrient Distributions and Energy Intakes, 1909–2006 (Males Only)

Years	Total Energy (kcal)	Percentage of Total Energy		
		Carbohydrate	Fat	Protein
1909–1919	3,300	58	31	11
1930–1939	3,200	55	34	11
1950–1959	3,100	50	38	12
1970–1979	3,200	49	39	12
1990–1999	3,600	51	37	12
2006	3,900	48	41	11

Reproduced from U.S. Department of Agriculture, Center for Nutrition Policy and Promotion. Nutrient Content of U.S. Food Supply, Developments Between 2000–2006. Home Economics Research Report Number 59, July 2011. Available at: www.cnpp.usda.gov/Publications/FoodSupply/Final_FoodSupplyReport_2006.pdf.

FIGURE 4.3 Hydrocarbon Chain. A portion of carbon and hydrogen bonds making up a hydrocarbon chain.

FIGURE 4.4 Long-Term Storage of Energy as Fat. Fat molecules can be formed from energy derived from carbohydrates.

fasting and starvation. The focus of this chapter is on the dietary sources of energy and how macronutrient chemical bonds are converted into cellular energy (i.e., ATP). The energy equivalents of each macronutrient, known as Atwater equivalents, are also defined. How energy is extracted from the food we eat follows next.

Dietary Energy

Why is dietary energy needed? For what purpose is it used? The energy in the C-H organic **hydrocarbon chains** of the macronutrients has the potential to be converted into high-energy **phosphate bonds** of ATP in all living cells within the cytoplasm and mitochondria. A hydrocarbon chain, in part, is shown in FIGURE 4.3. The C-H bonds permit points of saturation in fatty acid molecules. Not all of the chemical energy supplied by carbohydrates and fats in food generates energy in cells immediately after ingestion, although the energy extraction process is quite efficient. Some of the energy goes into long-term storage as fat in adipose tissue (see FIGURE 4.4); some goes into short-term storage as **glycogen**, a molecule similar to plant starch that keeps blood glucose concentration at normal levels between meals in hepatocytes (i.e., liver cells); and some of the energy is lost as heat. The amino acids from ingested protein are partly used for protein synthesis by cells and partly for the energy contained in their C-H bonds. Alcohol (ethanol) molecules may also generate ATP. Therefore, cellular energy (ATP) can be derived from the three macronutrients in foods; obtained from body stores; or, to a limited extent, generated from small amounts of alcohol.

About 80% to 85% of our energy is derived from major foods, such as starches, sugars, fats, and oils. Plant foods, including cereal grains, potatoes, pastas, and root and stalk foods, primarily provide starches, whereas fats and oils are obtained from butter or

hydrocarbon chain The carbon backbone of organic molecules that typically contains only hydrogen (H) atoms attached to each carbon in the chain; the hydrocarbon portion of fatty acids and amino acids is hydrophobic.

phosphate bond High-energy bond found in ATP and other molecules. ATP has three phosphate bonds.

glycogen A storage form of starch (a polysaccharide) found in almost all human tissues, especially the liver. It serves to keep the blood glucose concentration near normal between meals.

Key terms appear in bold and are defined in the margin for easy reference.

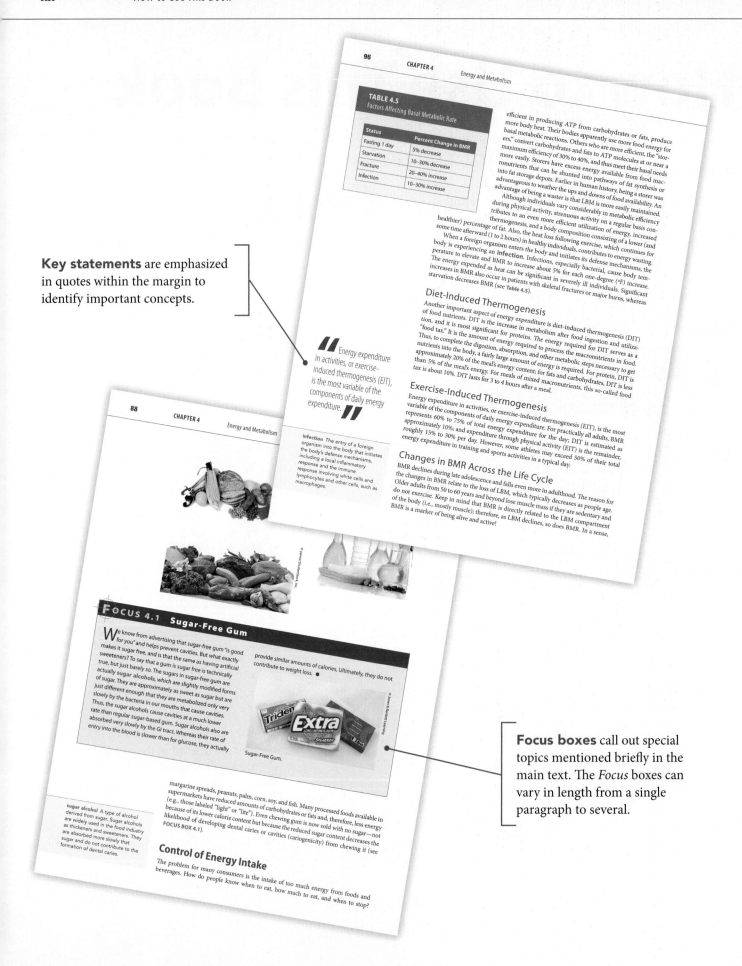

Key statements are emphasized in quotes within the margin to identify important concepts.

Focus boxes call out special topics mentioned briefly in the main text. The *Focus* boxes can vary in length from a single paragraph to several.

The following text appears within the book-page images shown:

96 — CHAPTER 4 — Energy and Metabolism

TABLE 4.5
Factors Affecting Basal Metabolic Rate

Status	Percent Change in BMR
Fasting 1 day	5% decrease
Starvation	10–30% decrease
Fracture	20–40% increase
Infection	10–30% increase

efficient in producing ATP from carbohydrates or fats, produce more body heat. Their bodies apparently use more food energy for basal metabolic reactions. Others who are more efficient, the "storers," convert carbohydrates and fats to ATP molecules at or near a maximum efficiency of 30% to 40%, and thus meet their basal needs more easily. Storers have excess energy available from food macronutrients that can be shunted into pathways of fat synthesis or into fat storage depots. Earlier in human history, being a storer was advantageous to weather the ups and downs of food availability. An advantage of being a waster is that LBM is more easily maintained.

Although individuals vary considerably in metabolic efficiency during physical activity, strenuous activity on a regular basis contributes to an even more efficient utilization of energy, increased thermogenesis, and a body composition consisting of a lower (and healthier) percentage of fat. Also, the heat loss following exercise, which continues for some time afterward (1 to 2 hours) in healthy individuals, contributes to energy wasting.

When a foreign organism enters the body and initiates its defense mechanisms, body is experiencing an **infection**. Infections, especially bacterial, cause body temperature to elevate and BMR to increase about 5% for each one-degree (°F) increase. The energy expended as heat can be significant in severely ill individuals. Significant increases in BMR also occur in patients with skeletal fractures or major burns, whereas starvation decreases BMR (see **Table 4.5**).

Diet-Induced Thermogenesis

Another important aspect of energy expenditure is diet-induced thermogenesis (DIT) of food nutrients. DIT is the increase in metabolism after food ingestion and utilization, and it is most significant for proteins. The energy required for DIT serves as a "food tax." It is the amount of energy required to process the macronutrients in food. Thus, to complete the digestion, absorption, and other metabolic steps necessary to get nutrients into the body, a fairly large amount of energy is required. For protein, DIT is approximately 20% of the meal's energy content; for fats and carbohydrates, DIT is less than 5% of the meal's energy. For meals of mixed macronutrients, this so-called food tax is about 10%. DIT lasts for 3 to 4 hours after a meal.

Exercise-Induced Thermogenesis

Energy expenditure in activities, or exercise-induced thermogenesis (EIT), is the most variable of the components of daily energy expenditure. For practically all adults, BMR represents 60% to 75% of total energy expenditure for the day; DIT is estimated as approximately 10%; and expenditure through physical activity (EIT) is the remainder, roughly 15% to 30% per day. However, some athletes may exceed 50% of their total energy expenditure in training and sports activities in a typical day.

Changes in BMR Across the Life Cycle

BMR declines during late adolescence and falls even more in adulthood. The reason for the changes in BMR relate to the loss of LBM, which typically decreases as people age. Older adults from 50 to 60 years and beyond lose muscle mass if they are sedentary and do not exercise. Keep in mind that BMR is directly related to the LBM compartment of the body (i.e., mostly muscle); therefore, as LBM declines, so does BMR. In a sense, BMR is a marker of being alive and active!

> **❝** Energy expenditure in activities, or exercise-induced thermogenesis (EIT), is the most variable of the components of daily energy expenditure. **❞**

infection The entry of a foreign organism into the body that initiates the body's defense mechanisms, including a local inflammatory response and the immune response involving white cells and lymphocytes and other cells, such as macrophages.

---

88 — CHAPTER 4 — Energy and Metabolism

FOCUS 4.1   Sugar-Free Gum

We know from advertising that sugar-free gum "is good for you" and helps prevent cavities. But what exactly makes it sugar free, and is that the same as having artificial sweeteners? To say that a gum is sugar free is technically true, but just barely so. The sugars in sugar-free gum are actually sugar alcohols, which are slightly modified forms of sugar. They are approximately as sweet as sugar but are just different enough that they are metabolized only very slowly by the bacteria in our mouths that cause cavities. Thus, the sugar alcohols cause cavities at a much lower rate than regular sugar-based gum. Sugar alcohols also are absorbed very slowly by the GI tract. Whereas their rate of entry into the blood is slower than for glucose, they actually provide similar amounts of calories. Ultimately, they do not contribute to weight loss. ●

Sugar-Free Gum.

margarine spreads, peanuts, palm, corn, soy, and fish. Many processed foods available in supermarkets have reduced amounts of carbohydrates or fats and, therefore, less energy (e.g., those labeled "light" or "lite"). Even chewing gum is now sold with no sugar—not because of its lower calorie content but because the reduced sugar content decreases the likelihood of developing dental caries or cavities (cariogenicity) from chewing it (see FOCUS BOX 4.1).

sugar alcohol A type of alcohol derived from sugar. Sugar alcohols are widely used in the food industry as thickeners and sweeteners. They are absorbed more slowly that sugar and do not contribute to the formation of dental caries.

Control of Energy Intake

The problem for many consumers is the intake of too much energy from foods and beverages. How do people know when to eat, how much to eat, and when to stop?

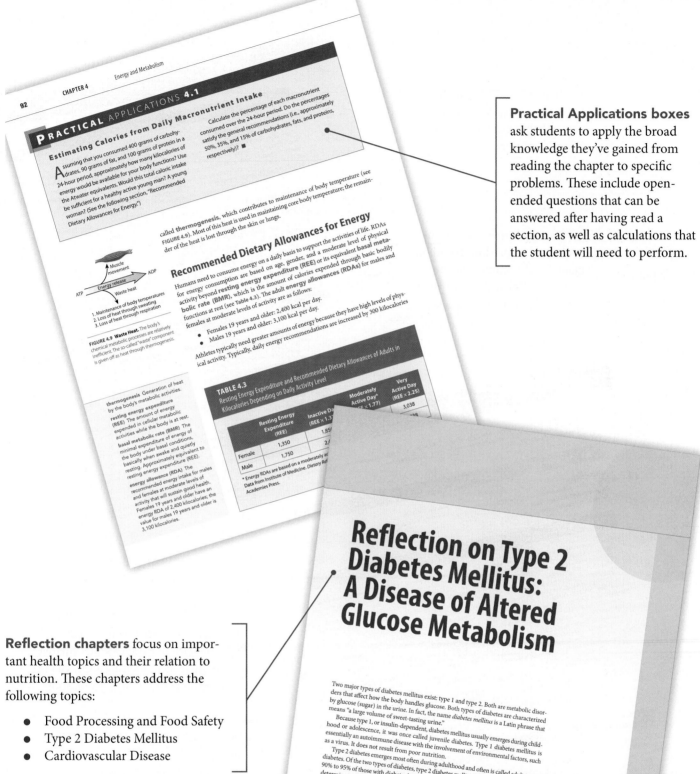

Practical Applications boxes ask students to apply the broad knowledge they've gained from reading the chapter to specific problems. These include open-ended questions that can be answered after having read a section, as well as calculations that the student will need to perform.

Reflection chapters focus on important health topics and their relation to nutrition. These chapters address the following topics:

- Food Processing and Food Safety
- Type 2 Diabetes Mellitus
- Cardiovascular Disease

PRACTICAL APPLICATIONS 4.1

Estimating Calories from Daily Macronutrient Intake

Assuming that you consumed 400 grams of carbohydrates, 90 grams of fat, and 100 grams of protein in a 24-hour period, approximately how many kilocalories of energy would be available for your body functions? Use the Atwater equivalents. Would this total caloric intake be sufficient for a healthy active young man? A young woman? (See the following section, "Recommended Dietary Allowances for Energy.")

Calculate the percentage of each macronutrient consumed over the 24-hour period. Do the percentages satisfy the general recommendations (i.e., approximately 50%, 35%, and 15% of carbohydrates, fats, and proteins, respectively)? ■

called **thermogenesis**, which contributes to maintenance of body temperature (see FIGURE 4.9). Most of this heat is used in maintaining core body temperature; the remainder of the heat is lost through the skin or lungs.

FIGURE 4.9 Waste Heat. The body's chemical metabolic processes are relatively inefficient. The so-called "waste" component is given off as heat through thermogenesis.

Recommended Dietary Allowances for Energy

Humans need to consume energy on a daily basis to support the activities of life. RDAs for energy consumption are based on age, gender, and a moderate level of physical activity beyond **resting energy expenditure (REE)** or its equivalent **basal metabolic rate (BMR)**, which is the amount of calories expended through basic bodily functions at rest (see Table 4.3). The adult **energy allowances (RDAs)** for males and females at moderate levels of activity are as follows:

- Females 19 years and older: 2,400 kcal per day.
- Males 19 years and older: 3,100 kcal per day.

Athletes typically need greater amounts of energy because they have high levels of physical activity. Typically, daily energy recommendations are increased by 300 kilocalories

thermogenesis Generation of heat by the body's metabolic activities.

resting energy expenditure (REE) The amount of energy expended in cellular metabolic activities while the body is at rest.

basal metabolic rate (BMR) The minimal expenditure of energy of the body under basal conditions, basically when awake and quietly resting. Approximately equivalent to resting energy expenditure (REE).

energy allowance (RDA) The recommended energy intake for males and females at moderate levels of activity that will sustain good health. Females 19 years and older have an energy RDA of 2,400 kilocalories; the value for males 19 years and older is 3,100 kilocalories.

TABLE 4.3
Resting Energy Expenditure and Recommended Dietary Allowances of Adults in Kilocalories Depending on Daily Activity Level

	Resting Energy Expenditure (REE)	Inactive Day (REE × 1.3)	Moderately Active Day* (REE × 1.77)	Very Active Day (REE × 2.25)
Female	1,350	1,850	2,4	3,038
Male	1,750			

* Energy RDAs are based on a moderately ac
Data from Institute of Medicine. Dietary Ref
Academies Press.

Reflection on Type 2 Diabetes Mellitus: A Disease of Altered Glucose Metabolism

Two major types of diabetes mellitus exist: type 1 and type 2. Both are metabolic disorders that affect how the body handles glucose. Both types of diabetes are characterized by glucose (sugar) in the urine. In fact, the name *diabetes mellitus* is a Latin phrase that means "a large volume of sweet-tasting urine."

Because type 1, or insulin-dependent, diabetes mellitus usually emerges during childhood or adolescence, it was once called juvenile diabetes. Type 1 diabetes mellitus is essentially an autoimmune disease with the involvement of environmental factors, such as a virus. It does not result from poor nutrition.

Type 2 diabetes emerges most often during adulthood and often is called adult-onset diabetes. Of the two types of diabetes, type 2 diabetes mellitus is far more common, with 90% to 95% of those with diabetes having this type. Type 2 diabetes has a strong genetic determinant, and it does tend to run in families. Type 2 diabetes is one of the 10 leading causes of death in the United States.

The focus of this diet-related disease feature is on type 2 diabetes mellitus because of its significant nutritional **etiology**. Etiology consists of the causation of a disease, which is usually based around several risk factors. In the case of type 2 diabetes mellitus, these risk factors are associated with excessive energy intake, especially from carbohydrates. Approximately 80% or more of those with type 2 diabetes mellitus are overweight or obese. The role of adipose and muscle tissue in contributing to insulin resistance and metabolic abnormalities involving elevations of both circulating insulin and glucose are described.

etiology The causation of a disease. Often based on one or more risk factors that contribute to the development of a disease. The etiology of most chronic degenerative diseases involves multiple risk factors.

119

The chapter **Summary** highlights important concepts from the chapter, helping students focus on key chapter material.

Student Activities consist of short-answer questions based on key material from that chapter. An Answer Key will be provided as part of the Instructor Resources.

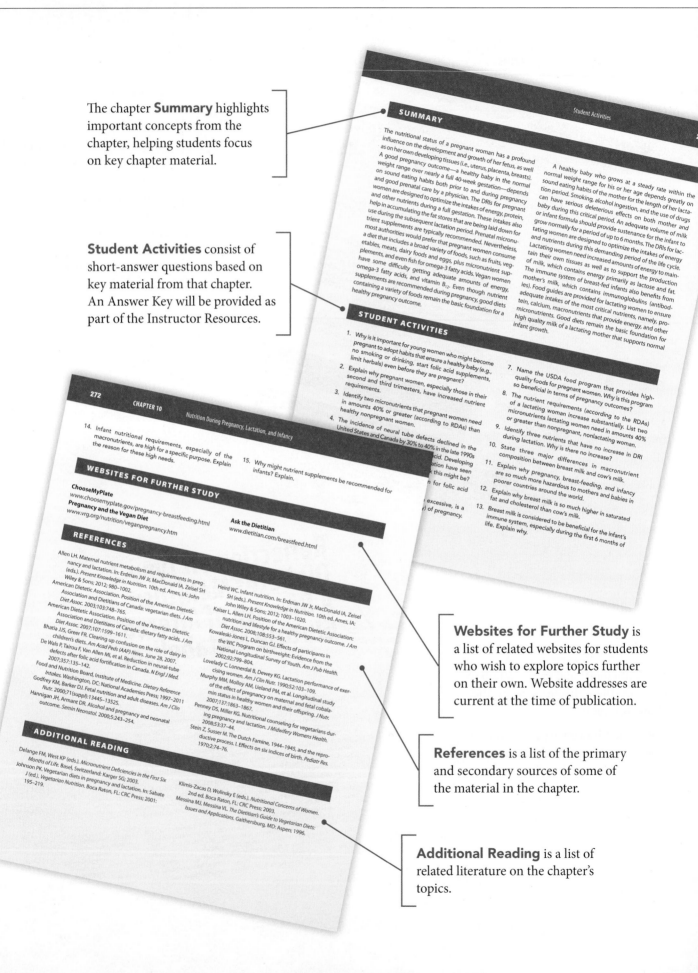

Websites for Further Study is a list of related websites for students who wish to explore topics further on their own. Website addresses are current at the time of publication.

References is a list of the primary and secondary sources of some of the material in the chapter.

Additional Reading is a list of related literature on the chapter's topics.

Student and Instructor Resources

For Students

The Navigate Companion Website, **go.jblearning.com/AndersonCWS**, offers a collection of study aids and learning tools to help students prepare for class and for their upcoming exams. Resources include

- Glossary
- Flashcards
- Matching Exercises
- Web Links
- Chapter Quizzes
- Nutrition Links

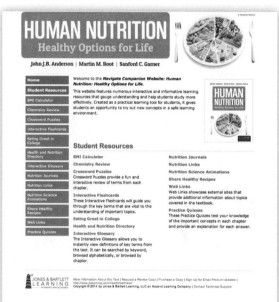

For Instructors

- **PowerPoint Lecture Slides**, more than 500 total, cover highlights of each chapter and serve as instructional aids.
- A **PowerPoint Image Bank** of all the figures from the book to which Jones & Bartlett Learning holds copyright or has permission to reproduce digitally.
- A **Test Bank** with more than 750 questions tests student knowledge with multiple choice, true/false, and essay questions.
- An **Instructor's Manual,** providing classroom activities, teaching points, a sample syllabus, and an answer key for end-of-chapter Student Activities can assist instructors in preparing their courses.

CHAPTER 1

An Introduction to Foods, Nutrients, and Human Health

Consumption of foods and fluids must occur on a regular basis for survival. Populations throughout the course of history, however, have survived despite poor nutrition and erratic eating patterns. The history of humankind has been shaped to a large degree by the varying success of cultures in producing, gathering, and securing foods. For tens of thousands of years, hunter-gatherer and similar societies survived rather precariously, barely increasing their population numbers, because the sporadic availability of uncultivated food was a critical limiting factor for survival. Only in the last 10,000 years of human history has the development of agriculture permitted the population growth that characterizes the modern world. The successful cultivation of cereal crops, the staples of life, has been a key element in the growth of most civilizations and today's global population (see **FIGURE 1.1**).

People do not automatically think of their foods as sources of energy and nutrients; rather, foods are eaten to satisfy hunger, a physiologic need that helps keep the body's functions operating. In today's world, however, many occasions of eating are social as well. Moreover, the foods consumed on both ordinary and special occasions, such as weddings and celebrations, often take on special meanings (see **FIGURE 1.2**). Economic factors also are significant in determining the kinds and amounts of foods that can be cultivated, purchased, and consumed. The food habits of a society are influenced by a variety of cultural, social, psychological, economic, and environmental factors. Supplying enough food to meet the body's needs, promote health, and prevent disease is key to a society's survival.

Foods, and the nutrients derived from them, serve many ends, not the least of which are meeting the body's needs. The body's needs are met by consuming the essential nutrients, both macronutrients and micronutrients, and newly recognized important phytochemicals, in amounts sufficient to maintain health. Macronutrients—fats, carbohydrates, and proteins—are those nutrients that provide energy for the body's systems. Micronutrients are nutrients that are required in small quantities for survival. They include vitamins and minerals. Phytochemicals (sometimes referred to as

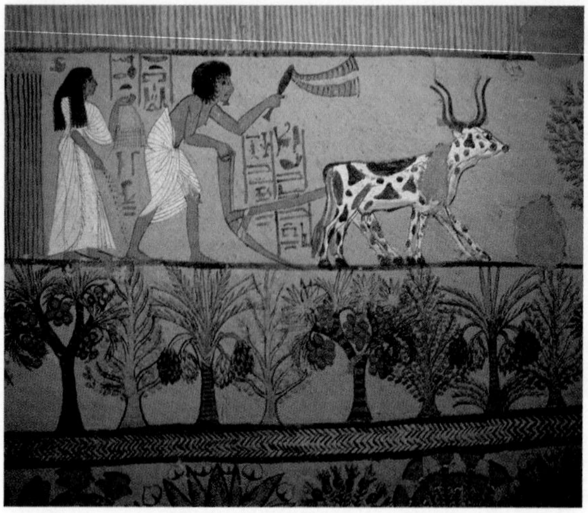

FIGURE 1.1 **Emergence of Agriculture.** The development of agriculture approximately 10,000 year ago permitted the increases in human population growth that characterize the modern world.

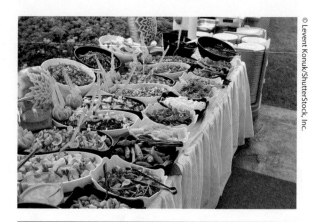

FIGURE 1.2 **Ample Food Availability.** Advances in agriculture and food processing have produced an abundance of food in many parts of the world. In many societies, food plays a key role in the celebration of special occasions.

phytomolecules) are plant-derived molecules that are increasingly being noted for their role in maintaining human health.

Nutrition, as a field of study, represents a broad area of knowledge encompassing information from the basic sciences, behavioral sciences, and other fields of investigation. Because of new findings from current research investigations, nutrition is evolving quite rapidly, but putting the new information into clinical practice or incorporating it into public policy takes time, often decades. New research findings are not rapidly implemented into clinical practice, even though the findings may be encouraging. This chapter examines several important nutrition topics in order to lay the foundation for additional study.

Food and Nutrients

The body's needs for macronutrients, micronutrients, and water relate to metabolic requirements and the role these nutrients play in forming biological compounds. Other dietary components that impact health are alcohol, dietary fiber, and phytochemicals. **Table 1.1** lists the **nutrients** and **non-nutrients** that are required across the human life cycle. As you learn more about nutrition, keep in mind the increasingly important roles of non-nutrient plant molecules that promote health.

Macronutrients

The **macronutrients**—carbohydrates, fats, and proteins—exist mainly as polymers or long chains. They provide energy, expressed as kilocalories (kcal), plus a few other unique structures required in human tissue. Fats and carbohydrates provide the bulk of energy, whereas proteins provide a smaller amount. The primary energy-providing macronutrients—carbohydrates and fats derived from plants and animals—provide approximately 85% of energy (expressed as kilocalories or kilojoules) intake by humankind in the Western world and perhaps 90% or more in other parts of the world. Protein provides nearly all of the remaining energy consumed on a daily basis. In addition to

nutrition The branch of science dealing with foods, nutrient composition, eating habits, nutritional status, and health and diseases of individuals and populations.

nutrient Essential or nonessential molecules or minerals derived from foods that are used by cells in the body to complete diverse functions.

non-nutrient Food molecules that are not considered nutrients because they are not essential for cellular or tissue needs. However, they may be important for other aspects of human health; for example, dietary fibers and many phytomolecules may protect against cancer and other chronic diseases.

macronutrient Class of nutrients that generate energy (carbohydrates, fats, proteins) and provide nitrogen (N) and amino acids (protein). Sometimes other molecules, such as dietary fiber and water, are included in this class because they are consumed in large amounts.

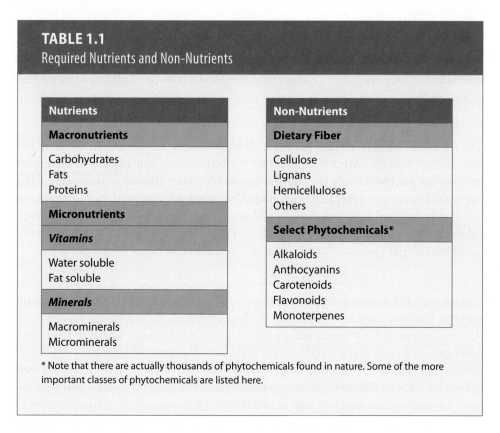

TABLE 1.1
Required Nutrients and Non-Nutrients

Nutrients	Non-Nutrients
Macronutrients	**Dietary Fiber**
Carbohydrates Fats Proteins	Cellulose Lignans Hemicelluloses Others
Micronutrients	**Select Phytochemicals***
Vitamins	Alkaloids Anthocyanins Carotenoids Flavonoids Monoterpenes
Water soluble Fat soluble	
Minerals	
Macrominerals Microminerals	

* Note that there are actually thousands of phytochemicals found in nature. Some of the more important classes of phytochemicals are listed here.

> The body's needs for macronutrients, micronutrients, and water relate to metabolic requirements and the role these nutrients play in forming biological compounds.

their constituent amino acids, proteins are essential because they provide nitrogen that is needed for the synthesis of deoxyribonucleic acid (DNA) and related molecules.

Micronutrients

The **micronutrients** are represented by vitamins and minerals, which have specific roles in metabolism. The micronutrients are needed in small quantities each day. **Vitamins** are categorized as water soluble or fat soluble. The distinction between these two types of vitamins lies in their solubility in water or in organic solvents, including fats and oils. Vitamins are needed for a large number of cellular and extracellular chemical reactions. For example, vitamins A and D are fat-soluble vitamins. Vitamin A plays a role in growth and vision; vitamin D, obtained from either the diet or synthesized when skin is exposed to the sun, has an important role in calcium metabolism.

Minerals are used in chemical reactions as well as in structural components of cells and tissues. For example, calcium is a critical component of hard tissues such as bone and teeth and plays a variety of other roles. Macrominerals are needed in daily amounts greater than 100 milligrams per day. Microminerals are needed in amounts of less than 100 milligrams per day. Water often is considered with minerals.

Energy

Food **energy** is measured in kilocalories, often simply referred to as calories or kcals. This energy is derived from the breakage of hydrocarbon bonds, often written as C-H bonds, in macronutrients (i.e., carbohydrates, fats, proteins). Energy is not a nutrient per se; rather, energy is derived from macronutrients. Therefore, when energy is classified with the macronutrients, it is correctly called a dietary variable rather than a nutrient.

micronutrient Class of nutrients that includes vitamins and minerals; nutrients consumed in small amounts each day.

vitamin An essential organic micronutrient needed in the diet in small amounts; consists of both water-soluble and fat-soluble vitamins.

mineral Elements in the earth's surface that are needed by the human body, such as calcium and iron.

energy (calorie) A physical unit of energy that is derived from food macronutrients and alcohol; 1 kilocalorie is the amount of heat required to raise the temperature of a gram of water 1°C. Energy also can expressed in joules, where 1 kilocalorie is equal to 4.2 kilojoules.

> Energy is not a nutrient per se; rather, energy is derived from macronutrients.

The recommended energy contribution of macronutrients to the diet by percentage typically breaks down to approximately 50% or more for carbohydrates, 35% or less for fats, and 15% or more for proteins. The percentage of energy from alcohol varies substantially, but the percentage for those who consume alcohol on a regular basis may be as high as 5%.

Atwater Equivalents

The **Atwater equivalents** system is used to provide a rough estimate of the available energy in foods. Atwater equivalents are estimates of the amount of energy in each of the macronutrients and alcohol (ethanol). These estimates are based on the energy in kilocalories generated when the hydrocarbon backbones of the molecules are completely oxidized to carbon dioxide and water. The Atwater system uses the average values of 4 kilocalories per gram for protein, 4 kilocalories per gram for carbohydrate, and 9 kilocalories per gram for fat. Alcohol is calculated at 7 kilocalories per gram.

The Problem of Too Much Energy

The greatest problem in the American diet today is the inability to maintain a healthy **energy balance**, which is the balance between energy intake and energy expenditure. Americans consume too much energy (calories) via the excessive intake of foods and beverages. Although average adult energy intake has decreased slightly since 2000, our energy expenditure for work and other activities has decreased even more! This energy imbalance leads to storage of excess calories in fat stores (adipose tissue deposits) scattered throughout the body as well as weight gain. Obesity, which reached epidemic proportions among American adults and children in the 1990s, results from the overconsumption of food energy coupled with a sedentary lifestyle. Although jogging and other sports activities have become popular with some health-conscious individuals, they have had relatively little effect on the U.S. population as a whole because of the high percentage of inactive individuals and because of the great amount of physical activity needed to balance energy intake, especially from excessive calories in the diet. This latter point—balancing energy intake with expenditure—is not readily embraced by most people.

Non-Nutrient Phytochemicals

No new nutrients have been discovered since the mid-twentieth century, but scientists continue to identify new, beneficial, non-nutrient phytochemicals. Because these molecules are derived from plants, they are logically referred to as **phytochemicals** or phytomolecules. Phytochemicals are found only in plant-based foods. Plants produce phytochemicals to serve a variety of diverse functions. For example, fiber, which in human nutrition is referred to as dietary fiber, serves as a structural component of plant cell walls and provides rigidity to plant tissues.

Thousands of different of phytochemicals exist, each with a unique chemical structure and purpose. Many of these molecules are polyphenols. Some of these molecules have rather simple structures, such as phytate, whereas others, such as polyphenols, have more complex structures (see **FIGURE 1.3**).

Phytochemicals do not provide energy (i.e., calories) to humans, but they do play important roles in maintaining human health (see **FIGURE 1.4**). Returning to our example of fiber, in humans, fiber molecules play a role in maintaining the health of the gastrointestinal tract. Other phytochemicals act as antioxidants that protect cells against free radicals or highly reactive chemicals produced as a result of cell metabolic pathways (see **FOCUS BOX 1.1**). Because phytochemicals are made by plants to meet their own needs, not those of humankind, the assumption that all phytochemicals are beneficial to human health is incorrect. In fact, some phytochemicals are actually toxic and must be avoided.

Atwater equivalent The energy equivalent per gram of macronutrient or alcohol (ethanol): 1 gram of carbohydrate yields 4 kilocalories, 1 gram of fat yields 9 kilocalories, 1 gram of protein yields 4 kilocalories, and 1 gram of alcohol (pure or 200 proof) yields 7 kilocalories.

energy balance The balance between energy intake and energy expenditure. Energy imbalance represents either higher intake than expenditure or the reverse. Positive (+) energy balance results in weight gain. Negative (–) energy balance results in weight loss.

phytochemical (phytomolecule) Non-nutrient molecules made by plants and found in diverse fruits, vegetables, grains, nuts, and seeds. Many of these molecules, especially antioxidants, are thought to protect against cancer.

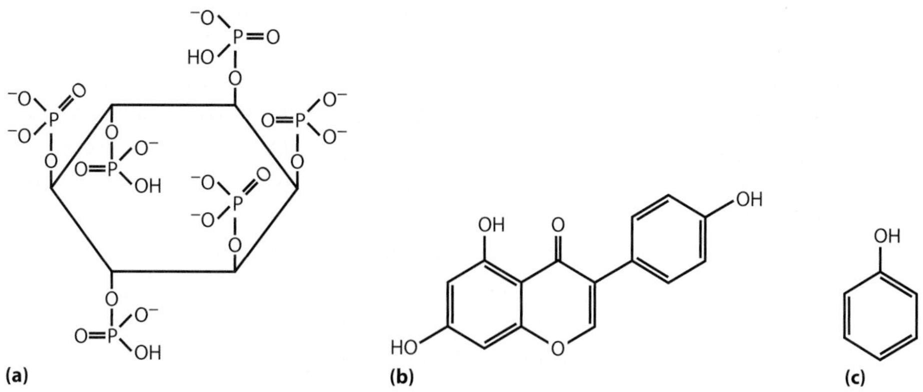

(a)

(b)

(c)

FIGURE 1.3 Phytochemicals. The molecular structures of phytochemicals vary. The molecular structure of three phytochemicals are shown: (a) phytate, (b) phytosterol, and (c) phenol. The ring in (a) is equivalent in size to those in (b) and (c).

FOCUS 1.1   Free Radicals

What are **free radicals**? Why should people be concerned about them? Free radicals are atoms that have an unpaired electron. Atoms with unpaired electrons can bond easily with other atoms with unpaired electrons, which means they are highly reactive! Many types of radicals are possible, but those of most concern in the human body are derived from oxygen. Collectively, the oxygen radicals are called reactive oxygen species. Damage to the body's cells and tissues occur when free radicals bond with other molecules or atoms. In particular, free radicals can do a lot of damage if they interact with cellular DNA or the cell membrane. However, the body has a way to fight the damage from reactive oxygen species: antioxidants. Antioxidants are molecules that can inactivate or neutralize free radicals, thus preventing them from causing cellular damage. Many of the phytochemicals in plants also act as antioxidants. ●

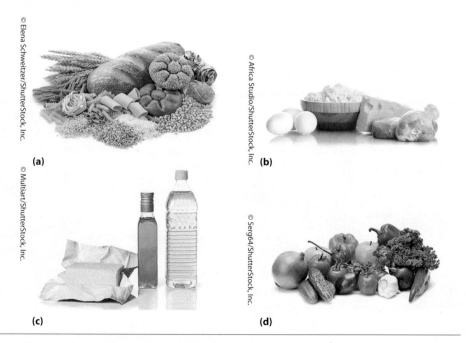

© Elena Schweitzer/ShutterStock, Inc.

© Africa Studio/ShutterStock, Inc.

© Multiart/ShutterStock, Inc.

© Serg64/ShutterStock, Inc.

(a)

(b)

(c)

(d)

FIGURE 1.4 Food as a Source of Energy and Phytochemicals. Food provides energy due to the breakage of chemical bonds in (a) carbohydrates, (b) proteins, and (c) fats. Phytochemicals found in fruits and vegetables (d) are important to human health, but they do not supply energy.

free radical A highly reactive chemical species (of very short life)—typically oxygen atoms containing an extra electron—that combine with a carbon atom of an unsaturated fatty acid (at the double bonds) or of other molecules, including proteins and DNA. This can result in an alteration at the point of the unsaturation as well as damage to DNA and mutations.

Guidelines and Recommendations

Healthy dietary patterns provide all of the essential nutrients, energy, and phytochemicals. For good health, the diet should include mostly nutrient-dense or nutrient-rich foods because they contain many micronutrients in addition to modest amounts of macronutrients for energy and protein. In contrast, energy-dense or calorie-dense foods are generally not recommended because they contain too much energy and too few micronutrients. In addition, diets that contain the amount of calories needed for good health help maintain a healthy body weight.

But what actually determines what people eat? The three major **determinants of food intake** are availability of foods, purchasing power (money or barter), and social and cultural values placed on specific foods (see **FIGURE 1.5** and **FOCUS BOX 1.2**). The first two factors are more important in developing countries, whereas the third becomes more important in developed countries where purchasing power and a wide availability of foods permit the selection of specific foods. (In these countries, food marketing and advertising may also contribute substantially to the consumption of specific food products, especially processed items such as chips, dips, soft drinks, and convenience foods.) **Food availability** is highly determined by one's geographic location due to production, distribution, and cultivation being dependent on an area's climate, infrastructure, and economy. **Social and cultural values** have historically been major factors contributing to food intake, and they remain so in many low-income nations, but they have become less influential in more affluent nations where markets have most foods available almost the entire year for those who can afford them.

Information, and even misinformation, on the nutritional quality of foods can be obtained from the **food composition table**. Though only in the last century has this been recognized as a standard for good health, it is gradually becoming a fourth determinant of food intake. In general, a growing interest in the role of food in health and the wide prevalence of nutritional labeling on food packaging have fostered this new determinant of food intake. Foods supply the nutrient requirements and non-nutrient phytochemicals that are critical for both health promotion and disease prevention. Governments around the world, in particular the United States, offer dietary guidelines and recommendations to improve the health of their populations.

> ❚❚ The three major determinants of food intake are availability of foods, purchasing power (money or barter), and social and cultural values placed on specific foods. ❚❚

determinants of food intake The major factors that drive people to choose the foods that they consume: purchasing power (money or barter), social and cultural factors, and food availability.

food availability The availability of food or foods in a particular geographic region because of production, distribution, or cultivation of the foods for human consumption. It is one of the basic determinants of food intake, particularly in poorer nations.

social and cultural values Values applied to foods by a group, culture, or society; in the United States, societal food values exist, but they have been greatly affected by the marketing of a tremendous array of processed foods. A major determinant of food habits.

food composition table A table or database that contains data on the nutrient content of foods. Such tables are published by U.S. government agencies, such as the USDA, and in other sources, such as *McCance and Widdowson's The Composition of Foods.*

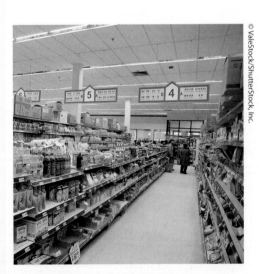
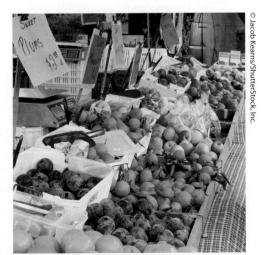

(a)   (b)

FIGURE 1.5 Food Availability. In developed countries, a wide variety of foods is available in supermarkets (a) and farmers' markets (b), offering consumers many options for both healthful and unhealthful eating.

FOCUS 1.2   Money and Food

An old quote states that "Money makes the world go round"; in some cases money also can determine whether a person is able to maintain a healthful diet. **Purchasing power**, or money, is a major determinant of food intake. In some poor nations, food choices may be limited due to limited food availability and inadequate purchasing power. For example, people who do not have money or who are living in a war zone may find it difficult to obtain a variety of nutrient-rich foods, or even any food. Typically, people with limited financial resources have less healthy eating patterns because their limited funds do not permit them to purchase more costly meats, dairy foods, fruits, and vegetables. Their diets consist primarily of foods derived from low-cost grains. Over time, such a diet will result in disorders caused by inadequate intake of certain macronutrients and micronutrients. To compound the problem, in many underdeveloped countries the poor must also contend with polluted water and unsanitary living conditions, which can exacerbate diseases resulting from malnutrition.

Money does not have as strong an influence on the dietary habits of populations in middle-income countries and in developed nations such as the United States and Canada. In the United States and other rich nations, a lower percentage of family income is spent on food by the vast majority of the population. Therefore, food habits are based less on purchasing power than on nutritional awareness, convenience, and cultural and family traditions. In the United States, in particular, poor eating habits are often associated with lower incomes and lower education levels. Lower-income consumers often exhibit relatively poor food habits. Middle- and upper-income consumers tend to consume more luxury items, more variety, more convenience foods, and more low-fat alternative foods. Because of their generally poor food habits, lower-income individuals have a substantially greater burden of obesity, hypertension, diabetes, and disorders associated with nutritional excesses and inadequacies. One solution is to provide better education on diet and exercise for low-income Americans. ●

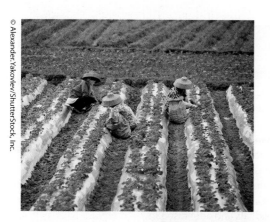
© Alexander.Yakovlev/ShutterStock, Inc.

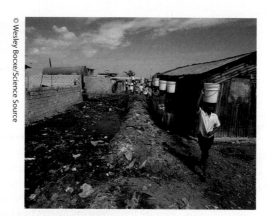
© Wesley Bocxe/Science Source

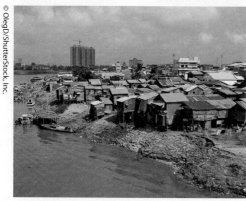
© OlegD/ShutterStock, Inc.

purchasing power (money) The economic capability of a family (or individual) to purchase items for a family unit. A major determinant of food habits.

Dietary Guidelines for Americans

The **Dietary Guidelines for Americans**, a report jointly produced by the U.S. Department of Agriculture (USDA) and Department of Health and Human Services (DHHS), provides the U.S. population with general recommendations for food consumption that will result in good health and will reduce the burden of diet-related chronic diseases. The *Guidelines* emphasizes the benefits of eating a variety of foods; consuming less sugar and salt; eating more fruits and vegetables and low-fat dairy products; and balancing energy intake with expenditure. The *Guidelines* also discourages the consumption of foods low in complex carbohydrates and high in saturated fats. A current selection from the *Dietary Guidelines for Americans* is provided in **Table 1.2**. Note that the *Guidelines* provides an up-to-date summary of what foods should be consumed, but not the amounts or numbers of servings.

MyPlate

The plant and animal foods commonly consumed in the United States and other developed countries are clustered into five general groups—grains, vegetables, fruits, meats and proteins, and dairy foods—as well as an additional miscellaneous group. The groups contain related foods and their products resulting from minimal processing of the raw foods. Food pyramids and food guides utilize these groups for making recommendations of the number of servings from each group on a daily basis. The USDA's **MyPlate** (see ChooseMyPlate.gov) is an example of such a food guidance system (see **FIGURE 1.6**). With MyPlate, food groups are represented as proportions on a plate relative to the recommended daily amounts. The plate shown in Figure 1.6 is the most recent visual diagram prepared by the USDA to convey important dietary information to the U.S. population. Note that MyPlate and the older **MyPyramid** (see **FIGURE 1.7**) replace the old USDA food pyramid.

Dietary Guidelines for Americans Document prepared by a committee representing both the USDA and the Department of Health and Human Services that provides guidelines that Americans should follow to ensure a healthy diet. The guidelines stress reductions in the consumption of fat, cholesterol, and sodium; increased consumption of complex carbohydrates, dietary fiber, and fruits and vegetables; maintenance of a desirable body weight; and limited alcohol consumption. The guidelines are updated every 5 years.

MyPlate The food guidance system developed by the USDA for the U.S. population. It includes five food groups: grains, proteins, vegetables, fruits, and dairy. It uses an icon that shows a plate and drink to provide a pictorial display of how much of a meal should be represented by each food group. It provides an entire website with menus, a food composition table, and many other dietary tools.

MyPyramid An update on the earlier U.S. food guide pyramid that was replaced by MyPlate. It stressed activity and moderation along with a proper mix of food groups in one's diet. MyPyramid was designed to educate consumers about a lifestyle consistent with the *2005 Dietary Guidelines for Americans*.

TABLE 1.2
Examples from the *Dietary Guidelines for Americans*

- Prevent and/or reduce overweight and obesity through improved eating and physical activity behaviors.
- Reduce daily sodium intake to less than 2,300 milligrams (mg) and further reduce intake to 1,500 mg among persons who are 51 and older and those of any age who are African American or have hypertension, diabetes, or chronic kidney disease.
- Consume less than 10% of calories from saturated fatty acids by replacing them with monounsaturated and polyunsaturated fatty acids.
- Reduce the intake of calories from solid fats and added sugars.
- Limit the consumption of foods that contain refined grains, especially refined grain foods that contain solid fats, added sugars, and sodium.
- Increase vegetable and fruit intake.
- Eat a variety of vegetables, especially dark-green and red and orange vegetables and beans and peas.
- Increase intake of fat-free or low-fat milk and milk products, such as milk, yogurt, cheese, or fortified soy beverages.

Data from U.S. Department of Agriculture and U.S. Department of Health and Human Services. *Dietary Guidelines for Americans 2010*. 7th ed. Washington, DC: U.S. Government Printing Office, 2010.

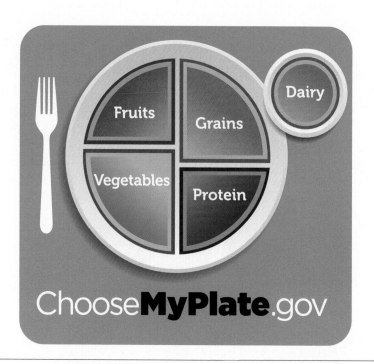

FIGURE 1.6 MyPlate. Released in 2011, MyPlate is a visual guide that helps consumers implement the principles of the *Dietary Guidelines for Americans, 2010* and other nutritional standards.

Courtesy of the U.S. Department of Agriculture.

Dietary Reference Intakes

Dietary needs are typically met by the consumption of a variety of foods in a balanced manner over a period of approximately a week, not necessarily every day. Nutrients, energy, and phytochemicals are needed for good health throughout the life cycle, but nutritional needs are typically higher during childhood and adolescence as well as pregnancy and lactation. Growth and development of the body and its organs early in life represent the first major challenges for obtaining sufficient amounts of all the essential nutrients. Maintenance and active functioning of the fully grown adult body require these same nutrients. Finally, nutrient requirements later in life typically decline as lean body mass (i.e., the mass of the body minus body fat) also declines. Foods provide all the nutrients, but all foods are not equal in their nutrient composition. Thus, it is important to choose a variety of foods each day to ensure that all the essential nutrients are consumed in a 24-hour period. Eating a variety of foods should supply the macronutrients and micronutrients needed by our cells and tissues at all stages of the life cycle.

Recommendations for the intake of different nutrients across the life cycle, including pregnancy and lactation, have been established for the populations of the United States and Canada. These recommendations are known as **Dietary Reference Intakes (DRIs)** (see **FIGURE 1.8**). The DRIs represent a set of recommended intakes for nutrients, energy, water, and dietary fiber that support health and prevent disease across the various stages of the life cycle, from birth to old age and during pregnancy and lactation. The DRIs serve as the standards for specific dietary recommendations as well as the upper limits of safe intakes. Four new categories have been added to the terminology of the DRIs in an effort to broaden understandings of how the DRIs are established. The four new categories and their acronyms are: **Estimated Average Requirement (EAR), Recommended Dietary Allowance (RDA), Adequate Intake (AI)**, and **Tolerable Upper Limit (UL) of Safety** (safe intake). Intakes of nutrients beyond their UL are not considered safe.

Dietary Reference Intake (DRI) Recommended intakes of nutrients that are presented in a series of books from the Institute of Medicine. Each nutrient either has a Recommended Dietary Allowance (RDA) or an Adequate Intake (AI), depending on the availability of information upon which to make a recommendation.

Estimated Average Requirement (EAR) The amount of intake of a nutrient needed by the average individual to maintain good health. If a nutrient has an EAR, its Recommended Dietary Allowance (RDA) is based on the mean (average) +2 standard deviations above the mean.

Recommended Dietary Allowance (RDA) Recommended intakes of specific nutrients; generally the Estimated Average Requirement (EAR) plus an additional safety factor specific for each nutrient. Age-gender groups are considered for different RDAs, as are women who are pregnant or lactating.

Adequate Intake (AI) A designation under the Dietary Reference Intakes (DRIs) of recommended intakes for several nutrients that do not have an Estimated Average Requirement (EAR). Usually used with nutrients where not enough information is available to set a more exact requirement (RDA).

Tolerable Upper Limit of Safety (UL) The safe upper limit of intake of a nutrient from foods and supplements; determined when establishing the Dietary Reference Intake (DRI) of a nutrient.

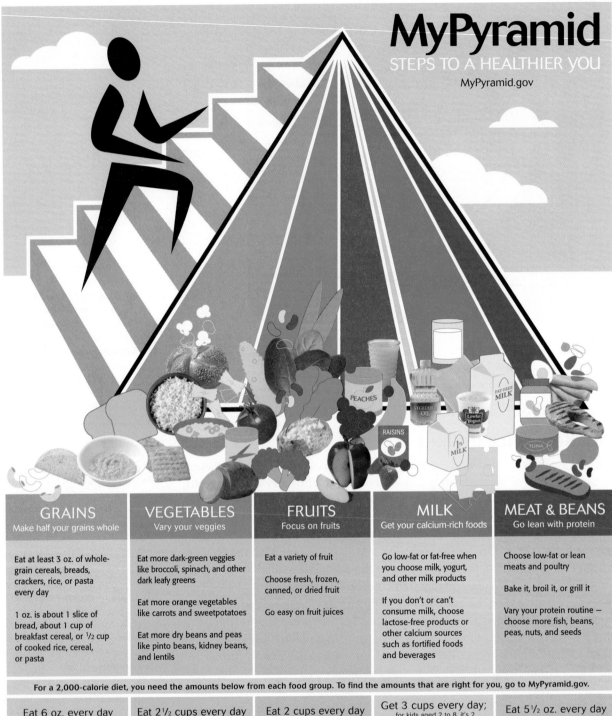

FIGURE 1.7 MyPyramid. Released in 2005, MyPyramid is an Internet-based educational tool that helps consumers implement the *Dietary Guidelines for Americans* and other nutritional standards.

Courtesy of the U.S. Department of Agriculture.

These measures have resulted from advances in our knowledge of the amounts of each nutrient needed to support human functioning at optimal levels. The RDA is the average daily dietary intake level that would adequately meet the nutritional needs of nearly all healthy persons. An EAR, which is the amount of a certain nutrient needed by an average individual, must be established for each age group and gender across the life cycle before an RDA for the nutrient can be estimated. Typically, an RDA is two standard deviations (SDs) greater than the EAR. These two standard deviations are considered a safety factor so that approximately 97.5% of the population at each age and gender will meet their requirements for the nutrient. For example, the EAR for protein for an adult male (18 to 50 years) is approximately 48 grams per day; two standard deviations of the EAR is ~15 grams per day; thus, the RDA for protein is 63 grams per day. Similarly, the RDA for protein for adult females (18 to 50 years) is set at 50 grams per day. In general, the RDAs for the other nutrients have been established in a similar manner. Note that the RDA for energy has no safety factor added; the RDAs are the same as the EARs for each gender across the life cycle.

For a few nutrients, however, less is known about their metabolism in the body and the amount required in the diet each day. Therefore, an EAR cannot be established, and thus no RDA can be estimated. For these few nutrients, AIs have been assigned because of the inability to establish EARs over the life cycle. AIs are essentially "guesstimates" arbitrarily selected by a panel of investigators as safe intake that will support all functions for the nutrient. Other countries and the World Health Organization (WHO) also have established recommendations for nutrient intakes, but the rationales behind these guidelines often differ from those used in the United States and Canada. In reality, the same set of guidelines should probably fit all populations of the world.

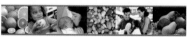

FIGURE 1.8 Dietary Reference Intakes. The Dietary Reference Intakes (DRI) publication is a system of nutritional recommendations from the Institute of Medicine. The DRI system is used by both the United States and Canada and is intended for the general public and health professionals.

American Eating Trends

Americans have access to the *Dietary Guidelines for Americans*, and many are familiar with the USDA's MyPlate as well as how to read a Nutrition Facts panel. These are labels on packaged food and provide information on serving size, calories, nutrients, and ingredients. Despite this new information, what do most Americans actually eat, and how have **American eating trends** changed over time? The traditional or so-called standard American diet has historically been based on the consumption of meats and dairy products, with cereals, vegetables, and fruits being used to provide the remaining energy and bulk. This "meat and potatoes" eating pattern, however, has undergone major changes in recent decades. Dietary trends since World War II include increased macronutrient consumption, the rise of fast foods, the emergence of fortified and functional foods, and the use of nutrient supplements. These are primarily U.S.-specific consumption patterns, but many of these trends have also emerged to some degree in other Western nations and even in some Asian countries.

> *The traditional or so-called standard American diet has historically been based on the consumption of meats and dairy products, with cereals, vegetables, and fruits being used to provide the remaining energy and bulk.*

Trends in Macronutrient Intake

Since 1960, five trends in macronutrient intake, as reported by the USDA, have revealed notable changes in American eating patterns (see **Table 1.3**). The first trend is a decrease in the consumption of animal fat, largely from meats and dairy products (see **FOCUS BOX 1.3**). This trend is encouraging because of the established association between intake of saturated animal fats (and cholesterol) and the incidence of obesity, type 2 diabetes mellitus, coronary heart disease, and other chronic diseases. However, major concerns have been voiced over our high intakes of salt and sugar and our relatively low intakes of vegetables, fruits, and whole grain cereals that supply many micronutrients and dietary fiber in addition to unsaturated fats.

American (U.S.) eating trends Trends since 1980 include decreases in the consumption of animal fats, cholesterol, meats, eggs, and dairy products, especially whole milk, and increases in the consumption of vegetable oils, poultry, fish, vegetables, fruits, low-fat dairy products, and whole grain products.

TABLE 1.3
Current U.S. Food Consumption Trends

The USDA has reported notable changes in U.S. eating patterns since 1960:

1. Decline in consumption of animal fat.
2. Increased consumption of processed vegetable oils (fats).
3. Decline in intake of complex carbohydrates and dietary fiber.
4. Increased consumption of animal protein (small increase).
5. Increased consumption of sugar.

Data from U.S. Department of Agriculture and U.S. Department of Health and Human Services. *Dietary Guidelines for Americans, 2010*. 7th ed. Washington, DC: U.S. Government Printing Office; 2010.

FOCUS 1.3   Vegetarian Eating Patterns

A survey conducted by Harris Interactive found that in 2012 approximately 9 million Americans were vegetarian and that many others were following a vegetarian-inclined diet. People adopt a **vegetarian eating pattern**, which entails removing meat from their diet, for a number of reasons. First, some view eating meat as environmentally unsustainable due to the low energy efficiency in raising animals for their meats from grains. Second, many believe that consumption of meat is not healthful. Third, some consider the raising and slaughtering of animals for their meat to be inhumane and a form of animal cruelty.

With regard to health concerns, many consumers and scientists think that most meats contain too much saturated fat and cholesterol. Meat consumption may also contribute to overnutrition because of large portion sizes and to undernutrition because of the avoidance of plant foods, which typically contain many essential micronutrients, plus phytochemicals and dietary fiber. Research has shown that high serum cholesterol concentrations are more likely to result from overconsumption of meats and other animal products.

An **omnivorous eating pattern** entails eating both plant and animal foods, whereas vegetarians emphasize plant foods (i.e., vegetables, fruits, cereals). Vegetarian eating practices actually vary quite widely. A list of the different types of vegetarian eating patterns is provided in **Table A**. The most liberal form allows eggs and dairy products (lacto-ovo-vegetarian), whereas the most conservative type (vegan) permits only plant foods—fruits, vegetables, cereals, nuts, and seeds. About two to three million people in the United States are vegans. In general, the term *vegetarian diet* includes all the types of vegetarians mentioned in Table A.

Vegetarians, in general, have learned to select and prepare mostly plant foods so that they consume virtually all the required nutrients in the appropriate quantities to ensure good health. Vegetarians who consume some egg and dairy products are, in general, healthier than the rest of the U.S. population, as evidenced by disease rates of Seventh-day Adventists, a Christian denomination that advocates a vegetarian eating pattern. Vegetarians have lower rates of most chronic diseases, such as heart disease, cancer, hypertension, and type 2 diabetes mellitus. Aspects of the vegetarian lifestyle other than diet may also contribute to their better health,

(continues)

vegetarian eating pattern A diet in which no meats are consumed. The strictest type of vegetarian diet, the vegan diet, does not include any animal products. Other types of vegetarian eating patterns allow consumption of dairy products and eggs.

omnivorous eating pattern Dietary pattern where an individual eats food from both plants and animals.

FOCUS 1.3 Vegetarian Eating Patterns (*continued*)

TABLE A
Different Types of Vegetarians, by Animal Products Permitted, Compared to Omnivores

Type of Diet	Animal Foods Allowed
Omnivore	No limits
Flexitarian	Limited in white meats, fish, dairy, eggs
Vegetarian	Generally no animal foods
Lacto-ovo-vegetarian	Dairy and eggs only
Pescatarian	Fish only
Vegan	No animal foods at all

but diet remains a very significant contributor to lower rates of obesity and other chronic diseases among vegetarians.

Many plant foods are sufficiently rich in calcium, nonheme iron, and riboflavin to provide adequate amounts of these micronutrients in the vegan diet. Micronutrient-rich plant-based foods include dark-green, leafy vegetables (e.g., broccoli, kale, collard and mustard greens, bok choy); beans (e.g., pinto, garbanzo, navy, kidney, black); soybeans; and black strap molasses. Fruits also are typically rich in micronutrients.

However, because vegans avoid all animal foods, their diets may be low in several important micronutrients, whereas macronutrient intakes can typically be kept at comparable intake levels as in omnivorous diets. Concerns have been raised regarding the nutritional status of vegans because of potentially marginal intakes of micronutrients such as iron, zinc, vitamin B_{12} (cobalamin), calcium, and riboflavin, which are found in good amounts in animal products. Thus, vegan diets must be supplemented with vitamin B_{12} and other micronutrients.

Vegetarian diets that include dairy foods and eggs may be safer and healthier than strict vegan diets because the broader selection of foods provides more opportunities to obtain all the essential nutrients. However, this has not been substantiated by research evidence. (Adding fish and other seafoods to a vegetarian diet would ensure that practically all trace elements would be consumed in sufficient amounts, but by definition seafoods are not part of a vegetarian diet.) Despite the few concerns raised, the health benefits of vegetarian diets need to be emphasized: Those adhering to vegetarian diets typically use raw or minimally processed foods only; they consume good amounts of fruits, vegetables, grains, nuts, and seeds; their meals almost always contain a wide variety of foods; and they generally limit intakes of excessive amounts of energy-rich macronutrients typically consumed in the standard American diet. Their protein intakes are adequate, phytochemical and fiber intakes are high, and their diets provide the essential amino acids needed for growth and tissue repair. In sum, the evidence suggests that vegetarian diets generally confer health benefits that start early and continue late in life. ●

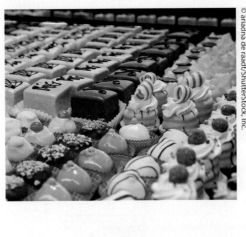

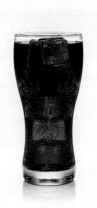

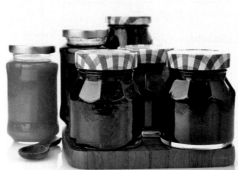

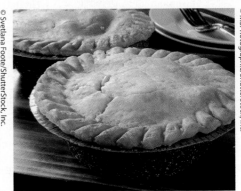

❝❝ Trans fats have largely been removed from processed foods, especially fast foods. **❞❞**

trans fat A type of fat added to vegetable oil products through the chemical process known as hydrogenation (adding hydrogen) in order to prevent these oils from spoiling. They are harmful to health because they raise bad cholesterol more so than other types of fats.

The second trend is a corollary to the first: an increase in the consumption of vegetable oils (i.e., fat from plant sources). Earlier, this trend reflected an increase in the consumption of trans fats, but the consumption of trans fats leveled out around 2000 and has since declined to very minimal amounts. Many vegetable oil products, such as margarines, contain these trans fats, which today are recognized as being detrimental to human health. Most **trans fats** result from the chemical modification (i.e., hydrogenation, or the addition of hydrogen) of plant oils that makes products containing trans fats more stable, giving them a longer shelf life. Trans fats were once common in processed foods such as margarine, baked goods, french fries, and snack foods. However, in recent years, due to concerns about their negative effects on health, trans fats have been removed from many processed foods, especially fast foods, in the United States and Europe.

A third trend has been the decline in complex carbohydrate intake from vegetables, particularly potatoes. This third trend has resulted in a substantial reduction in the intake of dietary fiber, which is found within plant cells, particularly plant cell walls.

A fourth trend is a slight (10%) rise in the consumption of animal protein, bringing protein consumption up to approximately 17% of total daily calories. This trend results primarily from increased use of poultry and, less so, of fish and other seafoods.

A fifth trend is the increase in sugar consumption, which was first observed in the 1950s, more than half a century ago. Although total carbohydrate intake has been decreasing, mainly because of the declining use of grains, vegetables, and fruits, which contain the complex carbohydrates, our appetite for the sweet simple carbohydrates, especially in snack foods and soft drinks, has become voracious. What this portends for future disease risk remains uncertain. Increased dietary sugar may elevate the total amount of energy consumed, thus contributing to the increased incidence of obesity.

According to the Institute of Medicine (IOM) of the National Academies of Science, the current contribution of macronutrient sources to total food energy for U.S. adults is approximately 50% carbohydrates, 35% fats, and 15% proteins (see **FIGURE 1.9**). This macronutrient distribution is based on the current recommended percentages for healthy living. The percent contribution of macronutrients in the U.S. population remains fairly constant across the life cycle, but total energy intake decreases with each decade beyond 60 years, as expenditure of energy in activities also decreases.

Over the last 30 years or so, the incidence of adult and child **obesity** has steadily increased in the United States. Total caloric intake rose gradually over the last few decades of the twentieth century; this, in turn, gave rise to the gradual increase in obesity during the same time frame (see **FIGURE 1.10**). Contributing to these trends is a major change in where meals are prepared and eaten. Currently, more than one in every three meals is consumed away from home, and this figure is growing. Institutional cafeterias, restaurants, and fast-food establishments supply the bulk of these meals. Fast-food

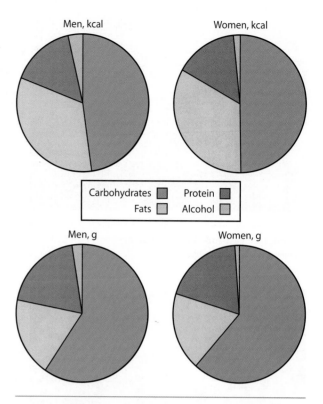

FIGURE 1.9 Distribution of Macronutrients in the U.S. Diet by Calories and Weight.

Data from Austin GL, Ogden LG, Hill JO. Trends in carbohydrate, fate, and protein intakes and association with energy intake in normal-weight, overweight, and obese individuals: 1971–2006. *Am J Clin Nutr*. 2011;93:836–843.

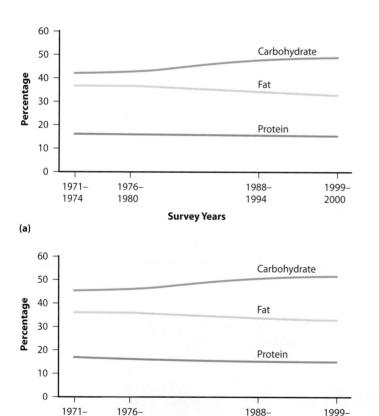

(a)

(b)

FIGURE 1.10 Trends in Calorie Consumption in the United States from 1971 to 2000. The increase in calories consumed since the 1970s is correlated with the gradual rise in obesity prevalence. (a) NHANES data for men. (b) NHANES data for women.

Reproduced from Wright JD, Kennedy-Stephenson J, Wang CY, McDowell MA, Johnson CL. Trends in intake of energy and macronutrients—United States, 1971–2000. *MMWR*. 2004;53(4):80–82.

obesity Excess accumulation of body fat mass. By definition, an individual is obese when his or her BMI is 30 or greater.

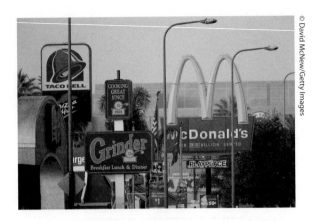

FIGURE 1.11 Fast-Food Restaurants. Fast-food outlets have dramatically grown in number and have influenced the eating patterns of many Americans.

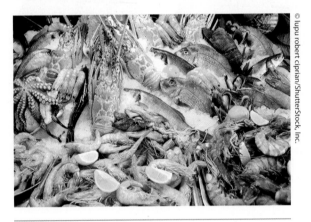

FIGURE 1.12 Seafood Products. The nutrient content of most seafood products is largely unaffected by commercial food processing. Thus, broiled or grilled seafood products can be a good choice at fast-food outlets.

> **❝ Fast foods generally provide large amounts of energy from fats and sugars and too little in the way of complex carbohydrates, phytochemicals, and dietary fiber. ❞**

fast foods Foods obtained quickly from outlets that typically are designed to prepare food rapidly and often for takeout. Many fast foods are high in calories and low in nutrients. There are many fast-food chains in the United States.

outlets, in particular, have grown in number and today have a strong influence on U.S. eating patterns (see **FIGURE 1.11**).

Fast Foods

Fast foods generally provide large amounts of energy from fats and sugars and too little in the way of complex carbohydrates, phytochemicals, and dietary fiber. The widespread satisfaction with fast foods, in general, is due to their convenience, taste and flavor, and reasonable prices, not their nutritional quality. An occasional meal at a fast-food outlet doesn't hurt, but a steady diet of fast foods provides, for the average person, excessive energy and sodium and too little vitamin A, iron, phytochemicals, and dietary fiber, leading to a nutritionally unbalanced pattern of eating.

Certain food items, such as meat-containing items like pizza, Mexican foods, and chili, provide a better balance, in general, than fast-food sandwiches, but they still remain fairly high in saturated fats from the cheese and sour cream often used in these dishes. Also, more salt is consumed with cheese because of the processing. The amounts of protein and most micronutrients appear to be adequate in fast foods. However, many of the processed foods used by fast-food vendors are lacking in a variety of trace minerals. An exception to this rule holds for most seafood products, the nutrient content of which is almost unaffected by commercial processing (see **FIGURE 1.12**).

The major nutritional disadvantages of the offerings of fast-food chains are the limited choice of foods, large serving sizes, the large amounts of animal fat from beef and other meats, the presence of saturated fats, and high amounts of salt. In addition, many fast foods, especially "nonmilk" shakes and soft drinks, are high in sugar. Large portion sizes tend to be the rule for fast foods. Fast foods also contain much less of the micronutrients and fiber provided by plant foods. As a consequence of the narrow choices of food items, the development of healthy individual food habits is difficult to achieve when relying on fast foods. The taste, flavor, and convenience of fast foods have had a powerful influence on the food-related behaviors of Americans. These new behaviors, and the accompanying decline in traditional food habits (i.e., the consumption of balanced meals with adequate servings of fruits, grains, and vegetables), may have long-term negative health risks (see **FIGURE 1.13**).

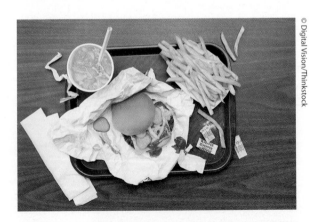

FIGURE 1.13 Fast-Food Meal. Most fast foods are high in saturated fat, sugar, and salt and low in dietary fiber.

TABLE 1.4
Advantages and Disadvantages of Fast Foods

Advantages	Disadvantages
High-quality protein	High in energy
Adequate in iron	High in fat, especially saturated fat
Good salads	High in sugar and high-fructose corn syrup
Good coffee	Limited offerings of fruits and vegetables
Convenient	Low in calcium
Cheap	Typically nutritionally unbalanced
Predictable	High in salt

Data from US DHHS and USDA, 2010.

Because of the high prevalence of obesity in the United States, fast-food providers have been coming under increasing attack for selling high-fat, high-energy foods that are prepared in extra-large servings. Of course, fast foods are not totally responsible for the great increase in body size over the last few decades, but the fast-food nation that we have become is probably a major contributor to our becoming a "fat nation." **Table 1.4** lists several of the advantages and disadvantages of fast foods.

PRACTICAL APPLICATIONS **1.1**

Compare the Energy and Protein Content of McDonald's Big Mac vs. Wendy's Grilled Chicken Sandwich

Using a fast-food nutrient content table, find the total energy (kilocalories), total fat (grams), and protein (grams) content for a McDonald's Big Mac and a Wendy's grilled chicken sandwich. How do these sandwiches differ with regards to total energy, fat, and protein? How healthy do you consider each sandwich to be? Explain.

	McDonald's Big Mac	Wendy's Grilled Chicken Sandwich
Energy (kcal)		
Total fat (g)		
Protein (g)		

For each sandwich, can you estimate total carbohydrate intake as a percentage of total energy intake? ■

Fortification of Foods

The **fortification of food** provides additional nutrients to ensure consumption of all essential micronutrients (i.e., vitamins and minerals). Food fortification is the process of adding **fortificants** (i.e., essential trace elements and vitamins) to food during processing. These extra nutrients are beneficial to the consumer of the food because public health policy aims to reduce the amount of people with dietary deficiencies in a population. A good example of the benefits of nutrient fortification is the use of folic acid, or folate, which has been added to flours, cereals, and other grain products since the late 1990s. Women who are or may become pregnant are encouraged to consume folate-containing foods because it has been shown to reduce the risk of neural tube defects, such as spina bifida, in children. Other nutrients are also used in fortifying foods and as components of supplements; for the most part, such fortification is generally considered to be healthful.

> **❦❦** Fortification of foods with folate has led to a decrease in neural tube defects in children. **❦❦**

PRACTICAL APPLICATIONS 1.2

Fortification of a Ready-to-Eat Breakfast Cereal

Obtain a box of Cheerios cereal and look at the Nutrition Facts panel. Find the listing of vitamins and minerals. Note that most of these are added to the raw cereal during processing. The following vitamins and minerals are fortificants: iron, zinc, vitamin C, B vitamins (niacin, pyridoxine, riboflavin, thiamin, folic acid, and cobalamin [B₁₂]), vitamin A, and vitamin D. Examine the Nutrition Facts panel of a different cereal and identify all the vitamins and minerals used to fortify the cereal. Which ingredient weighs the most? (See the first ingredient in the list.) ■

> **❦❦** Functional foods are specially designated as having health benefits or having advantages in reducing the risks of one or more chronic diseases. **❦❦**

fortification of food The addition of nutrients to foods for the purpose of improving intakes of nutrients that are not consumed in adequate amounts.

fortificant The specific nutrient added to a food during fortification.

functional food A food that contains, in addition to normal amounts of nutrients and non-nutrients, other molecules that promote health or prevent disease. Functional foods are often rich in phytochemicals. Examples include blueberries, broccoli, and salmon. They also are referred to as pharmfoods or neutraceuticals.

Functional Foods

Functional foods are specially designated as having health benefits or having advantages in reducing the risks of one or more chronic diseases. The U.S. Food and Drug Administration (FDA) permits several specific foods to be classified as functional foods because of the quantitatively large amount of a particular nutrient or phytochemical contained in one serving of the food. The designation functional food can be applied to a food that naturally contains a bioactive ingredient (i.e., nutrient or phytochemical) with major benefits to health beyond basic nutrition, especially for promoting health and preventing disease. The health benefit of the specific nutrient or ingredient (molecule) of interest must be supported by published research.

The focus is on the health effects of individual foods. Typically, a health claim for a functional food is made on the label or carton of a specific food, including fortified foods. The term *functional food* does not generally refer to additives, supplements, or herbals (botanicals). Examples of functional foods include blueberries, cranberry juice, tomatoes, spinach, broccoli, garlic, soybeans, green tea, fish, nuts, and oats. Red wine also may be considered a functional food. Epidemiologic studies have demonstrated health benefits of these foods for humans, such as reduction of cardiovascular diseases. An example of a "super" functional food, the blueberry, is highlighted in **FOCUS BOX 1.4**.

The view taken by the authors is that functional foods can be a great way to meet daily nutrient requirements. A food-based approach for meeting nutrient requirements, rather than focusing on supplements or herbals/botanicals that are not truly foods, is critical for healthy eating patterns. Nutrient-rich foods and plant foods also rich in phytomolecules support body functions better than nutrient-poor, energy-dense foods.

FOCUS 1.4   A Phytochemical Powerhouse: The Blueberry

Functional foods are foods that have a potentially positive effect on health beyond basic nutrition. A good example of a functional food is the blueberry (see **FIGURE A**), which is not only a good source of vitamins and minerals, but is also rich in phytochemicals. Blueberries are good sources of phytochemicals such as flavonoids, resveratrol, and anthocyanins (and their sugar-containing derivatives, the anthocyanidins). The phytochemicals in blueberries have considerable antioxidant properties; that is, they help reduce the presence of highly reactive oxygen molecules (species) in the cells, thereby protecting cells from oxidative damage. Specifically, studies on animals have found blueberries may help to protect the brain from oxidative stress, reducing the effects of age-related conditions such as Alzheimer's disease or dementia. Similar to cranberries, blueberries make it more difficult for bacteria to adhere to the mucosa of the urethra and bladder, thus reducing the risk of urinary tract infections. Many other berries have similar antioxidant properties because of their phytochemical content. The strong antioxidant properties of blueberries make them an excellent example of a functional food. ●

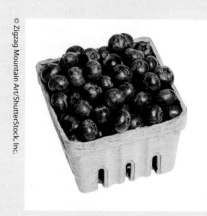

FIGURE A Blueberries. Blueberries are a major functional food, offering a variety of proven health benefits due to their high phytochemical content.

Nutrient Supplements

Nutrient supplements, typically pills containing multiple nutrients, provide an easy way for consumers to obtain almost all of the essential micronutrients (i.e., vitamins and minerals) they need each day (see **FIGURE 1.14**). Note that a supplement may not contain all of the required essential nutrients. Some supplement formulations are targeted to specific age groups (e.g., children, adult women, pregnant women, adult men, and older adults). In the future, nutrient supplements may be formulated to meet the needs of specific individuals, especially those who have genetic-related nutrient deficits!

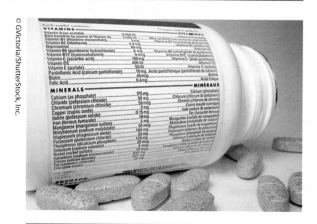

FIGURE 1.14 Supplement Label. The label on a supplement package lists all the vitamins and minerals as well as the amounts they supply.

Nutritional Status and Health

What does all of this nutrition information mean for individuals? How can people apply the guidelines and recommendations to achieve better health? How can governments assess the health of their populations to determine whether diet is a concern for the population? **Nutritional status** is important to both an individual's and nation's health surveillance. A number of different tools are available to evaluate the health and nutritional status of both individuals and populations. Two of the tools that are particularly useful are nutrition assessments and body mass index (BMI). These tools are used by nutritionists, registered dietitians, physicians, and personal trainers—basically anyone seeking to gain insight into a person's nutrition and health status.

nutrient supplement A product that provides nutrients in pill, tablet, or powder form for the purpose of improving nutritional status. Many micronutrients are available in pill form. Protein and energy also may be obtained through specific macronutrient supplements.

nutritional status The health of an individual with respect to nutrient intake. Also known as nutritional state.

Nutritional Assessment

A **nutritional assessment** is an in-depth evaluation of both objective and subjective data related to an individual's food and nutrient intake, lifestyle, and medical history. Once the data on an individual are collected and organized, the nutritional status of that person can be assessed and evaluated. An assessment can lead to the development of a plan to help the individual either maintain the assessed status or attain a healthier status.

Nutrition assessment can be achieved by completing a 24-hour food recall or a quantitative food frequency questionnaire. Current methods used to assess daily intake of nutrients and phytochemicals analyze all foods and beverages consumed during a day or over several days, and then the nutrient content of the diet is calculated using food composition tables. The USDA website, ChooseMyPlate.gov, offers a useful tool that enables a person to perform a nutrition analysis of his or her 24-hour intake.

Health Assessment

Various tools are currently used to assess health, including **body mass index (BMI)** and serum measurements of important molecules or biomarkers. BMI has become a standard assessment calculation based on weight and height to establish overweight and obesity as well as underweight ranges. Other measurements—for example, those resulting from whole-body scans (e.g., CAT scans, MRIs, X-rays)—also can be used, but these generally have less association with nutritional intake. In addition, simple measurements of girth can be useful. For example, waist and hip circumferences can be used to calculate a waist-to-hip ratio, an index of visceral (abdominal) body fat. Visceral fat is considered to be more metabolically active than fat around the buttocks and thighs; hence, this type of fat distribution (i.e., android or visceral) is considered to increase an individual's risk for chronic diseases more than the common female fat distribution (i.e., gynoid or hips; see **FIGURE 1.15**). The BMI ranges for underweight, normal weight, overweight, and obesity are listed in **Table 1.5**.

> *BMI has become a standard assessment calculation based on weight and height to establish overweight and obesity as well as underweight.*

nutritional assessment A complete nutritional assessment of an individual includes the ABCDs: anthropometric measurements, biochemical measurements, clinical evaluation for physical signs and other changes from normal, and dietary assessment (dietary questionnaires).

body mass index (BMI) An estimation of body fatness based on the equation of weight (kg)/height (m)^2 that is used to delineate overweight and obesity. Also referred to as the Quetelet index.

PRACTICAL APPLICATIONS **1.3**

Calculate Your BMI

It is easy to calculate your BMI. Just grab a calculator!

1. Convert your weight in pounds to kilograms by dividing by 2.2.
2. Convert your height in inches to meters by multiplying by 0.0254.
3. Square your height in meters (m).
4. Divide your weight in kilograms by meters squared to determine your BMI.

Consider an example. An adult male weighs 198 pounds and is 6 feet tall (72 inches). The metric conversions result in a weight of 90 kilograms and a height of 1.83 meters. Squaring of 1.83 equals 3.35, resulting in a BMI of 90/3.35, or 29.9. This man's BMI places him in the overweight category; in fact, he is almost obese! However, he is a weightlifter with large muscle mass. Would you still consider him to be overweight? ■

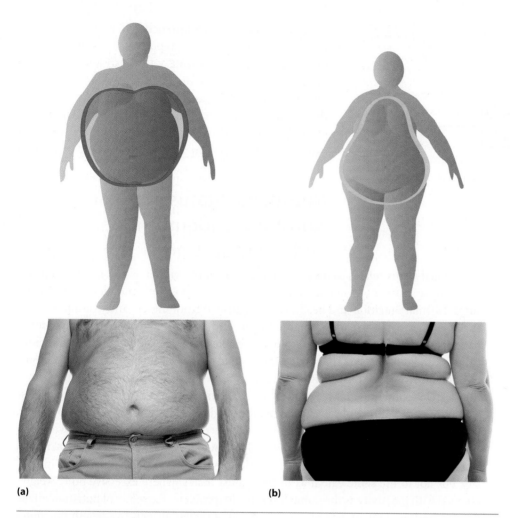

(a)

(b)

FIGURE 1.15 Obesity. (a) Android obesity is characterized by an excess of fat around the abdomen. (b) Gynoid obesity is characterized by an excess of fat around the hips and thighs.

(left) © kurhan/ShutterStock, Inc.; (right) © hartphotography/ShutterStock, Inc.

Excessive macronutrient intake contributes to four conditions that may lead to chronic disease: hypertension, hypercholesterolemia, impaired glucose tolerance, and obesity. The theory that unhealthy eating patterns involving excessive energy intake from all macronutrients plus too little physical activity contribute to the development of

> Excessive nutrient intakes contribute to four risk factors for the development of chronic disease: hypertension, hypercholesterolemia, impaired glucose tolerance, and obesity.

TABLE 1.5 Body Mass Index (BMI) Classifications	
Classification	**BMI Range**
Underweight	< 18.5
Normal	18.5–24.9
Overweight	25–29.9
Obesity	≥ 30

BMI = weight (in kg)/height (m)^2

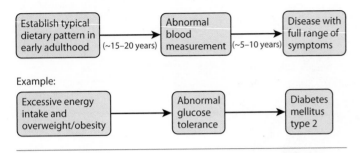

FIGURE 1.16 Diet–Disease Linkage. Dietary patterns established in early adulthood that may contribute to the development of a chronic disease, such as type 2 diabetes mellitus, later in life.

Reproduced from Anderson JJB. *Nutrition and Health: An Introduction.* Durham, NC: Carolina Academic Press; 2005.

" Nutritional status relates to the overall health of an individual or of a nation, as determined by assessment of nutritional intake, body composition, and biochemical measures. "

chronic disease has been instructive to researchers studying diseases such as stroke, type 2 diabetes mellitus, and diet-related cancers. **FIGURE 1.16** illustrates the linkage between dietary risk factors and type 2 diabetes mellitus. Other diet-related diseases, such as hypertension and cardiovascular diseases, may also follow obesity. All of these examples show **diet-disease linkage**, where one's diet can adversely affect him or her and possibly result in a disease.

Nutritional Status: Normal Nutrition, Undernutrition, and Overnutrition

Nutritional status relates to the overall health of an individual or of a nation, as determined by assessment of nutritional intake, body composition, and biochemical measures. Normal nutrition and health is distinguished from under- and overnutrition by specific types of information obtained from body weight and height; dietary intake patterns; biochemical measures of blood variables, such as fasting glucose; and clinical assessment of the skin, hair, and other visible or measurable features. The National Health and Nutrition Examination Survey (NHANES) provides this detailed information for U.S. subpopulations. For individuals, physicians and other healthcare professionals provide routine physical examinations and related tests. Prior to World War II, undernutrition was a serious problem that affected many; today, however, overnutrition—as evidenced by high rates of overweight and obesity—dominates the nutritional status of the nation. Other Western countries have also experienced increases in obesity, but not to the same extent as in the United States, where excessive body weight, coupled with inactivity, is the number one health problem. Extremes of nutrition intake (under- and overnutrition) are associated with a variety of negative health outcomes (see **FIGURE 1.17**).

Nutritional Intake

← Under   Normal   Over →

Poor Nations		Wealthy Nations
Economically unstable		Economically stable
Poor sanitation		High living standard
Limited food		Excess calorie consumption

Common Diseases	**Common Diseases**
Infant mortality	Obesity
Infections	Hypertension
Tuberculosis	Cardiovascular diseases
Single nutrient	Diabetes
deficiencies	Cancer
Marasmus	Osteoporosis
Kwashiorkor	Chronic obstructive
Parasites	pulmonary disease
	Congestive heart failure
	Renal failure

FIGURE 1.17 Nutrition and Health. Over- and underconsumption of nutrients both lead to negative health outcomes.

Reproduced from Anderson JJB. *Nutrition and Health: An Introduction.* Durham, NC: Carolina Academic Press; 2005.

diet–disease linkage The linkage between a long-term dietary pattern and the development of a chronic disease.

The assessment of the nutritional status of individuals and populations involves both measurements and observation, as undertaken by the periodic NHANES in the United States. Nutrition assessment often includes four components, sometimes referred to as the ABCDs of assessment:

- *Anthropometry*: Includes measurements of height and weight.
- *Biochemical assessment*: Includes biochemical measurements of blood or urine.
- *Clinical assessment*: Includes observations of the skin, hair, tongue, and mouth to look for abnormal physical signs.
- *Dietary assessment*: Involves estimations of dietary intake through 24-hour recalls or food frequency instruments.

TABLE 1.6
Physical Characteristics of Good Health

Characteristic	Description
Body size and shape	Appropriate weight for height (BMI)
Skin	No rashes or abnormal swelling
Hair	Shiny and not falling out
Lips and mouth	Not swollen, smooth, good color
Teeth	Not missing, no cavities, no pain
Eyes	Clear and shiny, pink membranes

These approaches, and other measurements of body composition, are used to try to determine the health of individuals as related to their usual nutritional intake.

A person's health status may be visually assessed by closely observing the body surface, skin, and hair and noting any excess fat accumulation in the body, including girth from abdominal fat or fat distribution on the buttocks and thighs (see **Table 1.6**). Undernutrition was widespread throughout the United States during the Great Depression of the 1930s, as illustrated by thin, hungry adult males waiting in line for food handouts (doles) (see **FIGURE 1.18**).

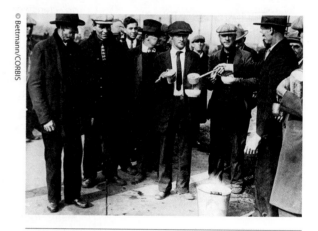

© Bettmann/CORBIS

FIGURE 1.18 Undernourished Men During the Great Depression. Undernutrition was common in the United States during the Great Depression of the 1930s.

Changing Understandings Based on Nutrition Research

The great change in the field of nutrition over the last few decades has been the enormous increase in overweight and obesity in the U.S. population, primarily among adults but also among children and adolescents. For example, in 2005 approximately 60% to 70% of all adults were either overweight or obese. A huge question for nutritionists is how nutrition is contributing to this enormous epidemic, an epidemic of relative affluence that also is affecting the rest of the industrialized world.

This increase in overweight and obesity is negatively influencing health and rates of **chronic diseases**, which are diseases typically diagnosed in adulthood as a result of dietary patterns, environmental risk factors, hormonal factors, or heredity. In fact, a cluster of chronic diseases or conditions is emerging that derives from obesity: high blood glucose, hypertension, abnormal blood lipids, and a large waist measurement. This cluster of conditions is commonly called metabolic syndrome because so many of the changes involve metabolic parameters, especially insulin resistance, resulting from excessive energy consumption and too little physical activity.

Scientific advances, whether from the laboratory, clinical research units, or epidemiological investigations, are being made at a fairly rapid pace. New studies often cast doubt on the validity of earlier studies. They also often complicate simpler interpretations of disease causation by uncovering additional complexities in diet–disease relationships. Re-evaluation of our knowledge base and disease concepts is an ongoing process.

chronic disease A disease typically diagnosed in adulthood as a result of suboptimal dietary intake patterns, environmental risk factors, hormonal factors, or heredity. Common chronic diseases include cardiovascular disease, type 2 diabetes, chronic obstructive pulmonary disease (COPD), and cancer.

" A cluster of chronic diseases or conditions is emerging that derives from obesity: high blood glucose, hypertension, abnormal blood lipids, and a large waist measurement. This cluster of conditions is commonly called metabolic syndrome because so many of the changes involve metabolic parameters, especially insulin resistance, resulting from excessive energy consumption and too little physical activity. **"**

Consumers need to keep an open mind that the most recently published report does not necessarily contradict earlier reports and understandings. In addition, consumers need to keep an eye open for fantastical claims by new fad diets or supplements (see **FOCUS BOX 1.5**). Typically, scientific studies need to be replicated at least once to be certain that the first study was not a "fluke" and that the subsequent studies corroborate the findings of the first report on the same study question.

FOCUS 1.5 Nutritional Science vs. Quackery

The difficulty for many consumers, at least in the United States, is recognizing the difference between legitimate scientific results and **quackery** based on poor or ill-conceived studies or testimonials. In a society that permits freedom of speech, almost anything on a nutrition topic can be written and published, whether based on science or not. When specific programs for improving health, such as a weight-loss program based on a fallacious concept of human biology, are advertised to consumers, the FDA or the Federal Trade Commission (FTC) has the authority to step in and stop the advertising and sale of the product. Keep a wary eye on advertisements that sound too good to be true! They most likely are. Quackery is just as alive today as it was in the past. In the late 1800s, an old-fashioned liquid elixir known as Lydia Pinkham's Vegetable Compound (see **FIGURE A**) was sold with claims that it could heal all manner of dysfunction and illness (it did not). Public awareness of the potential for quackery should be based on better understandings of foods, food ingredients, supplements, food labeling, and the roles of nutrients in health. This text should help you gain these understandings.

With obesity at an all-time high, people are so willing to try anything to lose weight that they are spending millions of dollars on every kind of product and program that promises results, especially quick results. So much money and effort are being put into the programs aimed at weight reduction that many wacky schemes have been invented to convince people that by using them they will accomplish their weight loss. Quackery and gimmicks that have no scientific validity abound in the realm of weight-loss products. ●

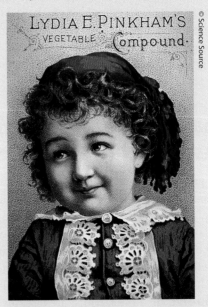

© Science Source

FIGURE A Quackery in Nutrition. Lydia Pinkham's Vegetable Compound was a quack remedy popular in the late 1800s. Today, quack remedies are just as widespread, and just as ineffective, for maintaining health.

quackery The distribution and promotion of false and misleading information. In the nutrition world, this consists of programs for health improvement and weight-loss and fad diets that are not backed in scientific data.

SUMMARY

Nutrients derived from foods must be consumed to maintain healthy human body tissues. The development of agriculture enabled human civilizations to develop because a steady supply of food was available to meet the population's needs. The body requires macronutrients (fats, proteins, and carbohydrates) and micronutrients (vitamins and minerals) to meet the body's energy needs and form biological compounds. The human body also requires water, dietary fiber, and phytochemicals, which are plant-based chemicals that have been found to be beneficial for human health. The energy in food is released from the breakage of hydrocarbon bonds and is measured in kilocalories. The recommended energy contribution for the macronutrients is 50% carbohydrates, 35% fats, and 15% proteins. Most Americans meet this distribution of macronutrients but consume too many calories, which often leads to overweight and obesity.

The three major determinants of food intake are availability of foods, purchasing power (money or barter), and social and cultural values placed on specific foods. More and more Americans are trying to make better food choices based on the nutritional quality of different foods. Various agencies in the U.S. government provide guidelines and tools to help Americans make better choices with regard to their nutrient intake. The *Dietary Guidelines for Americans* offers guidelines for making better food choices. The USDA's MyPlate is a visual tool to remind people to eat in the right proportions from the food groups. The Dietary Reference Intakes are guidelines for the intake of different macronutrients and micronutrients with the goal of meeting the health needs of approximately 98% of the U.S. population.

Dietary trends since World War II include increased macronutrient consumption, the rise of fast foods, the emergence of fortified and functional foods, and the use of nutrient supplements. These are primarily U.S.-specific consumption patterns, but many of these trends also have emerged to some degree in other Western nations and even in some Asian countries. In addition, more and more Americans are adopting vegetarian dietary patterns.

A variety of tools are available for evaluating the nutrition and health of both populations and individuals. Nutrition assessment is an in-depth evaluation of an individual's nutrient intake, lifestyle, and medical history. These data can be analyzed to find areas for improvement. Health assessments can be made by using BMI and serum measurements of biomarkers. Unhealthy dietary patterns can contribute to the development of chronic disease. In particular, obesity and overweight can lead to heart disease, high blood pressure, and type 2 diabetes. Diseases of overnutrition are becoming serious problems in developed countries. Diseases associated with undernutrition afflict the populations of poor countries. Nutrition research is continuing at a rapid pace to untangle the complexities of diet-related diseases.

STUDENT ACTIVITIES

1. List the three major determinants of food intake.

2. What are the three macronutrients? Which two macronutrients contribute the most energy to the diet?

3. What is the most common explanation for the current high rates of overweight and obesity in the United States?

4. What are phytochemicals? What is one of the major roles of phytochemicals in the human body?

5. What are the Atwater equivalents for the three macronutrients?

6. How do food guidelines and food pyramids differ? Briefly state the main difference between them, especially in terms of purpose and general content.

7. List recent trends (1970–2000) in consumption of macronutrients in the United States. Which macronutrient has seen increased consumption over this period?

8. List the advantages and disadvantages of fast foods.

9. Define the term *nutrient fortification*. Give an example.

10. Define *functional food*. How does a functional food differ from other foods?

11. Define *nutrient supplement*. Give an example. How does a nutrient supplement differ from adding nutrients (i.e., additives) to foods?

12. What is BMI? How is it calculated?

13. In the United States, prior to 1950 most nutrition-related problems, conditions, or diseases were of one type, whereas since 1950, they have been of another type. Explain why.

WEBSITES FOR FURTHER STUDY

Academy of Nutrition and Dietetics
www.eatright.org

American College of Nutrition
www.americancollegeofnutrition.org

American Society for Nutrition
www.nutrition.org

Centers for Disease Control and Prevention
www.cdc.gov

Food and Drug Administration
www.fda.gov

Canada's Food Guide
www.healthcanada.gc.ca/foodguide

Office of Dietary Supplements, NIH: Background Information on Dietary Supplements
http://ods.od.nih.gov/factsheets/DietarySupplements.asp

The Nutrition Society (British)
www.nutritionsociety.org

United States Department of Agriculture (USDA)
www.usda.gov

Vegan Health
www.veganhealth.org

Vegetarian Nutrition Resource, National Agricultural Library/USDA
http://snap.nal.usda.gov/resource-library/eat-healthy-every-day/vegetarian-nutrition

Vegetarian Resource Group
www.vrg.org

Position of the American Dietetic Association: Food and Nutrition Misinformation
www.eatright.org/WorkArea//DownloadAsset.aspx?id=8450

Nutrition and Well-Being A to Z from faqs.org: Quackery
www.faqs.org/nutrition/Pre-Sma/Quackery.html

Top 10 Tips to Identify Nutrition Quacks from Ask the Dietitian®
www.dietitian.com/quack.html

REFERENCES

American Dietetic Association. Position of the American Dietetic Association and Dietitians of Canada. Vegetarian diets. *J Am Diet Assoc.* 2003;103:748–765.

American Dietetic Association. Position of the American Dietetic Association: food and nutrition misinformation. *J Am Diet Assoc.* 2006;106:601–607.

Dwyer J, Picciano MF, Raiten DJ. Estimation of usual intakes: what we eat in America—NHANES. *J Nutr.* 2003;133:609S–623S.

Institute of Medicine. *Dietary Reference Intakes.* Washington, DC: National Academies Press; 1997–2004 (several volumes).

Institute of Medicine. *Dietary Reference Intakes for Calcium and Vitamin D.* Washington, DC: National Academies Press; 2011.

Levy D, ed. *50 Years of Discovery: Medical Milestones from the National Heart, Lung, Blood Institute: Framingham Heart Study.* Hackensack, NJ: Center for Bio-Medical Communications; 1999.

Stahler C. How Often Do Americans Eat Vegetarian Meals, and How Many Adults in the U.S. Are Vegetarian? Vegetarian Resource Group. May 18, 2012. Available at: www.vrg.org.

U.S. Department of Agriculture and U.S. Department of Health and Human Services. *Dietary Guidelines for Americans 2010.* 7th ed. Washington, DC: U.S. Government Printing Office; 2010.

U.S. Department of Health and Human Services. *Healthy People 2010: Understanding and Improving Health.* Washington, DC: U.S. Government Printing Office; 2000.

ADDITIONAL READING

Anderson JJB. *Nutrition and Health: An Introduction.* Durham, NC: Carolina Academic Press; 2005.

Fraser GE. *Diet, Life Expectancy, and Chronic Disease.* New York: Oxford University Press; 2003.

Havala Hobbs S. *Get the Trans Fat Out.* New York: Three Rivers Press; 2006.

Keiple K, Orneleas KC, eds. *The Cambridge World History of Foods.* New York: Cambridge University Press; 2000.

Mahan K, Escott-Stump S. *Krause's Food, Nutrition, and Diet Therapy.* 11th ed. Philadelphia: Saunders; 2004.

Pollan M. *Omnivore's Dilemma.* New York: Penguin Press; 2006.

Russell SA. *Hunger: An Unnatural History.* New York: Basic Books; 2005.

Sabate J, ed. *Vegetarian Nutrition.* Boca Raton, FL: CRC Press; 2001.

Schmidl MK, Labuza TP, eds. *Essentials of Functional Foods.* Gaithersburg, MD: Aspen Publishers; 2000.

Weil A. *Healthy Aging.* New York: Knopf; 2005.

Willett WC. *Eat, Drink, and Be Healthy.* New York: Free Press; 2001.

Williams JA. *Appalachia: A History.* Chapel Hill, NC: University of North Carolina Press; 2002.

2

Food Labels, Food Groups, and Phytochemicals

Although foods have social purposes, such as in celebrations and the welcoming of friends, they are consumed primarily because they contain the nutrients essential for sustaining life; that is, they contain the macronutrients, micronutrients, and phytochemicals required to maintain body tissues and biological functions. Knowledge of the nutrient composition of foods and beverages is important in planning meals for healthful living. Wise **food selection** each day, especially a variety of foods from the basic food groups, including fruits, vegetables, and other plant foods, ensures adequate intake of all the required macronutrients, micronutrients, and phytochemicals (see **FIGURE 2.1**). This chapter provides an overview of food labeling and food databases, food groups, and phytochemicals. Knowledge of the nutritional content of various foods is essential to developing and maintaining a healthy diet because planning balanced meals and sustaining good **food habits** are the foundation of long-term health and disease prevention.

> " Wise food selection each day, especially a variety of foods from the basic food groups, including fruits, vegetables, and other plant foods, ensures adequate intake of macronutrients, micronutrients, and phytochemicals. "

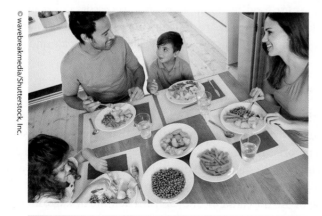

FIGURE 2.1 Healthy Meal Planning. A healthful diet includes all of the macronutrients, micronutrients, and phytochemicals the body needs to maintain health.

food selection Choosing foods from the basic food groups to ensure adequate intake of all the required macronutrients, micronutrients, and phytochemicals to maintain health.

food habit The usual selection of foods by an individual or a defined population on a long-term basis that characterizes a pattern of eating that reflects traditions, culture, and availability.

Food Labels

American supermarkets carry many processed foods that are packaged. These foods are required by law (Fair Packaging and Labeling Act of 1967) to be labeled. The purpose of food labeling is to provide the consumer with information about the nutrient content of the product in quantities that can be readily understood and, for perishable products, with information regarding how long the product can be safely kept on the shelves.

Required Information

All packaged foods must have a **Nutrition Facts panel** and an ingredients list of specific foods and additives. The manufacturer must also follow rules regarding statements made about the functionality of a specific ingredient or nutrient that may make the food item a "functional food." The information on food labels is intended to help consumers select nutritious foods as part of a healthy dietary pattern. The following information is required on all food labels:

- Serving or portion size.
- Amount of energy (in calories) per serving.
- Amount of fat, cholesterol, sodium, carbohydrate, and protein per serving.
- Percent Daily Value (%DV) of essential nutrients and dietary fiber, except for protein, per serving.
- An ingredients list of all ingredients in the food in order from high to low in mass units of each component or nutrient.

> *Each package is required to have a Nutrition Facts panel on the label that includes basic information about a serving of the food.*

Each package is required to have a Nutrition Facts panel on the label that includes basic information about a serving of the food. A sample Nutrition Facts panel of a breakfast cereal, Shredded Wheat, is provided in **FIGURE 2.2**. Information is required for macronutrients, saturated fat, cholesterol, trans fat, sodium, dietary fiber, sugars, vitamin A, vitamin C, calcium, and iron. (Trans fats have largely been removed from the food supply by action of the FDA.) Regulations do not require data on monounsaturated and polyunsaturated fats to be included on food labels, but many manufacturers provide this information. Other essential nutrients in the food are optional on a Nutrition Facts panel. The %DVs of any required nutrients and energy (based on a 2,000-calorie diet) must be on the panel. Additional information on the panel is given on the micronutrient content. Nutrient information about fat, cholesterol, and sodium content in a serving of a food also is given in terms of 2,000- and 2,500-calorie diets. An **ingredients list** is also required on packaging.

Additional food labeling regulations of the FDA went into effect in 1994. These specific guidelines for food manufacturers and processors cover practically all foods sold in the marketplace, and they are designed to provide clearer information about the nutritional content of food items. Mandatory labeling of meats and poultry went into effect in 2000.

Health Claims on Food Labels

Current regulations strongly limit the health messages conveyed by food companies on their labels, primarily to eliminate health claims that cannot be substantiated by published research reports. The FDA has approved several types of health claims. A **health claim** is a statement that establishes a beneficial association between a nutrient or food ingredient and a disease or health condition. A health claim must be reviewed and approved by the FDA. The claim must establish a definite linkage; for example, that calcium may help prevent osteoporosis or that soy protein may help prevent heart disease. These statements help food manufacturers market their products. Not all nutrients have claims associated with them, but manufacturers will be applying for additional

Nutrition Facts panel A label on packaged food that provides information about the serving size, calories, nutrients, and ingredients contained in the food product. Most provide information on saturated fats, trans fats, calories, sodium, and beneficial nutrients such as calcium, iron, and fiber.

ingredients list A list of all ingredients in a food item in order from high to low in mass units of each component or nutrient. It is required on all food labels in the United States.

health claim A statement that establishes a beneficial association between a nutrient or food ingredient and a disease or health condition. The claim must be reviewed and approved by the FDA and must establish a definite linkage (e.g., calcium may help to prevent osteoporosis).

Nutrition Facts
Shredded Wheat Cereal
Serving Size: 2 biscuits (47g)
Servings Per Container: 9

Amount Per Serving	2 Biscuits	2 Biscuits with 1/2 cup Skim Milk
Calories	160	200
Calories from Fat	10	10
	% Daily value**	
Total Fat 1g*	2%	2%
Saturated Fat 0g	0%	0%
Trans Fat 0g		
Polyunsaturated Fat 0.5g		
Monounsaturated Fat 0g		
Cholesterol 0mg	0%	0%
Sodium 0mg	0%	3%
Potassium 180 mg	5%	11%
Total Carbohydrate 37g	12%	14%
Dietary Fiber 6 g	24%	24%
Soluble Fiber <1g		
Insoluble Fiber 5g		
Sugars 0g		
Other Carbohydrate 31g		
Protein 5g		
Vitamin A	0%	4%
Vitamin C	0%	0%
Calcium	2%	17%
Iron	6%	6%
Thiamin	8%	13%
Riboflavin	0%	10%
Niacin	15%	15%
Phosphorus	15%	25%
Magnesium	15%	19%
Zinc	10%	15%
Copper	8%	10%

* Amount in cereal. One-half cup skim milk contributes an additional 40 calories, 65 mg sodium, 200 mg potassium, 6g total carbohydrate (6g sugars), and 4g protein.
** Percent Daily Values are based on a 2,000 calorie diet. Your daily values may be higher or lower depending on your calorie needs:

	Calories	2,000	2,500
Total Fat	Less than	65 g	80 g
Saturated Fat	Less than	20 g	25 g
Cholesterol	Less than	300 mg	300 mg
Sodium	Less than	2,400 mg	2,400 mg
Potassium		3,500 mg	3,500 mg
Total Carbohydrate		300 g	375 g
Dietary Fiber		25 g	30 g

FIGURE 2.2 Nutrition Facts Panel for Shredded Wheat. This panel illustrates the Percent Daily Values (%DVs) for two biscuit as well as two biscuits with 1/2 cup of skim milk. Protein has no %DV.

Reproduced from Anderson JJB. *Nutrition and Health: An Introduction.* Durham, NC: Carolina Academic Press; 2005.

approvals in the future. Examples of health claims authorized by the FDA are the following, according to the beneficial aspects of the nutrient(s):

- Calcium and osteoporosis: *high calcium*
- Sodium and hypertension: *low sodium*
- Dietary fat and cancer: *low total fat*
- Dietary fat and cholesterol and risk of coronary heart disease: *low amounts*
- Fiber-containing grain products, fruits, and vegetables and cancer: *high amounts*
- Fruits, vegetables, and grain products that contain fiber, particularly soluble fiber, and risk of coronary heart disease: *high amounts*
- Fruits and vegetables and cancer: *high amounts of several nutrients*
- Folate and neural tube defects: *high folate*

> *A health claim is a statement that establishes a beneficial association between a nutrient or food ingredient and a disease or health condition. A health claim must be reviewed and approved by the FDA.*

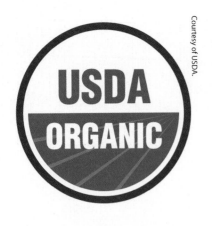

Courtesy of USDA.

FIGURE 2.3 The USDA's Organic Food Logo. This logo can only be used on food labels if the method of cultivation and production meets the USDA's criteria for "Organic."

Common household units of measurement are easier to use for everyday food preparation and consumption.

organic food An additive-free food that has been grown on soil that has not been treated with chemicals and that has been fertilized with natural fertilizers. The USDA's Certified Organic label carries specific requirements, including that the food has not been genetically modified.

food composition table A table or database that contains data on the nutrient content of foods. Such tables are published by U.S. government agencies, such as the USDA, and in other sources, such as *McCance and Widdowson's The Composition of Foods.*

- Dietary sugar alcohol and dental caries (cavities): *lack of sugar*
- Dietary soluble fiber, such as that found in whole oats and psyllium seed husk, and coronary heart disease: *high amounts*
- Soy protein and coronary heart disease: *high amounts of soy protein*
- Stanols/sterols and risk of coronary heart disease: *high amounts*

Organic Foods

In essence, all foods are organic in that they are composed of carbon, but a definition of **organic foods** implies that no synthetic chemicals—that is, no synthetic chemical fertilizers, herbicides, insecticides, or other products—have been used in the cultivation of the plants producing the foods, the rearing of livestock, or the packaging of the products. This definition applies to both plant and animal foods. Organic foods are often more expensive than traditional foods grown using chemicals, and much of the cost is related to transportation, especially for fossil fuels, from sites of production to markets. An alternate food source, such as locally produced crops and animals, is less expensive, but, of course, chemicals are sometimes used to grow local foods. Organic foods use their own logo (in green and white) if they meet the USDA's criteria for organic labeling (see **FIGURE 2.3**). Organic foods also are not derived from genetically modified organisms, or GMOs.

Food Composition Tables

Nutritionists and dietitians often need to know the specific nutrients and their relative quantities in certain foods. Several examples of the nutrient composition of items from the different food groups are provided in this chapter. This information is readily available in a variety of commercial and government tables and databases. The nutrient values of most foods found in food composition tables are usually presented in two different formats: (1) the amount of nutrient per 100 grams of the food and (2) in common household units of measurement, such as cups or ounces. In most cases, common household units are easier to use for everyday food preparation and consumption. Most food composition tables are incomplete because they typically lack information on all the micronutrient content of foods, especially trace elements. As chemical analytic techniques improve, however, future editions of such tables should provide more detailed information on the micronutrients.

The USDA maintains a database called the National Nutrient Database for Standard Reference. This important database contains nutrient information on more than 8,000 foods (see **FIGURE 2.4**). The information in the database is used as the foundation for most of the food and nutrition databases in the United States. The database can be accessed at http://ndb.nal.usda.gov. Note that this database is updated regularly as new foods become available and additional nutritional information is obtained.

Food composition tables and databases, including those provided by the USDA, provide data on the nutrient content of foods. Practically all the foods available in supermarkets have been analyzed and their composition listed in these tables or databases. Consumers can use these tables (plus the Nutrition Facts panel) to obtain reasonably good estimates of the amounts of nutrients they consume in a day (24 hours) or over longer periods. Information on fiber and a few phytochemicals is usually included in the food composition tables. When a specific food is not listed in a food composition table, nutrient values can be imputed or estimated from those listed for a similar food.

Food composition tables usually contain the following information about the content of each food: moisture (water), energy, protein, fat, carbohydrate, vitamins, minerals, fiber, and a few phytochemicals. Fats are further broken down by the specific types of fatty acids (i.e., saturated, monounsaturated, polyunsaturated). Information also may be provided on the amount of amino acids (almost 20), sugar, starch, dietary fiber (soluble, insoluble), cholesterol, alcohol, and specific biologically active phytochemicals.

Note that when looking at total carbohydrate values on food labels it is necessary to distinguish between utilizable carbohydrates such as starches and sugars and nonutilizable carbohydrates such as dietary fibers. Utilizable carbohydrates can be converted to energy in our bodies for use in cellular processes; nonutilizable components cannot.

Mixed foods, such as casseroles, pizzas, soups, and salads, contain a variety of specific ingredients, and each ingredient has its own specific nutrients. Prepackaged foods or meals, such as those in the frozen food section, are also examples of mixed foods. Some mixed foods are included in nutrient databases, others are not. For those that are not included in the databases, you need to have a fairly good idea of the specific foods consumed (and their amounts) and then find their composition in the food tables. The package labeling also may be helpful because all food manufacturers must provide nutrient analyses in their documentation for the FDA. In any event, read the labels!

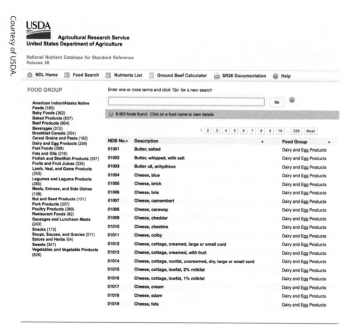

FIGURE 2.4 National Nutrient Database for Standard Reference. This important database maintained by the USDA contains nutrient information on more than 8,000 foods. As new food products are developed, they are added to the database.

P RACTICAL APPLICATIONS **2.1**

Food Composition Tables

Use a food composition table or database to determine the energy (kilocalories) provided by one serving of each of the following foods: cooked hamburger patty (3 ounces), cooked medium potato (whole with skin), and soy milk (8 ounces). Which food has the most total energy per serving? For each food, which macronutrient (carbohydrate, fat, or protein) contributed the most energy? What percentage of the food's energy was provided by that macronutrient? Would you classify any of these foods as calorically dense? ■

" Food composition tables usually contain the following information about the content of each food: moisture (water), energy, protein, fat, carbohydrate, vitamins, minerals, fiber, and a few phytochemicals. "

Plant Versus Animal Foods

At the most basic level, foods can be classified based on whether they come from plants or animals. Almost all foods are derived from either plants or animals. Foods from other sources, such as mushrooms, although packed with nutrients, make up a much smaller portion of the human diet.

Plant and animal foods differ in a number of ways. First, plant foods, especially when unprocessed, contain considerable amounts of dietary fiber. Second, plant foods generally provide most of the unsaturated fats (i.e., monounsaturated and polyunsaturated fatty acids) in the diet. Third, only plant foods provide phytochemicals. Finally, plants are good sources of many of the B vitamins, as well as vitamin C, vitamin K, vitamin E, beta-carotene, magnesium, potassium, and other minerals and trace elements.

Animal foods are the only food sources that provide vitamin B$_{12}$ (cobalamin). Also, animal foods provide much of the calcium, iron, and zinc in our diets in addition to a few B vitamins, vitamin D, and vitamin A. **Table 2.1** highlights the differences between plant and animal foods.

" Plant foods, especially when unprocessed, contain considerable amounts of dietary fiber, generally provide most of the unsaturated fats (i.e., monounsaturated and polyunsaturated fatty acids) in the diet, and provide phytochemicals. "

TABLE 2.1

General Composition of Plant and Animal Foods: Macronutrients and Micronutrients

Nutrient	Plant Foods	Animal Foods	Specific Food Items
Fats			
Total fats	Low	High	
Saturated fatty acids	Low	High	
Monounsaturated fatty acids	Moderate	Low	Very high in olive oil
Polyunsaturated fatty acids	High	Very low	Very high in vegetable oils
Trans fatty acids	None	None	High in processed foods
Cholesterol			
Total cholesterol	None	Moderate	High in liver
Proteins			
Total protein	Low	High	
Carbohydrates			
Total carbohydrate	High	Very low	
Starch	High	Very low	
Sugar	Low	None to low	High in fruit; high in candies and soda; low in milk
Dietary fiber	High	None	High in whole grains and dried beans
Water-Soluble Vitamins			
Total water-soluble vitamins	Moderate	Moderate	
Cobalamin	None	High	
Vitamin C	Moderate to high	Very low	High in fruit juices
Fat-Soluble Vitamins			
Total fat-soluble vitamins	Moderate	None to high	
Vitamin A	High (as beta-carotene)	Low	High in liver
Vitamin D	Low	Low	Also produced by skin upon exposure to sunlight
Vitamin E	High	None	
Macrominerals			
Total macrominerals	Low to high	Low to high	
Calcium	Low; moderate (dark greens)	Low; high (dairy)	Fortificant in orange juice
Magnesium	Moderate (dark greens)	Moderate	

(continues)

TABLE 2.1

General Composition of Plant and Animal Foods: Macronutrients and Micronutrients (*continued*)

Nutrient	Plant Foods	Animal Foods	Specific Food Items
Macrominerals			
Sodium	Low	Low	High (processed foods)
Potassium	High	High	Low (processed foods)
Trace Minerals			
Total trace minerals	Low to moderate	Low to high	
Iron	Low to moderate	Low to high	Moderate in dried fruit; low in dairy foods; high in meat; fortificant in cereals
Zinc	Low to moderate	Low to high	Moderate in cereals; low in dairy; high in meats
Selenium	Low to moderate	Moderate to high	Moderate in cereals; high in seafoods; varies with soil type where plant was grown or animal grazed
Iodine	Low to moderate	Low to high	High in seafoods; many foods are fortified with salt; varies with soil type where plant was grown or animal grazed
Fluoride	Low to high	Low to high	High in tea and seafoods; added to water supplies

MyPlate

Many **food groups** have been used over the last 60 years to aid consumers in the wise selection of a variety of foods to meet the body's needs and to maintain health. Shortly after World War II, the U.S. government began using four food groups (meat, milk and dairy products, cereals and breads, and fruits and vegetables) for consumer education. Although highly simplified, the traditional approach of the basic four food groups attempted to provide diversity in the diet as well as all essential nutrients each day. In the 1970s, a fifth group of miscellaneous foods (fats, sweets, alcohol, cooking oils, and others) was added. In the early 1990s, the vegetables and fruits were separated into two groups as part of the generic food guide or food pyramid, which has now been replaced by MyPlate, which was developed by the USDA (see ChooseMyPlate.gov). This revised food guidance system includes five groups of foods—grains, vegetables, fruits, protein (meats and beans or legumes), and dairy—for dietary planning (see **FIGURE 2.5**). The USDA also has developed MyPlate on Campus specifically for college students (see www.ChooseMyPlate.gov/MyPlateOnCampus).

Several features of the new food guidance system are highlighted in the MyPlate graphic. With the rapid increase of obesity and overweight in recent years, more attention has been given to appropriate energy intake. Consumers can go to the MyPlate website and enter their age, gender, and exercise level to obtain an estimate of their recommended caloric (energy) need. The website also offers consumers a tool to create a personalized plate that recommends the number of servings from each food group. For example, the site recommends that a 120-pound (55-kilogram), 21-year-old female who

> *This revised food guidance system [MyPlate] includes five groups of foods—grains, vegetables, fruits, protein (meats and beans or legumes), and dairy foods—for dietary planning.*

food groups Groupings of foods that are used to aid consumers in the wise selection of a variety of foods to meet the body's needs and to maintain health. The USDA's ChooseMyPlate food guidance system currently includes five groups of foods: grains, vegetables, fruits, protein (meat and beans or legumes), and dairy foods.

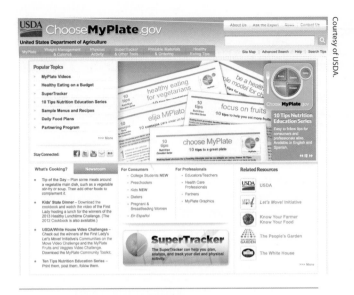

FIGURE 2.5 MyPlate at ChooseMyPlate.gov. The USDA's most recent food guidance system categorizes foods as fruits, vegetables, grains, proteins, dairy, and other. It also emphasizes the importance of physical activity in maintaining a healthy body weight.

exercises less than 30 minutes a day should consume 2,000 calories per day. The recommended daily intakes of food servings for this young adult female are illustrated in **FIGURE 2.6**.

Although the graphics and specific recommendations have changed over the last 60 years, the original goals of the food guidance systems to encourage a varied, balanced, and nutritious diet each day remain the same. MyPlate encourages consumption of whole grains. It also recommends consumption of whole fruits over fruit juices. Low-fat dairy foods are stressed, and fish and vegetable protein sources (i.e., beans and legumes) are emphasized. Another important new emphasis of MyPlate is the importance of drinking water. MyPlate recommends that consumers drink water instead of sugar-filled juices or soft drinks. Finally, salt reduction, consuming leaner animal protein sources, and cooking with vegetable oils rather than solid fats are recommended.

Physical activity is also an important component of MyPlate. It recommends moderate to vigorous exercise of more than 30 minutes most days of the week to help maintain weight. It recommends more than 60 minutes most days in order to lose weight. MyPlate provides consumers information on how to improve their diets, such as reducing portion sizes, making the plate about half fruits and vegetables, and consuming less fat from dairy foods.

> For those who wish to decrease their caloric intake and their weight, fewer and smaller servings will need to be selected from the major food groups, but they should still consume from all food groups to maintain healthy intake.

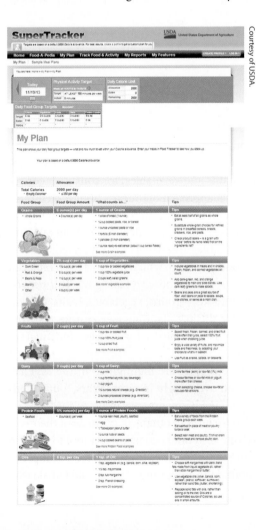

FIGURE 2.6 Recommended Food Servings for a 21-Year-Old Female. Note that a young male would typically require more servings to meet his energy needs. Keep in mind that the young adult female and male calorie recommendations are approximately 2,000 and 2,500 calories, respectively, as used on food labels.

The sample daily meal plan shown in **Table 2.2** shows a fairly healthy selection of foods. Practically all of these items are available at food services, cafeterias, and other eating establishments. Coupled with the *Dietary Guidelines for Americans, 2010*, MyPlate recommends healthy intakes that encourage individuals to maintain their current body weights, not to increase or decrease their weight. For those who wish to decrease their caloric intake and their weight, fewer and smaller servings will need to be selected from the major food groups, but they should still consume from all food groups to maintain healthy intakes. In order to achieve weight loss and then maintain a healthy diet, consultation with a dietitian or other health professional may be needed. The recommended range of fat intake is between 20% and 35% of total calories; thus, any diet selected for weight reduction needs to have its fat percentage fall within

TABLE 2.2

One-Day MyPlate Plan: A Sample One-Day Meal Plan Illustrating a Fairly Healthy Selection of Foods

	Grains	Vegetables	Fruits	Dairy	Meat and Beans	Others
Breakfast	1 oz Rice Krispies (1)		8 oz orange juice (1)	1 cup 1% milk (1)		1 cup coffee
Lunch	2 slices whole grain bread (2)	3 slices tomato (1), lettuce (0)		1½ oz Swiss cheese	3 oz sliced ham (1)	1 tbsp mayo, sweetened ice tea
Supper	1½ cup brown rice (3), 1 dinner roll (1)	1 cup cooked zucchini (1)		1½ oz shredded cheese	3 oz chicken patty	1 cup ice cream
Snack		1 carrot (1)	1 cup canned fruit cocktail (1)			3 cookies
Total number of servings	7 oz	3 cups	2 cups	3 cup equivalents	6 oz	Extra energy sources

The numbers in parentheses note the number of servings. This menu is based on information from www.chooseMyPlate.gov. This diet is intended for a 20-year-old woman who is 5 feet, 8 inches tall (173 cm) and weighs 130 pounds (59 kilograms) and is physically active (30 to 60 minutes of exercise a day). She requires 2,200 calories a day to maintain her current weight.
Data from the USDA.

PRACTICAL APPLICATIONS **2.2**

Macronutrient Composition of a Meal

Consider the following sample breakfast meal, eaten at home: orange juice (4 oz), Cheerios (1 serving), half a cup of skim milk, and one-half of a banana (medium size). Use a food composition table to find the energy (kilocalories), protein (grams), fat (grams), carbohydrate (grams), and cholesterol (milligrams) found in each food. Enter this information into a table. Calculate the percentage of total calories of the entire breakfast for each macronutrient. Sum each column in your table.

Then, using the Atwater energy equivalents, calculate the percentage of each macronutrient out of the total energy (kilocalories) in the meal. If you sum the amount of energy from each food, the total will be a good approximation of your caloric intake for your meal, but you need to sum the gram amounts of each macronutrient to obtain the total energy for the entire meal. This alternate method for calculating your energy intake from the meal is to multiply the gram amounts of each macronutrient in your food by the Atwater equivalent for each macronutri-

ent. (This sum may differ slightly from the sum of energy [kilocalories] derived from the food composition table.) The total kilocalories obtained by the two methods will differ somewhat but typically only by a trivial amount.

Using the Atwater equivalents, calculate the total calories from each macronutrient. Sum these three values, and use total calories as the divisor to find the percentage of each macronutrient (i.e., do not use the total energy directly from the food table in this activity because this value differs from the sum of the three macronutrient values). Also, total calories from meals may be estimated for a day using the Atwater equivalents. Remember that the miscellaneous group of calorie-dense foods (fats, sweets, and alcoholic beverages) typically add energy (calories) in sizeable quantities but not sufficient amounts of micronutrients (i.e., these foods are considered to be of low nutrient density). In general, the more processed the foods, the less nutritious they become because of the loss of micronutrients in processing. ■

> The food guidance systems are intended to help consumers choose foods wisely so that they meet their nutrient needs every day, while avoiding too many calories, salt, and other less healthy constituents of foods.

pyramid A food guidance tool used to help consumers choose foods wisely so that they meet their nutrient needs every day but do not consume too many calories, salt, and other less healthy constituents of foods; examples include the Mediterranean pyramid and the vegetarian pyramid.

alternate dietary pattern Diets that do not contain red meats (the standard American diet) or diets in which the protein is primarily obtained from legumes. Some consumption of eggs and dairy products may be permitted; various types of alternate diets exist, including vegan diets, but they are all assumed to be balanced diets.

Mediterranean diet A food guidance system inspired by the traditional dietary patterns of Greece and Italy. It recommends proportionally high consumption of olive oil, legumes, unrefined cereals, fruits, and vegetables, moderate to high consumption of fish, moderate consumption of dairy products (mostly as cheese and yogurt), moderate wine consumption, and low consumption of meat and meat products. Some studies have found that this diet may reduce the risk of coronary heart disease, possibly because of the high amounts of monounsaturated fats this diet provides.

vegetarian diet In general, a diet that does not include meat or meat products. The strictest type of vegetarian diet, the vegan diet, does not include any animal products. Other types of vegetarian eating patterns allow consumption of dairy products and eggs.

this range of total calories. Cutting dietary carbohydrates, such as sugar, also helps in weight control.

Alternate Food Guides or Pyramids

Alternate food guides or **pyramids** have been published, such as those for the Mediterranean diet, vegetarians, older adults, and so on. The USDA food guidance system, MyPlate, is used in this text, but other food guidance systems also may be useful. The food guidance systems are intended to help consumers choose foods wisely so that they meet their nutrient needs every day, while avoiding too many calories, salt, and other less healthy constituents of foods.

Examples of two **alternate dietary patterns** to USDA's MyPlate are the Mediterranean diet and the vegetarian diet practiced by many, including some Seventh-day Adventists (see **FIGURE 2.7**). The **Mediterranean diet** is based around seafoods, vegetables, fruits, olive oil, and wine (see **FIGURE 2.8**). Traditionally, it has contained limited servings of animal-based foods such as red meats and dairy products. The **vegetarian diet** contains only plant foods, such as whole grains, beans and other legumes, soy milk, and nuts and seeds, as well as limited dairy and egg consumption, if desired. Another food guidance system, the Dietary Approach to Stop Hypertension (DASH) diet, emphasizes whole grains, fruits, vegetables, low-fat dairy products, low-fat meats, and low-salt foods, with the goal of reducing hypertension and promoting cardiovascular health. This diet can be useful in managing diet-related chronic diseases. The Okinawa diet emphasizes seafoods and vegetables and fruits along with rice.

Overview of the Five Food Groups

The USDA's MyPlate recognizes five food groups: fruits, vegetables, grains, protein foods, and dairy. Each type of food has its own unique nutrient composition but,

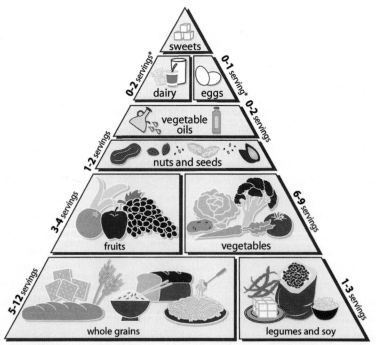

FIGURE 2.7 Vegetarian Food Pyramid. The vegetarian food guidance system shown here focuses on plant foods.

© 2008 Loma Linda University, School of Public Health, Department of Nutrition.

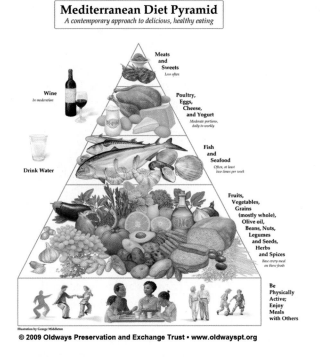

FIGURE 2.8 Mediterranean Food Pyramid. The Mediterranean food pyramid shows that the focus of this dietary plan is on seafoods, vegetables, fruits, and olive oil.

© 2009 Oldways Preservation & Exchange Trust.

P RACTICAL APPLICATIONS 2.3

Protein and Energy Content of Different Food Guidance Systems

Examine the MyPlate, Mediterranean, and vegetarian food guidance systems. For each, select the two groups of foods that provide (1) the most energy and (2) the most protein. Comment on the specific food items that are needed within each group to provide the energy and protein. Do the specific foods in the three plans differ? Explain any major differences between the three dietary plans. ∎

---

within a food group, the specific composition of nutrients tends to be similar, such as in the dairy group, where most of the foods are derived from animal milk and are good sources of calcium.

Fruits

The **fruit group** includes the fruits of any plant or 100% fruit juice. In addition to the wide variety of fruits available, fruits may be fresh, canned, frozen, or dried. **Table 2.3** lists some of the more commonly eaten fruits in the United States. In other parts of the world, diets will include fruits that are commonly grown in those areas.

MyPlate recommends that half your plate be fruits and vegetables. Specifically, most adult men and women should strive to consume at least two cups of fruit each day to maintain good health. Most fruits are naturally low in fat and sodium and are generally low in calories. They are good sources of potassium, dietary fiber, vitamin C, and folate. Fruits also are very rich in phytochemicals.

fruit group One of the basic food groups of the MyPlate food guidance system. This food group includes the fruits of any plant or 100% fruit juice. In addition to supplying macronutrients, fruits are rich in micronutrients, dietary fiber, and phytochemicals.

TABLE 2.3
Fruits Commonly Eaten in the United States

- Apples
- Apricots
- Bananas
- Blueberries
- Cantaloupe
- Cherries
- Grapefruit
- Grapes
- Honeydew melon
- Kiwi fruit
- Lemons
- Limes
- Mangoes
- Nectarines
- Oranges
- Peaches
- Pears
- Papaya
- Pineapple
- Plums
- Prunes
- Raisins
- Raspberries
- Strawberries
- Tangerines
- Watermelon

Reproduced from U.S. Department of Agriculture, Center for Nutrition Policy and Promotion. Food Groups: MyPlate. Available at: www.chooseMyPlate.gov/food-groups/fruits.html.

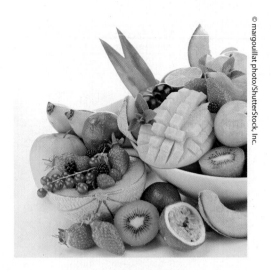

© margouillat photo/ShutterStock, Inc.

Diets high in fruits have been found to be protective against certain types of cancers and may reduce the risk of heart disease, obesity, and type 2 diabetes. Potassium is thought to play a role in maintaining a healthy blood pressure. Dietary fiber helps to reduce cholesterol levels, reducing the risk of heart disease. It also helps to prevent constipation. Vitamin C is critical for the growth and repair of body tissues and wound healing. Folic acid is needed in the formation of red blood cells and can help to prevent neural tube defects in fetal development.

Vegetables

The **vegetable group** includes any vegetable or 100% vegetable juice. Vegetables can be consumed raw or cooked. The vegetable group can be divided into five subgroups based on nutrient content. **Table 2.4** lists the five subgroups and commonly eaten vegetables in each subgroup.

MyPlate recommends that half your plate be fruits and vegetables. Specifically, most adult men and women should strive to consume at least 2 to 3 cups of vegetables each day to maintain good health. Most vegetables are naturally low in fat and calories. They are good sources of potassium, dietary fiber, vitamin C, vitamin A, and folate. Vegetables are also very rich in phytochemicals.

Dark green, leafy vegetables tend to be much more nutritious than those that are light or pale green. Broccoli, spinach, kale, dark varieties of lettuce, and other greens are especially high in several micronutrients, including vitamin C, beta-carotene and other

> Legumes represent a special subset of vegetables and, because of their high protein content, they often are grouped with other protein-rich foods, such as meats.

vegetable group One of the basic food groups of the MyPlate food guidance system. This food group includes any vegetable or 100% vegetables juice. Can be divided into five subgroups based on nutrient content: dark green, leafy vegetables, starchy vegetables, beans and peas (legumes), red and orange vegetables, and other. In addition to supplying macronutrients, vegetables are rich in micronutrients and dietary fiber.

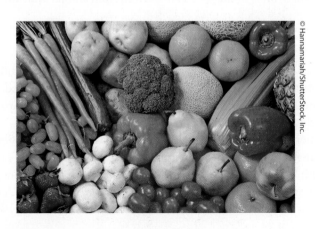

© Hannamariah/ShutterStock, Inc.

TABLE 2.4
The Five Vegetable Subgroups and Frequently Consumed Vegetables

Dark Green Vegetables	Starchy Vegetables	Beans, Peas, and Legumes	Red and Orange Vegetables	Other
• Bok choy	• Cassava	• Black beans	• Acorn squash	• Artichokes
• Broccoli	• Corn	• Black-eyed peas (mature, dry)	• Butternut squash	• Asparagus
• Collard greens	• Fresh cowpeas, field peas, or black-eyed peas (not dry)	• Garbanzo beans (chickpeas)	• Carrots	• Avocado
• Dark green, leafy lettuce	• Green bananas	• Kidney beans	• Hubbard squash	• Bean sprouts
• Kale	• Green peas	• Lentils	• Pumpkin	• Beets
• Mesclun	• Green lima beans	• Navy beans	• Red peppers	• Brussels sprouts
• Mustard greens	• Plantains	• Pinto beans	• Sweet potatoes	• Cabbage
• Romaine	• Potatoes	• Soy beans	• Tomatoes	• Cauliflower
• Spinach	• Taro	• Split peas	• Tomato juice	• Celery
• Turnip greens	• Water chestnuts	• White beans		• Cucumbers
• Watercress				• Eggplant
				• Green beans
				• Green peppers
				• Iceberg (head) lettuce
				• Okra
				• Onions
				• Turnips
				• Wax beans
				• Zucchini

Reproduced from U.S. Department of Agriculture, Center for Nutrition Policy and Promotion. Food Groups: MyPlate. Available at: www .chooseMyPlate.gov/food-groups/vegetables.html.

carotenoids, calcium, magnesium, and often iron. See **FOCUS BOX 2.1** for information about one of the most nutritious groups of vegetables—the Brassica family.

As with fruits, diets high in vegetables can reduce the risk of heart disease and protect against certain types of cancers. Vegetable consumption can also reduce the risk of obesity and type 2 diabetes. The potassium in vegetables helps to maintain a healthy blood pressure. Dietary fiber can help to reduce cholesterol levels and reduce the risk of heart disease. It can also prevent constipation and contribute to feelings of fullness with a meal. Vitamin A is essential to good vision and enhances immune system function. Vitamin C plays an important role in wound healing and maintaining connective tissues health. Vitamin C also aids in the absorption of iron.

Legumes represent a special subset of vegetables and, because of their high protein content, they often are grouped with other protein-rich foods, such as meats. Legumes include a variety of beans, peas, and soybeans (see **Table 2.5**). The macronutrient composition of legumes differs from other vegetables, especially their protein and fat content.

Grains

Grains, such as cereals, breads, pastas, and rice, have provided humans with most of their dietary carbohydrates since the dawn of agriculture. The **grain group** includes any food made from wheat, rice, oats, cornmeal, barley, or other cereal grain. Grains can be divided into two subgroups: whole grains and refined grains. Whole grains include the whole grain kernel: the bran, germ, and endosperm. Refined grains are

legume A special subset of vegetables that includes a variety of beans, peas, and soybeans. The macronutrient composition of legumes differs from other vegetables, especially their protein and fat content. Because of their high protein content, they are often grouped with other protein-rich foods, such as meats.

grain group One of the basic food groups of the MyPlate food guidance system. This food group includes any food made from wheat, rice, oats, cornmeal, barley, or other cereal grains. Grains can be divided into whole grains and refined grains. Grains are an important source of macronutrients as well as dietary fiber and B vitamins.

FOCUS 2.1   The Brassica Family: Vegetable Superfoods

The **Brassica family** of plants provides vegetables such as broccoli, cauliflower, Brussels sprouts, cabbage, and others. Members of this plant family are not only micronutrient rich and good sources of fiber, but they also contain indoles, a family of phytochemical molecules that may help to prevent cancer. These vegetables may be the best natural food sources of antioxidant nutrients, including beta-carotene, vitamin C, vitamin E, and selenium. An example of the nutrient content of broccoli is seen in **Table A**. Just one serving of cooked broccoli meets almost 50% of the RDA for adult women for vitamin C! ●

TABLE A
Nutrient Content of Broccoli as Percentage of RDA for Adult Female

Nutrient	One-Half Cup Broccoli (cooked, chopped)	RDA for Females (19–30 Years)	Percentage of RDA
Fiber	3 g	25 g	12%
Potassium	131 mg	4,700 mg	3%
Selenium	0.6 µg	55 µg	1%
Vitamin C	37 mg	75 mg	49%
Folate	52 mg	400 mg	13%
Vitamin E	1.2 mg	15 mg	8%
Vitamin A (as beta-carotene)	47 retinol activity equivalents (RAE)	700 RAE	7%

TABLE 2.5
Nutrient Content of Various Legumes

Legume (cooked, 1 cup)	Dry Weight (g)	Energy (kcal)	Carbohydrate (g)	Protein (g)	Fat (g)	Fiber (g)
Green beans	12	38	9	2	Trace	4
Greens peas	33	125	23	8	Trace	9
Navy beans	66	255	47	15	1	19
Lentils	60	230	40	18	1	16
Soybeans	64	298	17	29	15	10

Data from the USDA. National Nutrient Database for Standard Reference. Available at: www.ars.usda.gov/main/site_main.htm?modecode=12354500.

Brassica family Family of plants that includes broccoli, Brussels sprouts, cabbage, cauliflower, collards, horseradish, kale, mustard, radish, turnip, and watercress. Members of the Brassica family contain good quantities of many essential nutrients plus non-nutrient phytochemicals, especially indoles, that may help to prevent cancer.

those grains that have been processed so the bran and germ (and many micronutrients along with them) have been removed. Refined grains have a longer shelf life than whole grains, but the removal of the bran and germ removes much of the dietary fiber, iron, and B vitamins from the food. Because of this, many foods made from refined grains are fortified in order to add back these nutrients. **Table 2.6** lists examples of whole grain and refined grain foods.

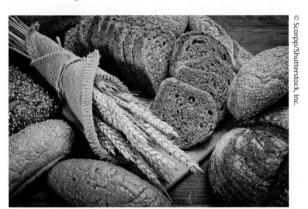

© Scorpp/Shutterstock, Inc.

MyPlate emphasizes that at least half the grains consumed each day should be whole grains. Adult men and women should consume 6 to 8 ounces of grains each day, with 3 to 4 ounces being whole grains.

Grains are important sources of dietary fiber and several of the B vitamins, including **fortified B vitamins**, i.e., thiamin, riboflavin, niacin, and folate. They are also rich in iron (fortified), magnesium, and selenium. The B vitamins are important in various metabolic processes and play a key role in maintaining nervous system function. Iron is needed to carry oxygen in the blood. Magnesium is important for bone health, and selénium in an important antioxidant. Focusing on consumption of whole grains rather than refined grains can also help in maintaining a healthy weight.

Ready-to-eat breakfast cereals, introduced in the marketplace through the pioneering work of W. K. Kellogg, have diverse compositions, depending on what nutrients (fortificants), sugar, and preservatives have been added. Look carefully at cereal labels, especially the Nutrition Facts panel, to determine their macronutrient and micronutrient composition.

> Whole grains include the whole grain kernel: the bran, germ, and endosperm. Refined grains are those grains that have been processed so the bran and germ (and many micronutrients along with them) have been removed.

> Focusing on consumption of whole grains rather than refined grains can also help in maintaining a healthy weight.

fortified B vitamins Vitamins that are important in various metabolic processes and that play a key role in maintaining nervous system function; examples include thiamin, riboflavin, niacin, and folate.

TABLE 2.6
Whole Grain and Refined Grain Foods

Whole Grains	Refined Grains
• Whole-wheat flour	• White flour
• Bulgur (cracked wheat)	• De-germed cornmeal
• Oatmeal	• White bread
• Whole cornmeal	• White rice
• Brown rice	

Reproduced from U.S. Department of Agriculture, Center for Nutrition Policy and Promotion. Food Groups: MyPlate. Available at: www.chooseMyPlate.gov/food-groups/grains.html.

PRACTICAL APPLICATIONS 2.4

Nutrient Composition of Two Ready-to-Eat Cereals

Shredded Wheat and Total are very different ready-to-eat cereals in their macronutrient and micronutrient content. One has almost no additives, whereas the other has many additives, including nutrient fortificants. One cereal also has a fairly high sugar content as part of its total carbohydrate content. Make a brief table for each cereal, similar to the Nutrition Facts panel, and then list the nutrients separately for each cereal and the % Daily Value for each nutrient. Which cereal do you think is a better choice? Explain why. ■

Proteins

The **protein group** contains a variety of foods that share one feature—they are very rich sources of high-quality proteins. This group contains **animal protein foods (muscle proteins)** such as meat, poultry, seafood, and eggs. It also includes **plant protein foods**, like legumes such as beans, peas, and soy products, and nuts, and seeds. Note that beans and peas are also part of the vegetable group.

According to MyPlate, most adults should consume 5 to 6 ounces of high-quality protein a day to maintain good health. Historically, meats have been the basis of the traditional American approach to meal planning. Although the idea that each meal has to contain at least one protein-rich animal product has been changing, the tradition remains deeply rooted and is clearly reflected in the nation's overall protein intake, which is considerably greater than the gender-specific RDAs!

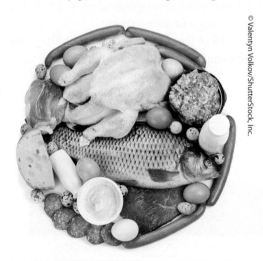

© Valentyn Volkov/ShutterStock, Inc.

protein group One of the basic food groups of the MyPlate food guidance system. This food group includes foods that share one feature—they are very rich sources of protein. Includes both animal and plant sources of proteins.

animal protein foods (muscle proteins) Dietary protein from animal sources, such as meat, poultry, seafood and eggs. Animal proteins typically provide greater quantities of specific amino acids, such as arginine, that give rise to hormones that stimulate insulin and glucagon release following a meal. Animal proteins are usually more complete than those obtained from plants.

plant protein foods Proteins obtained from plant sources, including cereal grains, vegetables, nuts, and seeds. Protein quality typically is lower for plant proteins than for animal proteins, with legumes having the highest quality plant proteins.

Proteins are essential for the maintenance of good health. They are the building blocks for bones, muscles, cartilage, skin, and blood. Proteins also are essential components of enzymes, hormones, and vitamins. The foods in this group also are good sources of B vitamins, vitamin E, iron, zinc, and magnesium. By now you are aware of the importance of B vitamins. They serve important roles in metabolic pathways, nervous system function, and tissue maintenance. Iron is needed because it is part of the hemoglobin used to carry oxygen to the body's tissues and myoglobin. Magnesium is used in building bones, releasing energy for muscles, and in metabolic synthesis of many molecules. Zinc is essential for a variety of biochemical reactions and helps the immune system function properly. Seafood, another protein-rich source, should be a dietary staple because it is rich in omega-3 fatty acids, which may protect against heart disease.

Although proteins are vital to good health, it is important to choose foods that are low in saturated fat and cholesterol. Consumption of large amounts of red meat, and the fat it contains, can contribute to high cholesterol and heart disease. It is better to choose lean cuts of meat or poultry when consuming animal proteins. All of the skin and fat should be removed to reduce the saturated fat content of the meat.

Dairy

The **dairy group** contains milk and foods made from milk, such as cheese, sour cream, and yogurt. Foods in this group are generally very high in calcium, with the exception of butter and ice cream. **Table 2.7** lists some of the more commonly consumed dairy products in the United States.

MyPlate recommends that adults consume 3 cups of foods from the dairy group each day. Milk and dairy products are rich in macronutrients and micronutrients, including calcium, phosphorus, riboflavin, thiamin, cobalamin, sodium, potassium, and magnesium. Some types of milk are fortified with vitamins A and D. Many modifications have been made to make milk more palatable, healthier, and more digestible (see **FOCUS BOX 2.2**). **Table 2.8** compares the nutrient composition of whole milk, 2% milk, 1% milk, and skim milk. In addition to low-fat milks, low-fat cheeses are now available. Many yogurts are available that have almost no fat. Note that these low-fat foods typically are not fortified with vitamins A and D.

Calcium is the critical nutrient in dairy products. In American diets, dairy products are the primary source of calcium, which is essential for building bones and teeth and in maintaining bone mass. Diets that provide 3 cups or the equivalent of dairy products per day help maintain bone mass after growth ceases. Consumption of calcium-rich dairy products has been linked with good bone health and a possible decreased risk of osteoporosis. Vitamin D in dairy products also aids in bone health by helping the body maintain needed levels of phosphorus and calcium. It also may have other beneficial effects, such as lowering the risk of type 2 diabetes.

> Seafood, another protein-rich source, should be a dietary staple because it is rich in omega-3 fatty acids, which may protect against heart disease.

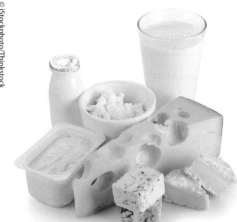

© iStockphoto/Thinkstock

TABLE 2.7
Commonly Consumed Dairy Products in the United States

Fluid Milk	Cheese	Milk-Based Desserts	Yogurt
• Fat-free (skim) • Low fat (1%) • Reduced fat (2%) • Whole • Flavored milks (chocolate, strawberry) • Lactose-reduced milks • Lactose-free milks	• Cheddar • Mozzarella • Swiss • Parmesan • Ricotta • Cottage cheese • American	• Puddings • Ice milk • Frozen yogurt • Ice cream	• Fat-free • Low fat • Reduced fat • Whole milk yogurt

Reproduced from U.S. Department of Agriculture, Center for Nutrition Policy and Promotion. Food Groups: MyPlate. Available at: www.chooseMyPlate.gov/food-groups/dairy.html.

dairy group One of the basic food groups of the MyPlate food guidance system. This food group includes milk and foods made from milk, such as cheese, sour cream, and yogurt. Foods in this group are generally good sources of calcium.

TABLE 2.8
Nutrient Composition of Various Types of Milk

Nutrient	Whole Milk (3.25% fat)	Low-Fat Milk (2% fat)	Low-Fat Milk (1% fat)	Skim Milk (0.1% fat)
Calcium (mg)	260	285	290	306
Phosphorus (mg)	222	229	232	247
Magnesium (mg)	24	24	27	27
Potassium (mg)	349	366	366	382
Iron (μg)	70	70	70	70
Zinc (μg)	980	1050	1020	1030
Vitamin A (RAE)	68	134	142	149
Vitamin D (IU)	98	105	127	100
Vitamin E (μg)	150	70	20	20
Thiamin (μg)	107	95	49	110
Riboflavin (μg)	447	451	451	446
Niacin (μg)	261	224	227	230
Pyridoxin (μg)	88	93	90	91
Folic acid (DFE)	12	12	12	12
Cobalamin (μg)	1.07	1.12	1.07	1.30
Pantothenic acid (μg)	883	869	881	875

Data from U.S. Department of Agriculture. National Nutrient Database for Standard Reference. Available at: www.ars.usda.gov/main/site_main .htm?modecode=12354500.

lactose intolerance The inability to digest milk sugar (lactose) after the consumption of milk or other lactose-containing products. Consumption of products containing lactose can cause adverse effects in people who do not produce enough lactase, the enzyme required to break down lactose in the small intestine.

lactose-free milk products Milks and other dairy foods that have been treated with lactase to degrade most of the lactose in the food. Lactose causes adverse effects in people who have low lactase enzyme production in their small intestine (i.e., lactose intolerance). These products enable people with lactose intolerance to consume dairy products.

FOCUS 2.2 Lactose Modification of Cow's Milk

Milk contains lactose, a sugar, as its only carbohydrate source of energy. Some people are unable to break down this sugar, a condition referred to as lactose intolerance. Symptoms of **lactose intolerance** include bloating, abdominal cramps, gas, diarrhea, and even vomiting. Some lactose-intolerant individuals might have to drink a quart of cow's milk or more before symptoms appear. Individuals with lactose intolerance (also called milk intolerance) might want to try lactose-modified milk. Lactose in cow's milk can be converted to glucose and galactose by the addition of the enzyme lactase. In the marketplace, several types of lactose-modified milks can be found. The trade name of one of these **lactose-free milk products** is Lact-Aid. ●

Phytochemicals

The macronutrients and micronutrients in foods are the focus of the bulk of nutrition information presented by government agencies to the U.S. population. However, evidence has emerged in recent years on the importance of other molecules in foods—phytochemicals—in maintaining, and perhaps even improving, human health. Phytochemicals (or phytomolecules) are non-nutrient substances found in plants. Phytochemicals are synthesized by plants to serve specific functions in the plants. Varying amounts are found in practically all fruits, vegetables, grains, nuts, and seeds. The energy-producing organelles (i.e., chloroplasts, mitochondria) in plant cells generate highly reactive oxygen free radicals. Buildup of free oxygen radicals can cause cell damage over time. Many of the phytochemicals produced by plants act as **antioxidants**, reducing the amount of oxygen free radicals.

Antioxidants and Human Health

In humans, as in plants, the normal metabolic activities of cells involving oxygen, especially mitochondrial reactions, produce free radicals. Free radicals, such as superoxides ($^{.}O_2$) and hydroxyl radicals ($^{.}OH$), are potent species that can react with DNA and other macromolecules within cells and initiate the changes that may eventually lead to cancer (see **FIGURE 2.9**). Free radicals are normally rapidly neutralized or quenched in cells by enzyme systems that use **antioxidant nutrients** such as vitamin C, beta-carotene, vitamin E, and selenium. These nutrient antioxidants and other plant phytochemicals may also act as nonenzymatic antioxidants, eliminating free radicals by directly neutralizing them. Thus, consumption of phytochemicals from plants can play an important role in preventing the accumulation of cellular damage over time. Some research suggests that phytochemicals can help to prevent or delay cancer, cardiovascular diseases, brain neuronal changes, and other conditions. Diets rich in phytomolecules are considered to be healthy, even though these molecules are not classified as nutrients.

Although RDAs have not been set for phytochemicals (aside from dietary fiber), an increasing emphasis is being placed on the consumption of sufficient amounts of fruits, vegetables, and whole grains in the diets of Americans and Canadians for reducing the risks of chronic diseases. A common test used to measure antioxidant activity in foods is known as oxygen radical absorbance capacity, or ORAC. Berries tend to have the highest ORAC scores (see **Table 2.9**).

Health Benefits of Phytochemicals

The health benefits of phytochemicals that are delivered as integral parts of the foods that humans consume are generally small, but nevertheless they are typically positive and may help prevent disease if consumed on a regular basis as part of a healthy dietary pattern. As described earlier, phytomolecules are considered to be beneficial to human health because of their antioxidant activities. Consuming combinations of phytomolecules may be even more beneficial because they typically act synergistically in the prevention of the common chronic diseases. The major benefits of phytomolecules include antioxidant and anticancer actions of these chemicals that help prevent cardiovascular disease, cancer, type 2 diabetes mellitus, cataracts, and other age-related declines in organ function. The antioxidative role of most phytochemicals in cells, as stated earlier, protects against damage to DNA, which contributes to their anticancer role, and other large molecules. Other antioxidant phytomolecules may also help reduce inflammation in peripheral arteries, which may trigger adverse cardiovascular events.

> Evidence has emerged in recent years on the importance of phytochemicals in food for maintaining and improving human health.

> Diets rich in phytomolecules are considered to be healthy, even though these molecules are not classified as nutrients.

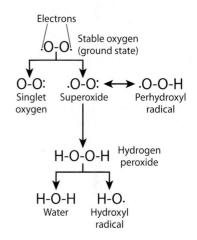

FIGURE 2.9 Free Radicals. Highly reactive free radicals are produced in all cells. Protective mechanisms, such as enzymes, help in quenching the free radicals, but certain nutrients also play key roles in this antioxidation process.

Reproduced from Anderson JJB. *Nutrition and Health: An Introduction.* Durham, NC: Carolina Academic Press; 2005.

antioxidant A molecule that prevents the reaction between an oxygen free radical and macromolecules of cells (e.g., unsaturated fatty acids, proteins, nucleic acids).

antioxidant nutrient Nutrient that acts as an antioxidant in the body, such as vitamin C, vitamin E, beta-carotene, and selenium.

TABLE 2.9
Antioxidant Capacity of Common Foods

Food	Antioxidant Capacity in ORAC Units*
Raspberry, black	19,220
Pecan	17,940
Wild blueberry	9,621
Cranberry	9,090
Red kidney bean, raw	8,606
Black bean, raw	8,494
Prune	8,059
Pinto bean, raw	8,033
Black plum, with peel	7,581
Artichoke, boiled	6,552
Blackberry	5,905
Raspberry	5,065
Blueberry	4,669
Strawberry	4,302
Apple, Red Delicious, with skin	4,275
Apple, Granny Smith, with skin	3,898
Sweet cherry	3,747
Apple, Gala, with skin	2,670
Potato, Russet, cooked	1,680

* ORAC units per 100 grams of food.
Data from U.S. Department of Agriculture, Agricultural Research Service. Oxygen Radical Absorbance Capacity (ORAC) of Selected Foods, Release 2. 2010. Available at: www.orac-info-portal.de/download/ORAC_R2.pdf.

The major benefits of phytomolecules include antioxidant and anticancer actions of these chemicals that help prevent cardiovascular disease, cancer, type 2 diabetes mellitus, cataracts, and other age-related declines in organ function.

Dietary components of plant foods, especially fiber molecules, have been investigated for their effects on human health for a half-century or more. Epidemiologic studies suggest that the consumption of sufficient fruits and vegetables each day is protective against heart diseases, stroke, and certain cancers, especially those of the prostate, breast, and colon. Several phytomolecules have been identified in the last few decades that in animal models appear to have protective roles against cancer and other chronic diseases. Human experimental data are just beginning to appear in the scientific literature. This research area is greatly expanding because pure preparations of these cancer-protective molecules have been developed and are available for clinical trials. Although a few of these phytomolecules are available as pills, obtaining small amounts of them from foods in everyday consumption is preferable. The smaller amounts in foods can be absorbed slowly with a meal as opposed to larger amounts in a pill, which when consumed all at once, may rapidly increase blood concentrations and lead to adverse effects.

Almost all plant foods contain phytochemicals called polyphenols that possess antioxidant properties. Thousands of molecules can be classified as **polyphenols**. All polyphenols have a chemical structure of several hydroxyl groups on aromatic rings (see **FIGURE 2.10**). Polyphenols are derived from one amino acid, phenylalanine, and are metabolized to thousands of different chemical structures in plants. These molecules help defend against the production of free radicals by ultraviolet light as well as free radicals generated by cellular pathways of metabolism. Other health benefits of phytochemicals, such as anti-inflammatory activity, have also been identified. The functions performed by phytochemicals in protecting against development of cancer include enhancement of detoxifying mechanisms leading to excretion of potential carcinogens, stimulating antioxidant mechanisms, providing direct interference with actions of carcinogens on cells, and inhibiting tumor growth. Several types of important phytochemicals and food sources of each are listed in **Table 2.10**.

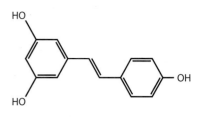

FIGURE 2.10 Generic Structure of Polyphenols. Polyphenols, which are derived from the amino acid phenylalanine, consist of aromatic rings plus hydroxyl groups. These phytochemicals have antioxidant properties and may offer protection against the development of cancer.

TABLE 2.10
Phytomolecules and Their Plant Sources

Phytochemicals	Food Sources*
Allyl sulfides	Garlic, onions, scallions, leeks, chives
Dithiolthiones	Broccoli, cabbages, bok choy, and other crucifers
Isothiocyanates and thiocyanates	Collards, bok choy, watercress, and other crucifers
Indoles	Rutabaga, turnips, Brussels sprouts, and other crucifers
Limonenes	Oranges, lemons, grapefruits, tangerines
Ellagic acid	Cherries, strawberries, grapes
Protease inhibitors	Soybeans, other legumes
Carotenoids (lycopene)	Carrots, squash, yellow peppers, tomatoes
Catechins	Teas, especially green teas
Isoflavones (genistein, daidzein, other)	Soybeans and other legumes, tofu, miso, pea pods, radishes, potatoes
Lignans**	Whole grains, especially flaxseed, fruits, vegetables
Anthocyanins	Grapes, grape juice, red wines, prunes, cranberries, blueberries, blackberries, strawberries, red apples
Resveratrol	Grapes and wines, especially reds
Saponins	Lentils, red beans, soybeans
Sulforaphanes	Broccoli, other crucifers
Coumarins	Citrus fruits, crucifers
Curcumins	Ginger, especially curry powders

* Plant foods not listed here typically have low amounts of phytochemical content (but not zero).
** Lignans are different chemically from lignins, a type of insoluble fiber
Data from Steinmetz KA, Potter JD. Vegetables, fruit, and cancer. I. Epidemiology. *Cancer Causes Control.* 1991;2(5):325–357; and Steinmetz KA, Potter JD. Vegetables, fruit, and cancer. I. Mechanisms. *Cancer Causes Control.* 1991;2(6):427–442.

> Several phytochemicals have been identified in the last few decades to have preventive roles against cancer and other chronic diseases in animal models. Human experimental data are just beginning to appear in the scientific literature.

polyphenol Group of molecules with a chemical structure of several hydroxyl groups on aromatic rings. They are derived from the amino acid phenylalanine and are metabolized to thousands of different chemical structures in plants. Many of these molecules act as antioxidants.

Dietary Fiber

Dietary fibers also are categorized as structural phytomolecules, but they do not function like other phytochemicals. Dietary fiber is a collective term for the many structural molecules in plants that are consumed in the diet from plant foods, including whole grains, fruits, vegetables, nuts, and seeds. In general, insoluble fiber molecules travel down the gastrointestinal (GI) tract with little or no modification by human secretions or enzymes, but other more soluble molecules may be partially digested by gut bacteria and have healthy effects within the lumen of the GI tract. Both types of fiber molecules, insoluble and water-soluble, however, are considered beneficial. **Table 2.11** lists the water-soluble and water-insoluble fiber molecules and their role in human health, so far as is known. One established beneficial health effect of dietary fiber, which appears to be related to its water solubility, is the cholesterol-lowering effect of whole grain oats found in breakfast cereals. Whole grain oats are a good source of dietary fiber. Regular servings of whole grain oats have been found to lower serum LDL-cholesterol, and thereby total cholesterol.

The AIs for dietary fiber are 38 grams per day for males aged 19 to 50 years and 25 grams per day for females aged 19 to 50 years. Fiber is provided by all plant foods, but berries, legumes, and bran cereals are especially rich in these molecules.

> *Both types of fiber molecules, water insoluble and water soluble, are considered beneficial.*

TABLE 2.11
Fiber Molecules and Their Possible Roles in Humans' Health

Fiber Molecule	Role in Human Body
Insoluble	
Cellulose	Slows gastric emptying; speeds colonic transit
Lignin	Slows gastric emptying; speeds colonic transit
Hemicellulose	Adsorbs water and dilutes contents of the stomach
Soluble*	
Pectins	Dilutes contents and protect mucosa
Gums	Dilutes contents and protect mucosa
Mucilages	Dilutes contents and protect mucosa

* The soluble fiber molecules are generally partially degraded by gut bacteria.

PRACTICAL APPLICATIONS 2.5

Dietary Fiber

List each food you consumed yesterday that contained fiber. A variety of sources is available that you can use to find the dietary fiber content of various foods. Determine how many servings of dietary fiber you consumed and then estimate your total fiber intake in grams (g).

Comment on how you did in terms of the current DRIs for your age and gender: very good ($\geq$ AI), good (>25 grams for men/20 grams for women), fair (>15 grams for men/12 grams for women), or poor ($\leq$ 15 grams for men/12 grams for women). ■

Increasing Your Consumption of Phytochemicals

Plants foods come in a wide variety of colors. Dark green, red, purple/blue, and yellow/ orange plant foods are considered to be particularly rich in antioxidants. One dietary strategy is to consume plants of each of the four different colors in meals each day for their antioxidant content. In addition to their antioxidative effects, many of the phytochemicals found in these colorful plant foods have other health benefits, such as reducing inflammation, improving vision, protecting heart muscle, reducing cancer, and enhancing the capabilities of brain neurons that help delay Alzheimer's dementia and other abnormal conditions. (White foods, like processed cereals and rice, are not considered as healthful.)

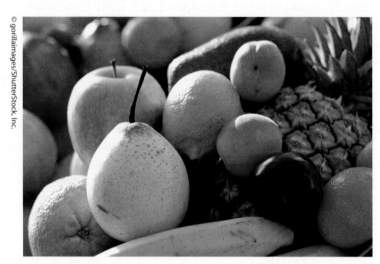

© gorillaimages/ShutterStock, Inc.

> **"** Life expectancy is higher in Greece and other Mediterranean nations with diets high in fruits and vegetables than it is for many non-Mediterranean countries. **"**

The diet common in many Mediterranean countries contains many plant foods rich in phytochemicals. A usual daily intake in Greece might contain tomatoes, greens, beans, olives, red wine, and two fruits, such as berries and citrus—approximately nine servings of fruits and vegetables a day! Mediterranean diets or eating patterns also include cereal grains and fish and other seafood almost on a daily basis and less red meat and dairy than in other **Western diets**. Researchers have found that such a diet is associated with lower rates of heart disease and other cardiovascular diseases, type 2 diabetes mellitus, obesity, hypertension, diet-related cancers, and metabolic syndrome. In addition, life expectancy is higher in Greece and several other Mediterranean nations with diets high in fruits and vegetables than it is in many non-Mediterranean countries.

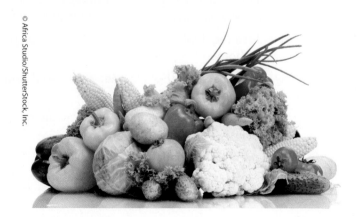

© Africa Studio/ShutterStock, Inc.

Western diet A dietary habit chosen by many people in some developed countries, and increasingly in developing countries. It is characterized by high intakes of red meat, sugary desserts, high-fat foods, and refined grains. It also typically contains high-fat dairy products, high-sugar drinks, and higher intakes of processed meat. This diet has been found to be correlated with obesity, heart disease, and cancer.

SUMMARY

Food labels provide consumers with information so that they can make informed choices about the foods they eat. All processed and packaged foods are required to have a Nutrition Facts panel that provides information on the product's serving size; calorie content; the amount of fat, cholesterol, sodium, carbohydrate, and protein per serving; the %DV of essential nutrients and dietary fiber; and an ingredients list. Manufacturers are also allowed to include preapproved health claims on the food label or packaging. A health claim is a statement that establishes a beneficial association between a nutrient or food ingredient and a disease or health condition. Organic foods may also be labeled as such. Manufacturers must meet USDA regulations in order to state that a food is organic.

Food composition tables and databases are an invaluable source of nutrition information on various foods. Most of these databases contain information on a food's macronutrient and micronutrient content. Some also include information on phytochemicals. The USDA maintains the National Nutrient Database for Standard Reference, which contains nutrient information on more than 8,000 different foods.

Most foods can be classified as either coming from plants or animals. Plant, but not animal, foods contain dietary fiber and are the primary source of unsaturated fats. Animal foods are the only food sources that provide cobalamin. Both types of foods are rich in vitamins and minerals.

The USDA's MyPlate food guidance system was developed to help Americans make better dietary choices. MyPlate recommends that half the plate be fruits and vegetables and that fatty foods be eaten in moderation. MyPlate also recommends daily exercise as part of a healthy lifestyle. Other food guidance systems have been developed for vegetarians and those wishing to follow the Mediterranean eating plan. MyPlate focuses on five food groups: grains, vegetables, fruits, protein, and dairy foods. The foods in each group have similar nutrient composition, and foods from all the food groups are needed to maintain optimal health.

Evidence has emerged in recent years on the importance of phytochemicals in food for maintaining and improving human health. Phytochemicals (or phytomolecules) are non-nutrient substances found in plants. Phytochemicals are synthesized by plants to serve specific functions. Many of the phytochemicals produced by plants act as antioxidants that reduce the amount of oxygen free radicals. In humans, nutrient antioxidants and other plant phytochemicals may also act as nonenzymatic antioxidants, eliminating free radicals by directly neutralizing them. Thus, consumption of phytochemicals from plants can play an important role in preventing the accumulation of cellular damage over time. Some research suggests that phytochemicals can help prevent or delay cancer, cardiovascular diseases, brain neuronal changes, and other conditions. Diets rich in phytomolecules are considered to be healthy, even though these molecules are not classified as nutrients.

STUDENT ACTIVITIES

1. List the information that must be included on the Nutrition Facts panel.

2. What is a health claim placed on a food package? How is a claim regulated?

3. What does the FDA's organic food label signify?

4. How can nutrient databases be used to assess the nutrient content of a meal?

5. State three ways that the nutritional content of plants and animals differ.

6. What is the purpose of a food guidance system? According to MyPlate, what food groups should be primary in any diet (i.e., make up "half the plate")?

7. Name three vegetable *sub*groups and list one example of each subgroup.

8. Why are beans and other legumes considered both vegetables and proteins?

9. With regard to grains, why should the focus be on whole grains?

10. Why are proteins essential to human health?

11. Which types of foods are high in phytochemicals?

12. How can phytochemicals aid in improving or maintaining human health?

13. Distinguish between the typical western (US) pattern of eating and a Mediterranean diet?

14. Explain why plant protein foods differ from animal protein foods.

15. Speculate on why partial vegetarians typically have better odds of being healthier and living longer than those consuming diets that contain plenty of meats and dairy.

WEBSITES FOR FURTHER STUDY

DASH Diet
www.dashdiet.org
Food and Drug Administration
www.fda.gov
My Food Guide, Canada
www.healthcanada.gc.ca/foodguide
Nutrient Ingredients Organization
www.nutraingredients.com

USDA MyPlate
www.choosemyplate.gov
www.choosemyplate.gov/MyPlateOnCampus
USDA and USDHHS, *Dietary Guidelines for Americans, 2010*
http://health.gov/dietaryguidelines/2010.asp

REFERENCES

Arab L, Steck S. Lycopene and cardiovascular disease. *Am J Clin Nutr.* 2000;71(suppl):1691S–1695S.

Bellur P, Lakkanna S, Joshi J, Cornelius J, Tripodi F, Boddupalli S. Food biofortification: breeding and biotechnology approaches to improve nutrients in vegetables and oil quality in soybeans. In: Erdman JW Jr, MacDonald IA, Zeisel SH (eds.). *Present Knowledge in Nutrition.* 10th ed. Ames, IA: John Wiley & Sons; 2012: 1903–1929.

Briefel RR, McDowell MA. Nutrition monitoring in the United States. In: Erdman JW Jr, MacDonald IA, Zeisel SH (eds.). *Present Knowledge in Nutrition.* 10th ed. Ames, IA: John Wiley & Sons; 2012: 1690–1715.

Cheynier V. Polyphenols in foods are more complex than often thought. *Am J Clin Nutr.* 2005;81(suppl): 222S–229S.

Coates PM, Nicastro H, Milner JA. Bioactive components in foods and supplements for health promotion. In: Erdman JW Jr, MacDonald IA, Zeisel SH (eds.). *Present Knowledge in Nutrition.* 10th ed. Ames, IA: John Wiley & Sons; 2012: 1930–1952.

Dwyer JT. Dietary standards and guidelines: Similarities and differences among countries. In: Erdman JW Jr, MacDonald IA, Zeisel SH (eds.). *Present Knowledge in Nutrition.* 10th ed. Ames, IA: John Wiley & Sons; 2012: 1716–1749.

Dwyer J, Picciano MF, Raiten DJ. Estimation of usual intakes: What we eat in America—NHANES. *J Nutr.* 2003;133:609S–623S.

Fowke JH, Morrow JD, Bostick RM, Ness RM. Brassica vegetable consumption reduces urinary F2-isoprostane levels independent of micronutrient intake. *Carcinogenesis.* 2006;27:2096–2102.

Kris-Etherton PM, Hecker KD, Bonanome A, et al. Bioactive compounds in foods: Their role in the prevention of cardiovascular disease and cancer. *Am J Med.* 2002;113(9B):71S–88S.

Liu RH. Health benefits of fruit and vegetables are from additive and synergistic combinations of phytochemicals. *Am J Clin Nutr.* 2003;78 (suppl 5):517S–520S.

Potter JD, Steinmetz K. Vegetables, fruits, and phytoestrogens as preventive agents. *IARC Sci Publ.* 1996;139:61–90.

Thomasset SC, Berry DP, Garcea G, et al. Dietary polyphenolic phytochemicals—promising cancer chemopreventive agents in humans? A review of the clinical properties. *Int J Cancer.* 2007;120:451–458.

U.S. Department of Agriculture and U.S. Department of Health and Human Services. *Dietary Guidelines for Americans, 2010.* 7th ed. Washington, DC: U.S. Government Printing Office; December 2010.

Vartanian LR, Schwartz MB, Brownell KD. Effects of soft drink consumption on nutrition and health: a systematic review and meta-analysis. *Am J Public Health.* 2007;97:667–675.

Weisell R, Albert J. The role of United Nations agencies in establishing international dietary standards. In: Erdman JW Jr, MacDonald IA, Zeisel SH (eds.). *Present Knowledge in Nutrition.* 10th ed. Ames, IA: John Wiley & Sons; 2012;1750–1771.

ADDITIONAL READING

Food and Nutrition Board, Institute of Medicine. *Dietary Reference Intakes*, 6 volumes. Washington, DC: National Academies Press, 1997–2004.

Fraser GE. *Diet, Life Expectancy, and Chronic Disease*. New York: Oxford University Press; 2003.

Gilani GS, Anderson JJB, eds. *Phytoestrogens and Health*. Champaign, IL: AOCS Press; 2002.

Gussow JD. *The Feeding Web*. New York: Bull Publishing; 1978.

Heber D. *What Color Is Your Diet?* New York: Regan; 2002.

Matalas A-L, Zampelas A, Stavrinos V, Wolinky I, eds. *The Mediterranean Diet: Constituents and Health Promotion*. Boca Raton, FL: CRC Press; 2001.

Nestle M. *What to Eat*. New York: North Point Press; 2006.

Pollan M. *Omnivore's Dilemma*. New York: Penguin Press; 2006.

Sabate J, ed. *Vegetarian Nutrition*. Boca Raton, FL: CRC Press; 2001.

Schmidl MK, Labuza TP, eds. *Essentials of Functional Foods*. Gaithersburg, MD: Aspen Publishers; 2000.

Weil A. *Healthy Aging*. New York: Knopf; 2005.

Willcox BJ, Willcox DC, Suzuki M. *The Okinawa Program*. New York: Three Rivers Press; 2001.

Willett, WC. *Eat, Drink, and Be Healthy*. New York: Free Press; 2001.

Reflection on Food Processing and Food Safety

In food processing, nutrients and chemicals, such as salt, sugar, and additives, may be added to a food to lengthen its shelf-life and improve its palatability, texture, and color. Nutrients and phytochemicals also may be removed during food processing, impacting the nutritional quality of the food. In some types of food processing, nutrients are added to a food (fortification) in order to enhance its nutritional content. Food safety is another important component of the commercial food system, whereby foods are brought from farms and fields to supermarkets. This feature provides an overview of food processing and food safety and the two major federal agencies that oversee the safety of the food supply, the U.S. Department of Agriculture (USDA) and the Food and Drug Administration (FDA).

Food Processing

Food processing, or the modification of a food by physical or chemical means, may be minimal, as practiced in ancient times, or more extensive, as practiced today. For many processed foods it may be difficult to know what the original raw food looked like or tasted like. The techniques used by food processors enable foods to be brought efficiently and economically from fields and barns to our tables (see **FIGURE 1**).

Food processing has both advantages and disadvantages. Food processing offers the following advantages:

- Seasonal foods can be supplied to consumers throughout the year.
- It provides a degree of uniform quality and attractiveness of foods.
- Waste is reduced by more efficient processing of foods than could be carried out in the home.
- Foods can be distributed to all parts of the country, even remote areas.
- It destroys many pathogens that may be found in raw food products.
- It increases the shelf-life or storage capacity of food products.
- It enhances the nutritional content of foods through fortification and enrichment.

food processing The modification of a food by physical or chemical means. With extensive food processing, it may be difficult to know what the original raw food looked or tasted like. The techniques used by food processors enable foods to be brought efficiently and economically from fields and barns to our tables.

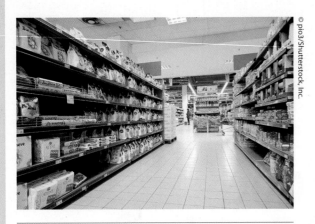

FIGURE 1 Processed Foods. Without food processing, many of the foods we take for granted would not be available.

Food processing, depending on the specific process, results in the following disadvantages:

- Processing may result in some quality loss (i.e., in taste and texture).
- Micronutrients may be lost during processing (e.g., in the milling of flour and canning of fruits and vegetables).
- Processed foods require chemical additives.
- The diminished dietary fiber in processed plant foods may have potentially deleterious effects, including increased energy intake that leads to overweight and obesity.

Food Preservation

Today, food manufacturers rely on both ancient and modern practices to preserve food products, increasing their shelf life, portability, and safety. These methods are summarized in **Table 1**. Salt and sugar have been used as **food preservatives** for millennia. Newer methods, though more technologically advanced, serve the same general purpose: controlling the growth of microorganisms in food by modifying their **water activity (A_w)**, temperature, and acidity (pH). Certain yeasts, molds, and bacteria that grow (culture) on foods cause spoilage. Still other microorganisms might be pathogenic by causing illness in the person consuming the affected food. These microorganisms need water to multiply. Agents such as salt and sugar reduce the water activity of the food, and hence reduce spoilage. Food irradiation also destroys these organisms and preserves food well.

TABLE 1 Common Food Preservation Methods: Traditional and Recent	
Traditional	**Recent Technologies**
• Drying • Heating, including smoking • Salting and sugaring • Cooling	• Refrigeration (mechanical) • Freezing • Pasteurization • Ultra-pasteurization (high temperature, short time) • Freeze-drying • Irradiation • Canning

food preservative A food additive that increases the shelf-life of foods and controls bacterial growth, thus increasing a food's shelf life, portability, and safety. For example, sulfur dioxide is used to preserve lettuce on salad bars of restaurants and salt is used to inhibit the growth of microorganisms in meats and vegetables.

water activity (A_W) The amount of water that is available to support the growth of bacteria, yeast, or mold. It is based on a scale of 0 to 1.0, with water having a value of 1.0. Products that have lower water content have lower water activity. Foods with low water activity are more resistant to spoilage by bacteria.

FOCUS 1   Water Activity

Water activity (A_w) is the amount of water that is available to support the growth of bacteria, yeast, or mold. Water activity is based on a scale of 0 to 1.0, with water having a value of 1.0. Products that have lower water content have lower water activity. For example, foods such as raisins and dried pastas have low water activity. Foods with low water activity are more resistant to spoilage by bacteria. The water activity of a food can be decreased by adding ingredients to bind the water, making it unavailable to microorganisms. Sugar and salt are often used to preserve foods because they decrease the water activity of the food item, thus increasing the product's shelf-life. ●

Enzymes in raw foods can cause food deterioration by inducing changes in the food's flavor, color, or texture (such as overripening of fruit). Certain spontaneous, nonenzymatic chemical reactions may occur in foods before they are harvested or during storage. Some of these nonenzymatic reactions cause browning in fruits, rancidity in fats, and flavor changes in a variety of foods.

Food technologists today try to improve food processing through modifications of the four traditional preservation methods, which remain the backbone of the food industry. These traditional methods of food preservation are drying, heat treatment, refrigeration, and, though more recent, freezing.

Drying

Drying is a centuries-old technique of preservation that reduces the water content of a variety of food crops as well as meats, thereby preventing the growth of microorganisms (see **FIGURE 2**). The amount of water available for microbial action (i.e., A_w) is significantly reduced by drying, but some water still remains in the foods. Generally, the first spoilage of dried foods, such as breads, is through the growth of molds (yeasts). Thus, whereas moist foods undergo bacterial decay relatively quickly, even "dried" foods may spoil under humid conditions.

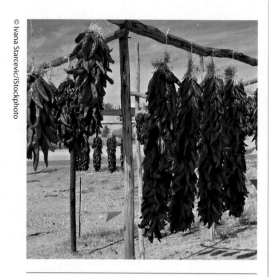

FIGURE 2 Drying. Drying of foods reduces the water content of a food, reducing the amount of moisture available to microorganisms.

Drying can be accomplished in several different ways, including using the heat of the sun, hot air driers, rotating drums, freeze-drying, and spray-drying chambers. The nutrient content of foods is altered very little by these techniques unless temperatures become high enough for a long enough period of time to destroy vitamins. Home drying methods are typically less efficient and result in greater losses of nutrients, primarily vitamins.

Heat Treatment

Heat treatment is generally used for the canning of certain foods (fruits, vegetables, meats, soups, and many mixed-food products) and the pasteurization of milk (see **FIGURE 3**). Heating under atmospheric pressure or under pressurized steam has a bactericidal or killing action. With heat treatment, nearly all microorganisms, including most pathogens, are killed or rendered inactive for the shelf-life of the food product. Milk **pasteurization** has a bactericidal action because it kills the pathogenic bacteria responsible for tuberculosis, typhoid fever, cholera, poliomyelitis, and brucellosis. **Ultra-pasteurization** at high temperatures (600°F) kills all microorganisms in milk.

drying A traditional method of food preservation to remove moisture and thereby preserve a food. This method is often used to preserve cereal grains and legumes.

heat treatment A traditional food preservation method where a food is heated to a high enough temperature to kill microorganisms, including most pathogens.

pasteurization Heating of milk or other beverages at high temperature (161 °F) for 20 seconds in order to kill pathogenic bacteria.

ultra-pasteurization Heating of milk or other beverages at a high temperature (600 °F) for a second or so to kill all bacteria and other microorganisms.

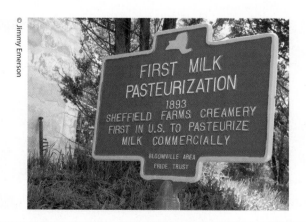

FIGURE 3 Pasteurization. Pasteurization is the process of heating a food to a specific temperature for a certain period of time in order to reduce the number of disease-causing organisms in the food product.

In most canning procedures, foods are blanched, and oxygen and other gases are removed. **Blanching** is the steam-heating, scalding, or cooking of fresh foods, especially vegetables, to sufficiently high temperatures in order to inactivate enzymes and their potential for spoiling foods. Foods that are blanched are then usually frozen or canned. In all of these heating processes, the temperature-labile nutrients (i.e., water-soluble vitamins such as thiamin and vitamin C) are partially destroyed by the heat. In ultra-pasteurization, no organisms survive and little vitamin damage occurs because of the shorter exposure time at the higher temperatures.

Mechanical Refrigeration

Mechanical **refrigeration (cooling)** as we know it today is a relatively modern method of food preservation, but cool places like root cellars have long been used to keep certain foods for long periods. Low temperatures in the range of 32°F to 40°F (0°C to 4°C) slow down the metabolic activity of fruits and vegetables and also inhibit the enzymatic activities of microorganisms. However, the ability to store meats, poultry, and fish by low-temperature methods is limited because bacterial growth is never totally inhibited. The retention of nutrient quality is high in processed foods that remain refrigerated unopened in sealed containers. Refrigeration has its limits in preserving foods, but it has probably had the greatest health impact on economically advanced societies by increasing the year-round availability of fruits and vegetables (see **FIGURE 4**). It also has reduced the need for consumers to shop every day for fresh foods.

Freezing

Freezing lowers the temperature of foods below water's freezing point (0°C) to about –18°C, stopping the growth of most microorganisms. Vegetables are usually blanched by heating them to over 200°F (93°C) for several minutes and then quick-frozen to –10°F (–22°C). Nutrient loss is generally minimal; for example, water-soluble vitamins retain nearly 100% of their activity. However, the proteins of meats, poultry, fish, and milk tend to be partially denatured through the formation of large crystals of ice, depending on the temperature used for freezing. This type of denaturation has relatively little or no effect on the nutrient quality of the food, and the altered product remains wholesome for consumers. **Denaturation** is the partial or total unwinding of globular or other proteins resulting from the breakage of chemical bonds that help maintain the structure of the molecules. The formation of smaller crystals of ice, which cause less denaturation, can be achieved by more rapid freezing. **Freeze-drying** is a modification of food freezing involving removal of water and freezing temperature simultaneously.

blanching The heating of fresh vegetables and other foods with steam or boiling water (scalding) in order to inactivate the enzymes that potentially cause food spoilage. In commercial food processing, foods that are blanched are either canned or frozen.

refrigeration (cooling) A traditional method of food preservation in which foods are stored at cool temperatures in order to slow the metabolic activity of fruits and vegetables and to inhibit the enzymatic activities of microorganisms.

freezing A method of food preservation whereby the food is stored below water's freezing point, which stops the growth of most microorganisms.

denaturation Disruption of the three-dimensional structure of a protein resulting from chemical or physical treatment of the molecule; for example, heat will denature the protein of egg white (albumen).

freeze-drying A method of food preservation that freezes foods and removes water in a vacuum chamber.

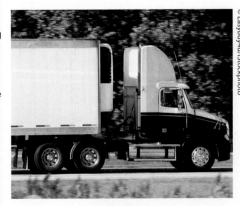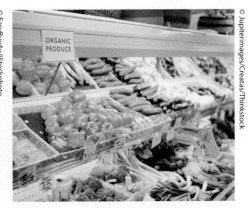

© EasyBuy4u/iStockphoto

© Jupiterimages/Creatas/Thinkstock

FIGURE 4 Refrigeration. Refrigeration greatly increases the shelf-life of fruits and vegetables, making it possible to transport them great distances without risk of spoilage.

Food Irradiation

A newer method of food preservation is **food irradiation**. This method has been controversial because of the widely mistaken fear that the irradiated food is radioactive. However, this method is very safe and has been used to preserve military rations for the last several decades with no adverse effects. Bacteria are eliminated from foods that are irradiated with x-rays or gamma rays, eliminating any possible negative effects from pathogens. A disadvantage of this method is the partial inactivation of vitamins, especially those sensitive to free radicals. Food irradiation is now approved for use in preserving ground beef and is considered the best method for increasing the safety of meats. In the United States, all foods that have been irradiated must contain the words "Treated with Radiation" or "Treated by Irradiation" and display the irradiation logo, the Radura (see **FIGURE 5**).

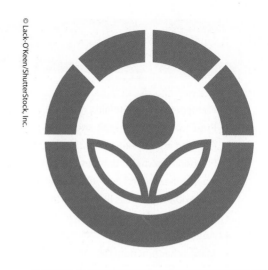

FIGURE 5 The Radura. The Radura logo must appear on the packaging of all irradiated foods.

Modified Atmospheric Packaging

Modified **atmospheric packaging** uses oxygen-free gases such as nitrogen or carbon dioxide to replace oxygen-containing air so that certain foods, such as salads, pastas, and breads, can be stored for longer than normal. Shelf-life is enhanced by the sealed plastic wrapping that is impermeable or selectively permeable to the gases. Pull dates listed on food labels are typically earlier than actual shelf-life, but they are so set for safety purposes. Nutrient loss is nil or low over the specified shelf-life of a food.

Nutrient Preservation or Losses

Of all the preservation methods, freezing and canning are best for maintaining the nutrient quality of foods. Approximate nutrient losses of 10% for freezing and 20% for canning occur over a period of a few weeks. Additional but smaller losses will follow over subsequent months of storage. The nutrients most susceptible to heat loss and storage loss are the vitamins, including thiamin, other water-soluble B vitamins, and vitamin C.

Nutrient losses in the consumers' kitchen are typically greater than all the other processing steps combined! Refrigeration of fresh foods permits only short-term storage, and it is accompanied by significant losses of nutrient quality, as much as 50% for many vitamins, after several days. Keeping fresh fruits at room temperature, as most consumers prefer, may lead to even greater nutrient losses. During cooking, nutrient losses tend to be small, but they increase with longer cooking times, such as in baking and in preparing stews and soups. Microwave cooking will lead to smaller losses because of the shorter times needed for cooking. Nutrient losses can be reduced by keeping raw foods refrigerated and storing leftover food in special bags or containers as soon as possible.

Food Additives

Food additives are nutrients or chemicals added to a food to maintain or preserve its desirable qualities, including color, flavor, appearance, and nutrient content. They may be organic molecules or inorganic minerals. In general, food additives are used to improve the quality of a specific processed food or to lengthen its shelf-life. Common additives used in the United States in foods are sugar, salt, phosphates, and other chemicals that have properties or functions that help preserve the food or maintain its appearance. **Table 2** lists a number of different food additives.

food irradiation The use of penetrating x-rays or gamma rays to kill all microorganisms in a food. It has been used successfully by the military to preserve foods. More recently, it has been approved for use with meats, such as hamburger, to reduce *E. coli*.

atmospheric packaging The use of oxygen-free gases such as nitrogen and carbon dioxide to replace oxygen-containing air so that certain foods, such as salads, pastas, and breads, can be stored for longer than normal.

food additive A chemical added to a food to maintain or preserve its desirable qualities, including color, flavor, appearance, and nutrient content.

TABLE 2
Food Additives, Including Fortificants

- Nutrients such as vitamins, minerals, and amino acids
- Preservatives such as salt, sugar, and phosphate salts
- Coloring agents, both natural and synthetic
- Flavoring agents, both natural and synthetic
- Agents that control acid–base balance
- Antioxidants, such as BHT and BHA
- Lubricants, such as glycerides
- Anticaking agents
- Many other functional agents

Nutrient Additives

Nutrient additives are added to enhance the nutritional quality of a product. Nutrient additives are generally put in foods to fortify them, which may help replace nutrients lost in processing or increase the amount of a nutrient that is commonly not consumed in adequate amounts. In the latter type of fortification, added nutrients may be used as a marketing advantage, as well as a correction of low content of the specific nutrient in the food.

Nutrient fortification of processed foods in the United States has had a significant positive impact on the nutritional status of the population. Starting early in World War II, cereals, breads, and other baked goods were fortified with thiamin, riboflavin, niacin, and iron. This early form of fortification resulted because of the poor nutritional status of many young military volunteers in the late 1930s and early 1940s. More recently, some foods, including cereals, are now fortified with folate (folic acid) because of the low intakes of this vitamin in the United States. Other foods, such as milk, bread, baby foods, and orange juice, are fortified with still other nutrients. **Table 3** lists several examples food fortificants used in the United States.

In recent years, microbials—that is, probiotic bacteria—have been added to some yogurts for the purpose of improving the digestion of the milk constituents. Yogurt is a good example of a food that contains probiotics.

Chemical Additives

Food manufacturers may add chemicals to a food product to increase its **shelf-life**, improve its taste or consistency, or alter its appearance (e.g., food dyes; see **FIGURE 6**).

nutrient additive A food additive used in the enrichment, fortification, or restoration of foods. For example, iron, thiamin, riboflavin, niacin, and folate are nutrient additives used to enrich wheat and corn flours and cereals. Vitamins A and D are added back to milk products following processing. Calcium, iron, and vitamin C also are added to many food items.

shelf-life The maximum time a processed food product is allowed to be on the shelf of a food market.

TABLE 3
Nutrient Fortification of Foods

Nutrient	Examples of Fortification
B vitamins and iron	Fortification of wheat and corn flours
Vitamin C	Packaged fruit-flavored drinks
Vitamin A	Restoration for low-fat milks and for dairy products
Vitamin D	Restoration for low-fat dairy milks, orange juice
Folate	Newest fortification of flour
Iron	Infant formula and breakfast cereal
Zinc	Infant formula and breakfast cereal
Amino acids	Sports drinks and protein powder
Iodine	Salt
Omega-3 fatty acids	Infant formula and granola bars

The issue of benefits versus risks of chemical additives was contentious through the 1970s and 1980s because of a clause in the food laws that stated that any chemical additive that increased the risk of human (or animal) disease, especially cancer, had to be removed—100% removed! The controversy over this issue has been greatly reduced by a compromise whereby small amounts of chemical additives that have little or no known effect on human health are now permitted. This issue focused on sugar substitutes like saccharin. Nevertheless, a few chemical additives, such as red dye #2, were removed from the safe lists of additives many years ago.

The so-called **Generally Recognized as Safe (GRAS) list** represents approximately 300 chemicals added to foods that have been determined by the FDA as being safe because of their long-time use and limited concerns about their effects on human health. The FDA also has a more flexible or interim list of additives that may represent as many as 5,000 different chemicals. This list occasionally has an additive removed or an additive moved to the GRAS list, but more likely it includes new additives as modern chemistry creates more potential food preservatives. Similar lists of additives are maintained by agencies in other nations.

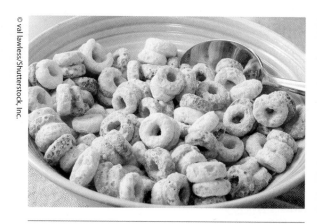

FIGURE 6 Food Dyes. Dyes are used in many processed foods to make them more appealing to consumers.

Government Agencies Involved in Food Safety, Food Distribution, and Food Security

Several federal agencies are involved with **food safety** because they have been tasked by laws governing U.S. food production, storage, processing, and cleanliness. Although jurisdictions may overlap on some issues, interagency cooperation is the rule. The **Food and Drug Administration (FDA)** oversees food safety, but the U.S. Department of Agriculture (USDA), the Centers for Disease Control and Prevention (CDC), and other state and federal agencies also have roles in maintaining the safety of the U.S. food supply. For example, the USDA has a major role in the inspection of produce and meats, poultry, and eggs. The Bureau of Fisheries in the Department of Commerce provides inspection services of fish and other seafood, especially marine fish.

Food and Drug Administration

Of all the U.S. federal agencies, the FDA is primarily responsible for the safety of the food supply, especially processed foods (see **FIGURE 7**). The FDA has several food-related functions that are not so apparent to consumers. For example, food labeling and packaging health claims fall under the jurisdiction of the FDA. Also, the FDA conducts a food basket survey of foods from various markets throughout the United States to measure the nutrient content of commonly consumed foods to ensure that adequate amounts of nutrients may be obtained from these foods by consumers. Finally, consumer education regarding the safety of foods falls under the province of the FDA.

U.S. Department of Agriculture

The USDA is responsible for overseeing farming, agriculture, forestry, and food production, particularly meat and egg production (see **FIGURE 8**). The USDA also is involved in ensuring safety in the production of genetically modified (GM) foods. Besides its food inspection responsibilities, the USDA also manages several food programs for

Generally Recognized as Safe (GRAS) list The food additives on the FDA's GRAS list have stood the test of time and scientific evaluation and have been determined by scientists and health experts to be safe for human consumption.

food safety Protection of the food supply so that it is safe for human consumption. Many laws and regulations exist to ensure the safety of foods. The Food and Drug Administration (FDA) oversees most food safety regulations, but the U.S. Department of Agriculture (USDA) and a few other federal agencies are also involved in the safety of the U.S. food supply.

Food and Drug Administration (FDA) The federal agency that regulates the safety of the U.S. food supply and mandates food labeling. It also is responsible for all drug safety and licensing issues.

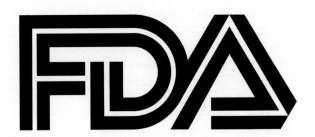

FIGURE 7 The FDA. The FDA is part of the U.S. Department of Health and Human Services. This agency is responsible for protecting and promoting human health through the supervision of food safety, dietary supplements, and medications.

Courtesy of U.S. Food and Drug Administration.

Supplemental Nutrition Assistance Program (SNAP) A federal food aid program, more commonly referred to as food stamps, that provides food assistance to low-income individuals and families. It is funded through the U.S. Department of Agriculture and administered through the states.

School Lunch Program A federal program that reimburses schools for serving low-cost and free lunches to qualifying students. The program uses surplus and low-cost foods to the benefit of the U.S. agricultural market. Standards recently have been raised to improve the nutritional quality of the meals provided. Many of these students also qualify for the Summer Food Service Program.

Women, Infants and Children (WIC) Food Program A federal food-assistance program that provides nutrition education and certain high-quality foods free for medically qualified mothers and their children. Is considered the most cost-effective of the U.S. Department of Agriculture's food programs due to the strong gains in birth weights and growth of infants and children.

Centers for Disease Control and Prevention (CDC) A federal agency within the Public Health Service charged with investigating disease outbreaks, maintaining health statistics, mounting prevention programs, and conducting periodic National Health and Nutrition Examination Surveys (NHANES).

the U.S. population. These federal programs include food stamps (the **Supplemental Nutrition Assistance Program [SNAP]**); cash assistance for the poor; several school food programs for children of all ages, including preschoolers; **School Lunch Programs**; and the **Women, Infants, and Children (WIC) food program**. The WIC program, which has been evaluated several times since the early 1970s, has been found to be the most cost-effective of all the USDA's food programs. This is because of the recommended provisions of specific healthy foods that have resulted in gains in birth weights, the growth of infants, and the improved iron and nutrient status of the children and mothers who medically qualify to participate. These USDA programs are efforts by the government to foster food security, but many nonprofit organizations also contribute to assure food security.

Centers for Disease Control and Prevention

The **Centers for Disease Control and Prevention (CDC)** investigates illness outbreaks related to foods. Sickness from foods contaminated with microorganisms (i.e., food-borne bacteria, viruses, molds) is much more prevalent than the number of cases reported each year to the CDC in Atlanta. Only an estimated 25% to 50% of cases are reported, whereas many more people may become ill from a contaminated food for only a short period and never see a physician.

FIGURE 8 The USDA. The USDA is the agency that is primarily responsible for ensuring the safety of the meat and egg supply in the United States.

Courtesy of the USDA

Foodborne Illness

Foodborne illness, which is sometimes referred to as food poisoning, is an illness resulting from the consumption of foods contaminated with pathogenic bacteria, viruses, or natural toxins. Most foodborne illnesses arise due to insufficient cooking (i.e., not cooking food to a high enough temperature to kill microorganisms); poor sanitation (especially hand-washing), which transmits pathogenic microorganisms; and inadequate storage, especially cold storage (picnic foods). Outbreaks of illnesses related to consumption of uncooked (raw) or poorly cooked shellfish in the summer and early fall are common in the southeastern United States because of contaminated waters in organic fertilizer–enriched estuaries that produce the seafoods. Both bacteria and viruses can be the culprits in these cases.

Clostridium botulinum is a bacteria that produces the botulinum toxin that, when consumed by humans, can cause paralysis or death. *C. botulinum* can live in improperly canned or preserved foods. Because botulism can be deadly, its prevention is critical. Some foods, such as meats (ham, bacon), are treated with **nitrites** or **nitrates** to protect against contamination by *C. botulinum* (see **FIGURE 9**). Too much nitrite, however, may contribute to stomach cancer from the increased production of nitrosamines in the stomach. Because nitrite additives in foods can be too high, a compromise upper limit was established in the 1980s in the United States, which has resulted in substantially lower rates of gastric cancer.

The biggest concern about food safety within the U.S. in recent years has been bacteria, especially *Escherichia coli* (see **FIGURE 10**), and viral contamination in meat and poultry processing plants. A few hamburger processing plants have been shut down because of serious disease outbreaks and deaths. Chicken processors have also come under great scrutiny because of widespread bacterial contamination. Concern remains about the bovine spongiform contamination (mad cow disease) in beef cattle. **Food spoilage** also may result from contamination by microorganisms.

The potential for food poisoning may be minimized by rinsing foods, if possible, prior to use, and by using clean cutting surfaces (not wood) and clean utensils. Adequate heating temperatures for meats are a must. Prompt refrigeration of foods requiring cold storage cannot be overemphasized.

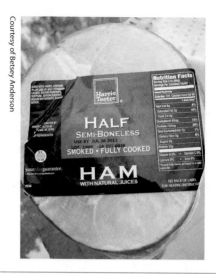

Courtesy of Betsey Anderson

FIGURE 9 Nitrites in Ham. The ingredients list includes nitrites that help protect against *Clostridium* contamination.

foodborne illness An illness resulting from the consumption of foods contaminated with pathogenic bacteria, viruses or natural toxins. Most foodborne illnesses are caused by insufficient cooking, poor sanitation, and inadequate storage. Characteristic symptoms include diarrhea and other disturbances, such as vomiting and cramping; elevated body temperature; and fluid losses.

nitrite (NO$_2$) A food additive used to cure meats and meat products, especially ham, bacon, frankfurters, and related products. It combines with the amines of meat proteins to form nitrosamines, which are potential carcinogens.

nitrate (NO$_3$) A nitrogen-containing food additive used in the curing of meats, hot dogs, and luncheon meats that inhibits bacterial growth. It combines with the amines of meat proteins to form nitrosamines, which are potential carcinogens.

food spoilage The breakdown of food products that can occur by browning reactions, oxidation reactions, and by contamination with microorganisms, such as molds and bacteria.

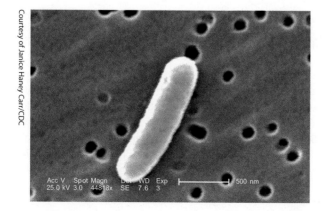

Courtesy of Janice Haney Carr/CDC

FIGURE 10 *E. coli.* An *E. coli* bacterium in the intestinal tract. Note its elongated, dowel-like shape.

SUMMARY

Food processing is the modification of a food by physical or chemical means. The techniques used by food processors enable foods to be brought efficiently and economically from fields and barns to our tables. Food processing provides many benefits, including the availability of seasonal foods throughout the year, increased shelf-life, and increased nutritional quality for fortified foods. However, food processing may also decrease the micronutrient content of foods and increase the use of chemical additives.

Food preservation techniques increase the shelf-life of foods. A number of food preservation techniques that have long been used by humans include drying, heating, salting and sugaring, and cooling. More recent techniques include mechanical refrigeration, freezing, pasteurization, and irradiation. The nutrient content of food may be affected by the type of preservation technique. Without food preservation techniques, consumers would have a very limited supply of foods from which to choose.

A variety of additives can be introduced to processed foods. Nutrient additives are nutrients that are added to enhance the nutritional content of a food item or to replace nutrients that may have been lost during processing. Chemical additives are added to foods to increase their shelf-life, improve their palatability, or enhance their color. The addition of chemical additives is regulated by the FDA, which maintains a list of additives that are considered safe for human health.

The FDA is the primary government agency tasked with the safety of the U.S. food supply, although the USDA plays a significant role in ensuring the safety of the meat and egg supply. The CDC monitors the U.S. population for outbreaks of foodborne illnesses. Foodborne illness results from the consumption of foods contaminated with pathogenic bacteria or viruses or natural toxins. Botulism and disease outbreaks resulting from *E. coli* are of particular concern in the United States. Most foodborne illnesses arise due to insufficient cooking (i.e., not cooking food to a high enough temperature to kill microorganisms); poor sanitation (especially handwashing), which transmits pathogenic microorganisms; and inadequate storage, especially cold storage (picnic foods).

STUDENT ACTIVITIES

1. List three advantages and three disadvantages of food processing.

2. What is water activity? Why does decreasing the water activity of a food increase its shelf-life?

3. Describe the effect of each of the following on the nutrient content of a food product: freezing, canning, irradiation.

4. How might the processing of tomatoes (raw) to tomato sauce or juice affect the quantity of vitamin C in the final product? Explain in terms of what type(s) of processing is involved. Speculate if you cannot find the specific information in this chapter.

5. What is purpose of the GRAS list of food additives?

6. State three specific roles of the FDA and two of the USDA in relation to food safety.

7. What is the role of the CDC regarding the safety of the U.S. food supply?

8. List three causes of foodborne illness.

REFERENCES

Bellur P, Lakkanna S, Joshi J, Cornelius J, Tripodi F, Boddupalli S. Food fortification: breeding and biotechnology approaches to improve nutrients in vegetables and oil quality in soybeans. In: Erdman JW Jr, MacDonald IA, Zeisel SH (eds.). *Present Knowledge in Nutrition*. 10th ed. Ames, IA: John Wiley & Sons; 2012: 1903–1929.

Tauxe RV, Neill MA. Foodborne infection and food safety. In: Erdman JW Jr, MacDonald IA, Zeisel SH (eds.). *Present Knowledge in Nutrition*. 10th ed. Ames, IA: John Wiley & Sons. 2012:1856–1880.

Wu X, Beecher GR, Holden JM, Haytowitz DB, Gebhardt SE, Prior RL. Lipophilic and hydrophilic capacities of common foods in the United States. *J Agric Food Chem*. 2004:52:4026–4037.

3

Digestion of Foods and Absorption of Nutrients

Human digestion encompasses a series of complex physical and chemical processes that free the nutrients—sugars, fatty acids, amino acids, vitamins, minerals, and other molecules—from foods for their absorption by the small intestine. Nutrients, of course, are needed for building and maintaining tissues, providing energy, and many other uses. Mastery of the basics of digestion, absorption, and delivery of these nutrients to cells helps in understanding nutrient metabolism.

Digestion is the chemical degradation, or breakdown, of foodstuffs, especially macronutrients, into forms that the body can absorb. Proteins are degraded to small peptides and amino acids; fats to fatty acids, glycerol, and monoglycerides; and carbohydrates to individual sugar units (monosaccharides). Only a limited digestion of a few vitamin micronutrients occurs. Digestion of foods containing the macronutrients yields or frees up other molecules, such as vitamins and minerals, which become available for absorption across the absorbing cells of the gut epithelium into the body. Plant foods also contain essentially indigestible fiber and other phytochemicals. The final products of macronutrient digestion are listed in **Table 3.1**. These molecules are taken up by the absorbing cells of the gastrointestinal (GI) tract for use by cells of the body.

TABLE 3.1
Final Products of Macronutrient Digestion

Carbohydrates	Triglycerides (Fats)	Proteins
Glucose	Free fatty acids	Amino acids
Fructose	Glycerol	Short peptides
Galactose	Monoglycerides	

digestion The physical and chemical (enzymatic) degradation of foods that results in the release of nutrients, especially macronutrients (i.e., proteins, fats, carbohydrates), so the digestion products can be absorbed across the gut mucosa. The major role of digestion in the stomach and small intestine is to create many small absorbable molecules from the large macronutrient molecules.

❝❝ Nutrient absorption is a complex process whereby molecules or ions are transferred from the lumen (open channel) within the GI tract into the absorbing cells (a special type of epithelial cell) that line the intestinal tract, mainly the small intestine (and other tracts of the body). These absorbing cells then pass water-soluble nutrients into the blood and fat-soluble nutrients into the lymph. **❞❞**

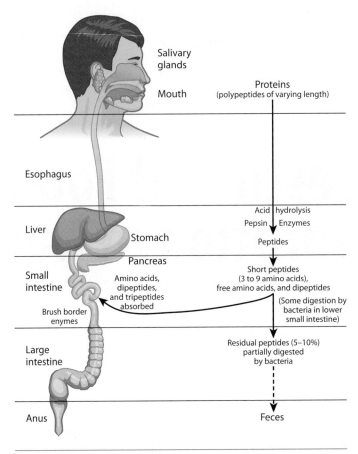

FIGURE 3.1 Protein Digestion. Dietary proteins are broken down by enzymes into amino acids and short peptides as they travel through the digestive system.

Reproduced from Anderson JJB. *Nutrition and Health: An Introduction.* Durham, NC: Carolina Academic Press; 2005.

absorption A complex process whereby molecules or ions are transferred from the lumen within the GI tract into the absorbing cells that line the intestinal tract, mainly the small intestine and other tracts of the body.

lumen The open channel within the GI tract.

epithelial cell Cells that line tubes and cavities in the body. They have rapid turnover or renewal and are typically susceptible to carcinogens and mutagens.

digestive tract Also known as the gastrointestinal (GI) tract, alimentary tract, or gut. This organ system consists of the tube that runs from the mouth to the anus and the associated organs, such as the salivary glands, pancreas, liver, and glands of the tube itself. Although the fluids in the lumen of the gut are technically part of the external environment, they are significantly modified by secretions of the contents of the various glands to allow for digestion and then absorption of nutrients.

An illustration of the steps of digestion of dietary proteins to amino acids is provided in **FIGURE 3.1**.

Nutrient **absorption** is a complex process whereby molecules or ions are transferred from the **lumen** (open channel) within the GI tract into the absorbing cells (a special type of **epithelial cell**) that line the intestinal tract, the small intestine, and other tracts of the body. These absorbing cells then pass water-soluble nutrients into the blood and fat-soluble nutrients into the lymph. The water-soluble nutrients cross the cytoplasm of the absorbing cells and then travel through the basolateral membrane where they are then transferred into the blood by a membrane carrier or porter. Absorbed fat-soluble nutrients exit into the lymphatic circulation as part of chylomicrons, a type of lipoprotein made by the absorbing cells of the small intestine.

In this chapter, the digestion and absorption of the macronutrients and micronutrients are detailed. Also, the various organs, glands, and enzymes involved in digestion, absorption, and utilization of nutrients are presented.

Basics of Digestion

The **digestive tract**, also called the gastrointestinal (GI) tract, is a long tubular structure (30 feet long!) that begins at the mouth and extends to the anus (see **FIGURE 3.2**). The mouth, esophagus, stomach, small intestine, large intestine, and rectum make up the GI tract. Several glands and other organs, such as the pancreas and liver, are associated with it.

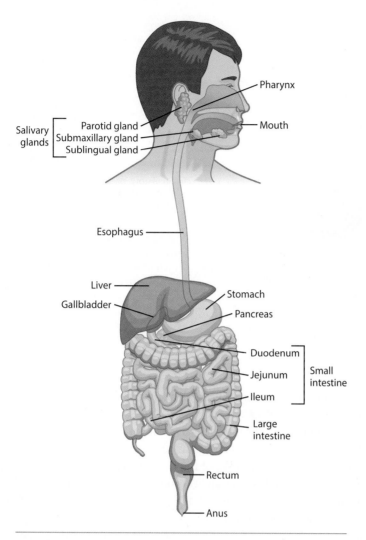

FIGURE 3.2 Major Anatomic Structures of the GI Tract. The major anatomic structures of the GI tract are the mouth, esophagus, stomach, small intestine, large intestine, and rectum.

Reproduced from Anderson JJB. *Nutrition and Health: An Introduction*. Durham, NC: Carolina Academic Press; 2005.

mucosa or mucosal layer The epithelial layer that contains the columnar absorbing cells, such as those in the small intestine. This layer extends into the lumen of the small intestine, and it serves as the barrier to nutrients entering the blood. The absorbing cells of this layer have mechanisms for transporting nutrients from the lumen to the blood.

smooth muscle Nonstriated muscle that exists in the middle layers of arterial walls, the intestinal tube, and other epithelial tissues of the body.

serosa The outer layer of the gastrointestinal tract that is in contact with the venous and lymphatic collection vessels. It surrounds the middle muscular layer, which, in turn, surrounds the mucosal layer of the gastrointestinal tract.

brush border The microvilli on the luminal surfaces of absorbing cells. They look like microscopic paint brushes with lengthy, well-organized cytoplasmic extensions. Similar to the villi, these membrane modifications of the epithelial cells of the small intestine greatly increase the surface area available for absorption.

basolateral membrane The anchoring surface of the absorbing epithelial cells.

Throughout the GI tract, three distinct layers are observed: (1) an inner **mucosa** of epithelial cells, which line the lumen, or inside of the tube, (2) a middle layer consisting of two sheets of **smooth muscle** that contract to produce peristaltic waves that move the digested food along the entire tube, and (3) an outer **serosa** containing connective tissue, capillaries, lymphatics, and nerves (see **FIGURE 3.3**). In real life, the structural components of the three layers are not so easy to recognize as in Figure 3.3 and vary significantly along the whole length of the GI tract. The surface of the small intestine can be referred to as the **brush border**, luminal membrane, or mucosal membrane. The anchoring surface of the absorbing epithelial cells is the **basolateral membrane**. The projections of the

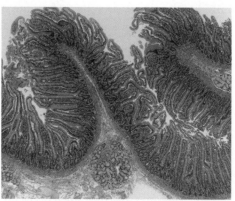

© Donna Beer Stolz, PhD, Center for Biologic Imaging, University of Pittsburgh Medical School.

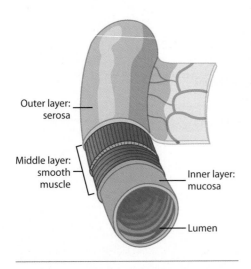

FIGURE 3.3 Cross Section of the Small Intestine. The small intestine, like the rest of the GI tract, has three layers: serosa, smooth muscle, and mucosa.

Reproduced from Anderson JJB. *Nutrition and Health: An Introduction.* Durham, NC: Carolina Academic Press; 2005.

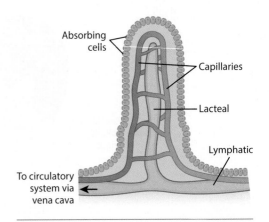

FIGURE 3.4 Villus. The villi of the small intestine project into the lumen of the small intestine, greatly increasing the surface area available for absorption of nutrients.

Reproduced from Anderson JJB. *Nutrition and Health: An Introduction.* Durham, NC: Carolina Academic Press; 2005.

> ❝ The surface of the small intestine can be referred to as the brush border, luminal membrane, or mucosal membrane. The anchoring surface of the absorbing epithelial cells is the basolateral membrane. ❞

food bolus A mass of chewed food that is swallowed from the mouth and moves down the esophagus to the stomach.

gastric acid Produced by the stomach lining cells, this denatures proteins and enhances chemical actions of the enzyme pepsin.

pH Hydrogen ion concentration in body fluid and other solutions in logarithmic units. A pH of 7.0 is neutral. Solutions with a pH less than 7.0 are acidic, and those with a pH greater than 7.0 are basic (or alkaline).

mucosal layer into the lumen are called villi and greatly increase surface area for nutrient absorption (see **FIGURE 3.4**).

The inside or interior of the intestine, also known as the lumen, is connected to the outside of the body at both ends, and so material in the GI tract is still, in one sense, part of the outside world. A number of food components, including indigestible fiber, are not absorbed at all, and pass straight through. When nutrients enter the epithelial cells of the gut lining, they become part of the body, except that these cells themselves (as we shall see in a later section of this chapter) die and are periodically released into the lumen and lost to the body. However, when a molecule or ion has passed through the cell and across the basolateral membrane, it immediately enters into the blood or lymph and is carried away from the GI tract. At this point the molecule or ion is fully absorbed and is available for the body to use. The absorption of nutrients—that is, entry from the gut, movement across the epithelial cell, and transfer to the blood or lymph—is a unidirectional process that occurs either by active transport (see **FIGURE 3.5A**), facilitated diffusion (see **FIGURE 3.5B**), or passive diffusion.

Digestion involves three major processes: mechanical digestion, chemical digestion, and bacterial digestion. First, large pieces of food must be broken into little pieces by mechanical digestion. This process begins in the mouth, where the food is chewed and mixed with salivary secretions, forming multiple boluses. These **food boluses** are swallowed from the mouth or oral cavity and move down the esophagus to the stomach. Mechanical digestion concludes with the churning action that occurs at the same time as chemical digestion in the stomach.

Second, some food macronutrients (and other components) are chemically degraded in the stomach through the actions of gastric acid and digestive enzymes produced by the stomach lining cells. **Gastric acid** denatures proteins and enhances the chemical actions of the enzyme pepsin in the stomach, which is responsible for most of the degradation of proteins. Gastric fluid's **pH**—which is the measure of how acidic or basic a fluid is based on its hydrogen ion concentration—is between 1 and 2, which is very acidic! The small intestine, the pancreas, and other GI-associated glands also secrete digestive enzymes into the lumen of the GI tract. In the small intestine, the degradative

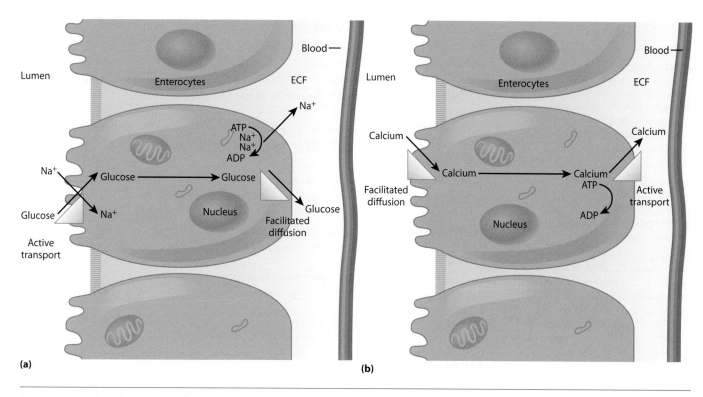

FIGURE 3.5 Unidirectional Flow of Nutrients. Nutrient absorption into the blood or lymph is a one-way process. Nutrients are absorbed into the absorbing cells at the brush border of the mucosa by (a) active transport or (b) facilitated diffusion and then move into the blood or lymph at the basolateral membrane of the serosa. ECF = extracellular fluid.

Reproduced from Anderson JJB. *Nutrition and Health: An Introduction.* Durham, NC: Carolina Academic Press; 2005.

enzymes operate at a near-neutral pH 7.0. The cells of the glands of the small intestine and the pancreas and liver secrete a basic (alkaline) fluid to neutralize the acidic **chyme** (partially digested food) entering from the stomach. Therefore, the slightly basic pH of the fluid medium of the intestines allows the intestinal enzymes to function and makes available for absorption the molecules and ions generated in the digestive process. Fluids secreted by the segments of the GI tract aid significantly in both digestion and absorption.

Enzymes play key roles in digestion, absorption, and metabolism of foods. Many enzymes are secreted by glands existing within the intestinal tract itself or by glands, such as the pancreas, associated with the intestinal tract. Enzymes have very specific

> The slightly basic pH of the fluid medium of the intestines allows the intestinal enzymes to function and to make available for absorption the molecules and ions generated in the digestive process.

chyme The viscous mixture of partially digested food contents and water in the lower stomach and small intestine. This partially digested material (i.e., digesta) is distinguished from a food bolus, which is essentially undigested.

enzyme A protein or protein complex that acts as a biological catalyst that speeds up a chemical reaction. Also a type of food additive used in the processing of foods.

FOCUS 3.1 Digestive Enzymes

Macronutrients are chemically degraded by enzymes that are named for the substrates (molecules) they break down. A typical peptidase splits the peptide bonds of proteins or polypeptides, leaving as products free amino acids and shorter peptides that are then subject to degradation by other peptidases. Pepsin is the name specifically applied to gastric peptidases. Similarly, amylase degrades the bonds linking glucose molecules in long-chain starches (carbohydrates). Lastly, lipases found in many locations, including the gut lumen, break the ester bonds linking fatty acids to glycerol in fats (triglycerides). Many other digestive enzymes also exist, but only a few others are covered in this chapter. ●

pepsin An active enzyme that degrades peptide bonds of food proteins within the lumen of the stomach to smaller peptides and, to a lesser extent, to free amino acids. It is made and secreted as pepsinogen by the chief cells of the gastric glands.

peptidase A type of enzyme that attacks peptide bonds in proteins, starting at either the N-terminus (i.e., aminopeptidase) or the C-terminus (i.e., carboxypeptidase).

amylase Enzyme that hydrolyzes α-1,4-glycosidic bonds in starch molecules. It is secreted by the salivary glands, where it acts in the mouth and the stomach (until inactivated), and by the pancreatic (exocrine) gland as a proenzyme.

lipase Class of enzymes that are located in a variety of tissues (e.g., liver and adipose) as well as in gut lumen (e.g., pancreatic lipase) and in the capillary beds of the general circulation (e.g., lipoprotein lipase). Hormone-sensitive lipase is responsible for lipolysis in fat cells.

salivary glands Secretory glands located in the oral cavity that provide saliva that mixes food with water, mineral ions, and amylase enzymes. Also bathes the teeth with caries-preventing water and mineral ions.

saliva The fluid secreted by the salivary glands into the mouth to facilitate chewing and swallowing. Saliva is responsible for the initial digestion of complex carbohydrates (i.e., starches).

lower esophageal sphincter (LES) The muscular segment between the esophagus and the stomach that, when closed, prevents acid reflux from the stomach into the esophagus. Heartburn occurs when the LES does not close adequately and stomach acid enters the sensitive esophagus.

hydrogen ion (H⁺) Ion formed by removal of the electron from atomic hydrogen. Found in all aqueous solutions of acids. It can be formed by the dissociation of the carboxylic acid group in organic acids or from other sources, such as inorganic acids.

roles (actions), and the function of a particular enzyme can usually be discerned by the meanings of the prefix and the suffix of its name. For example, the enzyme sucrase breaks down a carbohydrate called sucrose. The prefix *sucr-* comes from the word *sucrose*, and the suffix *-ase* is typically used in naming most enzymes. Another suffix for an enzyme is *-sin*. For example, consider the names of the following enzymes:

- **Pepsin** and **peptidase**: The prefixes *pep-* and *pepti-* refer to proteins (from the word *peptide*). These enzymes degrade proteins within the stomach and small intestine.
- **Amylase**: The prefix *amyl-* refers to carbohydrate (from a starch called amylose). These enzymes principally degrade complex carbohydrates in the small intestine via the pancreas.
- **Lipase**: The prefix *lip-* comes from the word *lipid*, which refers to fat. Lipases act on fats primarily in the lumen of the small intestine.

Third, gut bacteria also digest macronutrients, especially in the large intestine, or colon. Bacteria may also synthesize small amounts of vitamin B_{12} (cobalamin) and vitamin K.

Oral Aspects of Digestion

The mouth, or oral cavity, is the beginning of the digestive tract. Here the teeth physically break down foodstuffs into smaller pieces by chewing. The **salivary glands** in the oral cavity secrete **saliva**, a water-based solution that contains amylase, a starch-degrading enzyme, to moisten the food and begin the chemical degradation of starches. Salivary gland secretions are affected by the taste, smell, or even sight of food, especially if a person is hungry or about to sit down to a meal. Saliva also contains minerals that provide protection for the surfaces of teeth; the continuous bathing of the teeth helps prevent cavities (caries).

At the back of the oral cavity is the pharynx, an open space where the digestive and respiratory tracts overlap between the nose and lungs. The esophagus transports the chewed food, called a bolus (literally a little ball), and any liquid from the mouth to the stomach for digestion. Mucosal cells of the esophagus secrete mucus, a fluid that provides for an efficient, nearly frictionless flow of each food bolus to the stomach. The **lower esophageal sphincter** is a valve that normally prevents backflow or reflux of food or acid from the stomach into the esophagus.

Gastric Digestion

The stomach further degrades the ingested food by churning it while secreting acid from its glandular cells and chemically digesting proteins via specific enzymes. A decrease in pH of the gastric contents is created by the **hydrogen ions** (acid) secreted by the gastric glands. The salivary amylase is eventually destroyed by the high acidity in the stomach. However, the stomach's acidic conditions favor catalytic enzymes, primarily pepsin (peptidase), that initiate digestion of proteins within the lumen. During fasting periods, the pH of an empty stomach is approximately 2.0, or about the same acidity as lemon juice. Although the stomach secretes acid during a meal, the gastric acid concentration decreases during fasting and the pH rises to about 3.0 because of the presence of neutralizing alkaline minerals and other basic components residing in the stomach.

Digestion and Absorption in the Small Intestine

The **pyloric sphincter**, the valve between the stomach and the small intestine, controls the movement of the partly digested food, also known as chyme; it is closed when food is in the stomach. When specific hormonal and nervous mechanisms cause it to open, small amounts of chyme (which is also called digesta) are propelled through the opening by the force of the stomach's contracting muscles. Once the partially digested food is in the small intestine, its low pH value signals the release of other intestinal hormones, causing the pyloric sphincter to close and for intestinal glands and the pancreas and liver to secrete buffering fluids into the gut lumen along with enzymes and proenzymes.

The **small intestine** is somewhat arbitrarily divided into three parts: the duodenum, jejunum, and ileum. The **duodenum** receives the digesta from the stomach and digestive fluids from the liver and from the pancreas. Most digestion occurs in the duodenum and **jejunum**, whereas most of the absorption occurs in the jejunum and ileum. The **ileum** empties into the large intestine. The appendix, according to new research, harbors "good" bacteria that help repopulate the lower small intestine and large intestine with good bacteria after bouts of diarrhea or other GI illnesses.

During transit along the small intestine, the pH of the chyme increases from the highly acidic state of the stomach to a neutral state of greater than 7 in the large intestine. The low pH of the stomach and the duodenum reduces the growth of intestinal bacteria in these regions of the GI tract. Bacteria in the intestine, called intestinal flora or **gut bacteria**, are first found in large concentrations in the ileum, the final segment of the small intestine, but their density is much greater in the large intestine. (*Helicobacter pylori* in the stomach contribute to gastric ulcers, but they typically exist in very low numbers in the high-acid stomachs of most people.) **FIGURE 3.6** illustrates the relative number of bacteria within the major segments of the GI tract. *E. coli* are commonly found in the ileum and the large intestine (see **FIGURE 3.7**).

The fingerlike projections, or **villi**, of the small intestine greatly increase the surface area. The brush border of the intestinal absorbing cells is aptly named because at the microscopic level it looks like bristles of a paintbrush (i.e., small protrusions into the lumen; see Figure 3.4). As an analogy, imagine the indented edges of a postage stamp that significantly increase the length of the edge of the stamp. In fact, if the surface of the intestine could be spread out flat, it would have a surface area approximately the size of a tennis court, or about 250 square meters. The absorbing epithelial cells themselves, called **enterocytes**, which cover the projecting villi, have similar

> *The stomach's acidic conditions favor catalytic enzymes, primarily pepsin (peptidase), that initiate digestion of proteins within the lumen.*

pyloric sphincter Thick muscular portion of the lower stomach that contracts and occasionally relaxes during gastric digestion. The closing permits gastric grinding and digestion of food molecules until small quantities of chyme are released into the duodenum.

small intestine The segment of gastrointestinal tract between stomach and large intestine that functions primarily in digestion and absorption. It consists of three segments: duodenum, jejunum, and ileum.

duodenum The first segment of the small intestine, approximately 12 inches in length, where intestinal absorption is typically highly efficient.

jejunum The segment of the small intestine between duodenum and ileum. It is approximately 8 feet in length. Some digestion occurs here.

ileum The final segment of the small intestine that joins the colon. It is responsible for the absorption of significant amounts of macronutrients, micronutrients, and bile acids. Large numbers of bacteria (gut flora) live within its lumen. The intrinsic factor (IF)–vitamin B_{12} complex combines with a receptor in the lower ileum prior to absorption.

gut bacteria The flora that normally exist only in the lower small intestine and the large intestine. The number of bacteria is much larger in the large intestine than in the ileum.

villi Fingerlike projections in the small intestine increase its surface area.

enterocyte The primary columnar absorbing cell type of the gut epithelium. Also used to refer to any cell type, including goblet cells, in the epithelial lining of the gastrointestinal tract.

	Flora
Stomach	10^1–10^4 bacteria/mL
Duodenum	10^3 bacteria/mL
Jejunum-ileum	10^4–10^7 bacteria/mL
Large intestine	10^{10}–10^{12} bacteria/mL

FIGURE 3.6 Bacteria in the Gut. Various species of bacteria inhabit the GI tract and aid in digestion. Bacteria in the large intestine, in particular, play an important role in the detoxification and fermentation of digested food.

> ❝ Bacteria in the intestine, called intestinal flora or gut bacteria, are first found in large concentrations in the ileum, the final segment of the small intestine, but their density is much greater in the large intestine. ❞

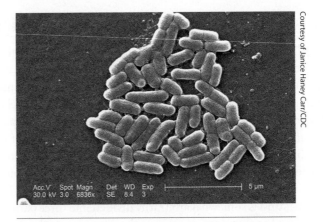

Courtesy of Janice Haney Carr/CDC

FIGURE 3.7 *E. coli*. The ileum of the small intestine and the large intestine harbor large numbers of *E. coli*.

subcellular protrusions called microvilli. The flow of nutrients across the absorbing cells and into blood or lymph supplies nutrients to the body's tissues and cells (see Figure 3.5).

The absorbing epithelial cells (enterocytes) that line the small intestine are especially well suited to absorb nutrients because of their microvilli (i.e., brush borders). The microvilli contain several types of molecular ferries (proteins), also known as porters, in their membrane structure that facilitate the entry of specific nutrients into the cells. Epithelial cells themselves are dynamic; they have a short and very active life before being removed. They are created through active cell division in the crypts of Lieberkuhn at the base of the villi, and they migrate up the villi as functioning cells. As the abrasive action of the intestinal contents wears down the cells, aging occurs, and subsequently the epithelial cells die and slough off at the tips of the villi as newly formed cells slowly follow them up the villi. After actively participating in the vital work of absorption for several days, these cells, in turn, die and are dislodged into the lumen. The nutrients in these sloughed dead cells are themselves digested and reabsorbed further down the GI tract. The cycle of new cells being formed in the crypts and progressing up the villi to the tips lasts about 6 days.

**epithelial sheet
(epithelium)** Epithelial tissue that consists of specialized epithelial cells that line the gastrointestinal tract (gut), respiratory tract, and the urogenital tract. These tissues act as barriers and as absorbing surfaces. They also contain cells that secrete mucus that coats the luminal surface and thereby protects the epithelia.

**absorption period
(postprandium)** The 3- to 4-hour period that follows the last ingestion of a meal during which the most nutrients are absorbed. This period is associated with wide swings in blood glucose and insulin concentrations, even under normal conditions.

prandium (meal or eating period) The period of eating a meal, typically lasting from 15 minutes to an hour. The eating period follows the early phase of the premeal period; it is followed by the absorption (postprandial) period.

FOCUS 3.2 Bidirectional Flow in Enterocytes

The absorbing cells in the intestine are part of an **epithelial sheet** that is only one cell thick! This epithelial layer contains small numbers of a few other cell types in addition to the absorbing cells. Following eating, gastric digestion, and the release of chyme into the small intestine, the absorbing cells take up nutrients from the gut lumen, move them across the cells, and finally transfer them to the blood or lymph. The nutrients cross two membranes: the brush border at the gut lumen and the basolateral membrane. This unidirectional flow represents absorption. At the same time, other cells of the epithelial surface of the gut are secreting water to maintain the appropriate osmotic concentration of the gut luminal fluids. During the roughly 3-hour **absorption period** (or post-prandium) following the meal (eating period or **prandium**), nutrients flow in one direction—from the lumen to blood or lymph. At the same time, water is secreted in the opposite direction—from the blood to the gut lumen. These two major intestinal functions, absorption and secretion, are essential for good health. ●

The Pancreas, the Liver, and Enterohepatic Circulation

Pancreas

Secretions from the exocrine **pancreas** contain numerous proenzymes (inactive enzyme precursors) that become activated enzymes capable of degrading proteins, fats, carbohydrates, and other molecules present in foods to their basic molecular components. Pancreatic proenzymes must be activated within the gut lumen by enterokinase, an enzyme secreted by absorbing cells before they are capable of enzymatic activity. The pancreas contains groups of cells that look like small grape clusters (acini); these cells create the proenzymes necessary for the further digestion of proteins, fats, carbohydrates, and many other nutrient components. **FIGURE 3.8** shows the grapelike clusters of exocrine secreting cells adjacent to the endocrine cells of the islets of Langerhans, which secrete the hormones insulin and glucagon. The clusters of pancreatic cells not only secrete proenzymes into the gut lumen but also secrete a basic (alkaline) solution that helps buffer acid within the lumen of the duodenum. The **pancreatic duct**, which carries buffering fluid and proenzymes, joins the common bile duct from the liver just prior to entering the upper duodenum. Once in the small intestine, the proenzymes are converted to active enzymes by enterokinase.

> Secretions from the exocrine pancreas contain numerous proenzymes (inactive enzyme precursors) that become activated enzymes capable of degrading proteins, fats, carbohydrates, and other molecules present in foods to their basic molecular components.

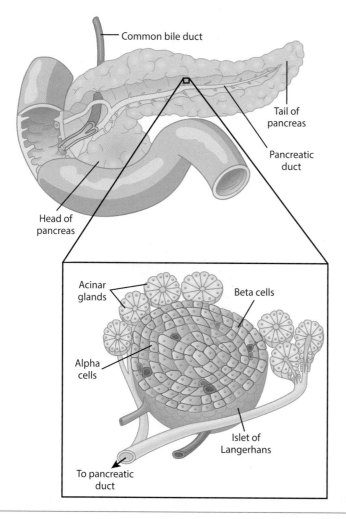

FIGURE 3.8 Pancreas. The pancreas includes grapelike clusters (acini) of proenzyme-secreting exocrine cells and the hormone-secreting endocrine cells of the islets of Langerhans.

pancreas (exocrine and endocrine) A large gland associated with the digestive system that produces enzyme precursors, such as trypsinogen, and fluids (pancreatic juice) that are secreted into the gastrointestinal tract, where the enzymes are then activated. The pancreas also has the islets of Langerhans, which produce insulin.

pancreatic duct The duct that carries the secretory products of the exocrine pancreas (buffering fluid and proenzymes) to the common bile duct before entering the upper duodenum. The pancreatic fluid is then secreted into the intestinal lumen.

liver A large organ that has many functions relating to energy and protein metabolism. It plays important roles in the urea cycle, the ketogenic pathway, bile acid synthesis, bile (fluid) production, and lipoprotein production (except for chylomicrons) and degradation. It is also responsible for the metabolism of alcohol, drugs, toxic chemicals, and vitamin D. Alcoholic liver has characteristic pathologic changes, including excess fatty deposits and cirrhosis.

common bile duct The duct that carries both bile and pancreatic juice into the lumen of the upper duodenum. If blocked, jaundice can result.

bile A secretion of the liver (and by the gallbladder after storage) containing water, bile salts, cholesterol, and phosphatidylcholine, in addition to fat-soluble waste products. It is secreted into the small intestine, where it is critical to the digestion and absorption of fats.

bile salts (bile acids) Synthesized by liver cells from cholesterol, the primary bile acids, such as cholic acid, aid in fat digestion and absorption by acting as detergents in forming micelles in the small intestine. Bile salts can be modified in the gastrointestinal tract by bacteria to secondary bile acids through the loss of one or more hydroxyl groups. Secondary bile acids are considered to be carcinogenic in the large intestine.

micelle A small complex of fat and bile formed in the lumen of the small intestine after the breakdown of large fat emulsions. The smaller micelles permit greater access of lipase enzymes to triglycerides and phospholipids for enzymatic degradation. They also serve to ferry the digestion products of lipid molecules to the brush-border surfaces for absorption.

gallbladder A muscular sac that collects and concentrates bile (fluid) released by the liver. During a meal, the gallbladder contracts periodically and releases some of its contents through the common bile duct into the lumen of the gastrointestinal tract to aid in the digestion and absorption of dietary fats.

Liver

The **liver** secretes a biliary fluid into the **common bile duct** that enhances both digestion and absorption of the products of lipid molecules, including fatty acids and cholesterol. Triglycerides are degraded to free fatty acids before they are absorbed with the help of bile. **Bile** is a secretion of the liver that consists of a watery solution of cholesterol, bile salts, phospholipids, and other components. **Bile salts** (formed from bile acids), which act like detergent in solubilizing lipids, are essential for the efficient breakdown of the fats and fat-soluble molecules in the lumen of the small intestine and their subsequent absorption.

A major role of bile is to solubilize large fat emulsions derived from foods by facilitating their physical breakdown into smaller spherical aggregates called **micelles** that contain both fats and bile components (see **FIGURE 3.9**). This degradation happens in much the same way as dish detergent solubilizes the greasy remnants of a meal and completely disperses and suspends them in the dishwater. A micelle essentially dissolves the fat in its fat-soluble core and allows the water-soluble components of the molecules (oxygen-containing groups) to float at the external surface of the outside layer. Micelles permit efficient attack by water-soluble digestive enzymes on the fat molecules and also make the absorption of the degradation products more efficient by serving as ferries that deliver the molecules directly to the luminal membranes of the absorbing cell.

The liver makes bile continuously; it is either used immediately in digestion or it is stored in the gallbladder for later use. Bile is carried in the common bile duct from the liver to the duodenum. The **gallbladder** stores bile between meals. When the gallbladder contracts after the ingestion of food, bile is released into the lumen of the duodenum for the purpose of dissolving fats from foods and forming micelles that are much smaller than emulsions. Refer to Figure 3.2, which shows the relationships among the pancreas, liver, and gallbladder.

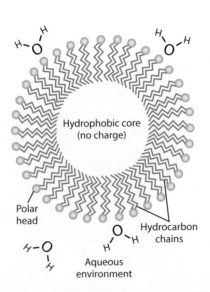

FIGURE 3.9 Micelle Structure. Water-insoluble fats incorporated by micelles are formed from the biliary secretions into the lumen of the small intestine. The oxygen-containing water-soluble groups of the dietary lipids face the water-lipid interface of the micelle, but the hydrocarbon chains extend into the core of the micelle.

Enterohepatic Circulation

The **enterohepatic circulation (EHC)** is the pathway taken by components of bile, particularly bile salts and cholesterol, after secretion into the duodenum and participation in the digestion of fats. The bulk of these molecules is then reabsorbed by the ileum and recycled for reuse in the liver. **FIGURE 3.10** illustrates the EHC of fat-soluble molecules. This pathway allows for the recycling of these important bile components along with other fat-soluble diet-derived molecules, such as cholesterol.

The liver cells, which are also called **hepatocytes**, make numerous molecules as well, such as albumin, which are secreted into the blood and serve useful functions

> The enterohepatic circulation is the pathway taken by components of bile, particularly bile salts and cholesterol, after secretion into the duodenum and participation in the digestion of fats.

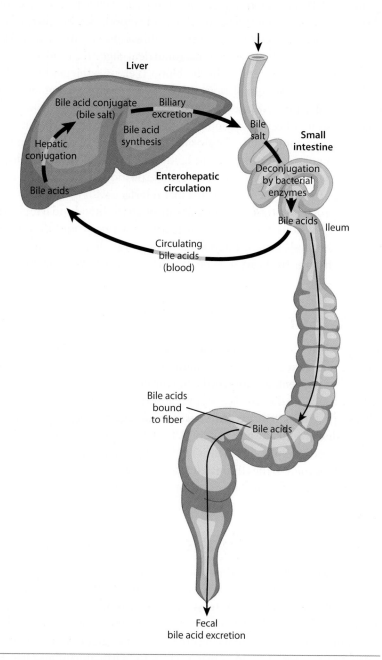

FIGURE 3.10 Enterohepatic Circulation. Note the directional relationships of the biliary secretions of the liver (or gallbladder) into the duodenum and the partial return of the bile components via the ileum to the liver.

enterohepatic circulation (EHC) The circulation of bile acids and salts and fat-soluble components of bile fluid from the liver (and gallbladder) into the gastrointestinal tract and then the absorption of a percentage of these molecules in the ileum for return to the liver for reuse.

hepatocyte The major cell type in the liver. The hepatocytes are responsible for most of the liver's synthetic and storage functions. It also is secreted into the blood and serves useful functions throughout the body.

throughout the body. The liver also stores a minimal amount of carbohydrate via the animal starch known as glycogen; it also stores some fat (triglycerides) and vitamin A. In addition, hepatocytes make two types of lipoproteins, very low-density lipoprotein (VLDL) and high-density lipoprotein (HDL), as part of the distribution of fat-soluble nutrients. Finally, liver cells make bile, which enhances fat digestion and absorption of their degradation products.

Hepatic Portal Circulation and Lymphatic Drainage

The large **hepatic portal vein** collects blood from the veins draining the small intestine and some of the large intestine and delivers the blood, rich in water-soluble nutrients following a meal, directly to the liver for utilization or further distribution (see Figure 3.10). An estimated 50% of the macronutrient digestive products are taken up by the liver! Nutrients that remain in the blood (i.e., unextracted by the liver) pass along to the general venous circulation and the heart to supply all other tissues of the body. Vessels involved in **lymphatic circulation** in contact with the absorbing cells in the small intestine collect the chylomicrons and their nutrient-rich, fat-soluble molecules as part of the lymph (fluid). **Chylomicrons** are a type of lipoprotein that consist of sphere-like complexes of proteins and lipids; like other lipoproteins, chylomicrons often are referred to as particles. The water-soluble portions of the proteins are exposed at the external surfaces of the lipoproteins that interface with the water of blood, thus permitting lipoproteins to transport their fats through the blood and lymph. The lymph is delivered to the venous collection of the heart via a long lymphatic vessel, the thoracic duct, which travels from the abdomen through the thorax to connect to a major vein from the left arm. The heart then pumps the chylomicrons throughout the body.

Large Intestine

The next organ of the GI tract is the **large intestine**, also known as the colon. Most of the remaining fluid and electrolytes (sodium, potassium, and chloride ions) and small amounts of other nutrients are absorbed from the lumen of the large intestine. The large intestine has a much smaller surface area for absorption than the small intestine.

The digesta passed on to the rectum consists of undigested materials such as cellulose, liver waste products, cellular waste materials, bacteria, and small amounts of undigested or unabsorbed food components, such as fat. Bile pigments secreted by the liver give the characteristic dark color to the eliminated feces. The rectum is the final compacting and temporary storage site of fecal contents prior to defecation (i.e., elimination).

Digestion and Absorption of Macronutrients

As has been discussed, the chemical and biochemical processes of digestion use enzymes to break down macronutrients. Enzymes are chemical catalysts that speed up reactions; they are practically always proteins. Several steps of digestion have already been outlined, such as the degradation of proteins in both the stomach and small intestine; starch digestion in the mouth, stomach (limited), and small intestine; and fat digestion in the small intestine with the aid of bile used for the formation of micelles. Except for protein, 90% or more of macronutrients are absorbed. This section summarizes the digestion and absorption of carbohydrates, proteins, and fats.

hepatic portal vein Large vein that runs from the intestines to the liver. It collects water-soluble nutrients absorbed across the gastrointestinal tract and carries them to the liver for initial processing and utilization.

lymphatic circulation The collection of lymph, or fluids basically devoid of cells, from the tissues and the return of albumin-rich and chylomicron-rich (only after meals) fluid from the body cavities to the blood vascular circulation.

chylomicron A type of lipoprotein made by intestinal absorbing cells after a meal to carry triglycerides around the body. After most of the lipid contents are removed by peripheral tissues, a chylomicron remnant is taken up by the liver for degradation.

large intestine Organ in the GI tract that is also known as the colon. Most remaining fluid and electrolytes (sodium, potassium, and chloride ions) and a small amount of other nutrients are absorbed from the lumen of the large intestine.

Absorption of Water- Versus Fat-Soluble Nutrients

During the 3 hours after a meal (i.e., the postprandial period), passively absorbed fat-soluble molecules are incorporated into chylomicrons prior to their exit from the enterocyte cytoplasm to the lymphatic system by passive diffusion. Chylomicrons are large packets (microscopically speaking) of fats secreted from the intestines and configured with specific structural proteins into ball-shaped structures that facilitate the movement of fat-soluble molecules through water-based blood.

Also following a meal, the concentration of water-soluble macronutrients in the gut lumen increases, and their degradation products enter the epithelial cells by facilitated diffusion. Adenosine triphosphate (ATP) is not required to accomplish this transfer of water-soluble nutrients from the gut lumen (higher concentration) into the cytosol of the absorbing cells (lower concentration). Water-soluble macronutrients are transferred across the cell cytosol by diffusion. Then, at the exit step, they are transferred by active transport to the blood for distribution throughout the body. The process of active transport is accomplished by a variety of molecular ferries or porters specific for different sugars and amino acids that requires energy (ATP).

Nutrients are absorbed from the gut lumen into the body by two distinct transport steps: (1) the entry step is the passage of the nutrient from the lumen across the brush border into the epithelial cells and (2) the exit step is the movement of the nutrient from these cells at the basolateral membrane to the blood or lymph. In between these two steps the incoming molecules move across the enterocyte cytosol from the brush border membrane to the basolateral membrane.

Molecules or minerals cross the brush border and basolateral membranes of absorbing cells by: (1) passive diffusion, (2) facilitated diffusion, or (3) active transport (see **FIGURE 3.11**). In the cases of passive diffusion and facilitated diffusion, transfer of nutrients requires no added energy (ATP). **Passive diffusion** of a water-soluble molecule along its concentration gradient (from high to lower) may occur around cells through gaps rather than across membranes and through cells! Passive transfer from a higher concentration to a lower concentration does not require energy. However, **active transport** does require ATP to energize the uphill movement of the molecule or ion from a low concentration across a membrane to a higher concentration. In addition, both **facilitated diffusion** and active transport mechanisms require specific protein carriers or porters for the movement of different classes of molecules or ions across the membrane. In the passive diffusion of fat-soluble molecules via micelles, the fat components of the membrane are critical for absorbing the molecules through the membranes and into the epithelial cells. (Membranes in our bodies are made mostly of a specialized type of fat.) Fat-soluble molecules move across the membrane by passive diffusion at both entry and exit steps; no energy and no carriers are needed. Micelles assist in passive transfer of fat degradation products at the entry step and chylomicrons assist at the exit step. In general, water-soluble nutrients are transported across membranes via specialized carriers in the brush border membranes and then across the basolateral membrane.

Carbohydrates

Carbohydrate digestion begins with the chewing of foods in the mouth. Starches are a type of carbohydrate that consists of long polymer chains of glucose molecules. The salivary glands secrete fluids into the oral cavity that aid in the digestive process by wetting the foodstuffs and by supplying the enzyme salivary amylase. Salivary amylase begins to break some of the bonds between adjacent monosaccharide (glucose) units of the starches in the mouth and continues its action until it is inactivated by acid in the stomach. Practically all starch digestion begins in the upper duodenum. For a complete list of digestive enzymes, see **Table 3.2**.

passive diffusion Intestinal absorption through or between epithelial cells that requires no energy (ATP) because of movement of nutrients from high concentration to low concentration.

active transport The movement of a molecule across a membrane from a region of lower to higher concentration (i.e., up a concentration gradient), which requires both a carrier (porter) and cellular energy (ATP). Uphill transport applies to water-soluble molecules and ions, including nutrient molecules and ions, that are not soluble in the lipophilic membranes of cells.

facilitated diffusion Transfer of solutes (molecules and ions) across a membrane down a concentration gradient (from high to low) through the use of a carrier molecule (protein), but without the expenditure of energy (ATP). Typical transport mechanism for water-soluble chemical species.

Passive Diffusion

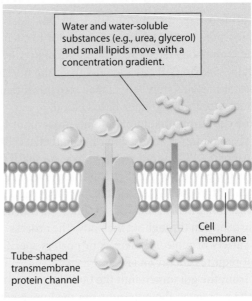

Water and water-soluble substances (e.g., urea, glycerol) and small lipids move with a concentration gradient.

Cell membrane

Tube-shaped transmembrane protein channel

(a)

Facilitated Diffusion

High

Concentration

Transmembrane protein carrier changes shape to facilitate entry and exit of some nutrients (e.g., fructose).

Low

(b)

Active Transport

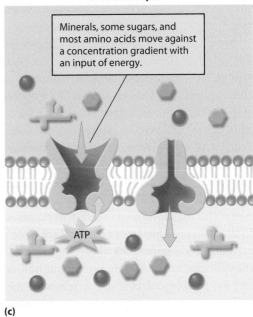

Minerals, some sugars, and most amino acids move against a concentration gradient with an input of energy.

ATP

(c)

FIGURE 3.11 Transport Mechanisms Across the Absorbing Cell. Depending on the particular substance, substances cross the membranes of absorption cells by (a) passive diffusion, (b) facilitated diffusion, or (c) active transport.

Carbohydrate digestion takes place mainly in the duodenum and jejunum. One of the enzymes, pancreatic amylase, which is secreted in the pancreatic fluid as a proenzyme, is activated in the lumen and attacks the bonds between the glucose units of starches. The final products of starch digestion in the small intestine are glucose molecules and short strands of glucose molecules (2 to 10 units in length) called dextrins. Digestion of these dextrins is completed at the brush border of enterocytes by enzymes attached to the brush border membrane itself.

TABLE 3.2
Digestive Enzymes

Origin	Enzyme	Substrate	Products
Salivary glands	Salivary amylase	Starches	Disaccharides, trisaccharides
Stomach	Pepsin	Proteins	Short peptides
Pancreas	Pancreatic amylase	Starches	Disaccharides (maltose)
Intestinal glands	Maltase	Maltose	Glucose
	Sucrase	Sucrose	Glucose, fructose
	Lactase	Lactose	Glucose, galactose
	Exopeptidases	Short peptides	Amino acids
Intestinal cells	Enterokinase	Proenzymes from pancreas	Active enzymes
Pancreas	Trypsin	Proteins	Short peptides
	Chymotrypsin	Proteins	Short peptides
	Lipase	Triglycerides	Diglycerides, fatty acids, and glycerol

Associated with these membrane surfaces, which remain in contact with fluids in the lumen, are several enzymes that are named for the substrates or molecules whose bonds they attack and split. These enzymes include: (1) **sucrase**, which splits sucrose (table sugar) into glucose and fructose; (2) **lactase**, which hydrolyzes lactose (milk sugar) into glucose and galactose; and (3) **maltase**, which degrades maltose (from digested starch) into two glucose molecules. Food starches contain only glucose units in their long polymers.

After sugars and starches are digested, the major product, glucose, is rapidly transferred by an ATP-requiring active transport mechanism across the brush-border membrane into the mucosal cell cytosol. Once inside the absorbing cells, glucose and other sugar molecules (fructose and galactose) are either used for intracellular metabolic pathways to generate ATP or they are translocated to the basolateral membrane where they are transported from the epithelial cell into the blood capillaries. The blood carries these monosaccharide sugar molecules via the hepatic portal circulation directly to the liver.

Some foods, particularly when not chewed adequately, are not accessible to digestive enzymes. An extreme example of incomplete digestion would be kernels of corn eaten off the cob that are swallowed whole and often found intact in stools; the kernels' waxy surface resists attack through the entire length of the gastrointestinal tract. For most fruits and vegetables, however, only small amounts of carbohydrates remain unavailable for attack by enzymes. Nevertheless, in diets with large amounts of complex carbohydrates and dietary fiber, the inefficiency of digestion may be greater, especially with high carbohydrate and low protein diets, such as consumed by strict vegetarians and by people living in much of the developing world. In general, carbohydrate digestion efficiency exceeds 90%.

In the ileum and especially in the large intestine, bacterial populations abound, and they utilize the residual small amounts of the carbohydrates passed on from the upper

sucrase An enzyme of the small intestine that degrades sucrose.

lactase An enzyme of the small intestine that metabolizes lactose, the milk sugar, to glucose and galactose. In infants, this enzyme is present in adequate amounts during the breastfeeding period, and thereafter it declines.

maltase Enzyme complex at the luminal surface of epithelial cells of the small intestine that degrades maltose (disaccharide) and dextrins (short chains containing 3 to 10 glucose units) derived from starches (polysaccharides) into glucose.

> Under normal circumstances no digestible carbohydrate appears in stools.

bowel. Bacterial flora populations, which are largely anaerobic (i.e., carry out their activities without oxygen), frequently form gases as by-products of their metabolism. A few of these gases are absorbed and exhaled through the lungs, whereas others can only be eliminated by exit through the anus. These bacteria feast on beans and other legumes, which contain some carbohydrates for which humans have no digestive enzymes. Under normal circumstances no digestible carbohydrate appears in stools. Indigestible fiber components that are predominantly carbohydrate in nature, however, are found in stools of healthy individuals who consume fruits, vegetables, nuts, seeds, and cereal grains.

Proteins and Amino Acids

The digestion of proteins involves both gastric and small intestinal phases. Proteins are long-chain polymers of amino acids. The gastric phase includes the action of pepsin in a highly acidic medium in the degradation of the bonds between the amino acids (i.e., peptide bonds). Peptides (i.e., fragments of proteins) of various lengths produced by the stomach are released into the small intestine for continuing digestion until mostly amino acids, dipeptides (two amino acids), and some tripeptides (three amino acids) remain. The digestion of proteins, also known as proteolysis, is completed in the small bowel through the action of pancreatic enzymes. These enzymes are **trypsin**, which hydrolyzes peptide bonds in dietary proteins in the small intestine, and chymotrypsin; both are initially secreted as proenzymes. Enterokinase, located on the brush-border surfaces of enterocytes, converts the inactive pancreatic proenzymes **trypsinogen** and chymotrypsinogen into the active enzymes trypsin and chymotrypsin, respectively, within the gut lumen. The *-ogen* suffix in the enzyme names indicates that these are inactive proenzymes. Digestion of short peptides (two and three amino acids) is completed by cytosolic enzymes within the intestinal absorbing cell rather than by pancreatic enzymes.

Absorption of individual amino acids occurs by at least four specific transport mechanisms in the epithelial surfaces at the brush border. Absorption of dipeptides and tripeptides is now also known to occur, and this mechanism may account for the absorption of a significant quantity of amino acids. Finally, if not used for the needs of the enterocytes in the small intestine, amino acids in the cytosol are transferred by active transport mechanisms across the basolateral membrane to the blood for immediate distribution to the liver via the hepatic portal vein.

In all, about 75% of the dietary proteins from mixed Western meals containing animal and plant sources are completely digested to their constituent amino acids or to dipeptides and tripeptides, which are then rapidly absorbed. The remainder (~25%) of the dietary protein exits the small intestine as fragments (long polypeptides) and passes into the large bowel. Bacteria degrade the remaining peptides and their amino acids, and they also generate diverse amines that are absorbed by epithelial cells in the large intestine and distributed throughout the body. Most gut amines are metabolized by the liver. No protein or free amino acids are normally found in stools.

> No protein or free amino acids are normally found in stools.

Lipids and Fats

Lipids are more difficult to digest than water-soluble molecules because of their water insolubility. Fats (triglycerides or triacylglycerols) are composed of three long hydrocarbon chains (fatty acids) attached to a glycerol molecule. The lipid (fat) solubility of these molecules prevents them from being dissolved in the watery environment of the GI tract. These highly water-insoluble molecules are incorporated into micelles in the intestinal lumen that are formed in the presence of bile from the liver. Lipases, which are secreted as prolipases, break down the fats with the assistance of colipases. These enzymes degrade specific bonds of the lipid molecules. For example, pancreatic lipase attacks triglyceride bonds, freeing the fatty acids from the glycerol backbone. The

trypsin An enzyme that hydrolyzes (splits with the addition of water) peptide bonds in dietary proteins in the small intestine.

trypsinogen A proenzyme secreted by the pancreas that must be partially cleaved within the small intestinal lumen to yield the active enzyme trypsin, which degrades peptide bonds.

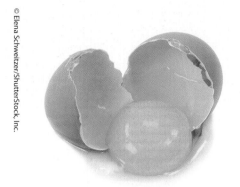

© Elena Schweitzer/ShutterStock, Inc.

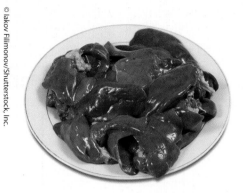

© Iakov Filimonov/Shutterstock, Inc.

> Cholesterol, mainly provided as cholesterol esters in animal-based foods such as eggs and liver, is digested and absorbed in a fashion similar to the triglycerides and is also incorporated into chylomicrons for distribution around the body.

micelles then carry the free fatty acids and other fat-soluble molecules, such as vitamins A, D, E, and K, to the surfaces of the epithelial cells where they are absorbed into the cells by passive diffusion. Greater than 90% of dietary fats are digested in individuals with healthy digestion.

After absorption, lipid components are carried from the small intestine by the lymphatic system. Newly synthesized triglyceride molecules, plus fat-soluble vitamins, are incorporated into chylomicrons within the enterocytes. These chylomicrons then move passively across the cell membrane into lymphatic lacteals. The chylomicrons are then carried by larger lymphatic vessels from the abdomen into the thorax and finally transferred to a major vein near the heart for distribution to all the tissues in the body. Chylomicron particles are large lipid-rich lipoproteins that allow triglycerides and other fat-soluble molecules to be carried from the small intestine through the **lipophobic** water-based environment of lymph and blood to tissues.

Cholesterol, mainly provided as **cholesterol esters** in animal-based foods such as eggs and liver, is digested and absorbed in a fashion similar to the triglycerides and also is incorporated into chylomicrons for distribution around the body. (Plant foods contain other sterol molecules known as phytosterols.) Recall that the components of bile are reabsorbed through the EHC. Some specific dietary fiber components reduce the efficiency of the EHC, especially by reducing the absorption or reabsorption of cholesterol from bile. The net effect is a lowering of the efficiency of the EHC and, therefore, the serum total cholesterol concentration. The water-soluble fibers found in oat bran, pectins in certain fruits, and other fiber molecules can also bind to cholesterol molecules, lower their absorption, and thereby lower the total cholesterol concentration in circulating blood. Although this beneficial cholesterol-lowering effect of a high-fiber intake is modest, it may be significant over a long period of time.

PRACTICAL APPLICATIONS **3.1**

Enterohepatic Circulation and Absorption of Lipids

Trace the pathways of the EHC with a paper-and-pencil diagram, starting at the liver where bile is secreted and ending at the liver where the major sterol components, especially cholesterol, are taken up via the path from the ileum. ■

lipophobic Adjective referring to the dislike of lipid molecules.

cholesterol ester A storage form of cholesterol formed by the addition of a fatty acid to cholesterol by an ester bond.

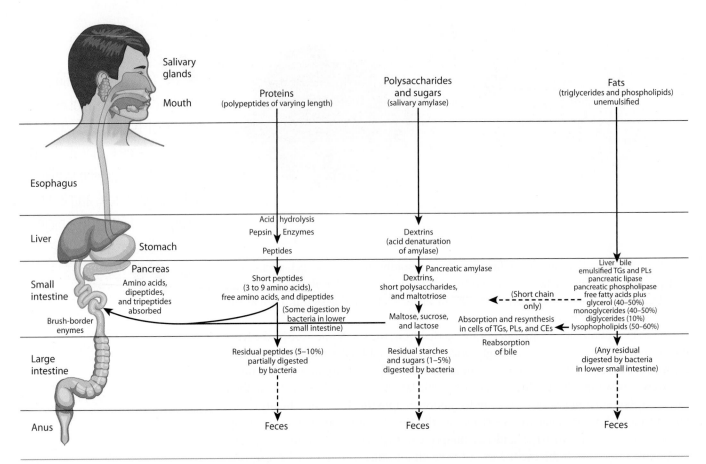

FIGURE 3.12 Macronutrient Digestion. The three macronutrients have different paths of digestion and preparation for intestinal absorption.

Adapted from Anderson JJB. *Nutrition and Health: An Introduction*. Durham, NC: Carolina Academic Press; 2005.

In summary, digestion of proteins results in intestinal absorption of free amino acids, dipeptides, or short peptides; digestion of polysaccharides and sugars results in formation of maltose, sucrose, and lactose for further digestion by brush-border enzymes; and digestion of fats results in absorption of free fatty acids, glycerols, and monoglycerides (see **FIGURE 3.12**).

Digestion and Absorption of Micronutrients and Water

Micronutrients

The two steps of absorption for most minerals are the same as those for the macronutrients. The entry step to the enterocyte is by facilitated diffusion and the exit step is by active transport. Generally, each vitamin and mineral has its own dedicated transport carrier in each of the two membranes and often its own binding protein within the cytoplasm as well as in the blood plasma.

The efficiency of absorption across the absorbing cell to blood (both steps of absorption) for some minerals is low: for calcium it is about 25% to 30%; for iron it is about 5% to 10%; for zinc it is about 10%; and for phosphate ions it ranges from 35% to 75%. (See Figure 3.5 for calcium absorption.) For macronutrients and most water-soluble vitamins, however, the absorption efficiencies range between 50% and 95%.

Most vitamins in foods are attached to proteins or otherwise trapped in food structures. As digestion progresses, these proteins and compartments are broken down and the vitamins are released. The digestive process also chemically modifies several vitamins into forms that are more readily absorbed. Water-soluble vitamins such as vitamin C and most B vitamins are absorbed by the enterocytes by special carriers unique for each vitamin. These vitamins are then transferred to the capillaries at the basolateral membrane. After digestion or separation from food cells, the fat-soluble vitamins, such as vitamin A, are held by, or dissolved into, the micelles containing fats and bile acids. Intestinal epithelial cells absorb the fat-soluble vitamins from the micelles at the entry step by passive diffusion along with the products of fat digestion. In the enterocyte, the fat-soluble vitamins are incorporated into chylomicrons, which are then released to the **lacteals** (vessels) of the lymphatic system.

Water molecules are absorbed mostly with the water-soluble macronutrients and micronutrients. Because water also is secreted into the gut lumen during digestion, typically enough water (fluid) is available for the cotransport entry steps along with other water-soluble nutrients during absorption.

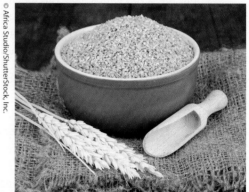

© Africa Studio/ShutterStock, Inc.

The Special Role of Dietary Fiber

Fiber, a unique class of food constituents, is not absorbed, and its beneficial effects occur primarily in the GI tract. **Dietary fiber** is a general term applied to the diverse components of plant foods that constitute the indigestible cell wall and other structures, including many polymeric molecules such as cellulose and pectin. Dietary fibers, because of their capacity to hold water and other molecules, add bulk to digested material and slow the digestion, absorption, and elimination of several dietary components. The laxative effect of high-fiber diets stimulates the rapid movement of material through the lower GI tract. A less rapid rate of flow of gut contents, especially in the large intestine, may exist in those individuals with low-fiber diets, such as the typical Western diet. Additional fiber may speed up this rate.

Many plant-based foods are good sources of dietary fiber. Wheat bran is high in water-insoluble fiber; oat bran is high in water-soluble fiber. Consumption of high-fiber foods or fiber supplements is used to treat certain intestinal disorders, such as diverticular disease, characterized by fingerlike projections of the colonic mucosa into the lumen as well as constipation and hemorrhoids. Fiber provides for bulky, soft stools and gentle laxation that eases defecation. Distinctions between water-soluble and water-insoluble fibers relate mainly to the capacity to dissolve in gut fluid and exert beneficial effects on the mucosal cells of the GI tract.

> Fiber provides for bulky, soft stools and gentle laxation that eases defecation.

Prebiotics and Probiotics

Prebiotics are nondigestible food ingredients that stimulate the growth and/or activity of bacteria in the digestive system in ways claimed to be beneficial to health. Prebiotic fibers are supplied in foods or as supplements, which are generally soluble in the gut fluid. Prebiotics provide a food source for the gut bacteria to attack with their enzymes. In contrast, **probiotics** are live bacteria that may confer a health benefit on those that consume them. Probiotics are most commonly introduced in food, such as some fermented cheeses and yogurts. The combination of prebiotics and probiotics may have potential benefits for the health of the GI tract, and research on these effects is continuing.

The premise behind the use of probiotics is that the human gut is inhabited by 10,000 species of bacteria. Most are helpful strains, but some are potentially harmful.

lacteal (vessel) A lymphatic vessel that collects lymph within the villi of the small intestine.

dietary fiber A broad class of indigestible plant polysaccharides and related molecules. Dietary fiber can be divided into water-soluble and water-insoluble fiber. Found in whole unrefined grains and fruits and vegetables, dietary fiber is part of a healthy diet and plays a role in reducing the risk of several chronic diseases.

prebiotic Nondigestable food ingredients that stimulate the growth and/or activity of bacteria in the digestive system in ways claimed to be beneficial to health.

probiotic Live bacteria (often found in fermented cheese and yogurt) that, when introduced to the stomach, may promote a balance between healthful and harmful bacteria.

PRACTICAL APPLICATIONS 3.2

Fiber: Soluble and Insoluble

Recall that dietary fiber is only found in plant-based foods. The two broad types of fiber are **soluble** and **insoluble**. Insoluble fiber is sometimes called crude fiber because it is relatively easy to measure the cellulose, insoluble hemicellulose (high molecular weight), and lignan in plant cell walls and other structures. It does not exert an osmotic force. The soluble fibers are smaller in molecular size and are water soluble. The water-soluble fibers include gums, pectins, mucilages, some hemicelluloses (low molecular weight), and algal derivatives. Soluble fibers often are used as chemical additives by the food industry to permit gel formation in some foods and to provide consistency in cold or frozen mixtures, such as ice creams. Soluble fibers are considered to benefit GI functions like laxation and defecation when used as prebiotics. Furthermore, both soluble and insoluble forms from unprocessed plant foods support gastrointestinal health when consumed on a daily basis. Some fiber products, such as Metamucil, are used as dietary supplements to aid GI functions. List three major roles of dietary fiber in the GI tract. ■

By occasionally encouraging the growth of the helpful strains, balance can be maintained between the healthful and harmful bacteria. Some diseases and conditions affecting the GI tract may benefit from an infusion of mixtures of bacterial strains as part of the healing process.

The best evidence for an effect of adding bacterial strains to the diet or supplementing with specific strains is limited to a few conditions at this point. When people take oral antibiotics, the balance of bacteria in the gut is dramatically altered for several days. Preliminary studies suggest that treatment with probiotics may speed the rebalancing of bacterial strains in people with antibiotic-induced diarrhea. Probiotics may also aid in the treatment of ulcerative colitis. Future studies will likely provide better understandings of the effects of different combinations of pre- and probiotics.

soluble fiber The components of dietary fiber that are soluble in water and that exert an osmotic force in body fluids, such as in the gut. A significant fraction of soluble fiber can be degraded (fermented) by gut bacteria, thereby improving a number of diverse bodily functions.

insoluble fiber The components of dietary fiber that are not soluble in water and do not, therefore, exert an osmotic force.

SUMMARY

Digestion and absorption are complex processes that proceed in stages over most of the length of the GI tract. Enzymes and other secretions of the stomach and pancreas digest proteins and carbohydrates. These water-soluble components are absorbed in the duodenum into the absorbing epithelial cells and then transferred into the portal vein. Fats and other fat-soluble molecules are digested with the help of bile from the liver and enzymes from the pancreas. Fats are broken down into small micelles that are absorbed through the microvilli and secreted into the lymph as chylomicrons. Several possible ways exist for transferring nutrients across the absorbing cells to blood and lymph. A summary of macronutrient digestion is provided. Bile acids and some cholesterol molecules are reabsorbed through the enterohepatic circulation. Bacteria of the ileum and large intestine assist in the final digestive processes. Macronutrient absorption occurs primarily in the small intestine. Minerals and vitamins are typically absorbed in the upper part of the small intestine. Water and some minerals are, however, absorbed in the large intestine where dietary fiber plays a key role in holding water and providing bulk. The two types of fiber molecules, water-soluble and water-insoluble, have different GI roles. Finally, waste material and water are excreted as feces via the anus.

STUDENT ACTIVITIES

1. How does the GI tract penetrate through the thorax or thoracic cavity? Name the structure.

2. Which organs secrete fluids into the GI tract? Consider the entire GI tract.

3. Which cells are responsible for nutrient absorption, and where in the GI tract are they located?

4. Name the three general types of enzymes involved in macronutrient digestion, i.e., of carbohydrates (starches only), fats (triglycerides), and proteins.

5. Explain how the enterohepatic circulation (EHC) functions. Why is it so important for health?

6. State why fiber components may be important for the health of the GI tract and the individual in general.

7. Which gland is able to extract large percentages of macronutrients right after their absorption into the blood vascular system?

8. Which gland associated with the GI tract secretes pro-enzymes essential for the digestion of the macronutrients within the GI tract? Which enzyme activates these pro-enzymes to enzymes?

9. Micronutrient absorption is similar in some ways to macronutrient absorption. Explain.

10. Fecal waste products rarely contain undigested macronutrients. Explain why.

WEBSITES FOR FURTHER STUDY

National Institutes of Health: Nutrition Tools and Resources
http://www.nhlbi.nih.gov/health/public/heart/obesity/wecan/tools-resources/nutrition.htm
USDA Food and Nutrition Information Center
http://fnic.nal.usda.gov/

National Institutes of Health: Institute of Digestive Diseases, Nutrition Site
www2.niddk.nih.gov/HealthEducation/HealthNutrition.htm

REFERENCES

Buchman AL, McClave SA. Nutrition and gastrointestinal illness. In: Erdman JW Jr, MacDonald IA, Zeisel SH, eds. *Present Knowledge in Nutrition*. 10th ed. Ames, IA: John Wiley & Sons; 2012;1360–1383.

Drewnowski A, Monsivais, P. Taste and food choices. In: Erdman JW Jr, MacDonald IA, Zeisel SH, eds. *Present Knowledge in Nutrition*. 10th ed. Ames, IA: John Wiley & Sons; 2012;1598–1626.

Erdman JW Jr, MacDonald IA, Zeisel SH, eds. *Present Knowledge in Nutrition*. 10th ed. Ames, IA: John Wiley & Sons; 2012.

Roberfroid MB. Prebiotics and probiotics: are they functional foods? *Am J Clin Nutr*. 2000;71(suppl):1682S–1687S.

Taylor SL, Baumert JL. Food allergies and intolerances. In: Erdman JW Jr, MacDonald IA, Zeisel SH, eds. *Present Knowledge in Nutrition*. 10th ed. Ames, IA: John Wiley & Sons; 2012;1881–1902.

ADDITIONAL READING

Netter F. *Netter's Atlas of Human Anatomy*. Philadelphia: Saunders/Elsevier; 2006.

CHAPTER 4

Energy and Metabolism

The primary purpose of hunger, the primal drive to eat, is to obtain energy from foods. Thus, the body's control system regulating food intake is directed by the amount of energy released from our food upon digestion and absorption. This energy largely comes from the breaking of chemical bonds linking carbon (C) and hydrogen (H) atoms in the macronutrients of our food. The **C-H bonds** contain energy that is converted by metabolic pathways in cells into other useful bonds, such as the energy-rich phosphate bonds in **adenosine triphosphate (ATP)** molecules. ATP molecules are responsible for synthesis and transportation of molecules across membranes. The macronutrients in food—carbohydrates, fats, and proteins—provide the energy and basic molecules that the body needs to form important structures and carry out all functions.

Complex metabolic processes in cells degrade the energy-rich molecules, such as fatty acids from fats and glucose from sugars and starches, after the arteries take them to where they are needed in the body. Most of this energy is used to support the basic synthetic functions of the liver, heart, brain, and other organs, whereas smaller amounts are used for the physical activities of life, such as walking, running, dancing, or gardening (see **FIGURE 4.1**). The body can adapt fairly well when too little energy intake is available (starvation or undernutrition), but it does not adjust in a healthy way when food intake provides an endless supply (chronic) of too much energy, which may lead to excessive fat accumulation and eventually to obesity.

Energy is measured in calories (cal) or kilocalories (kcal or Cal) or in **joules (j)** or **kilojoules (kj)**. A calorie is the amount of energy required to warm 1 gram of water 1 degree Celsius. A **kilocalorie** is 1,000 calories. Nutrition labels use kilocalories to denote the energy content in a certain food but express it simply using the term *calorie*. This is the only context in which calorie and kilocalorie are used interchangeably. It may seem puzzling to see the word "energy" in a nutrition text, as you would expect to read more about specific foods than about energy. When nutritionists talk about energy, they generally mean the energy existing in the chemical bonds of the macronutrients in the foods we eat or the molecules of our bodies. An example of a useful energy molecule is glucose, a carbohydrate molecule that circulates in the blood as a ready source of

C-H bond A carbon-hydrogen bond in organic compounds that is converted by metabolic pathways in cells into other useful bonds, such as the energy-rich phosphate bonds in ATP.

adenosine triphosphate (ATP) The major intracellular energy molecule that is used for the synthesis of many molecules and for active transport of molecules across membranes. It contains three high-energy phosphate bonds.

joule (j) (kilojoule [kj]) Metric unit of energy (as opposed to calorie and kilocalorie) used for calculating energy content of foods and energy consumption; 1 calorie = 4.18 joules.

kilocalorie (kcal) A unit of energy (calories) used to estimate both energy consumption from foods and energy expenditure in activities; 1 kilocalorie is the amount of energy required to raise the temperature of 1 kilogram of water 1 degree Celsius (1° C); 1 kilocalorie is often written as 1 Cal.

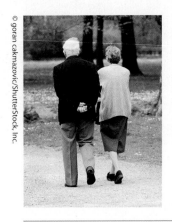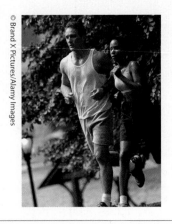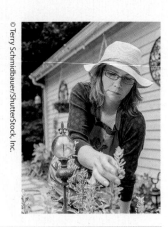

© goran cakmazovic/ShutterStock, Inc.

© Brand X Pictures/Alamy Images

© Terry Schmidbauer/ShutterStock, Inc.

FIGURE 4.1 Energy Uses in Physical Activities. Physical activity, including the activities of daily living as well as exercise, requires energy obtained from macronutrients.

> The carbon-hydrogen (C–H) bonds contain energy that is converted by metabolic pathways in cells into other useful bonds, such as the energy-rich phosphate bonds in adenosine triphosphate (ATP) molecules.

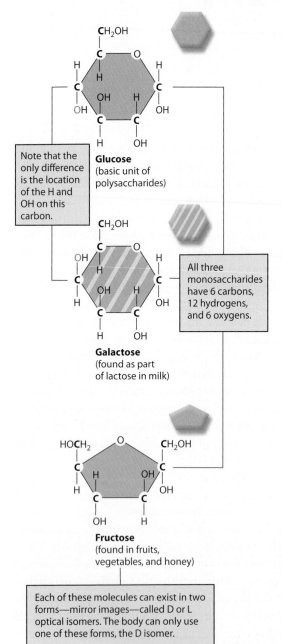

Note that the only difference is the location of the H and OH on this carbon.

Glucose (basic unit of polysaccharides)

All three monosaccharides have 6 carbons, 12 hydrogens, and 6 oxygens.

Galactose (found as part of lactose in milk)

Fructose (found in fruits, vegetables, and honey)

Each of these molecules can exist in two forms—mirror images—called D or L optical isomers. The body can only use one of these forms, the D isomer.

FIGURE 4.2 Glucose. Glucose is a carbohydrate molecule that circulates in the blood as a ready source of energy.

energy (see **FIGURE 4.2**). Another energy source that is stored is a fat or triglyceride molecule; when degraded, its fatty acids enter metabolic pathways to generate energy molecules (ATP) or to synthesize other molecules needed by cells. (The terms *fat* and *triglyceride* are interchangeable.) Another example of an energy molecule is creatine phosphate (CP), which is stored in muscle for use during physical activity. However, scientists often slip and instead of referring to the intake of energy-rich macronutrients in foods, for example, they refer simply to the intake of energy. This shortcut may bring to mind an image of physically getting plugged into an electrical outlet instead of just eating a roll or a doughnut. In this text, this shortcut of simply referring to energy as a nutrient is used to save us from always referring to the actual source of the energy from the chemical bonds of carbohydrates, fats, and proteins.

Keep in mind that a shift in the intake of the two major macronutrients, carbohydrates and fats, occurred in the United States over the latter part of the 20th century (see **Table 4.1**). This chapter considers topics relating to control of food intake, to the body's requirements for energy, and to

TABLE 4.1
Approximate Macronutrient Distributions and Energy Intakes, 1909–2006 (Males Only)

Years	Total Energy (kcal)	Percentage of Total Energy		
		Carbohydrate	Fat	Protein
1909–1919	3,300	58	31	11
1930–1939	3,200	55	34	11
1950–1959	3,100	50	38	12
1970–1979	3,200	49	39	12
1990–1999	3,600	51	37	12
2006	3,900	48	41	11

Data from U.S. Department of Agriculture, Center for Nutrition Policy and Promotion. *Nutrient Content of U.S. Food Supply, Developments Between 2000–2006.* Home Economics Research Report Number 59, July 2011. Available at: www.cnpp.usda.gov /Publications/FoodSupply/Final_FoodSupplyReport_2006.pdf.

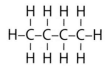

FIGURE 4.3 Hydrocarbon Chain. A portion of carbon and hydrogen bonds making up a hydrocarbon chain.

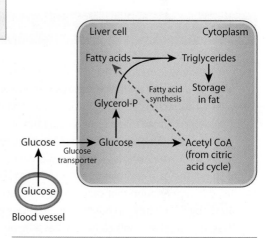

FIGURE 4.4 Long-Term Storage of Energy as Fat. Fat molecules can be formed from energy derived from carbohydrates.

fasting and starvation. The focus of this chapter is on the dietary sources of energy and how macronutrient chemical bonds are converted into cellular energy (i.e., ATP). The energy equivalents of each macronutrient, known as Atwater equivalents, are also defined. How energy is extracted from the food we eat follows next.

Dietary Energy

Why is dietary energy needed? For what purpose is it used? The energy in the C-H organic **hydrocarbon chains** of the macronutrients has the potential to be converted into high-energy **phosphate bonds** of ATP in all living cells within the cytoplasm and mitochondria. A hydrocarbon chain, in part, is shown in **FIGURE 4.3**. The C-H bonds permit points of saturation in fatty acid molecules. Not all of the chemical energy supplied by carbohydrates and fats in food generates energy in cells immediately after ingestion, although the energy extraction process is quite efficient. Some of the energy goes into long-term storage as fat in adipose tissue (see **FIGURE 4.4**); some goes into short-term storage as **glycogen**, a molecule similar to plant starch that keeps blood glucose concentration at normal levels between meals in hepatocytes (i.e., liver cells); and some of the energy is lost as heat. The amino acids from ingested protein are partly used for protein synthesis by cells and partly for the energy contained in their C-H bonds. Alcohol (ethanol) molecules may also generate ATP. Therefore, cellular energy (ATP) can be derived from the three macronutrients in foods; obtained from body stores; or, to a limited extent, generated from small amounts of alcohol.

About 80% to 85% of our energy is derived from major foods, such as starches, sugars, fats, and oils. Plant foods, including cereal grains, potatoes, pastas, and root and stalk foods, primarily provide starches, whereas fats and oils are obtained from butter or

hydrocarbon chain The carbon backbone of organic molecules that typically contains only hydrogen (H) atoms attached to each carbon in the chain; the hydrocarbon portion of fatty acids and amino acids is hydrophobic.

phosphate bond High-energy bond found in ATP and other molecules. ATP has three phosphate bonds.

glycogen A storage form of starch (a polysaccharide) found in almost all human tissues, especially the liver. It serves to keep the blood glucose concentration near normal between meals.

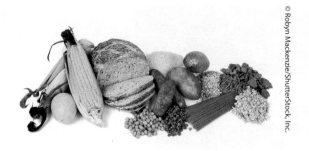

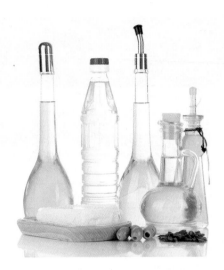

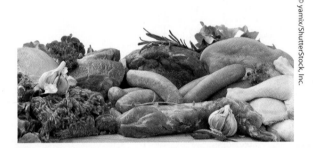

FOCUS 4.1   Sugar-Free Gum

We know from advertising that sugar-free gum "is good for you" and helps prevent cavities. But what exactly makes it sugar free, and is that the same as having artificial sweeteners? To say that a gum is sugar free is technically true, but just barely so. The sugars in sugar-free gum are actually **sugar alcohols**, which are slightly modified forms of sugar. They are approximately as sweet as sugar but are just different enough that they are metabolized only very slowly by the bacteria in our mouths that cause cavities. Thus, the sugar alcohols cause cavities at a much lower rate than regular sugar-based gum. Sugar alcohols also are absorbed very slowly by the GI tract. Whereas their rate of entry into the blood is slower than for glucose, they actually provide similar amounts of calories, Ultimately, they do not contribute to weight loss. ●

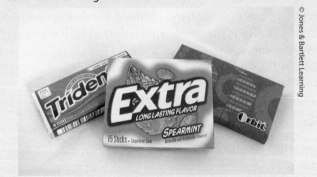

Sugar-Free Gum.

margarine spreads, peanuts, palm, corn, soy, and fish. Many processed foods available in supermarkets have reduced amounts of carbohydrates or fats and, therefore, less energy (e.g., those labeled "light" or "lite"). Even chewing gum is now sold with no sugar—not because of its lower calorie content but because the reduced sugar content decreases the likelihood of developing dental caries or cavities (cariogenicity) from chewing it (see **FOCUS BOX 4.1**).

sugar alcohol A type of alcohol derived from sugar. Sugar alcohols are widely used in the food industry as thickeners and sweeteners. They are absorbed more slowly that sugar and do not contribute to the formation of dental caries.

Control of Energy Intake

The problem for many consumers is the intake of too much energy from foods and beverages. How do people know when to eat, how much to eat, and when to stop?

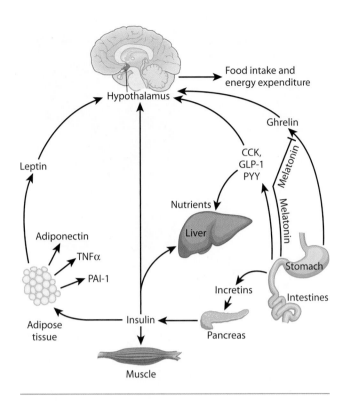

FIGURE 4.5 Control of Food Intake. Conscious control of food intake resides in the cerebral cortex, which influences the hypothalamus.

The conscious **control of food intake** resides in the **food intake center** of the cerebral cortex, the highest part of the brain, which, in turn, influences the older, more primitive parts of the brain, including the hypothalamus (see **FIGURE 4.5**). The survival functions that are partially regulated by the **hypothalamus**, including eating, drinking, and sexual behavior, are largely controlled at an unconscious level. Hormones from gut mucosa endocrine cells and fat cells throughout the body act on the hypothalamus to control food intake. Studies of serum glucose and insulin changes suggest that the hypothalamus may be able to monitor blood glucose concentration and, hence, the overall energy balance of the body. Other neuronal and hormonal pathways also have been found to be involved in the regulation of food intake. In fact, the overall mechanism governing food intake is quite complex and not completely understood.

The control of food intake is a complex physiologic process involving hormones secreted by the stomach and gut that then act on the brain (see **FIGURE 4.6**). Recently discovered hormones made by fat cells, such as leptin, adiponectin, and others, also serve as signals to the brain to either reduce or increase food intake. When adipose cells are full they secrete leptin, which binds to receptors in the brain, causing a reduction in appetite. When adipose cells are not full, they send other hormones to the brain to increase food intake. The complex interplay of these factors and other hormones from the GI tract help regulate the ingestion of food.

Although our knowledge of the biochemical control of food intake remains incomplete, psychological influences or cues acting on the higher brain centers are well recognized. Cues such as usual meal times, food odors, advertising messages, social activities, emotions, and other factors have influential roles in governing the consumption of food (see **FIGURE 4.7**). In affluent societies, hunger itself, as elicited by the physiologic signals that make us consciously aware of a need to eat, is a less important signal for food intake than the psychological cues or signals. The high prevalence of obesity (see **FIGURE 4.8**)

> The control of food intake is a complex physiologic process involving hormones secreted by the stomach and gut that then act on the brain.

control of food intake The regulation of the intake of food by the integrated actions of the feeding center and the satiety center in the hypothalamus.

food intake center An area of the brain in the lateral nucleus of the hypothalamus that controls food intake behavior. This feeding center is connected with the satiety center and other neuronal pathways in the lower brain.

hypothalamus The part of the brain that regulates food intake, satiety, water consumption, thirst, and other basic functions of life. It is where the feeding center and satiety center are located.

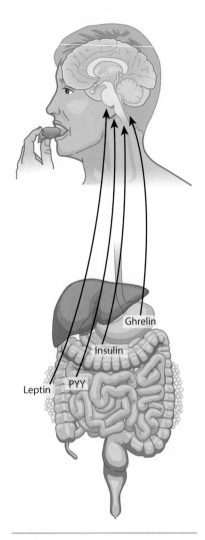

FIGURE 4.6 Hormonal Control of Food Intake. Hormones secreted by the stomach and brain are partly responsible for the control of food intake.

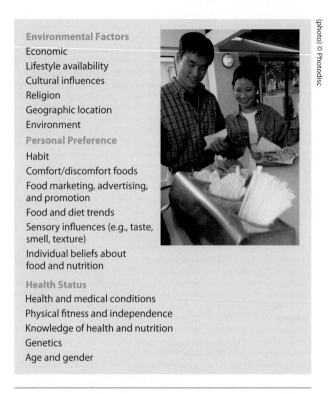

Environmental Factors
Economic
Lifestyle availability
Cultural influences
Religion
Geographic location
Environment

Personal Preference

Habit
Comfort/discomfort foods
Food marketing, advertising, and promotion
Food and diet trends
Sensory influences (e.g., taste, smell, texture)
Individual beliefs about food and nutrition

Health Status

Health and medical conditions
Physical fitness and independence
Knowledge of health and nutrition
Genetics
Age and gender

FIGURE 4.7 Cues that Control Food Intake. Cues such as usual meal times, food odors, advertising messages, social activities, emotions, and other factors have influential roles in governing the consumption of food.

citric acid cycle (Krebs cycle) The cyclic metabolic pathway in the mitochondria that begins with the combining of oxaloacetate and acetyl CoA and ends with the regeneration of oxaloacetate after the oxidation of two carbon units to carbon dioxide and water, along with the generation of ATP and heat. The citric cycle also generates water (metabolic) and carbon dioxide through the complete oxidation of glucose, fatty acids, amino acids, and alcohol.

partly attests to the power of these psychological determinants. Eating more slowly helps reduce the critical role of psychological cues.

Atwater Energy Equivalents

In addition to carbohydrates and fats, proteins and alcohol also provide energy. The macronutrients and alcohol yield different amounts of energy to the body after digestion, absorption, and metabolism according to the Atwater energy equivalent of the macronutrient (see **Table 4.2**). These conversion factors are useful in calculating the energy intake from a record of foods eaten by an individual. Note that fats are much more calorically dense (9 kilocalories per gram) than carbohydrates (both simple and complex) and proteins (both have 4 kilocalories per gram). The value of alcohol (7 kilocalories per gram) falls between that of fats and carbohydrates. A major nutrient component that is not included as a source of energy is dietary fiber, which certainly contains chemical energy in its carbohydrate-like structures, but the human body cannot absorb or break down fiber to yield energy.

The cellular breakdown of macronutrients yields carbon dioxide, water, urea (from the nitrogen in amino acids), energy molecules (ATP), and a significant amount of heat as a by-product of the metabolic pathways. Carbohydrates, fats, proteins, and alcohol are metabolized by specific chemical pathways in cells for the generation of ATP. The final biochemical pathway for all macronutrients and alcohol is the mitochondrial **citric acid cycle**, also known as the Krebs cycle for its discoverer. Because of the inefficiency of chemical metabolic processes, about half of the energy from the C-H chemical bonds is not converted to ATP. This so-called "waste" component is given off as heat by a process

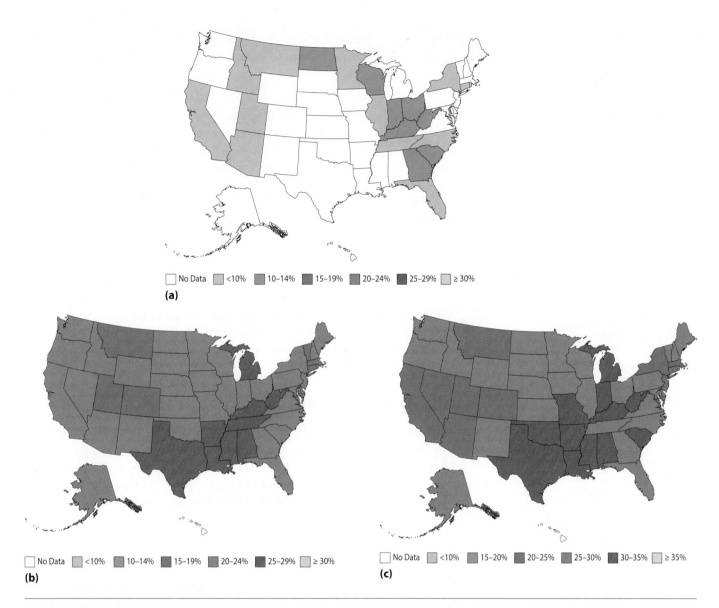

FIGURE 4.8 Prevalence of Obesity. The increasing incidence of obesity in U.S. adults is evident in these charts from the years 2000 (a), 2005 (b), and 2011 (c).

Reproduced from Centers for Disease Control and Prevention. Overweight and Obesity: Adult Obesity Facts—Obesity Prevalence in 2011 Varies Across States and Regions. Available at: www.cdc.gov/obesity/data/trends.html.

TABLE 4.2
Atwater Equivalents: Energy Derived from Macronutrients and Alcohol

Macronutrient or Alcohol	Net Energy Yield (kcal/g)
Carbohydrate	4
Fat	9
Protein	4
Alcohol	7

" The macronutrients and alcohol yield different amounts of energy to the body after digestion, absorption, and metabolism according to the Atwater energy equivalent of the macronutrient. "

PRACTICAL APPLICATIONS 4.1

Estimating Calories from Daily Macronutrient Intake

Assuming that you consumed 400 grams of carbohydrates, 90 grams of fat, and 100 grams of protein in a 24-hour period, approximately how many kilocalories of energy would be available for your body functions? Use the Atwater equivalents. Would this total caloric intake be sufficient for a healthy active young man? A young woman? (See the following section, "Recommended Dietary Allowances for Energy.")

Calculate the percentage of each macronutrient consumed over the 24-hour period. Do the percentages satisfy the general recommendations (i.e., approximately 50%, 35%, and 15% of carbohydrates, fats, and proteins, respectively)? ■

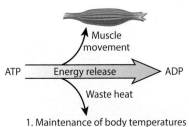

1. Maintenance of body temperatures
2. Loss of heat through sweating
3. Loss of heat through respiration

FIGURE 4.9 Waste Heat. The body's chemical metabolic processes are relatively inefficient. The so-called "waste" component is given off as heat through thermogenesis.

thermogenesis Generation of heat by the body's metabolic activities.

resting energy expenditure (REE) The amount of energy expended in cellular metabolic activities while the body is at rest.

basal metabolic rate (BMR) The minimal expenditure of energy of the body under basal conditions, basically when awake and quietly resting. Approximately equivalent to resting energy expenditure (REE).

energy allowance (RDA) The recommended energy intake for males and females at moderate levels of activity that will sustain good health. Females 19 years and older have an energy RDA of 2,400 kilocalories; the value for males 19 years and older is 3,100 kilocalories.

called **thermogenesis**, which contributes to maintenance of body temperature (see **FIGURE 4.9**). Most of this heat is used in maintaining core body temperature; the remainder of the heat is lost through the skin or lungs.

Recommended Dietary Allowances for Energy

Humans need to consume energy on a daily basis to support the activities of life. RDAs for energy consumption are based on age, gender, and a moderate level of physical activity beyond **resting energy expenditure (REE)** or its equivalent **basal metabolic rate (BMR)**, which is the amount of calories expended through basic bodily functions at rest (see **Table 4.3**). The adult **energy allowances (RDAs)** for males and females at moderate levels of activity are as follows:

- Females 19 years and older: 2,400 kcal per day.
- Males 19 years and older: 3,100 kcal per day.

Athletes typically need greater amounts of energy because they have high levels of physical activity. Typically, daily energy recommendations are increased by 300 kilocalories

TABLE 4.3

Resting Energy Expenditure and Recommended Dietary Allowances of Adults in Kilocalories Depending on Daily Activity Level

	Resting Energy Expenditure (REE)	Inactive Day (REE × 1.375)	Moderately Active Day* (REE × 1.77)	Very Active Day (REE × 2.25)
Female	1,350	1,856	2,400	3,038
Male	1,750	2,406	3,100	3,938

* Energy RDAs are based on a moderately active day (in approximate kcals).
Data from Institute of Medicine. *Dietary Reference Intakes.* Washington, DC: National Academies Press.

during pregnancy and 500 kilocalories during lactation. In general, the four main variables related to individual energy requirements are: (1) physical activity, (2) body size and composition, (3) age, and (4) climate and other environmental factors. (Note that body composition includes the three major tissue components—lean mass, fat mass, and bone mass—which are discussed later in this chapter.) Hormones, especially thyroid hormones, can also influence basal energy needs.

The energy RDAs for adult females and males are greater than those for children and adolescents. Energy recommendations for children and adolescents are estimated to meet the body's needs during growth and development and continue to increase up to age 19. Most adults are not sufficiently active to need the amounts of energy recommended. Even if they have decreased energy intake, many adults experience increases in body weight due to lack of physical activity. Keep in mind that zero energy balance (intake vs. expenditure) does not lead to weight gain!

Body Composition: Major Body Compartments

According to one popular model, **body composition** consists of three major compartments: **lean body mass** (or LBM), **fat mass**, and **bone mass (bone mineral content)**. The sum of the three compartments is total body weight or mass. (Water mass is included primarily in the lean compartment.) Lean mass is typically referred to as lean body mass (LBM), which largely consists of skeletal muscle mass, and is almost 67% of total body weight in healthy young adults. During growth, LBM reaches its maximum by about age 20. After age 20, LBM typically declines because of reduced activity levels. In older adults, muscle tissue (lean mass) declines even more through disuse. In addition to lean body mass, fat mass consists of all fat tissue and bone mass is the mineral content of one's bones.

FIGURE 4.10 shows changes in the three major body compartments resulting from increased energy intake. **FIGURE 4.11** shows general changes in body appearance with increased energy consumption over a long period of time.

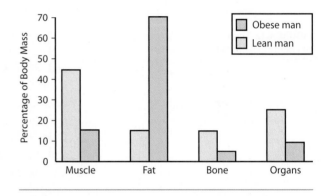

FIGURE 4.10 Body Composition of a Lean Man and a Morbidly Obese Man. Increased energy intake over time results in changes to the three major body compartments.

body composition Division of the body into two or more compartments, depending on the model used, based on the different chemical properties of those compartments. The two-compartment model consists of the fat tissue (compartment 1) and lean body mass (compartment 2). The three-compartment model consists of the fat compartment, lean body mass, and bone mass.

lean body mass (LBM) The compartment of the body that includes skeletal muscle and other tissues but excludes fat tissue and generally bone.

fat mass The body compartment consisting of all fat tissue, including subcutaneous fat, abdominal fat, and other stores of fat tissue.

bone mass (bone mineral content) The mineral phase of the entire skeleton, exclusive of the organic component of the skeleton; it consists primarily of hydroxyapatite.

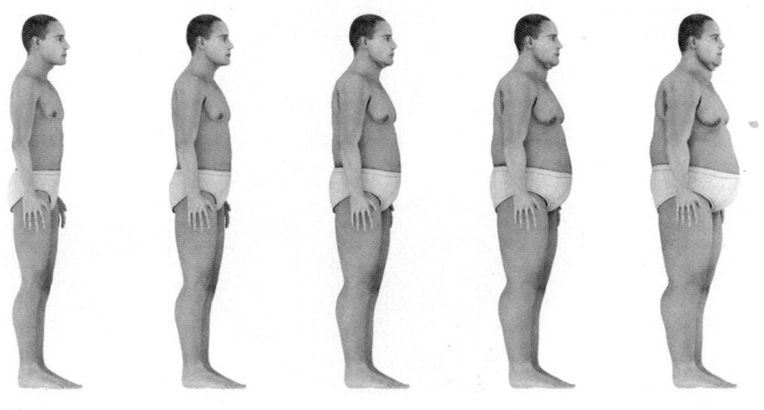

© Raycat/iStockphoto

FIGURE 4.11 Body Fat Accumulation with Excessive Energy Intake. Changes in body appearance occur with increased energy consumption relative to energy expenditure over a lengthy period of time.

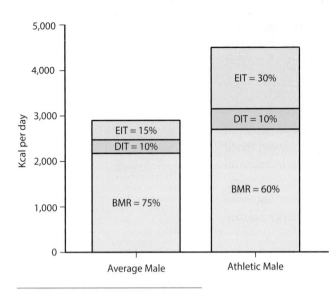

FIGURE 4.12 Three Major Components of Energy Expenditure. The contributions of BMR, DIT, and EIT to total energy expenditure in a male of average physical activity versus an athletic male.

Modified from Anderson, J.J.B. *Nutrition and Health: An Introduction.* Carolina Academic Press, Durham, NC, 2005.

Energy Uses, Metabolic Rate, and Thermogenesis

The body is a chemical factory, with the cells serving as the metabolic machines. Many reactions make or utilize energy to support the functions of life, which are collectively known as metabolism. The catabolic side of metabolism refers to the degradation of molecules, including macronutrients, especially carbohydrates and fats, which are the major sources for generating cellular energy (ATP). The anabolic side refers to the synthetic reactions of cells in which new molecules are generated with the use of cellular energy. For example, muscle cells continually synthesize proteins for repairing contractile fibers under the control of DNA.

The body expends its energy in three major ways:

1. The basal metabolic rate (BMR) or REE is the energy needed to keep our bodies active, including maintaining basic cellular functions and operation of the brain and other organs. This does not include energy expended in any physical activity or in eating, digesting, and absorbing nutrients from food. BMR is closely associated with the amount of lean body mass (LBM). BMR is measured while fasting and at rest.
2. **Diet-induced thermogenesis (DIT)** is the energy expended by the digestive and absorptive processes.
3. The energy expended in activities, sometimes called **exercise-induced thermogenesis (EIT)**, is the energy expenditure related to muscular contraction during activities over and beyond BMR (see **FIGURE 4.12**).

Basal Metabolic Rate

Basal metabolism is the amount of energy needed to maintain vital functions of the body. These consist of involuntary processes going on at all times in our bodies such as respiration, the pumping of the heart and circulation, and many other cellular metabolic functions (see **FIGURE 4.13**). The BMR is directly related to the amount of

diet-induced thermogenesis (DIT) Energy expended and waste heat generated as a result of processes required for macronutrient digestion and absorption. DIT for proteins represents approximately 20% of the energy contained in the protein in the meal; DIT is lower for carbohydrates and lowest for fats (triglycerides). The overall DIT for a mixed meal is approximately 10% of the calories the meal contains.

exercise-induced thermogenesis (EIT) Energy expended as heat by the body because of muscular activities; this energy is over and above the energy expended for basal metabolism (BMR).

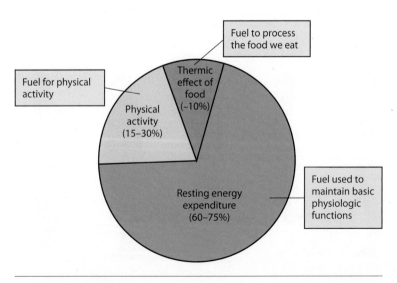

FIGURE 4.13 Basal Metabolism. Most of our daily energy intake is used to maintain basic physiologic functions.

TABLE 4.4
Harris-Benedict Equations to Estimate Resting Energy Expenditure (REE)*

Sex	Equation
Female	REE = 655 + (9.6 × Weight in kilograms) + (1.9 × Height in centimeters) − (4.7 × Age in years)
Male	REE = 66 + (13.8 × Weight in kilograms) + (5 × Height in centimeters) − (6.8 × Age in years)

* REE is measured in kilocalories per day.
Data from Harris JA, Benedict FG. *A Biometric Study of Basal Metabolism in Man* (publication no. 279). Washington, DC: Carnegie Institute of Washington; 1919.

metabolically active tissue in the body, which is referred to as LBM. LBM consists of muscle (about 50% to 60% of body weight) and other tissues exclusive of fat tissue. BMR is usually determined by indirect calorimetry (measurement of calories) while the individual is lying down, at least 12 hours after the previous meal. Another way to estimate the amount of energy needed by the body at rest is to calculate REE using a gender-specific equation, which is an equivalent estimate to BMR that is used more in clinical settings. The Harris-Benedict equations given in **Table 4.4** are used to estimate the REE of men and women. For example, a 21-year-old female who stands 160 centimeters (63 inches) tall and weighs 60 kilograms (132 pounds) would have an REE of 1,446 kilocalories. The equations assume a constant LBM for each unit of height, but this assumption may not be correct for the elderly.

BMR decreases throughout adult life, and also from early infancy through to puberty, during which time the number and size of fat cells become more significant. Beyond about age 50, the rate of decrease of BMR accelerates as muscle and other essential tissues continue to decrease in size and lost cells may not be renewed by cell division. Women, in general, have lower BMRs because of their lower LBM.

Thyroid hormones are considered to "set" a specific level of metabolic activity of cells and, hence, the BMR in individuals. Thyroid hormones thus control the relative amount of heat generated as well as the body temperature. Hyperthyroid individuals (i.e., those with too much thyroid hormone) tend to be thin, always seem to feel warm, and have little difficulty maintaining body weight. In contrast, hypothyroid subjects (i.e., those with too little thyroid hormone) tend to be lethargic, overweight, and always seem to feel cold (see **FIGURE 4.14**).

Thermogenesis, or the generation of heat while at rest, is one of the components of basal metabolism. The efficiency of the energy-generating steps of metabolism must differ to a small degree from individual to individual, and these differences are determined genetically. For example, the "wasters," who are less

> " Basal metabolic rate (BMR) or REE is directly related to the amount of metabolically active tissue in the body, which is referred to as lean body mass (LBM). "

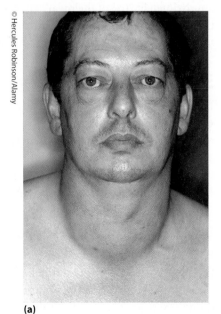
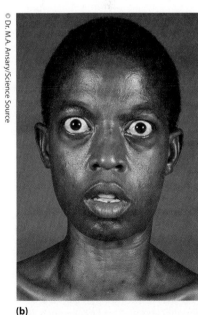

(a)   (b)

FIGURE 4.14 Hypothyroidism and Hyperthyroidism. Hypothyroidism (a) develops when the body does not produce enough thyroid hormone. Individuals with hyperthyroidism (b) produce too much thyroid hormone. Both conditions affect BMR.

TABLE 4.5
Factors Affecting Basal Metabolic Rate

Status	Percent Change in BMR
Fasting 1 day	5% decrease
Starvation	10–30% decrease
Fracture	20–40% increase
Infection	10–30% increase

efficient in producing ATP from carbohydrates or fats, produce more body heat. Their bodies apparently use more food energy for basal metabolic reactions. Others who are more efficient, the "storers," convert carbohydrates and fats to ATP molecules at or near a maximum efficiency of 30% to 40%, and thus meet their basal needs more easily. Storers have excess energy available from food macronutrients that can be shunted into pathways of fat synthesis or into fat storage depots. Earlier in human history, being a storer was advantageous to weather the ups and downs of food availability. An advantage of being a waster is that LBM is more easily maintained.

Although individuals vary considerably in metabolic efficiency during physical activity, strenuous activity on a regular basis contributes to an even more efficient utilization of energy, increased thermogenesis, and a body composition consisting of a lower (and healthier) percentage of fat. Also, the heat loss following exercise, which continues for some time afterward (1 to 2 hours) in healthy individuals, contributes to energy wasting.

When a foreign organism enters the body and initiates its defense mechanisms, the body is experiencing an **infection**. Infections, especially bacterial, cause body temperature to elevate and BMR to increase about 5% for each one-degree (°F) increase. The energy expended as heat can be significant in severely ill individuals. Significant increases in BMR also occur in patients with skeletal fractures or major burns, whereas starvation decreases BMR (see **Table 4.5**).

Diet-Induced Thermogenesis

Another important aspect of energy expenditure is diet-induced thermogenesis (DIT) of food nutrients. DIT is the increase in metabolism after food ingestion and utilization, and it is most significant for proteins. The energy required for DIT serves as a "food tax." It is the amount of energy required to process the macronutrients in food. Thus, to complete the digestion, absorption, and other metabolic steps necessary to get nutrients into the body, a fairly large amount of energy is required. For protein, DIT is approximately 20% of the meal's energy content; for fats and carbohydrates, DIT is less than 5% of the meal's energy. For meals of mixed macronutrients, this so-called food tax is about 10%. DIT lasts for 3 to 4 hours after a meal.

Exercise-Induced Thermogenesis

> Energy expenditure in activities, or exercise-induced thermogenesis (EIT), is the most variable of the components of daily energy expenditure.

Energy expenditure in activities, or exercise-induced thermogenesis (EIT), is the most variable of the components of daily energy expenditure. For practically all adults, BMR represents 60% to 75% of total energy expenditure for the day; DIT is estimated as approximately 10%; and expenditure through physical activity (EIT) is the remainder, roughly 15% to 30% per day. However, some athletes may exceed 50% of their total energy expenditure in training and sports activities in a typical day.

Changes in BMR Across the Life Cycle

infection The entry of a foreign organism into the body that initiates the body's defense mechanisms, including a local inflammatory response and the immune response involving white cells and lymphocytes and other cells, such as macrophages.

BMR declines during late adolescence and falls even more in adulthood. The reason for the changes in BMR relate to the loss of LBM, which typically decreases as people age. Older adults from 50 to 60 years and beyond lose muscle mass if they are sedentary and do not exercise. Keep in mind that BMR is directly related to the LBM compartment of the body (i.e., mostly muscle); therefore, as LBM declines, so does BMR. In a sense, BMR is a marker of being alive and active!

PRACTICAL APPLICATIONS 4.2

Energy Expenditure in Physical Activity

You may have been surprised to learn just how much of our energy is spent on basal metabolic functions and how little is spent on the rest of life, such as talking, walking, playing, or studying. It may also be discouraging to see how little energy our body burns during exercise. Find the wrapper from your favorite snack food, whether a candy or energy bar, chips, or cookie. Note the number of calories in a serving. Now consider how much energy is used in the exercises shown in the following table:

Using your own body weight in pounds and your favorite activity from this list, how many minutes of activity does it take to burn the calories in your favorite snack? Identify your snack. Calculate the kilocalories in a serving of your snack by using a food composition table or the snack's Nutrition Facts panel. ■

Activity	Kilocalories per Pound Body Weight per Minute
Soccer	0.097
Jogging	0.074
Swimming	0.032
Walking	0.035
Reading	0.011

FOCUS 4.2   Lean Body Mass and Basal Metabolic Rate

Muscle mass, especially skeletal muscle, represents the vast amount of LBM. Furthermore, BMR is directly related to LBM. Therefore, if LBM declines in later life from inactivity and less use of the muscles, then BMR also will decline. A reasonable BMR late in life, i.e., LBM, is associated with reduced risk of mortality. For this reason, continuing daily activities that require physical work in the adult and elder years helps maintain muscle tissue and BMR. This close relationship between LBM and BMR also holds for early life development of the musculoskeletal system: the more muscle mass accrued, the greater is the BMR. ●

Energy Balance, Starvation, and Overeating

Energy balance is the balance between energy intake and energy expenditure over a period of weeks or a month or two. An individual is said to be in energy balance if no difference exists between intake and expenditure of energy. Daily fluctuations in energy balance, as reflected by slight changes in weight (plus or minus 2 pounds, depending on water retention) are insignificant. Energy balance is partly under genetic control, but everyday patterns of activity and eating can override this control. Positive energy balance occurs when energy intake exceeds expenditure, whereas negative energy balance is the opposite condition (see **FIGURE 4.15**).

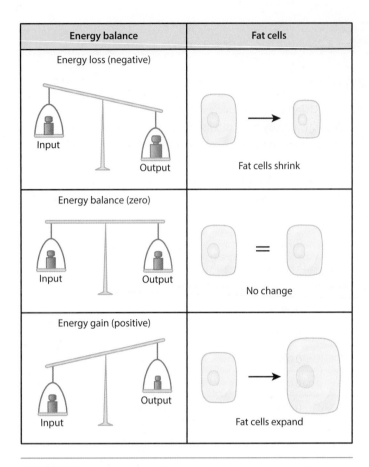

Energy balance	Fat cells
Energy loss (negative) Input / Output	Fat cells shrink
Energy balance (zero) Input / Output	No change
Energy gain (positive) Output / Input	Fat cells expand

FIGURE 4.15 Energy Balance. When energy intake exceeds expenditure, the result is a positive energy balance and the expansion of fat cells. When energy intake is less than expenditure, the result is negative energy balance and the shrinking of fat cells.

Reproduced from Anderson JJB. *Nutrition and Health: An Introduction.* Durham, NC: Carolina Academic Press; 2005.

Chronic undernutrition is usually an unintended consequence of limited food availability that leads to starvation or **marasmus**. With marasmus, the body literally consumes itself, with all body compartments losing mass. The wasted bodies of people with anorexia nervosa and late-stage cancer are both examples of marasmus, despite their different causes. **FIGURE 4.16A** shows a marasmic (starved) child with symptoms of wasting.

If dietary protein is very inadequate (well below the age- and gender-specific DRI) and energy intake is relatively more adequate over a long period, then the primary protein deficiency disease **kwashiorkor** may result. With kwashiorkor, a person develops edema and may look round and plump but in fact is seriously malnourished (see **FIGURE 4.16B**). The focus on weight loss in this chapter is on voluntary activities of individuals toward the goal of losing weight through negative weight balance.

Tissue losses, particularly of muscle and adipose tissues, occur when inadequate amounts of calories are consumed to maintain normal cellular energy needs. The body's adaptation to a hypocaloric diet is to degrade energy stores and functional components, namely structural proteins, to provide calories to meet the body's energy needs, leaving almost only "skin and bones." The liver plays a major role in this hormonal response to fasting through its generation of new glucose molecules via gluconeogenesis. This hormonal response is the opposite of the insulin response and leads to an increase of the blood glucose concentration. A major insulin counter-regulatory hormone is glucagon, which is also synthesized in the pancreas but by different

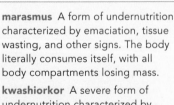

marasmus A form of undernutrition characterized by emaciation, tissue wasting, and other signs. The body literally consumes itself, with all body compartments losing mass.

kwashiorkor A severe form of undernutrition characterized by extremely low protein intake as well as inadequate energy intake. Changes to the skin and hair and edema are characteristic of this protein–energy deficiency disease.

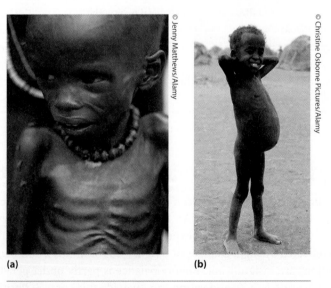

(a)   (b)

FIGURE 4.16 Characteristics of Marasmus and Kwashiorkor. Note the emaciated appearance of the child with marasmus (a) versus the bloating of the belly, arms, and face of the child with kwashiorkor (b).

cells than those that produce insulin. All tissue cells can use the newly generated glucose that is released from the liver to the blood. The brain, other neurons, and red blood cells, however, have an absolute requirement for glucose at all times; all other tissues can use other molecules for energy in addition to glucose.

Both under- and overconsumption of dietary energy result in changes in body composition. With excess energy intake, body fat mass increases substantially. LBM (i.e., skeletal muscle and related tissues) may increase as well to a much lesser extent to support the gain in fat mass. With underconsumption of energy, fat mass decreases substantially. LBM declines as well, but more slowly and to a lesser extent than fat loss. If extreme underconsumption of food continues, amino acids from muscle tissue will be used for gluconeogenesis (see **FIGURE 4.17**), and LBM will continue to decline until an individual becomes "skin and bones." Anorexia and starvation characterize the severest forms of reduction of energy intake, whereas overconsumption of energy is exemplified by either overweight or obesity—two ends of a continuum.

> **"** Tissue losses, particularly of muscle and adipose tissues, occur when inadequate amounts of calories are consumed to maintain normal cellular energy needs. **"**

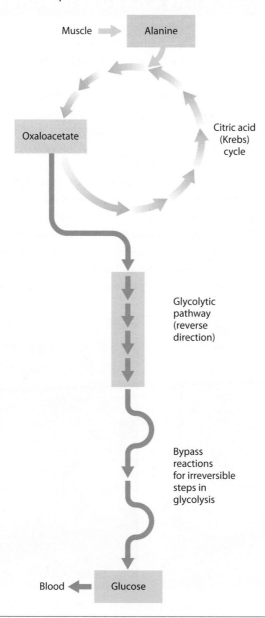

FIGURE 4.17 Gluconeogenesis. In the process of gluconeogenesis, new glucose molecules are formed from noncarbohydrate sources in the liver to help keep blood glucose concentrations within the normal range during fasting, long-term undernutrition, or semistarvation.

FOCUS 4.3 Energy Sources Utilized During Starvation

After the liver's glycogen stores have been depleted, the body starts to cannibalize its own tissues, namely lean tissues such as muscle, to generate new glucose molecules in the liver. This process of generating new glucose molecules from amino acids is known as gluconeogenesis. The brain and the red blood cells cannot function without glucose. During periods of starvation, the amino acids from the muscle tissues are used to generate glucose. The lean body mass can provide enough amino acid-derived glucose for survival of a totally starved individual for a period up to about 60 days, as long as water is consumed. A person who is partially fasting or semistarved can survive much longer, depending on the amount of LBM available for hepatic conversion to glucose. ●

FOCUS 4.4 Body Changes in Semistarvation

During World War II, several young healthy males volunteered for a study at the University of Minnesota to examine changes in body function and body composition during a 6-month period of **semistarvation**. The participants received about 67% of their normal daily energy requirements. As expected, they lost weight and stamina. In addition, their performance on the Harvard two-step test (up and down and switching legs on a stool) and other tests of strength declined after several months (see **FIGURE A**). Biochemical tests also showed decline in the functions of body tissues and organs.

After 6 months, the young men began a gradual, slow refeeding program to bring them back to health, similar to what prisoners of war would face when liberated after the war. The volunteers did not return to their prestudy weight until approximately 12 months later, and their biochemical measures took even longer to return to normal ranges. This study clearly demonstrated how semistarvation can ravage the body by using fat stores and degrading tissues, especially muscle, for energy and how slow the recovery process is for returning to normal health. ●

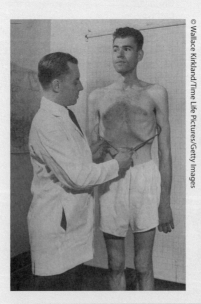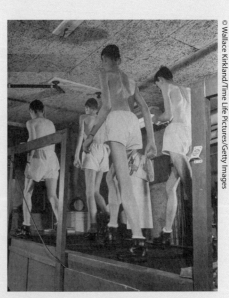

FIGURE A Starvation and Changes in Body Composition. The University of Minnesota study on semistarvation found that reduced caloric intake over a long period of time resulted in changes in body function and body composition.

semistarvation The deliberate consumption of less than the recommended number of calories for a period of time. A diet that has roughly 30% fewer calories than the normal diet.

A Day in the Life of Energy Molecules: Glucose and Fatty Acids

Bob, a 20-year-old college student, wakes up at 7:00 a.m. and is hungry. He has a bowl of cereal with milk for breakfast. The starches in the cereal are absorbed mainly as glucose. The milk sugar lactose is broken down into glucose, which is absorbed directly, and galactose, which after absorption is converted in the liver to glucose, causing blood glucose levels to rise. About half of these sugars are taken up and used by the liver and the other half are taken up by all other cells of the body under the influence of insulin. Much of the glucose remaining in the liver is converted to glycogen for temporary storage. Similar events are taking place in Bob's muscles. After glycogen stores are filled and cellular ATP levels become sufficient, excessive glucose in the liver is shunted into fatty acid synthesis for triglyceride storage in the liver or for triglyceride transport to other tissues of the body, mainly fat cells.

The triglycerides in the milk are digested and their fatty acids are absorbed and transported through the blood for use by liver and other cells or for storage. Some triglycerides are transferred to adipose tissue for long-term storage, whereas the remainder is taken up by the liver for storage, by fat cells for storage, and by muscles for endurance physical activities. (Note how important the liver is in the distribution of glucose and triglycerides for use in other parts of the body.)

Later in the morning, after Bob has been on his feet in the laboratory for several hours, liver glycogen is now being degraded as blood glucose levels drop because of uptake and use of glucose in his muscles and other tissues. After a late morning class, Bob has two doughnuts with a cup of coffee. The excess sugar is again converted to glycogen and triglycerides in the liver. Some of the triglycerides are packaged into VLDL complexes together with cholesterol from the cream in Bob's coffee that then circulate to adipose tissue where much of the fat is deposited. At lunch the process is repeated but, because Bob has a double cheeseburger, the amount of fat stored is much higher. Much of this dietary fat is dropped off directly at his adipose tissue by the chylomicrons during the meal and early postprandial period, causing Bob's waist to grow over time by a small but measurable amount.

Bob plays a game of basketball when he gets home later in the day after his classes. The readily available glucose in his blood is used quickly as a result of his intense activity, and glycogen in his muscles and liver is rapidly broken down for use as fuel. Stored fat in his muscles is also degraded for use during his energetic play. After about 30 minutes, Bob starts panting. Because oxygen is now limited, glucose is being metabolized in the relatively inefficient anaerobic glycolytic pathway. With limited oxygen getting to his muscles, glucose is no longer being utilized efficiently, and glucose sparing by the "burning" of triglycerides is no longer possible. Bob stops playing, and he gradually catches his breath. His next meal will help replenish his glycogen and fat stores. **FIGURE 4.18** summarizes the energy systems involved in using and replenishing the body's energy stores.

At home Bob has a simple dinner, watches some television, studies a few hours and heads to bed. Overnight while he sleeps, Bob's body slowly depletes its store of glycogen in the liver. His body begins to metabolize fats, using some of the triglycerides that were placed in the liver and fat stores during the day. Fatty acids are released to the blood and are picked up by all cells of functional organs and by the liver. As his blood glucose concentration falls slowly overnight, the liver starts generating glucose via gluconeogenesis from amino acids. Bob's liver also converts some fatty acids to ketones, which are released to the blood circulation. By the time Bob wakes up, he has "morning breath" from acetone, one of the ketones, and he is ready for breakfast.

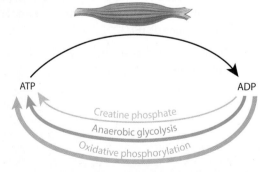

FIGURE 4.18 Metabolic Systems Required to Use and Replenish Energy Stores. A number of different metabolic systems are required to use and replenish the energy the body needs.

SUMMARY

The human body is adept at utilizing the available sources of dietary fuels—the three macronutrients—that are consumed on a daily basis. The majority of the body's dietary energy is derived from carbohydrates and fats. Fats provide a little over two times as much energy per gram as carbohydrates. Food intake is controlled through a complex web of hormonal messages that turn hunger off and on. The energy RDA for adult females is 2,400 kilocalories per day, and for adult males it is 3,100 kilocalories per day. Most of the energy expended by the body is to meet the basic maintenance functions of the basal metabolism, with lesser amounts supporting diet-induced thermogenesis and physical activity. Energy metabolism also produces heat and maintains body temperature.

A complex control mechanism makes available to the body a steady source of energy both in times of excess and during periods of starvation. After a meal, food-derived energy that is not used immediately is stored as glycogen and fat. During periods of fasting or insufficient intake of calories, these stores are metabolically degraded by diverse cells for body functions, including physical activities. If fasting becomes more extensive or starvation exists, then tissue protein, especially skeletal muscle, is degraded to amino acids for conversion in the liver to glucose by the process known as gluconeogenesis. In our modern, more affluent era, both excessive energy intake and minimal energy expenditure in activities have led to an imbalance in energy metabolism resulting in the increasing incidence of overweight and obesity in many populations.

STUDENT ACTIVITIES

1. State in general terms what energy is. Is energy a nutrient? Explain.

2. Which two macronutrients are the major sources of energy in our diets.

3. Where is the body's control center for food and energy intake located? Does it work well?

4. What is the importance of the C-H bond in macronutrients?

5. What are the Atwater energy equivalents for carbohydrates, fats, proteins, and alcohol? Use the Atwater equivalents to calculate the total kilocalories consumed in a 24-hour period for a daily intake of 250 grams of carbohydrates, 80 grams of protein, 60 grams of fat, and 20 grams of alcohol.

6. Define basal metabolic rate (BMR), diet-induced thermogenesis (DIT), and exercise-induced thermogenesis (EIT).

7. Distinguish between the ways that BMR and REE are determined and then used.

8. What is the relationship between lean body mass (LBM) and BMR? Why is maintaining LBM important?

9. In simple terms of energy balance, explain why people gain weight and lose weight.

10. During fasting and starvation, which two major tissue types are degraded to provide energy? In what way are the "energy" molecules transported to the liver? What two major types of energy molecules are used from outside the liver? Also, what is the name of the major energy-providing molecule that is needed for all cell functions during fasting and starvation?

11. List the three major body compartments. Which compartment is the primary energy storage one?

12. In the semistarvation study at the University of Minnesota, how long was the recovery period before the young male volunteers got back their normal weight and function?

WEBSITES FOR FURTHER STUDY

Fat Replacers
www.diet.com/g/fat-replacers

U.S. Department of Agriculture (USDA)
www.usda.gov

REFERENCES

American Dietetic Association. Position of the American Dietetic Association and Dietitians of Canada: Dietary fatty acids. *J Acad Nutr Diet*. 2007;107:1599–1611.

Casazza K, Nagy TR. Body composition evaluation. In: Erdman JW Jr, MacDonald IA, Zeisel SH, eds. *Present Knowledge in Nutrition*. 10th ed. Ames, IA: John Wiley & Sons; 2012:1447–1573.

Das SK, Roberts SB. Energy metabolism in fasting, fed, exercise, and re-feeding states. In: Erdman JW Jr, MacDonald IA, Zeisel SH, eds. *Present Knowledge in Nutrition*. 10th ed. Ames, IA: John Wiley & Sons; 2012:117–133.

Johnstone AM. Energy intake, obesity, and eating behavior. In: Erdman JW Jr, MacDonald IA, Zeisel SH, eds. *Present Knowledge in Nutrition*. 10th ed. Ames, IA: John Wiley & Sons; 2012:1627–1650.

Keys A. ed. *Biology of Starvation*, 2 volumes. Minneapolis; University of Minnesota Press; 1950.

Pedersen SB, Sjödin A, Astrup A. Obesity as a health risk. In: Erdman JW Jr, MacDonald IA, Zeisel SH, eds. *Present Knowledge in Nutrition*. 10th ed. Ames, IA: John Wiley & Sons; 2012:1127–1146.

Schwartz MW, Woods SC, Porte D Jr, et al. Central nervous system control of food intake. *Nature* 404: 661–671, 2000. [Classic]

Stein Z, Susser M, Saenger G, Marolla F. *Famine and Human Development: The Dutch Hunger Winter of 1944–1945*. New York: Oxford University Press; 1975.

Wang T, Hung CC, Randall DJ. The comparative physiology of food deprivation: from feast to famine. *Annu Rev Physiol*. 2006;68:223–251.

Wing RR, Gorin A, Tate DF. Strategies for changing eating and exercise behavior to promote weight loss and maintenance. Erdman JW Jr, MacDonald IA, Zeisel SH, eds. *Present Knowledge in Nutrition*. 10th ed. Ames, IA: John Wiley & Sons; 2012;1651–1671.

ADDITIONAL READING

Hobbs SH. *Get the Trans Fat Out*. New York: Three Rivers Press; 2006.

Russell SA. *Hunger: An Unnatural History*. New York: Basic Books; 2005.

Spindler, K. *The Man in the Ice*. New York: Harmony Books; 1994.

5

Carbohydrates

Carbohydrates are one of the most important sources of energy in our diets, providing almost half of an American's total caloric intake. Together, dietary fats and carbohydrates provide approximately 80% to 85% of our total caloric intake. Small amounts of carbohydrates are stored as glycogen (animal starch) in various tissues of the body. Excess dietary carbohydrate may be converted to triglycerides and stored in fat tissue, which is where most of the body's energy is stored. Besides their use in generating cellular energy (ATP), some carbohydrate molecules are used to synthesize structural components of cells and tissues throughout the body. This chapter provides information about the different types of carbohydrates and how they are metabolized to meet the body's needs.

Food Sources of Carbohydrates

Traditionally, carbohydrates in the form of starches have been the primary source of food energy. Simple sugars are provided by fruits, sweetened cereals, processed foods, and candy. Over recent decades, because of concerns about overweight and obesity, fat consumption has declined modestly, while that of carbohydrates, especially sugars, has increased. Today, carbohydrates provide nearly half of our total energy, whereas fats provide about a third. Protein consumption has remained fairly constant over the past few decades, contributing approximately a sixth of the energy in the typical American diet (see **Table 5.1**).

Major foods supplying carbohydrates include **starches** in cereals and grain products, potatoes and other starchy vegetable roots and stems, and **sugars** in fruits and fruit juices. A variety of other sweets, ice creams, candies, and soft drinks provides primarily simple sugars. Honey and maple syrup are two other foods rich in simple sugars (see **FIGURE 5.1**). Today, a manufactured sugar, **high-fructose corn syrup (HFCS)**, represents a large percentage of the monosaccharides used in processed convenience foods and beverages.

starch A complex carbohydrate (polysaccharide) consisting of amylose, amylopectin, or glycogen molecules.

sugar A monosaccharide or disaccharide that is characterized by a sweet taste; naturally occurring sugars include sucrose, fructose, and lactose; refined and processed sugars include high-fructose corn syrup (HFCS).

high-fructose corn syrup (HFCS) A sweetener made from corn starch through several enzymatic reactions and purification steps that has about the same concentration of fructose and sweetness as sucrose. A rather controversial product partially blamed for the increased intake of sweetened beverages and the rise in childhood obesity.

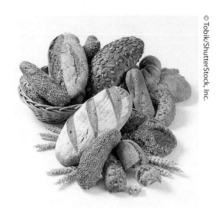

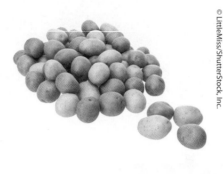

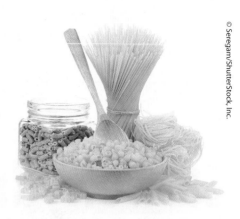

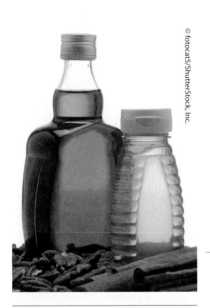

FIGURE 5.1 Foods Rich in Sugar. A number of foods found in nature are rich in simple sugars. Honey, which is made by bees using nectar from flowers, is composed primarily of the simple sugars glucose and fructose. Maple syrup is a syrup usually made from the xylem sap of sugar maple, red maple, or black maple trees. It consists largely of sucrose and water.

sweetener Food additive used to add sweetness to a food. May be a nutrient (sugar) or a non-nutrient compound, such as aspartame, saccharin, sucralose, and others.

TABLE 5.1
Changes in Contribution of Macronutrients to the U.S. Diet: 1971–2006

Macronutrient	Percent Contribution to Daily Calories	
	1971–1975	**2005–2006**
Protein	16.5%	15.7%
Carbohydrate	44.0%	48.7%
Fat	36.6%	33.7%

Data from Austin GL, Ogden LG, Hill JO. Trends in carbohydrate, fat, and protein intakes and association with energy intake in normal-weight, overweight, and obese individuals: 1971–2006. *Am J Clin Nutr.* 2011;93;836–843.

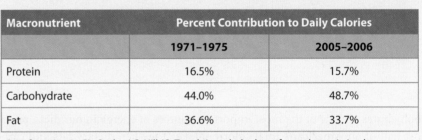

FOCUS 5.1 High-Fructose Corn Syrup

High-fructose corn syrup (HFCS), sometimes called corn sugar, is a chemically modified product of corn. One commonly used blend of two different HFCS extractions used as a food and beverage ingredient consists of 55% fructose and 45% glucose, and it has a sweetness equivalent to sucrose extracted from cane sugar. In the United States, HFCS is widely used in soft drinks, baked goods, sports drinks, and candies.

HFCS is made through the enzymatic degradation of corn starch (amylose, a linear starch), and a large percentage of the glucose molecules are converted to fructose. Health concerns have been raised about HFCS, but so far these have not been sufficiently supported by findings of clinical research using human subjects. HFCS blends have about the same chemical composition and the same nutritional quality as table sugar and honey. ●

Sugar Substitutes

Saccharin, sucralose, aspartame, and other related chemicals serve as important sugar substitutes or artificial **sweeteners** that are used extensively to provide sweetness without the calories of sugar. These synthetic molecules, marketed under different trade names, need only be present in small amounts in coffee, iced tea, soft drinks, or certain desserts to satisfy the desire for sweetness. Saccharin, which is very poorly absorbed, is basically an inert molecule that is approximately 400 times sweeter than sucrose.

Aspartame, though almost 200 times sweeter than table sugar, is actually a dipeptide (amino acids linked as aspartyl-phenylalanine) that is digested in the GI tract. The individual amino acids are absorbed, but because of their small quantity they yield only a few calories after their metabolism. Because people with the rare inherited disorder called phenylketonuria must limit their intake of phenylalanine, they must avoid products with this sweetener.

A newer sugar substitute is sucralose, a chlorinated sucrose. It is 600 times as sweet as sucrose and seems to have less of an aftertaste associated with the other artificial sweeteners. Because it is not digested in the intestine, sucralose provides no calories, and for this reason this sugar substitute has become widely used by those concerned with their body weight and diabetes.

Stevia, the newest sweetener on the market, is a chemical extract of the plant *Stevia rebaudiana*. Among the steviol glycosides, the most common derivative is ribaudioside, which is used in commercial products because it is about 250 times sweeter than sugar. Because stevia is also heat and acid stable, it can be used in cooked food products.

Carbohydrate Structure

Sugars and starches are the major energy-generating carbohydrates provided by foods. **FIGURE 5.2** shows the structures of common **monosaccharides** (one sugar molecule)

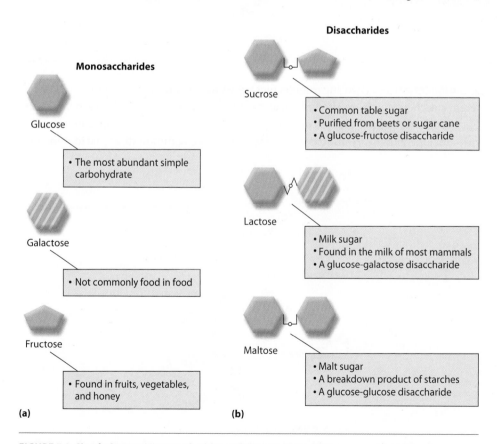

(a)   **(b)**

FIGURE 5.2 Simple Sugars: Monosaccharides and Disaccharides. (a) The monosaccharides—glucose, galactose, and fructose—are the most basic units of biologically important carbohydrates. They are the simplest forms of sugar. Monosaccharides are the building blocks of disaccharides (such as sucrose) and polysaccharides (such as cellulose and starch). (b) Common disaccharides include sucrose, lactose, and maltose.

monosaccharide Simple sugars. Glucose, galactose, and fructose are naturally occurring monosaccharides. The preferred molecular arrangement of these simple sugars in foods and in our bodies is a ring structure.

FOCUS 5.2   Lactose Intolerance

Lactose, a disaccharide containing glucose and galactose, requires the enzyme lactase to be broken down into two monosaccharides in the small intestinal lumen, where the enzyme operates at the luminal surface. If the enzyme is very low or practically absent, the lactose is not broken down into its component sugars, glucose and galactose. The lactose molecules then pass into the large intestine where millions of bacteria live by feasting on undigested food components, such as lactose. Bacterial degradation of lactose results in gas (carbon dioxide and others) and other products that cause the symptoms of loose stools, bloating, and intestinal pressure (pain) from gas buildup within the gut. Once the GI tract clears the lactose and bacterial degradation products, affected individuals begin to feel better and the uncomfortable effects disappear for the time being until additional milk is consumed.

Worldwide, the majority of people are intolerant of lactose; lactose tolerance is more common in those of Northern European ancestry. However, in most human populations, dairy products continue to be consumed, most commonly as yogurts and cheeses, as well as other fermented products, in which bacteria and other microorganisms have digested the lactose present in the original milk. The ability to metabolize lactose with lactase exists early in life in all babies and young children. However, as infants grow, lactase production by the cells in the small intestine declines, in some cases to very low amounts. Those children who develop symptoms of lactose intolerance following milk consumption (i.e., bloating, cramping, gas, diarrhea, general discomfort) often totally stop consuming milk. Today, lactase-treated milk is available in food markets and this milk contains little or no lactose. ●

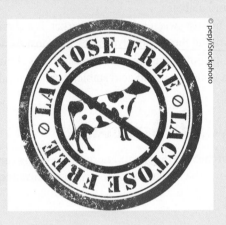

and **disaccharides** (two sugar molecules). **FIGURE 5.3** shows the structure of two different starches, which are also known as **polysaccharides** or complex carbohydrates. Each saccharide unit is glucose or a glucose-like molecule. The common monosaccharides include glucose, **galactose**, and **fructose**. The common disaccharides include

disaccharide A sugar consisting of two monosaccharide units. Examples include sucrose, lactose, and maltose.

polysaccharide Long carbohydrate molecules consisting of monosaccharide units joined together by glycosidic bonds. Examples include starch and cellulose.

galactose A monosaccharide similar to glucose. Lactose contains galactose and glucose as its two monosaccharides.

fructose A six-carbon monosaccharide. Also called fruit sugar, it has a very sweet taste. Together with glucose, it makes up sucrose, a disaccharide. It is an intermediary molecule in glycolysis. Often used as a sweetener, it may have adverse effects when consumed in large quantities.

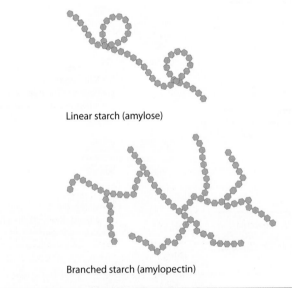

FIGURE 5.3 Starches: Linear and Branched Polysaccharides. Polysaccharides are long carbohydrate molecules of monosaccharide units joined together by glycosidic bonds. They range in structure from linear to highly branched.

PRACTICAL APPLICATION 5.1

Glucose Molecules

Essentially, all carbohydrates are glucose. This statement is based on the fact that following digestion in the gut or metabolism in the body all sugars and starches can be converted to glucose molecules. Thus, an understanding of the structure of glucose and its roles in the body is very important in the field of nutrition. In simple terms, a glucose molecule is made of 6 carbon atoms, 12 hydrogen atoms, and 6 oxygen atoms. The major energy source in a glucose molecule comes from the energy released in the breakage of the C-H bonds during metabolism that is then used to generate ATP.

Examine the two-dimensional ring structure of a glucose molecule. This **ring structure** provides stability to glucose in the body's water-based body fluids, such as serum, blood, and cytoplasm. Note that the ring has one oxygen atom and five carbon atoms. The sixth carbon branches off the fifth carbon of the ring. Count the number of C-H bonds in glucose. Notice all the OH groups. The OH groups make glucose very water soluble.

Glucose

In cellular metabolism, the first step of modification of glucose is the addition of a phosphate group at the sixth carbon to form glucose-6-phosphate. Once this **phosphorylation** step has occurred, glucose-6-phosphate zips through the different pathways that use it, especially those involved in ATP production. Practice writing the structure of glucose on paper to review these features. ■

---

sucrose (table sugar), **lactose** (milk sugar), and **maltose**. Lactose takes on greater importance for people who lack the enzyme lactase, which is needed to digest the disaccharide in the small intestine. The polysaccharides include linear and branched starches and the individual monosaccharides in starches are linked by **glycosidic bonds**. One important branched starch in our bodies is glycogen, the storage form of carbohydrates made in liver and other cell types. Relatively little glycogen is consumed from meats and other animal foods.

Regardless of the specific structure, each type of carbohydrate provides 4 kilocalories per gram. Although the carbohydrates are primarily used for generating energy (i.e., ATP), a few complex molecules containing carbohydrates are also used for synthesizing some structural components of cell membranes and complex molecules in connective and brain tissues.

Dietary Fiber

The dietary fiber molecules in plant foods are largely complex carbohydrates that are not absorbed across the gut barrier. Thus, both **water-insoluble** and **water-soluble fiber molecules** function only within the lumens of the stomach and small and large intestines. They do not enter the cytoplasm of the cells lining the gut. Dietary fibers may be fibrous, such as **celluloses** (a nondigestable polysaccharide found in cell walls of plants) or **hemicelluloses**, or gel-like, such as **gums**, **pectins**, and **mucilages**. Some of the gel-like fibers are chemically modified by gut bacteria, and the resulting new soluble components may aid in the digestion of nutrients. Some studies have found the dietary fiber may promote gastrointestinal health, but research is continuing in this

---

ring structure Provides stability to glucose in the body's water-based body fluids, such as serum, blood, and cytoplasm.

sucrose A disaccharide containing fructose and glucose. It is most well known as common table sugar.

lactose A disaccharide composed of glucose and galactose found in milk and milk products. The intestinal enzyme lactase metabolizes lactose to its monosaccharides.

maltose A disaccharide containing two glucose units that is derived from starch.

glycosidic bonds Bonds between the rings of disaccharide or polysaccharide molecules.

water-insoluble fiber molecule Dietary fibers that are not soluble in water. Because they are not soluble in the watery fluids of the GI tract, they are not subject to digestion by gut bacteria in the lower small intestine and large intestine. Examples include the celluloses, lignans, and most of the hemicelluloses.

water-soluble fiber molecule Dietary fibers that are soluble in water. Because they are soluble in the watery fluids of the GI tract, they can be digested by gut bacteria in the lower small intestine and especially in the large intestine. Include the gums, mucilages, pectins, algal polysaccharides, and some hemicelluloses of low molecular weight.

cellulose A nondigestible polysaccharide that makes up a large fraction of the dietary fiber in plant foods. It is classified as a water-insoluble fiber and is found mainly in the cell walls of plants.

hemicellulose A type of dietary fiber that contains both soluble and insoluble polysaccharides, depending on their length (i.e., molecular weight).

gum A type of water-soluble dietary fiber classified as a type of mucilage. It is a relatively small polysaccharide that is partially degraded by gut bacteria.

pectin A type of water-soluble dietary fiber that is used in the making of fruit jelly.

mucilage A type of dietary fiber that is soluble in water.

TABLE 5.2
Actions of Dietary Fiber in the Gastrointestinal Tract

Gut Function	Impact of Dietary Fiber
Transit rate	Slows gastric emptying; speeds up colonic movement.
Nutrient absorption	Some nutrients may be bound to fiber, which limits nutrient absorption.
Fermentation	Some fiber molecules are metabolized by colonic bacteria and increase healthy bacterial populations.
Enterohepatic circulation	Some fiber molecules interfere with colonic reabsorption of cholesterol and steroid hormones, such as estrogens.

" With a meal (also known as the prandium) that contains a reasonable amount of dietary carbohydrate (40% to 60% of the meal's total energy), the blood glucose concentration will peak approximately 30 to 60 minutes after the first bite. **"**

postprandium (absorption period) The 3- to 4-hour period that follows the last ingestion of a meal during which the most nutrients are absorbed. This period is associated with wide swings in blood glucose and insulin concentrations, even under normal conditions.

blood glucose The concentration of glucose in blood that changes from low fasting values to the higher values of the postprandial period in healthy normal individuals. High blood glucose levels are indicative of a potential disease state, such as diabetes.

serum The liquid fraction of blood remaining after clotting.

plasma The fraction of blood containing fluid and any dissolved molecules after centrifugation. Differs from serum because an anticlotting agent is added to the blood prior to centrifugation.

area. **Table 5.2** highlights some actions of fiber in the gastrointestinal tract. Fiber slows stomach emptying but it speeds up transit within the large intestine—seemingly opposite actions, but each has a major impact!

Intestinal Absorption of Glucose

With a meal (also known as the prandium) that contains a reasonable amount of dietary carbohydrate (40% to 60% of the meal's total energy), the blood glucose concentration will peak approximately 30 to 60 minutes after the first bite. Glucose absorption during the 3- to 4-hour absorption period or **postprandium** occurs by a special carrier-mediated process in the absorbing cells of the small intestine. The glucose then enters the blood and circulation on its way to the liver (see **FIGURE 5.4**). In normal individuals, the **blood glucose** concentration will rise by 25 to 50 milligrams per deciliter above the individual's base level and then return within 3 to 4 hours to the premeal or fasting glucose base level, which ranges from 70 to 100 milligrams per deciliter. The fasting blood glucose base level tends to creep up with each decade of adult life, typically in direct relationship to increasing body fat mass. **Table 5.3** provides normal fasting **serum**, or **plasma**, glucose concentrations as well as ranges for those with **prediabetes** and **diabetes** types 1 and 2.

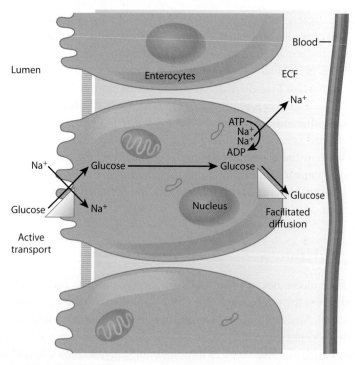

FIGURE 5.4 Glucose Absorption Across the Small Intestine. Movement of glucose from the lumen of the small intestine into the absorbing cells occurs by a special carrier-mediated process. Glucose moves across the absorbing cells and is then released into the blood.

Reproduced from Anderson JJB. *Nutrition and Health: An Introduction.* Durham, NC: Carolina Academic Press; 2005.

As the serum glucose concentration rises following a meal, so does the serum insulin concentration. **Insulin** is a hormone produced by beta cells (designated by β or B) in the pancreas that act on cells of the body to permit glucose entry into cells from blood and extracellular fluids. As insulin rises, it stimulates the uptake of glucose by insulin-responsive cells throughout the body, especially the muscles, and fat cells. Thus, the action of insulin causes the decline in blood glucose during the 3- to 4-hour postprandium (absorption period), returning it toward the usual fasting level. **FIGURE 5.5** shows postprandial changes in serum concentrations of glucose and insulin in individuals with normal **glucose tolerance** and in diabetic individuals after meals rich in either sugars or starches containing little or no dietary fiber. The potential health benefits of the fiber-rich dietary starches compared with dietary sugars result from the slower digestion of starches (see **FIGURE 5.6**) and the subsequent delay in and the lesser rise of blood glucose following a meal. The slower postprandial rise in blood glucose leads to a reduced rise in blood insulin and a longer time frame for glucose disappearance from the blood because of the slower glucose uptake by tissues of the body.

TABLE 5.3 Fasting Serum Glucose Concentrations: Normal, Prediabetes, and Diabetes*			
Glucose Units	**Normal**	**Prediabetic**	**Diabetic**
Milligrams per deciliter (mg/dL)	< 100	100–125	≥ 126
Millimoles per liter (mmol/L)	< 5.6	5.6–7.0	≥ 7.0

* The terms serum and plasma are used interchangeably. They differ from whole blood because the blood cells are removed in the process of obtaining either serum or plasma.
Data from American Diabetes Association. How to Tell If You Have Diabetes or Prediabetes. Available at: www.diabetes.org/diabetes-basics/prevention/pre-diabetes/how-to-tell-if-you-have.html.

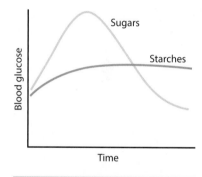

FIGURE 5.6 Postprandial Serum Glucose Concentration Changes. Starches and sugars elicit different blood glucose concentrations over time.

Data from Crapo PA. Theory vs. fact: Glycemic response to foods. *Nutrition Today*. 1984;19(2):6–11.

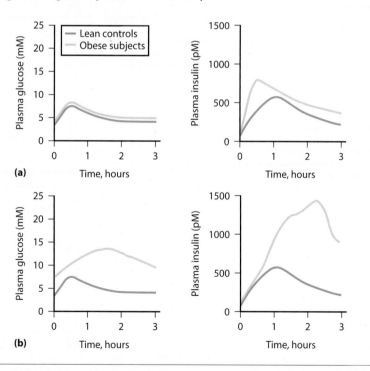

FIGURE 5.5 Normal and Abnormal Postprandial Glucose Tolerance Curves. The graphs in (a) show the glucose and insulin responses after glucose intake (i.e., drink, meal) for a normal individual (lower curves) and for a prediabetic, obese individual (upper curves). The graphs in (b) show the responses for the normal individual contrasted with those for a diabetic, obese individual with abnormal uptake of glucose by cells and very high, fasting glucose concentrations.

Modified from Anderson JJB. *Nutrition and Health: An Introduction*. Durham, NC: Carolina Academic Press; 2005.

insulin Hormone produced by beta (β) cells of the islets of Langerhans in the pancreas that primarily acts on cells of the body, especially liver, muscle, and fat cells, to permit glucose entry into cells from blood and extracellular fluids, especially during the postprandial (post-meal) period.

glucose tolerance The state of responding appropriately to a glucose challenge (oral load) by lowering the blood glucose concentration in a normal fashion. Glucose intolerance refers to not being able to appropriately lower the blood glucose concentration after a glucose or meal challenge.

Glycemic Index

Glycemic index (GI) refers to the rise in serum glucose concentration from baseline (fasting) following the ingestion of a single carbohydrate-rich food item (experimental food) in comparison with the glucose rise following the consumption of the same amount of glucose itself, which is arbitrarily assigned a GI value of 100%. **Table 5.4** lists the GI values of several foods in comparison with glucose. A few of the common processed cereal grains containing little or no dietary fiber have GI values similar to white bread. Carbohydrate-rich foods such as fruits and vegetables typically have lower GI values because they contain more dietary fiber, which modulates the spike in the blood glucose level. Excessive energy intake from carbohydrates as well as from other macronutrients and alcohol is a major dietary risk factor for various chronic diseases, including type 2 diabetes mellitus. High glycemic-index foods cause a rapid increase in

glycemic index (GI) Refers to the rise in serum glucose concentration from baseline (fasting) following the ingestion of a single carbohydrate-rich food item (experimental food) in comparison with the glucose rise following the consumption of the same amount of glucose itself, which is arbitrarily assigned a GI value of 100%. High GI foods cause a rapid increase in blood glucose concentration after ingestion.

TABLE 5.4
High Glycemic Index Foods

Food Item	Glycemic Index*
Fruit roll-ups	99
Bagel, white, plain	95
Corn flakes cereal	93
White rice, regular	89
Boiled white potatoes	82
Gatorade	78
Waffles	76
Watermelon	72
Whole wheat bread	71
White wheat flour bread	71
Sweet potato	70
Raisins	64
Cola drink	63
Raisin Bran	61
Honey	61
Ice cream	57
Snickers bar	51
Kidney beans	29

* Compared to glucose at 100%.
Data from Atkinson FS, Foster-Powell K, Brand-Miller JC. International tables of glycemic index and glycemic load values: 2008. *Diabetes Care.* 2008;31(12):2281–2283; and Harvard Medical School. Glycemic Index and Glycemic Load for 100+ foods. Available at: www.health .harvard.edu/newsweek/Glycemic_index_and_glycemic_load_for_100_foods.htm

FOCUS 5.3   Glycemic Load and Dietary Fiber

Glycemic load represents the total amount of carbohydrate in a meal; that is, the sum of all glucose sources, especially the high GI carbohydrates in a meal. A meal with a high glycemic load would be one that contains typically one or more high GI carbohydrate food items. For example, a meal with three glucose-rich foods would have the glycemic load shown below:

Roll (white bread)*	2 × 12 g carbohydrate (starch)	24 g × 0.77** = 18.6
Milk (low fat)	1 × 12 g lactose	12 g × 0.30** = 3.6
Pudding (milk)	1 × 28 g lactose + sucrose	28 g × 0.57** = 16.0
Glycemic Load		**Total 38.2 g**

* Equivalent to two slices of white bread.
** GI of each food

The total amount of highly available glucose in this meal is 38.2 grams, which when multiplied by 4 kilocalories per gram, is equivalent to a glucose load of 152.2 kilocalories! Such a high glucose load puts stress on the islet cells of the pancreas to produce more insulin. This rise in blood glucose from the sample meal is fairly robust, but the glucose response would be even greater if the meal provided 100% sugar with no dietary fiber at all!

Foods high in water-soluble dietary fiber, especially gums and mucilages, typically reduce the elevation of blood glucose concentration after a meal because the fiber molecules effectively lower the GI values of the carbohydrates in the same food. The reason for this effect relates to the drawing of water molecules to the water-soluble fiber molecules in the gastrointestinal tract and the subsequent slowing of gastric emptying. The partially digested food molecules enter the small intestine for further digestion prior to absorption at a slower rate. Because of the nondigestible fiber molecules present, the intestinal digestion of macronutrients in the lower half of the small intestine is slowed. As a result of both the delayed gastric emptying and the fiber-induced slower intestinal digestion, the entry of glucose molecules from the digested carbohydrates into the blood is delayed. This delaying of glucose entry contributes to a more normal and healthier blood glucose (tolerance) curve that also reduces serum insulin during the postmeal period. ●

blood glucose concentration after ingestion. Another tool used to analyze the carbohydrate content of a food or meal is glycemic load.

Blood Transport, Distribution, and Storage of Carbohydrates

During and following a meal, absorbed glucose and other monosaccharides are carried to the liver by the portal vein for use by liver cells (hepatocytes). Hepatocytes, however, only extract approximately 50% of the glucose from the portal blood and let the remainder pass on to all other organs of the body to satisfy energy requirements for metabolism and to provide raw materials for the synthesis of new molecules. The monosaccharides galactose and fructose are converted to glucose in the liver before entering the common energy pathways. Much of the fructose in high-fructose corn syrup (HFCS) also is converted to glucose. Red blood cells, the tubular cells in the kidney, brain cells, and other nerve cells throughout the body normally use only glucose for their energy needs. Excessive carbohydrate intake, and hence elevated serum glucose levels, adversely affects the insulin-producing cells in the pancreas over long periods.

> Red blood cells, the tubular cells in the kidney, brain cells, and other nerve cells throughout the body normally use only glucose for their energy needs.

glycemic load Represents the total amount of carbohydrate in a meal; that is, the sum of all glucose sources, especially foods with high glycemic indexes. A meal with a high glycemic load would be one that contains one or more foods with a high glycemic index.

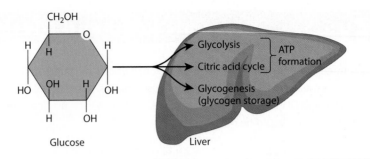

FIGURE 5.7 Liver Glucose Pathways After a Meal. Note the three major pathways taken by glucose in the liver: glycolysis, the citric acid cycle, or glycogenesis.

glycogenesis The synthesis of glycogen in the liver and in most other cells of the body.

anaerobic respiration Cellular respiration that does not require oxygen.

glycolysis An anaerobic respiration pathway in the cell cytoplasm that begins with glucose and ends with pyruvate or lactate and the generation of two ATPs.

aerobic respiration Cellular respiration that requires the presence of oxygen.

citric acid cycle (Krebs cycle) The cyclic metabolic pathway in the mitochondria that begins with the combining of oxaloacetate and acetyl CoA and ends with the regeneration of oxaloacetate after the oxidation of two carbon units to carbon dioxide and water, along with the generation of ATP and heat. The citric cycle also generates water (metabolic) and carbon dioxide through the complete oxidation of glucose, fatty acids, amino acids, and alcohol.

pyruvic acid (pyruvate) A three-carbon keto acid that allows entry of degraded carbohydrates and selected amino acids to the citric acid (Krebs) cycle for oxidative metabolism.

lactic acid (lactate) A derivative (reduced form) of pyruvate formed by the addition of two hydrogen atoms in the liver and other cells after glycolysis. In exercising skeletal muscle tissue deprived of oxygen, such as following physical exertion, lactate is released by the muscles to the blood circulation for return to the liver and use in the gluconeogenic pathway.

oxidative phosphorylation The linking of two processes in the electron transport chain of mitochondria with the end result being the oxidation of nutrients to produce adenosine triphosphate (ATP). Although this process is quite efficient, some of the energy generated is lost as heat.

The liver is the body's key organ in the parceling out of energy as either glucose or triglycerides to other body tissues, often referred to as peripheral tissue with respect to the liver being central (i.e., the body's metabolic control center). The liver and other cells in the body utilize glucose primarily for the generation of ATP. After ATP generation, the remainder of the glucose extracted from the portal blood by the liver after a meal is converted (1) to glycogen by a process called **glycogenesis** for storage in hepatocytes or (2) to triglycerides for both peripheral tissue use and for storage in the fat depots when carbohydrate intake is excessive (see **FIGURE 5.7**). These two functions are also carried out in muscle cells, and they generate modest stores of both glycogen and triglycerides that are readily available for bursts of activity. Unlike liver cells, muscle cells use these fuels only for their own metabolic needs.

Metabolic Pathways for Glucose Degradation by Cells

The two major catabolic pathways of the liver and muscle are: (1) **anaerobic respiration**, or **glycolysis**, which requires no oxygen, and (2) **aerobic (oxygen requiring) respiration**, which includes the **citric acid cycle** (also known as the Krebs cycle; see Figure 5.7). Glycolysis starts with a single glucose molecule and ends with two molecules (3 carbon) of **pyruvic acid (pyruvate)** or **lactic acid (lactate)**. The net result of this anaerobic pathway is the generation of two ATP molecules. Aerobic respiration takes these pyruvate molecules (three carbon atoms each) and metabolizes them in several steps, the last being **oxidative phosphorylation**, which oxidates nutrients to generate more than 30 ATPs. If a glucose molecule is completely degraded via acetyl CoA molecules, the final reaction products are carbon dioxide, water, about 38 ATP molecules with their high-energy bonds, and released heat (thermogenic). In addition to the liver, practically all other cells of the body, especially muscle, use these same two pathways for the generation of cellular ATP molecules with high-energy phosphate bonds. Only the liver cells, however, are capable of generating new glucose molecules for secretion to blood for use by all other cells and tissues of the body during periods of fasting.

Whereas glycolysis occurs in the cytoplasm of cells, the citric acid cycle and oxidative phosphorylation of ADP to ATP occur only in the mitochondria. The generation of ATP, the cellular energy source, from ADP is detailed in **FIGURE 5.8**. The addition of phosphate, a negatively charged ion (anion), to form ATP demonstrates one of the most important roles of phosphate in cellular functioning.

When the liver does not need to convert all the pyruvate (3-carbon structures) to CO_2 and H_2O for ATP production, the excess amounts are diverted from the citric acid

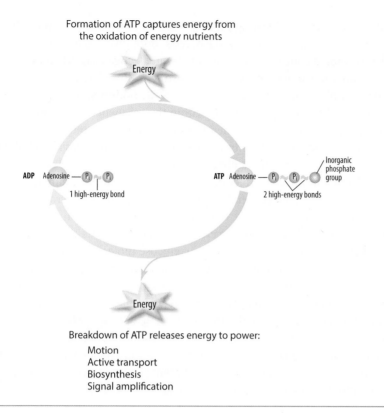

Formation of ATP captures energy from
the oxidation of energy nutrients

Energy

ADP   Adenosine — P_i ~ P_i

1 high-energy bond

ATP   Adenosine — P_i ~ P_i ~ P_i

Inorganic
phosphate
group

2 high-energy bonds

Energy

Breakdown of ATP releases energy to power:
    Motion
    Active transport
    Biosynthesis
    Signal amplification

FIGURE 5.8 Generation of Cellular ATP. The addition of a phosphate ion to ADP is required for the formation of ATP.

> The liver is the body's key organ in the parceling out of energy as either glucose or triglycerides to other body tissues, often referred to as peripheral tissue with respect to the liver being central (i.e., the body's metabolic control center).

> Carbohydrates can be used for the synthesis of fats when dietary carbohydrates are provided in greater quantities than the body can use.

cycle to the synthesis of fatty acids and triglycerides. Thus, carbohydrates can be used for synthesis of fats when dietary carbohydrates are provided in greater quantities than the body can use. During fasting or starvation, the liver also uses pyruvate and other small molecules, especially amino acids derived from proteins in the body, to produce new glucose molecules by the process of gluconeogenesis. These new glucose molecules also are used to maintain the normal blood glucose concentration.

During each meal, glycogen is synthesized from glucose in hepatocytes. During an overnight fast (typically 12 hours or more), approximately 75% to almost 100% of hepatic glycogen may be converted by glycogenolysis back to glucose, a process regulated mainly by the hormone **glucagon**, a product of alpha (designated as α or A) cells. Keep in mind that insulin is the hormone that governs most of the hepatic pathways during the postprandial period (after a meal) when glucose is being turned into glycogen and triglycerides. Glucagon dominates during periods of fasting when glycogen is being broken down and new glucose molecules are being made via gluconeogenesis to maintain blood glucose.

Formation and Breakdown of Glycogen

During the 1- to 2-hour period following a meal, new glycogen molecules are synthesized in the liver and in practically all other cells of the body from the excessive amount of glucose derived from the recently consumed foods. Glycogenesis occurs after every meal and, if enough carbohydrates are consumed, after every snack during a 24-hour period (see Figure 5.7).

Stored glycogen is gradually degraded at storage sites during fasting. Liver glycogen is used to keep the blood glucose concentration within a healthy range during fasting,

glucagon Hormone produced by alpha (α) cells of the islets of Langerhans that acts primarily on the liver to stimulate gluconeogenesis and glycogenolysis, especially during periods of fasting, to make glucose available to the body's cells.

During extended fasting, blood glucose concentration can be maintained by two different processes occurring simultaneously in the liver: glycogenolysis and gluconeogenesis.

especially during extended fasting periods, such as overnight (8 or more hours). The breakdown of glycogen is called glycogenolysis. Both glycogenesis and glycogenolysis are under hormonal control. Insulin dominates in glycogenesis, whereas glucagon and a couple of other hormones operate during fasting to stimulate glycogenolysis.

Almost all cells in the extrahepatic tissues of the body also store glycogen that can be broken down for use as glucose only within the cells where it is stored. Unlike liver cells, which degrade glycogen and then release glucose to the blood to supply all body tissues, these extrahepatic cells only use their own glycogen stores for cellular needs of glucose. Also, unlike liver-cell membranes, the membranes of other cells do not permit glucose molecules to exit to the blood. Skeletal muscle cells, for example, store considerably greater amounts of glycogen for use in physical activities/exercise than other cell types, but this glucose cannot leave the muscle cells for use by nonmuscle cells.

During an extended fast, such as overnight with no food intake, the liver also has the capability via gluconeogenesis to make new glucose molecules from the C-H components of amino acids. For example, skeletal muscle can break down some of its protein in muscle fibers to the amino acid, alanine, which can then be released to blood, carried to the liver, and then converted to glucose molecules that are, in turn, released to blood for use by all other cells of the body. This **alanine–glucose cycle** involves the process of gluconeogenesis in the liver (see **FIGURE 5.9**), and it operates during fasting to help replenish the glucose concentration in blood. So, during extended fasting, blood glucose concentration can be maintained by two different processes occurring simultaneously in the liver: glycogenolysis and gluconeogenesis.

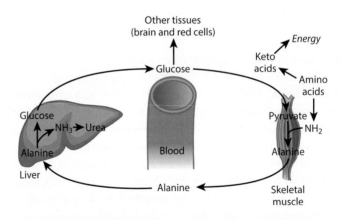

FIGURE 5.9 Alanine–Glucose Pathway. The alanine–glucose pathway helps to replenish glucose in the blood and tissues.

Reproduced from Anderson JJB. *Nutrition and Health: An Introduction*. Durham, NC: Carolina Academic Press; 2005.

alanine–glucose cycle Cycle whereby alanine moves from muscle via the blood to the liver and as glucose back to the blood. Provides hydrocarbon backbones for hepatic gluconeogenesis, after which glucose is delivered to tissues, especially to the brain and red blood cells, which have an essential requirement for it.

SUMMARY

Around the world, dietary carbohydrates are the major source of calories, meeting about half of the body's energy needs. Carbohydrates come in several forms, including the simple sugars, monosaccharides and disaccharides; the starches, both linear and branched; and fibers, both water soluble and water insoluble. Both types of fibers are found exclusively in plant foods. HFCS is a fructose and glucose mixture derived from corn and used in place of sugar in many applications. It has the sweetness of sugar and costs less. Several sugar substitutes are on the market, including saccharin, aspartame, sucralose, and stevia.

Sugars and starches are digested to monosaccharides before they are absorbed in the small intestine. Fiber is minimally digested and passes through the GI tract. A large share of the absorbed monosaccharides, primarily glucose, are taken up by the liver, under the influence of insulin, and converted into glycogen or fatty acids. The remainder of the glucose is taken up by other tissues, particularly muscle and fat, where it is similarly converted to glycogen and fatty acids. During fasting and between meals, glucose is solely released from the liver and taken up in the periphery, particularly by nervous tissues and red blood cells that require glucose.

STUDENT ACTIVITIES

1. Which food sources supply the bulk of carbohydrates in our diets? Do animal products provide much of the carbohydrate in our diets?

2. Give the number and types of atoms in glucose. How does glucose differ from a starch molecule?

3. Describe (or draw) the chemical ring structure of glucose.

4. Define the two types of dietary fiber and give an example of each type. How do most fiber molecules differ from starches?

5. Fasting serum glucose concentration is a health indicator. What does a high fasting glucose concentration mean in terms of health/disease?

6. Define glycemic index and glycemic load. How do they differ?

7. Explain why glycogen stored in the liver differs from glycogen stored in skeletal muscle or other cells.

8. The liver has several major pathways for metabolizing glucose derived from food sources. Explain the general meaning of the following: glycolysis, Krebs cycle/citric acid cycle, and glycogenesis.

9. Describe the alanine–glucose cycle and then explain gluconeogenesis.

10. Explain what lactose intolerance is and define the role of lactase (enzyme).

WEBSITES FOR FURTHER STUDY

Glycemic Index and Glycemic Load for 100+ Foods
www.health.harvard.edu/newsweek/Glycemic_index_and_glycemic_load_for_100_foods.htm
High-fructose Corn Syrup: Any Health Concerns?
www.mayoclinic.com/health/high-fructose-corn-syrup/AN01588

The Truth on Artificial Sweeteners
www.webmd.com/diet/features/truth-on-artificial-sweeteners
The World's Healthiest Foods: Fiber, Dietary
www.whfoods.com/genpage.php?tname=nutrient&dbid=59

REFERENCES

Barclay AW, Petocz P, McMillan-Price J, et al. Glycemic index, glycemic load, and chronic disease risk—a meta-analysis of observational studies. *Am J Clin Nutr.* 2008;87: 627–637.

Bhatnagar S, Aggarwal R. Lactose intolerance. *BMJ.* 2007; 334:1331–1332.

Chiu CJ, Liu S, Willett WC, et al. Informing food choices and health outcomes by use of the dietary glycemic index. *Nutr Rev.* 2011;69:231–242.

Food and Nutrition Board, Institute of Medicine, *Dietary Reference Intakes for Energy, Carbohydrate, Fiber, Fat, Fatty Acids, Cholesterol, Protein, and Amino Acids (Macronutrients).* Washington, DC: National Academies Press; 2002.

Jenkins DJ, Wolever TM, Taylor RH, et al. Glycemic index of foods: a physiological basis for carbohydrate exchange. *Am J Clin Nutr.* 1981;34:362–366.

Johnson IT. Dietary fiber. In: Erdman JW Jr, MacDonald IA, Zeisel SH, eds. *Present Knowledge in Nutrition*, 10th ed. Ames, IA: John Wiley & Sons; 2012;178–212.

Lattimer JM, Haub MD. Effects of dietary fiber and its components on metabolic health. *Nutrients.* 2010;2:1266–1289.

Sanders LM, Lupton JR. Carbohydrates. In: Erdman JW Jr, MacDonald IA, Zeisel SH, eds. *Present Knowledge in Nutrition*, 10th ed. Ames, IA: John Wiley & Sons; 2012:156–177.

Wiebe N, Padwal R, Field C, Marks S, Jacobs R, Tonelli M. A systematic review on the effect of sweeteners on glycemic response and clinically relevant outcomes. *BMC Med.* 2011;9:123.

Reflection on Type 2 Diabetes Mellitus: A Disease of Altered Glucose Metabolism

Two major types of diabetes mellitus exist: type 1 and type 2. Both are metabolic disorders that affect how the body handles glucose. Both types of diabetes are characterized by glucose (sugar) in the urine. In fact, the name *diabetes mellitus* is a Latin phrase that means "a large volume of sweet-tasting urine."

Because type 1, or insulin-dependent, diabetes mellitus usually emerges during childhood or adolescence, it was once called juvenile diabetes. Type 1 diabetes mellitus is essentially an autoimmune disease with the involvement of environmental factors, such as a virus. It does not result from poor nutrition.

Type 2 diabetes emerges most often during adulthood and often is called adult-onset diabetes. Of the two types of diabetes, type 2 diabetes mellitus is far more common, with 90% to 95% of those with diabetes having this type. Type 2 diabetes has a strong genetic determinant, and it does tend to run in families. Type 2 diabetes is one of the 10 leading causes of death in the United States.

The focus of this diet-related disease feature is on type 2 diabetes mellitus because of its significant nutritional **etiology**. Etiology consists of the causation of a disease, which is usually based around several risk factors. In the case of type 2 diabetes mellitus, these risk factors are associated with excessive energy intake, especially from carbohydrates. Approximately 80% or more of those with type 2 diabetes mellitus are overweight or obese. The role of adipose and muscle tissue in contributing to insulin resistance and metabolic abnormalities involving elevations of both circulating insulin and glucose are described.

etiology The causation of a disease. Often based on one or more risk factors that contribute to the development of a disease. The etiology of most chronic degenerative diseases involves multiple risk factors.

> ❝ Type 2 diabetes is characterized by abnormal glucose tolerance, hyperglycemia (significantly elevated fasting blood concentration of glucose), and glycosuria (sugar in the urine). ❞

> ❝ The way to determine an individual's tolerance to glucose is to perform an oral glucose tolerance test (OGTT). ❞

hyperglycemia Significantly elevated fasting blood concentration of glucose (i.e., beyond the range of normality of the laboratory measurement used). Often an indicator of diabetes mellitus or prediabetes.

glycosuria The presence of sugar (glucose) in the urine, which is not the normal condition. It is a warning sign of type 2 diabetes mellitus.

peripheral insulin resistance The resistance of peripheral tissues (e.g., muscle, adipose) to the action of insulin to take up glucose. This condition precedes the development of type 2 diabetes mellitus.

oral glucose tolerance test (OGTT) A test of glucose tolerance involving an overnight fast and fasting glucose measurement, followed by an oral challenge (load) of glucose (75 grams) or a meal and serial measurements of blood glucose at several times following the time of the load.

Abnormal Glucose Tolerance

Type 2 diabetes mellitus is characterized by abnormal glucose tolerance, **hyperglycemia** (significantly elevated fasting blood concentration of glucose), and **glycosuria** (sugar in the urine). In addition, severely altered glucose regulation occurs because of the elevation of serum insulin, which is sometimes referred to as insulin insensitivity or **peripheral insulin resistance**. Fat and muscle cells have reduced capabilities of taking up glucose from the blood. Also, elevated serum glucagon concentrations develop over time, and this hormone stimulates the liver to generate even more glucose via gluconeogenesis!

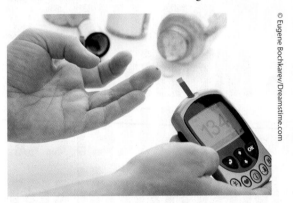

© Eugene Bochkarev/Dreamstime.com

The typical rise in blood glucose following a meal is referred to as normal glucose tolerance, whereas an abnormally elevated rise in blood glucose after a meal is referred to as glucose intolerance or abnormal glucose tolerance. Many stages of glucose tolerance or disposal of glucose after a meal exist between these two extremes (normal and extreme hyperglycemia). The way to determine an individual's tolerance to glucose is to perform an **oral glucose tolerance test (OGTT)**. This test requires a person to fast overnight and then to swallow a preset amount of glucose, usually 75 grams, in a flavored drink in the morning. A blood sample is taken from the individual prior to consuming the drink and then every 30 to 60 minutes thereafter in order to generate a glucose tolerance curve (i.e., plotting of serum glucose concentration versus time in hours). **FIGURE 1** illustrates an abnormal glucose tolerance curve compared to a normal curve. Sometimes a standard meal (typically a breakfast) is given instead of the glucose drink to determine glucose tolerance because the response after a meal is more typical of how the body will ingest sugar.

Abnormal glucose tolerance curves are altered either because blood glucose concentrations go too high (overshoot) or they extend too long at too high a concentration after an oral glucose load in an OGTT (see Figure 1). Each abnormal pattern following the three major meals of the day represents glucose intolerance. Blood glucose typically rises too high early after a meal, and then it may undershoot 3 hours or so later

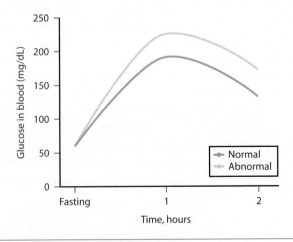

FIGURE 1 Abnormal Glucose Tolerance Curve Compared to a Normal Curve.

before returning to its fasting level. In severe cases of type 2 diabetes, the blood glucose concentration may go down from its peak by only a small amount several hours after a meal. Glucose concentration curves following a regular meal containing a variety of foods, including fiber sources, generally result in a lower peak in healthy individuals, but possibly a slightly more extended (and flatter) peak following because of fiber-induced delays in digestion and absorption.

Hormonal Actions: Insulin and Glucagon

During the period following a meal (or OGTT), the elevated concentration of blood glucose perfuses the beta cells located in the islets of Langerhans of the pancreas and stimulates insulin secretion. In healthy people, the amount of insulin released to the blood is roughly proportional to the rise (or change from fasting level) in the blood glucose concentration. Amino acids derived from a meal containing animal proteins also circulate in the blood at elevated concentrations, but they exert a more modest stimulation of insulin release by islet cells as long as glucose obtained from dietary carbohydrates also is elevated. Thus, a meal containing a potentially large quantity of glucose molecules and a fair amount of amino acids, especially those derived from more rapidly digested animal products, will have additive effects on insulin secretion. A variety of abnormal blood glucose patterns can result if insulin-secreting cells do not function appropriately in response to stimulatory molecules in a meal. Under normal conditions, an increase in insulin leads to an increased uptake of glucose by extrahepatic cells, which have normal numbers of **glucose porters**, or **carriers**, in their cell membranes that facilitate the transport of glucose over the plasma membrane. Therefore, insulin concentrations in blood serum tend to follow the same patterns as serum glucose. **FIGURE 2** is a schematic illustration of porters carrying glucose across the cell membrane.

Glucagon operates largely to oppose the actions of insulin. When blood glucose is low, glucagon is secreted by pancreatic islet alpha (α) cells to increase both hepatic glycogenolysis and gluconeogenesis. Other hormones, such as epinephrine and cortisol, also may be secreted under hypoglycemic conditions in order to increase blood sugar and mount a corrective hormonal response during fasting. Think of glucagon and the

> *Under normal conditions, an increase in insulin leads to an increased uptake of glucose by extrahepatic cells, which have normal numbers of glucose porters or carriers in their cell membranes that facilitate the transport of glucose over the plasma membrane.*

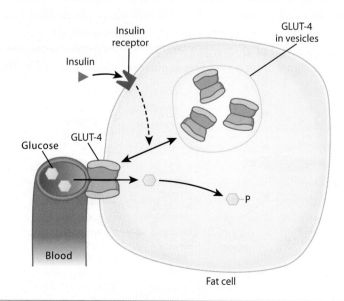

Insulin
Insulin receptor
GLUT-4 in vesicles
Glucose
GLUT-4
Blood
P
Fat cell

FIGURE 2 Transport of Glucose Across the Blood–Brain Barrier. GLUT-4 is a glucose porter or carrier in the membrane that is required for glucose entry.

glucose porter (carrier) A membrane protein that facilitates the transport of glucose across the plasma membrane. GLUT-4 is a glucose porter or carrier in the membrane that is required for glucose entry.

other hormones stimulating an increase in blood glucose as being counter-regulatory to insulin. Insulin tends to lower blood glucose, whereas glucagon and the other hormones tend to raise blood glucose.

Central Role of Peripheral Fat and Muscle Tissue in Insulin Resistance

Adipose (fat) tissue in peripheral regions of the body (e.g., under the skin, in the abdomen, and elsewhere) plays a significant role in the development of type 2 diabetes mellitus. This phenomenon is called peripheral resistance to insulin. The "insulin resistance" of peripheral fat cells, skeletal muscle cells, and other cell types occurs because insulin, the hormone that normally reduces the blood glucose concentration after a meal (or snack or sweet drink), cannot maintain an efficient transfer of glucose molecules from the blood into cells via the glucose porters. Blood glucose concentrations continue to rise above normal levels. Peripheral tissues loaded with fat, especially muscle and adipose cells, resist the stimulation of insulin to enhance glucose uptake by these cells. **FIGURE 3** illustrates the rise in serum insulin concentration that accompanies the increase in serum glucose concentration.

Peripheral resistance to insulin, an adaptive mechanism resulting from excessive fat stores within individual adipocytes and muscle cells, is the major reason for type 2 diabetes. All insulin-responsive cells are probably affected by obesity. Because of their increased size (**hypertrophy**) and increased number (**hyperplasia**), a large mass of fat cells represents a great source of this resistance. Fat cells must take up glucose from blood before they can make new triglycerides. To keep taking up glucose, fat cells must synthesize and then insert the glucose transporters (porters) in their membranes to allow ready glucose entry. When the fat cells become overloaded with triglycerides, they no longer make the transporters and insert them in their membranes for glucose uptake (see **FIGURE 4**). Blood glucose continues to rise, and the serum insulin concentration also increases with continuing body fat accumulation over a time period of years or decades. The blood is said to be rich in glucose, but the fat and muscle cells are poor in glucose.

With sustained insulin resistance, the blood glucose concentration continues to rise, even above the renal threshold (the upper level at which the kidney can reabsorb glucose back to the blood) of approximately 180 to 220 milligrams per deciliter (see **FIGURE 5**). Beyond this serum glucose concentration, some glucose molecules begin to appear in the urine, which is a sign of glucose intolerance. Serum insulin continues to increase in response to the signal of increased serum glucose, which is sensed by the beta cells.

> " Peripheral resistance to insulin, an adaptive mechanism resulting from excessive fat stores within individual adipocytes and muscle cells, is the major reason for type 2 diabetes. "

adipose (fat) tissue Fat storage tissue containing fat cells, or adipocytes, whose function is to store and mobilize fats (triglycerides).

hypertrophy Cells that are larger in size than normal. A characteristic of adipose cells of people with overweight and obesity.

hyperplasia An increase in production of new cells by mitosis (cell division). Common in growing and developing tissues in children and adolescents as well as in the adipose tissue of people with obesity.

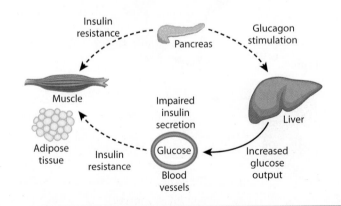

FIGURE 3 Peripheral Resistance to Insulin. Fat cells and muscle cells loaded with triglycerides resist the uptake of glucose. Glucagon release increases when glucose cannot readily enter alpha cells from blood, and the action of glucagon on liver cells is to stimulate both gluconeogenesis and glycogenolysis.

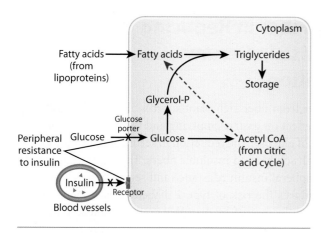

FIGURE 4 Fat Cells Become Insulin Resistant. Glucose cannot enter the overloaded fat cells because of a lack of glucose porters in the cells' outer membranes. Glucose entry into to cells requires a glucose-specific porter in the membrane.

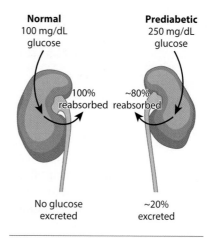

FIGURE 5 Renal Reabsorption of Glucose. Once serum glucose levels exceed the renal threshold of about 200 mg/dL, excess glucose begins to appear in the urine.

As insulin resistance becomes chronic, the beta cells of the pancreatic islet become less responsive to the high blood glucose concentration, hence secreting less and less insulin over time (years to decades). When the pancreatic islet beta cells wear out and can no longer produce insulin, insulin must be given by injection or by pump for survival. This long developing change represents a conversion from type 2 to type 1 diabetes and the need for insulin replacement.

The loss of glucose through the urine, or glycosuria, is accompanied by increased fluid (water) loss, a condition known as polyuria. This condition requires a person to consume more water to maintain the proper osmotic concentration of the blood. People with type 2 diabetes mellitus experience increased thirst and must consume more water to prevent dehydration.

> With sustained insulin resistance, the blood glucose concentration continues to rise, even above the renal threshold (the upper level at which the kidney can reabsorb glucose back to the blood) of approximately 180 to 220 milligrams per deciliter. Beyond this serum glucose concentration, some glucose molecules then begin to appear in the urine, which is a sign of glucose intolerance.

Practical Application 1

Elevation of Blood Sugar After a Meal

For this activity, assume that all the carbohydrates in a fast-food meal are completely digested and absorbed within 30 minutes of finishing a sandwich and shake. The meal contains approximately 100 grams of carbohydrate (assume all glucose) and it is low in fiber. The white roll and sugar (in the shake) are equivalent to the glycemic index of white bread, and these foods provide four equivalents of white bread slices. How much of a rise in serum glucose concentration would you expect to see at maximum peak (~60 minutes after starting to eat) in a young, healthy person who has normal weight (BMI 18.5 to 24.9) if you assume that the individual's fasting glucose prior to the meal was 70 milligrams per deciliter? This estimation applies to both females and males. [Hint: Use 50% of the total amount of carbohydrates as an additive factor to normal fasting blood glucose concentration.] For example, 50 grams of carbohydrate in a meal should increase the serum glucose concentration by 15% to 25% around 60 minutes after the meal is consumed in a healthy, fit young adult. What would the expected blood glucose concentrations be above the baseline value? ■

Benefit of Dietary Fiber in Reducing the Postprandial Rise in Serum Glucose Concentration

The consumption of dietary fiber from fiber-rich plant sources along with starch and sugars has a significant slowing effect on gastric emptying and the intestinal digestion of carbohydrates and absorption of glucose. The reduction in serum glucose concentration after a meal results from both soluble and insoluble fibers. This significant benefit has lowering effects on both peripheral insulin resistance and serum hemoglobin A1c concentration and, therefore, reduces the risk of type 2 diabetes onset. Hemoglobin A1c concentration also can be slightly lowered by diets that contain sufficient fiber.

Arterial Damage from High Blood Glucose

Type 2 diabetes develops slowly, typically over 5 to 10 years. However, this time frame may be reduced in children and adolescents, depending on the severity of excessive calorie consumption, bad eating habits, limited physical activity, and genetic factors.

If the blood glucose concentration becomes significantly elevated throughout the day (24 hours), and not just postprandially, pathologic changes will occur in the arteries. Recall that the gradual elevation of the serum glucose concentration is a result of the peripheral resistance to insulin primarily of fat cells and muscle cells. A consequence of elevated serum glucose concentration is **glycation** of tissue proteins, especially the proteins of arterial walls. Glycation is a nonenzymatic chemical reaction in which glucose binds to proteins in blood or tissue. This binding with glucose reduces the proteins' ability to function. This reaction is responsible for the degradation observed in arterial walls, especially those in the eyes, kidneys, and brain.

The long-term effects of high blood glucose levels include kidney failure, resulting in the need for dialysis treatment. Also, two types of serious damage resulting from glycation occur in other tissues: diabetic **retinopathy**, which may eventually cause blindness, and diabetic **neuropathy**, which may result in amputations of toes or the lower leg. These adverse effects stem from glycation of proteins in the small arteries and capillaries of the kidneys, eyes, and nerves. People with either type of diabetes mellitus are at much higher risk of both stroke and heart disease due to damage to the larger arteries of the heart and brain and the strong tendency to have increased blood pressure and higher blood cholesterol levels. In addition to these risks, people with diabetes often have other clinical dysfunctions. Glycation of proteins is detected clinically by the measurement of the amount of red blood cell hemoglobin bound to glucose (a hemoglobin A1c quantitative score). This measurement can determine the long-term effects of too high a concentration of serum glucose that results in glycation—an excellent marker!

Prevention of Type 2 Diabetes: Dietary and Exercise Recommendations

The best way to prevent type 2 diabetes is to maintain a healthy body weight (i.e., a BMI of 18.5 to 25) and to remain physically active. In addition to maintaining a healthy weight and an active lifestyle, caloric distribution of the diet should approximate the usual intake percentages (see **Table 1**). Carbohydrate intake at the lower limit (45%) may have a better preventive effect as part of a total reduction of caloric intake. In fact, excessive carbohydrate consumption may be more critical than excessive dietary fat in packing on the pounds that produce obesity and then diabetes!

> *If the blood glucose concentration becomes significantly elevated throughout the day (24 hours), and not just postprandially, pathologic changes will occur in the arteries.*

glycation A nonenzymatic chemical reaction in which glucose binds to proteins in blood or tissue, reducing the proteins' ability to function.

retinopathy A complication of diabetes that affects the eyes. It is caused by damage to the blood vessels of the light-sensitive tissue at the back of the eye (retina).

neuropathy A complication of diabetes caused by damage to the nerve fibers by high blood sugar. Most often damages nerves in the legs or feet, resulting in pain or numbness of the extremities.

TABLE 1
Dietary Recommendations for Diabetes Prevention

Nutrient Variable	Percentage of Total Calories	Comments
Energy	—	Achieve/maintain BMI in the normal range of 18.5–25.
Carbohydrate	45–55%	Consume complex carbohydrates with dietary fiber (little processed food). Reduce intake of sugar-rich juices and drinks.
Fat	15–30%	Consume low-fat dairy foods and reduce saturated and trans fats. Include sufficient mono- and polyunsaturated fatty acids, especially omega-3s.
Protein	15–18%	Reduce the number of servings of meat/fish/poultry by one to two per day. Increase legumes by 1 to 2 servings per day.
Alcohol	—	Only one drink per day for women or two drinks per day for men.
Dietary fiber	—	Consume ≥ 30 g per day from a variety of plant sources (legumes, whole grains, nuts, seeds, vegetables, and fruits)
Cholesterol	—	Consume ≤ 300 mg per day. Reduce consumption of animal foods.
Micronutrients	—	Consume five or more servings of fruits and vegetables per day (minimum), especially fresh citrus fruits and dark green, leafy vegetables.

Additionally, an optimal diet should be moderate in starches (complex carbohydrates) and dietary fibers and contain several servings each of fruits and vegetables (see Table 1). Ideally, it should include only limited amounts of processed foods. Thus, an optimal diet should be low in saturated fats (with no trans fats), animal proteins, salt, sugars (except naturally occurring ones present in dairy products and fruits), and alcohol, which contains largely "empty" calories. Avoidance of excessive amounts of fruit juice and other sugar-containing juices and beverages is recommended because of the high amounts of glucose in them. This wholesome diet not only may act to prevent the development of type 2 diabetes but also may offer protection against cancer, high blood pressure, arterial disease, and heart disease. The antidiabetic diet is one of the best all-round diets for all people.

> *The antidiabetic diet is one of the best all-round diets for all people.*

In addition to diet modification, an increase in physical activity is an equally important component in the prevention of type 2 diabetes. Participation in a regular exercise program for a minimum of 30 minutes most days of the week helps to reduce weight over a period of weeks and improves the effectiveness of insulin in moving glucose into skeletal muscle, fat tissue, and other tissues. The combination of these two approaches—diet and exercise—can be successful in reducing blood sugar and improving cell functions.

The key to reducing the risk of type 2 diabetes remains the maintenance of body weight in the normal range of BMI through dietary modification, portion control, and a regular exercise program.

Medical and Dietary Treatment of Type 2 Diabetes Mellitus

The focus in this text is on prevention rather than treatment, but a few comments about specific therapies are needed. Control of blood sugar requires major dietary modifications, but other treatments, especially drugs, may be needed.

> **With moderate caloric restriction, intake may be reduced only to 1,200 to 1,600 kilocalories per day, depending on the individual's sex, height, and weight.**

> **A loss of body weight (and its maintenance) typically indicates that the body is better able to handle glucose.**

hypocaloric weight-loss diet A diet low in calories (usually 1,200 to 1,600 kilocalories) that is followed for the purpose of weight reduction.

gradual weight loss Weight loss of 1 pound or so per week, based on decreasing daily intake by 500 kilocalories per day for 7 days, or 3,500 kilocalories.

The vast majority of people with type 2 diabetes are overweight or obese. Weight loss and regular physical activity can help regulate blood glucose levels and often eliminate the need for drug treatment of patients with type 2 diabetes. Comprehensive obesity treatment programs typically employ a combination of diet modification, physical activity, and behavior modification strategies. With moderate caloric restriction, intake may be reduced only to 1,200 to 1,600 kilocalories per day, depending on the individual's sex, height, and weight. Fat should be reduced on any low-calorie diet. A well-planned **hypocaloric weight-loss diet** at this daily caloric level (1,200 to 1,600 kilocalories) can provide the necessary nutrients and will usually result in **gradual weight loss** (1 pound or so per week, based on decreasing daily intake by 500 kilocalories per day for 7 days or 3,500 kilocalories, which is the calorie deficit required to lose 1 pound). Physical activities need to be tailored to the abilities of the individual and supervision may be required.

Typically, patients with type 2 diabetes are allowed to consume foods according to their own preferences, but are asked to keep carbohydrates at less than 50%, the same as those overweight or with obesity. Patients are instructed to count the number of carbohydrate servings each day and to keep the total at or below the allowable limit, depending on their weight (or BMI) and gender. A loss of body weight (and its maintenance) typically indicates that the body is better able to handle glucose. A decline of hemoglobin A1c, resulting from less binding of glucose, assures that the effects of the disease are also lessened. Long-term success of dietary modifications depends on the motivation and adherence to healthy eating practices, but most patients require drug therapy to achieve improvements in health.

Pharmacologic (drug) therapy is widely used in the treatment of severe type 2 diabetes when diet alone or diet and exercise become ineffective in keeping both blood glucose and hemoglobin A1c levels in the healthy ranges. Oral hypoglycemic drugs that help glucose molecules enter cells more efficiently are the first-line drugs in treatment. If these are not sufficiently effective in regulating blood glucose, then insulin injections or infusions (pump) may be needed.

Dietary approaches to improved glucose control with type 2 diabetes should be tried first, but drugs typically are necessary. Diet therapy usually requires long periods for the

FOCUS 1   Hemoglobin A1c

When the serum glucose concentration at baseline becomes greater than approximately 100 mg per dL, some glucose molecules become attached chemically (nonenzymatically) to circulating hemoglobin in red blood cells. The binding of glucose to a protein, including hemoglobin, is called glycation. At baseline serum glucose values of roughly 70 mg/dL, binding is normally about 5 units, but at a serum glucose of 100 mg/dL, the hemoglobin A1c binding increases to 5.5 to 6. At serum glucose concentrations greater than 120 mg/dL, hemoglobin A1c is typically greater than 6, a prediabetes condition. Once the hemoglobin A1c level is greater than 6.5, an individual enters the diabetic state from prediabetes. The hemoglobin A1c is a long-term marker of glucose status because its concentration changes little from day to day, but over a period of weeks to months it can be reduced by improved dietary selections and reduced amounts of foods consumed. If the hemoglobin A1c concentration continues to remain high or even increases above 7.0, the treatment of type 2 diabetes requires drugs to try to enhance glucose tolerance and to prevent arterial damage. ●

effective modification of eating patterns and gaining nutrition knowledge that contributes to the general improvement of health status. Drugs generally work much faster, but they have side effects. To obtain successful dietary modification, especially the acceptance of more plant foods in the diet, patients need to be willing to modify their diets. Health professionals, especially dietitians and diabetes educators, are needed to serve as change agents for motivated patients.

SUMMARY

Carbohydrates provide the bulk of energy in the form of starches and sugars. Dietary fiber provides no energy and influences the gastrointestinal digestion and absorption of glucose (and other monosaccharides) by slowing down each process and thereby slowing the entry of glucose from the intestine to blood after the meal (i.e., postprandial period). The rise in blood glucose following a meal stimulates the release of insulin, which, in turn, lowers the serum glucose concentration under normal conditions. The control of blood glucose is critical for the prevention or delay of the onset of type 2 diabetes.

Obesity, and the inactivity that often accompanies it, is the major predisposing factor for the development of type 2 diabetes because of the resistance of fat and muscle cells to the normal action of insulin that begins in a prediabetic state. Type 2 diabetes is a chronic disease affecting millions of U.S. adults. It contributes to mortality, especially as a contributing factor to heart disease and strokes. Hyperglycemia and glycosuria result from the abnormally altered metabolism of glucose, the major fuel source for the body's cells. The pathologic consequences of type 2 diabetes are caused by damage from high blood glucose concentrations in the arteries of susceptible organs, such as the eyes and kidneys. Prevention and treatment of type 2 diabetes primarily focus on weight loss, reasonable dietary modifications, and regular exercise.

STUDENT ACTIVITIES

1. Using the current definitions of BMI, define overweight and obesity. Which macronutrient contributes the most to enlarged fat cell storage of triglycerides?

2. Describe the biological process by which fat cells may increase in size (and possibly number) in the body over extended periods.

3. Diagram normal blood glucose responses after (a) consumption of sugar only and (b) consumption of starch only. How might the addition of a considerable amount of fiber to the starch affect the blood glucose response?

4. List the three abnormalities in glucose metabolism in the body that occur in type 2 diabetes mellitus.

5. Define glycation. How does glycation of proteins affect the body?

6. Hemoglobin A1c is a blood marker for poor serum glucose control. Explain why this marker is helpful.

7. Describe abnormal (impaired) glucose tolerance in terms of serum glucose concentration. Define insulin resistance and mention the role of glucose porters in insulin resistance.

8. Which specific cell types shut down the effectiveness of insulin activity when serum glucose remains elevated, as in type 2 diabetes or prediabetes.

9. Explain why type 2 diabetes may be so critical to the development of arterial damage and the specific organ complications of this disease in its continued development.

10. Create a table with two columns. In the left-hand column, list the dietary risk factors for type 2 diabetes mellitus. In the right-hand column, give a short explanation of how each may contribute to the development of type 2 diabetes mellitus.

WEBSITES FOR FURTHER STUDY

American Diabetes Association
www.diabetes.org/home.jsp
Diabetes on Medline Plus
www.nlm.nih.gov/medlineplus/diabetesmellitus.html
Type 2 Diabetes from Mayo Clinic
www.mayoclinic.com/health/type-2-diabetes/DS00585

National Institute of Diabetes and Digestive and Kidney Diseases
www2.niddk.nih.gov
Type 2 Diabetes on WebMD
http://diabetes.webmd.com

REFERENCES

Alberti KG, Eckel RH, Grundy SM, et al. Harmonizing the metabolic syndrome: a joint interim statement of the International Diabetes Federation Task Force on Epidemiology and Prevention; National Heart, Lung, and Blood Institute; American Heart Association; World Heart Federation; International Atherosclerosis Society; and International Association for the Study of Obesity. *Circulation.* 2009;120:1640–1645.

American Diabetes Association. Standards of medical care in diabetes—2012. *Diabetes Care.* 2012;35(supp 1):11S–63S.

Jaaks LM, Wylie-Rosett J, Mayer-Davis EJ. Diabetes. In: Erdman JW Jr, MacDonald IA, Zeisel SH, eds. *Present Knowledge in Nutrition.* 10th ed. Ames, IA: John Wiley & Sons; 2012;1278–1320.

Reaven GM. Role of insulin resistance in human disease: Banting Lecture 1988. *Diabetes.* 1988;37:1595–1607.

CHAPTER 6

Fats and Other Lipids

Fats, which are also referred to as triglycerides, are important energy sources in the human diet, comprising approximately 35% of total caloric intake. In addition to providing energy in their numerous C-H bonds, fats also supply different types of fatty acids, including essential polyunsaturated fatty acids. This chapter reviews the various categories of fats and provides information on the energy pathways of triglycerides.

Fats fit into the broad category of molecules known as **lipids**. A lipid is a molecule that can be extracted from a tissue with an organic solvent, but not with water. Lipids are considered to be **lipophilic** ("lover of fats," or fat-soluble molecules), as opposed to **hydrophilic** ("lover of water," or water-soluble molecules). Lipids represent a large class of molecules. Triglycerides are the major focus of this chapter, but phospholipids, cholesterol, steroids, and lipoproteins also are important lipids (see **Table 6.1**). All of these molecules are soluble in organic solvents. Many different types of lipids have diverse functions in the human body, but only those with major nutritional roles and adverse effects are covered in this chapter.

Foods high in fat include butter, margarine, and vegetable oils (see **FIGURE 6.1**). Many processed foods, such as desserts, cheese products, and luncheon meats, also contain "hidden" saturated fats that may contribute to cardiovascular diseases. Because fat intake has been implicated in the rise in overweight and obesity, food manufacturers have generated many low-fat or light (lite) products and fat substitutes, which are briefly noted in this chapter.

Basic Structures of Fatty Acids and Triglycerides

The C-H bonds of fats, as in carbohydrates, are one of the primary sources of energy in the human diet. **Triglycerides** are composed of fatty acids. Triglycerides, a subclass of lipids, come in a greater variety of structures than carbohydrates. A common triglyceride called triacylglycerol is composed of a glycerol molecule with three fatty acids attached (see **FIGURE 6.2**). The fatty acids in foods are typically long chains of

> " A lipid is a molecule that can be extracted from a tissue with an organic solvent, but not with water. "

fat A type of lipid molecule. Another name for triglyceride molecules containing glycerol and three fatty acids. The fatty acid composition determines whether it is solid or liquid at room temperature.

lipid A broad class of water-insoluble molecules that includes triglycerides, phospholipids, cholesterol, steroids, eicosanoids, waxes, fat-soluble vitamins, and many phytomolecules.

lipophilic Adjective that means "love of fats." Used to refer to fat- or lipid-soluble molecules or the portion of an organic molecule that is attracted to fat.

hydrophilic An adjective that means "love of water." Refers to the portion of an organic molecule that is attracted to water, such as the organic acid (COOH) portion of fatty acids and amino acids.

triglyceride A triacylglycerol or fat that contains glycerol linked to three fatty acids by ester bonds.

TABLE 6.1
Lipids: Fat-Soluble Molecules with Unique Functions

Fat-Soluble Molecules	Function
Fatty acids	Energy source, component of triglycerides and phospholipids, precursor of eicosanoids
Triglycerides	Energy storage in adipose tissue
Phospholipids	Major component of membrane bilayers, intracellular regulatory molecules
Cholesterol	Component of membranes, precursor for vitamin D and steroid hormones
Cholesterol Esters	Transportation and storage forms of cholesterol
Bile Acids and Bile Salts	Detergent function to aid fat digestion
Steroids	Sex hormones, adrenocortical hormones
Lipoproteins	Lipid transport in blood
Sterols	Chemical class to which cholesterol and phytosterols belong
Phytosterols	Sterol molecules in plant cell membranes
Fatty alcohols	Energy reserve and thermal insulator
Waxes	Sealant and protective molecule in plant walls
Eicosanoids	Hormones and tissue factors

Adapted from Anderson JJB. *Nutrition and Health: An Introduction.* Carolina Academic Press, Durham, NC, 2005. Figure 26-03, p. 492.

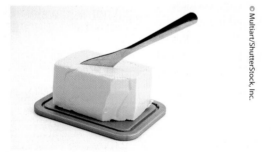
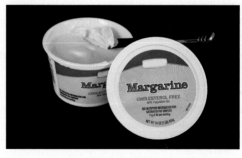
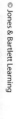
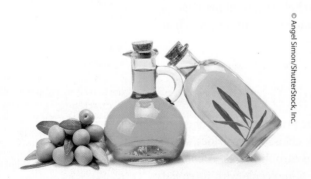
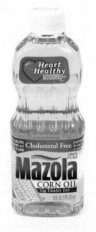

FIGURE 6.1 High-Fat Foods. Foods high in fat include butter, margarine, and vegetable oils.

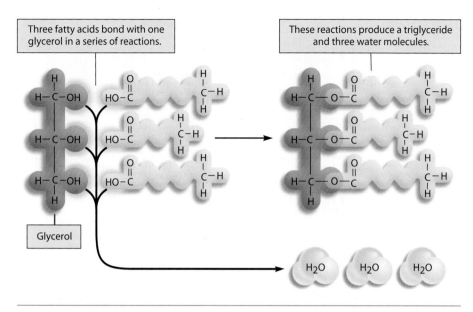

Three fatty acids bond with one glycerol in a series of reactions.

These reactions produce a triglyceride and three water molecules.

Glycerol

H_2O H_2O H_2O

FIGURE 6.2 Triglyceride Structure. Triacylglycerol is a simple fatty acid composed of glycerol plus three fatty acids.

carbon and hydrogen; these hydrocarbon chains are usually 16 to 20 carbons in length. The acid portion (or carboxyl group) of each fatty acid attaches to the hydroxyl (OH) groups of glycerol. Keep in mind that glycerol is a short-chain carbohydrate with three carbon atoms. Fatty acids in foods have about twice as many C-H bonds as are found in carbohydrates, and they therefore provide about twice as much energy per gram—9 kilocalories per gram (Atwater equivalent). The distinguishing characteristic of fats is that they are not water soluble; they are **hydrophobic**, which means that they are repelled by water. This physical property leads to the unique chemistry of fat digestion and transport of fats into the blood, which is a watery medium, and through the circulation.

Saturated, Monounsaturated, and Polyunsaturated Fatty Acids

Three major types of fatty acids are derived from plant and animal fats: saturated, monounsaturated, and polyunsaturated. These three types of fatty acids have different properties. Most of the fatty acids in our diets and in our bodies are more than 12 carbons in length and are referred to as long-chain fatty acids. A **saturated fatty acid (SFA)** has the full complement of hydrogen (H) atoms per carbon (C) atom in the hydrocarbon part of the molecule. Some fatty acids have carbon-to-carbon double bonds. Because these **double bonds** result in a fatty acid having less than its full complement of hydrogen atoms, it is referred to as an **unsaturated fatty acid (UFA)**. Those unsaturated fatty acids with only one double bond are called **monounsaturated fatty acids (MFAs or MUFAs)** and those with multiple (two or more) double bonds are called **polyunsaturated fatty acids (PFAs or PUFAs)** (see **FIGURE 6.3**).

Polyunsaturated fatty acids are important for human health. Humans are unable to synthesize a double bond at the third or the sixth carbon from the terminal carbon—the omega (n) end of the hydrocarbon—of fatty acids. **Omega-3 (n-3)** and **omega-6 (n-6) fatty acids** are essential fatty acids because, like vitamins, they are essential for human life, they cannot be made by the body, and they must be obtained from the diet.

Saturated fatty acids are common in animal products such as dairy products, meats, and poultry (see **FIGURE 6.4**). Monounsaturated fatty acids are present in large amounts

hydrophobic An adjective that means "fear of water." Refers to the portion of an organic molecule that is repelled by water, such as the hydrocarbon chain of fatty acids and amino acids.

saturated fatty acids (SFAs) Fatty acids with no double bonds (and no points of unsaturation). Common in meat and dairy products; excess consumption has been found to be a dietary risk factor for heart disease.

double bond A type of carbon-to-carbon atomic bond that involves two bonds (C=C) rather than one (C-C). Represents a point of unsaturation with respect to hydrogen atoms in a hydrocarbon.

unsaturated fatty acids (UFAs) Mono- or polyunsaturated fatty acids. The double bonds in these molecules represent points of unsaturated carbon atoms with respect to hydrogen atoms. The double bonds of monounsaturated fatty acids (MFAs) and polyunsaturated fatty acids (PFAs) are subject to oxidative attack by free radicals.

monounsaturated fatty acids (MFAs) Fatty acids with one point of unsaturation (double bond), usually at omega-9 position. Olive oil is a good source of MFA.

polyunsaturated fatty acids (PFAs or PUFAs) Fatty acids containing two or more double bonds (points of unsaturation). Two types exist in plants and animals: omega-6 and omega-3.

omega-3 (n-3) fatty acids Subclass of essential polyunsaturated fatty acids (PFAs) whose first double bond begins at the third carbon from the end (omega-3) in the hydrocarbon chain.

omega-6 (n-6) fatty acids Subclass of essential polyunsaturated fatty acids (PFAs) whose first double bond begins at the sixth carbon from the end (omega-6) in the hydrocarbon chain.

Type of fatty acid   **Name and chemical structure**

Saturated

Stearic acid

Monounsaturated

Oleic acid

Polyunsaturated

Linoleic acid

FIGURE 6.3 Fatty Acids. Fatty acids can be saturated, monounsaturated, or polyunsaturated.

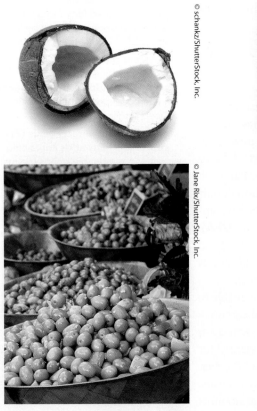

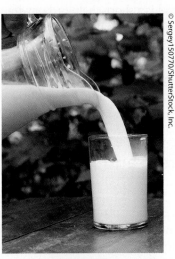

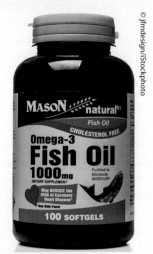

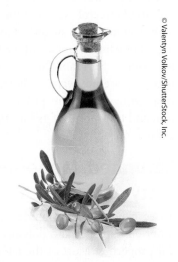

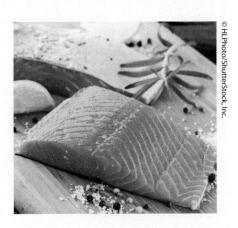

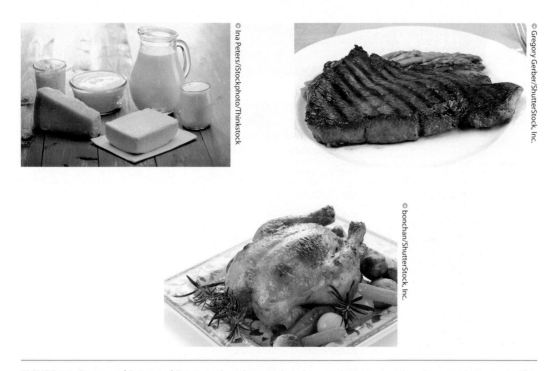

FIGURE 6.4 Sources of Saturated Fat. Animal products, such as dairy products, meat, and poultry, are rich in saturated fat.

in plant oils, such as in olive oil and canola oil, and in certain nuts. The polyunsaturated omega-3 fatty acids are found in some plant oils, such as flax seed oil, and in cold-water fish, such as salmon. Corn oil is rich in omega-6 fatty acids. All fatty acids with the same number of C-H bonds, whether saturated or unsaturated, generate the same amount of energy (ATP).

Polyunsaturated fatty acids that are 20 carbons or more in length, including both omega-3 and omega-6 fatty acids, can be converted into two different families of local tissue factors (hormone-like molecules) known as eicosanoids. **Eicosanoids** operate in many short-term signaling pathways in the body. Because of their differences in chemical structure, fats from different dietary sources (see **FIGURE 6.5**) often have different physical properties. **Table 6.2** lists various fatty acids, their sources, and the number of carbons they contain.

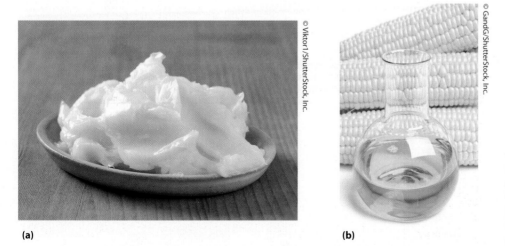

(a)

(b)

eicosanoids The general name of hormone molecules derived from specific 20-carbon (eicosa-) polyunsaturated fatty acids. Examples include arachidonic acid (AA, C20:4) found in vegetable oils and eicosapentaenoic acid (EPA, C20:5) found in fish oils.

FIGURE 6.5 Physical Properties of Fats. Because of the physical properties of different types of fats, some fats, such as lard (a) are solid at room temperature. Others, such as vegetable oils (b), are liquid.

TABLE 6.2
Common Fatty Acids, Their Food Sources, and Number of Carbons

Common Name	Food Sources	Number of Carbons: Number of Double Bonds (First Double Bond)
Capric	Milk, coconut	10:0
Lauric	Milk, coconut	12:0
Myristic	Milk, coconut	14:0
Palmitic	Milk and meat	16:0
Palmitoleic	Animal fat	16:1(n-9)
Stearic	Animal fat	18:0
Oleic	Olive oil	18:1(n-9)
Linoleic	Corn oil	18:2(n-6)[a]
α-Linolenic	Soybean oil	18:3(n-3)[b]
Arachidonic	Animal fat	20:4(n-6)
Eicosopentaenoic	Fish oil	20:5(n-3)
Docosahexaenoic	Fish oil	22:6(n-3)

[a] n-6, omega-6 polyunsaturated fatty acids.
[b] n-3, omega-3 polyunsaturated fatty acids.
Reproduced from Anderson JJB. *Nutrition and Health: An Introduction.* Durham, NC: Carolina Academic Press; 2005.

Trans Fats

Industrial food processing also produces an additional form of fatty acid, known as trans fatty acids, or simply trans fats, in the human diet (see **FIGURE 6.6**). The industrial process that produces trans fatty acids is **hydrogenation**, which is the addition

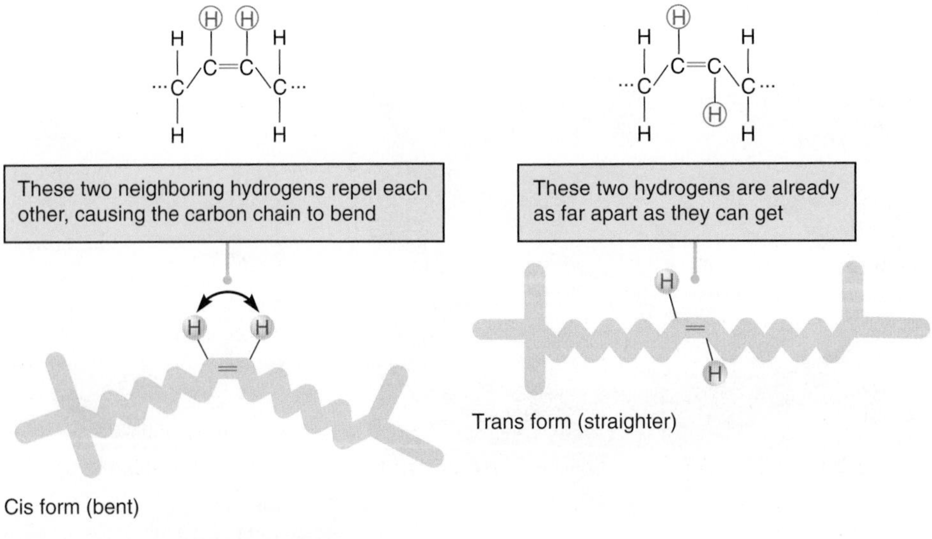

These two neighboring hydrogens repel each other, causing the carbon chain to bend

These two hydrogens are already as far apart as they can get

Cis form (bent)

Trans form (straighter)

hydrogenation The addition of hydrogen (H) atoms to double bonds, or points of unsaturation, in a hydrocarbon. This industrial process is usually done by passing hydrogen gas through liquid vegetable oils.

FIGURE 6.6 Fatty Acid Configuration. A *cis* fatty acid versus a *trans* fatty acid. Two different hydrocarbon conformations are possible around one double bond (one point of unsaturation) in the fatty acid molecule.

FOCUS 6.1   Food Oils and Fats

The fat in beef or pork is solid even at room temperature, whereas the fat extracted from corn and vegetables exists as a liquid (oil) at room temperature. The reason for this difference is the structure of the fatty acids in these foods. Animal fat is largely composed of long, straight-chain saturated fatty acids (see **Figure A**). These molecules nest together when cooled, like a stack of teaspoons, and readily form crystalline solids. The polyunsaturated fatty acids in corn oil and the monounsaturated fatty acids in olive oil have kinks in their long chains and become tangled instead of nesting as they cool. Therefore, they have to be cooled to quite a low temperature before becoming solids (i.e., converting from the liquid to the solid state). Even when kept in a refrigerator, corn oil does not solidify, though it becomes a bit hazy. These differences in properties can be drawn directly from an understanding of the diverse chemical structures of the constituent fatty acids. ●

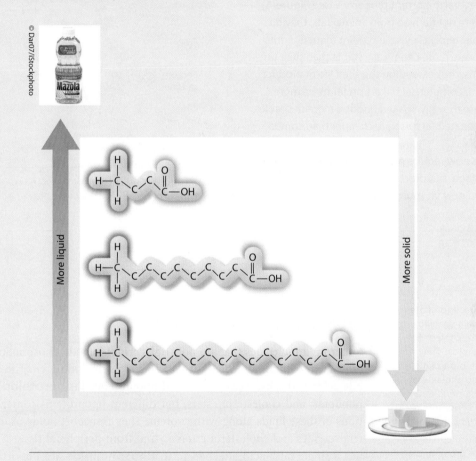

© Dar07/iStockphoto

FIGURE A   Effect of Fatty Acid Length on Transition of Fats from Liquid to Solid. As the chain length of saturated fatty acids increases, fats tend to becomes more solid at room temperature.

of hydrogen atoms. Trans fats result from the conversion of liquid polyunsaturated fatty acids to solid trans fats at room temperature. Trans fatty acids have an unusual unsaturated hydrocarbon configuration (i.e., *trans* form versus the normal *cis* form) such that they have chemical properties similar to saturated fatty acids. Because of this, they contribute to the development of atherosclerosis because their breakdown is more rapid than that of cis monounsaturated fatty acids, which bend back at the position of the double bond.

FOCUS 6.2 Hydrogenation

Partially hydrogenated oils were previously found in baked goods, snack foods, fried foods, margarines and shortening but are now banned from use in processed foods. The industrial food process that forms trans fats is called hydrogenation because it involves adding hydrogen atoms to unsaturated bonds to saturate them. The newly saturated fatty acids, and the small amount of trans fat produced as a byproduct, exist in a semisolid state. Margarines typically contain some trans fat. For food processors, these new fats have several important properties (see **Figure A**). Because they were not derived from animal fats, they do not contain cholesterol, a key selling point for margarine. In addition, they are more chemically stable than their unsaturated cousins, thus extending the shelf life of products containing them. Commercial bakers prefer these more solid fats because they give baked goods a more desirable texture. Hydrogenated fats also are cheaper than comparable animal fats.

Food labels now require processors to list the amount of trans fat in a food, but practically all food manufacturers have substituted new fat sources in products previously containing trans fats because of the adverse effects of trans fats on cholesterol and cardiovascular health. ●

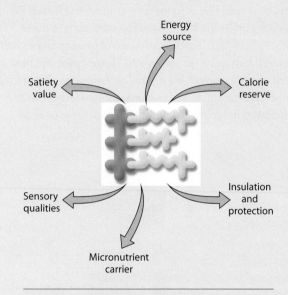

FIGURE A The Functions of Triglycerides. Fat performs a number of essential functions in the body.

---

lipoproteins Complex aggregates or particles that contain specific proteins, triglycerides, cholesterol esters, and phospholipids. They transport lipids in the blood and carry triglycerides and cholesterol esters to and from the peripheral tissues. The modified lipoproteins are taken up (cleared) by liver cells.

phospholipid A molecule that contains a phosphate group and a fat component.

cholesterol A lipid consisting of a characteristic four-ringed sterol structure that is used by the body for many functions. It is used either as is or after modification to cholic acid and other bile acids, steroid hormones, vitamin D, and other structures. Cholesterol can be produced by most cells and also obtained in the diet from animal products. Serum levels are routinely monitored because of linkage of high serum cholesterol with heart disease.

Other Lipid Molecules

Other lipid molecules that are not triglycerides include phospholipids; cholesterol (in ester form with an attached fatty acid); sterols, including vitamin D; steroids; waxes; bile acids and salts; eicosanoids; and lipoproteins. **Lipoproteins** contain fats, phospholipids, and cholesterol esters, but different lipoproteins contain different proportions of these lipids along with protein. They transport lipids in the blood and carry triglycerides and cholesterol esters to and from peripheral tissues. A cholesterol ester has a single fatty acid attached to it. **Phospholipids** are important components of cell membranes, containing a phosphate group and fat component (see **FIGURE 6.7**). **Cholesterol** has a four-ringed sterol structure and is a starting molecule for a variety of fat-soluble products in the body, including bile salts, steroid hormones, and vitamins (see **FIGURE 6.8**). Memorization of the structure of these compounds is not necessary, but it is important to understand how their conformations support their different roles in the human body.

Cholesterol and Phytosterols

Cholesterol, a type of lipid, is not used as an energy source. Cholesterol has four attached carbon rings, and serves as the starting molecule for the synthesis of sex hormones, adrenal steroids, vitamin D, and bile acids (see Figure 6.8). Cholesterol is found only in animals, and it is a major structural component of normal animal cell membranes.

Dietary cholesterol is obtained in modest amounts from membranes of meat, but it is richest in liver and other animal organs. Excessive consumption of cholesterol-containing foods can increase human serum cholesterol concentrations. Along with fat, cholesterol builds up in the arteries. Over time, this buildup can cause **atheromas** (fatty deposits) in arteries that can lead to **atherosclerosis**. This condition is characterized by plaque buildup in the arterial walls that interferes and even blocks blood flow through the vessels (leading to cardiovascular disease). Cholesterol may increase the risk of heart disease when its total concentration is high. Because cholesterol is a component of cell membranes, simply removing the visible fat from meat, though a healthy practice for lowering the intake of total fat, does not lower the meat's cholesterol content.

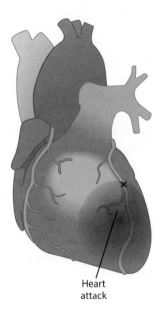

Heart attack

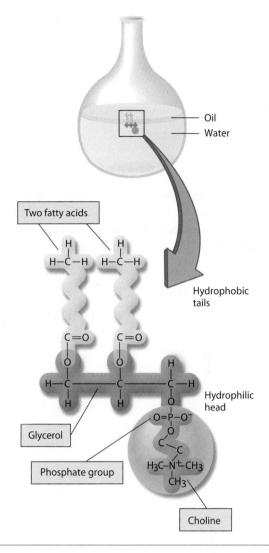

FIGURE 6.7 Phospholipids. Lecithin, also known as phosphatidylcholine, is a common phospholipid. It has glycerol plus two fatty acids and one phosphate linked to an organic base known as choline. Note the position of lecithin at the interface between the oil (hydrophobic tails) and water (hydrophilic head) layers.

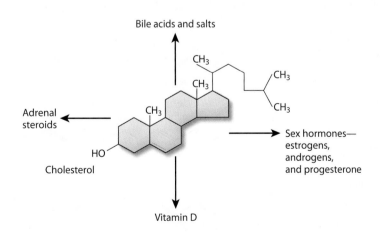

FIGURE 6.8 Cholesterol and Molecules Made from Cholesterol. A variety of complex molecules is formed from cholesterol, including sex hormones, adrenal hormones, vitamin D, and bile acids.

atheroma A fatty deposit (or plaque) on the wall of an artery or arteriole formed as part of the atherosclerotic process; less advanced in development than an atherosclerotic lesion. It is similar to a fatty streak but more defined.

atherosclerosis An early form of arteriosclerosis characterized by plaques or lipid accumulations (atheromas) in the arterial wall; any such lesion can become sufficiently extensive to interfere with or even to block blood flow through the vessel, causing a clot (thrombus) to form at the site of obstruction. Plaques contain cholesterol, triglycerides, other fatty molecules, and tissue debris, including mineralizations.

Plants make sterols for their membranes known as **phytosterols**, which are in the same chemical family as cholesterol. The phytosterols consumed in plant products are similar in structure and function to cholesterol, but when consumed they do not elevate the serum cholesterol concentration, but rather lower it.

PRACTICAL APPLICATIONS 6.1

Cholesterol Content of Foods

Create a table with three columns. In the first column, list three animal-based foods and three plant-based foods that you eat frequently. In the second column, place a checkmark beside each food that contains cholesterol.

In the third column, record the amount of cholesterol in a serving of that food. Consult a food composition table or ChooseMyPlate.gov to obtain the cholesterol information about the six foods you have selected. ■

Phospholipids

Phospholipids are partially water-soluble lipids that also serve as functional components of membranes and lipoproteins. They are similar in chemical structure to triglycerides in that they have a glycerol "backbone" to which two fatty acids are attached. In place of the third fatty acid of triglycerides, phospholipids contain ionized phosphate and one nitrogen-containing component (base), which helps make them more water soluble. One of these nitrogen-containing bases is choline, which combines to make phosphatidylcholine, also known as lecithin (see Figure 6.7). After digestion, the two fatty acids of phospholipids are metabolized in the same way as those in triglycerides.

Eicosanoids

Eicosanoids are local factors or hormones that act in practically all tissues of the body. Essential polyunsaturated fatty acids are used to synthesize eicosanoid molecules that act as hormones very close to where they are synthesized (i.e., locally). Omega-6 fatty acids, represented by arachidonic acid, and omega-3 fatty acids, represented by both eicosapentaenoic acid (EPA) and docosahexaenoic acid (DHA), are precursors of two different types of eicosanoids (see **FIGURE 6.9**). A balance between these two types of polyunsaturated fatty acids in the diet is considered healthy because they are *not* interchangeable in the body. An optimal dietary ratio has not been established, but some

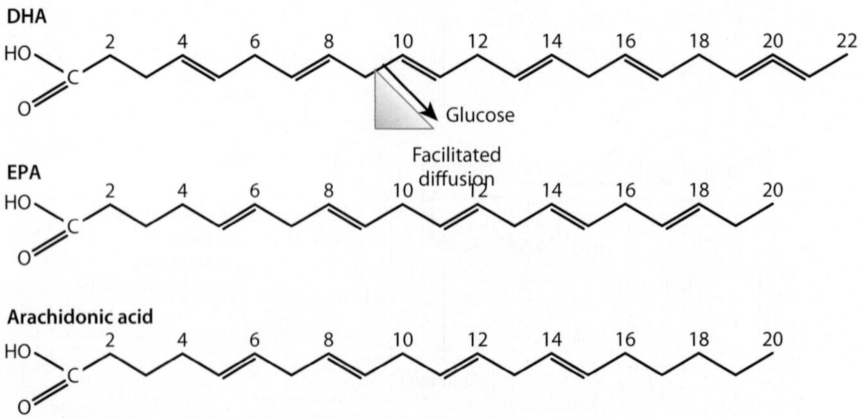

phytosterol A type of sterol made by plants that is in the same chemical family as cholesterol. However, unlike cholesterol, phytosterols do not elevate serum cholesterol concentrations when consumed.

FIGURE 6.9 Precursors to Eicosanoids. The dietary omega-3 (DHA and EPA) and omega-6 arachidonic fatty acids are modified to produce eicosanoids.

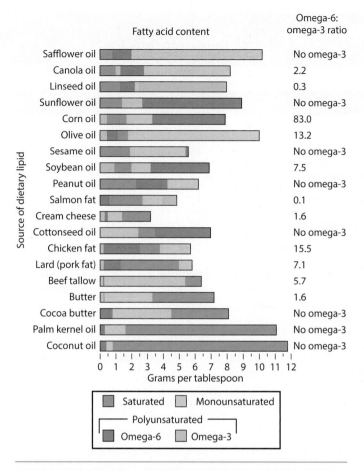

FIGURE 6.10 Ratio of Omega-6 to Omega-3 Fatty Acids in Different Foods. Less healthy foods have a omega-6 to omega-3 ratio of greater than 10:1. Healthier foods have ratios of less than 10:1.

Data from GBI Healthwatch.

researchers suggest that a 10 to 1 ratio of omega-6 to omega-3 is healthy, whereas others think the ratio should be as low as 4 to 1. **FIGURE 6.10** illustrates healthy and less healthy ratios in different foods.

Lipoproteins

Lipoproteins are essential molecular complexes that enable fat-soluble molecules to be transferred around the body in a water-based medium (i.e., blood). These small complexes consist of proteins, phospholipids, triglycerides, cholesterol, and a few other lipid-soluble molecules. The major components of lipoproteins relate to their different functions (see **Table 6.3**).

Lipoproteins are classified according to their density, which is directly related to how much protein (i.e., heavy components) and triglycerides (i.e., light components) they carry. **High-density lipoproteins (HDLs)** made by the liver have the greatest protein-to-lipid ratio, the smallest diameter, and the greatest density. **Very low density lipoproteins (VLDLs)** made by the liver have a low ratio of protein-to-lipid content, are less dense, and are also triglyceride rich. **Low-density lipoproteins (LDLs)** are intermediate in density between HDL and VLDL, and they carry most of the cholesterol. Triglyceride-rich chylomicrons are even less dense and are much larger than VLDLs. Chylomicrons have the greatest amount of triglycerides of all the lipoproteins but are found in the blood only after meals. The proteins found in lipoproteins, called **apolipoproteins**, are unique to each class of lipoprotein and act to hold the structure

high-density lipoproteins (HDLs) A type of lipoprotein that is protective against heart disease and stroke because it brings back cholesterol from the body tissues to the liver. Often referred to as the so-called good cholesterol.

very low density lipoproteins (VLDLs) The class of lipoproteins made by the liver for export to extrahepatic tissues. They contain triglycerides, cholesterol, and phospholipids in addition to protein. They are converted in the capillary beds to low-density lipoproteins (LDLs) through the action of lipoprotein lipase and other enzymes.

low-density lipoproteins (LDLs) A type of lipoprotein derived from very low density lipoproteins (VLDLs) in the capillary beds through the action of lipoprotein lipase and other enzymes. This lipoprotein has the highest concentration of cholesterol (as an ester) and the longest half-life. High circulating concentrations of LDL-cholesterol is a risk factor for cardiovascular disease.

apolipoprotein (apo) Class of proteins associated with plasma lipoproteins, such as very low density lipoproteins (VLDLs), chylomicrons, low-density lipoproteins (LDLs), and high-density lipoproteins (HDLs).

TABLE 6.3
Lipoprotein Classes: Different Compositions Relate to Different Functions

Composition	Chylomicrons	HDL	LDL	VLDL
Protein (%)	1	50	25	5
Lipids (%)	99	50	75	95
Cholesterol (%)	4	18	45	10
Triglycerides (%)	90	2	10	70
Phospholipids (%)	5	30	20	15
Origin	Intestine	Liver	VLDL	Liver
Function with regard to triglyceride or cholesterol delivery	Triglyceride delivery to tissues	Return of cholesterol to liver (reverse)	Removal of tissue cholesterol to liver	Triglyceride delivery to tissues

Reproduced from Anderson JJB. *Nutrition and Health: An Introduction.* Durham, NC: Carolina Academic Press; 2005.

> Lipoproteins are classified according to their density, which is directly related to how much protein (i.e., heavy components) and triglycerides (i.e., light components) they carry.

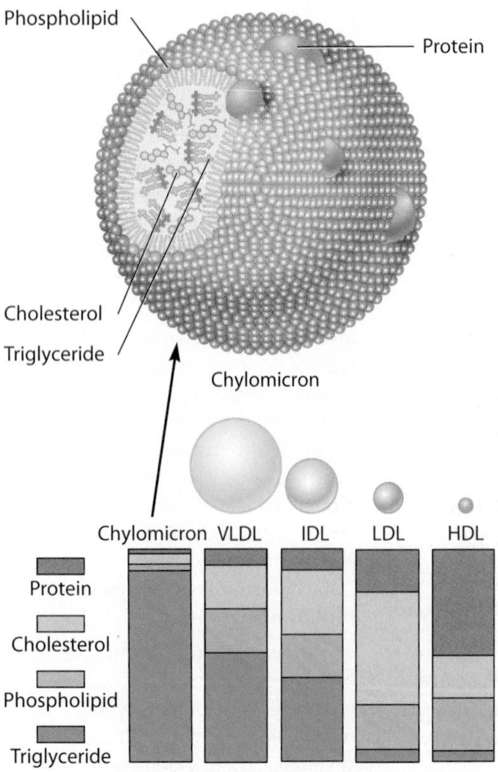

FIGURE 6.11 Lipoproteins. The composition of lipoproteins is related to their functions in the human body.

together in blood (water). The apolipoproteins also serve as signals, directing molecular interactions and metabolism. **FIGURE 6.11** illustrates the different lipoprotein classes and their composition. Note that, in addition to apolipoproteins, all lipoproteins contain phospholipids as part of their structures. Lipoprotein synthesis occurs only in the gut (chylomicrons) and the liver (VLDL and HDL).

Transport of Lipid Molecules by Lipoproteins

The metabolism of triglycerides is quite different from that of carbohydrates because of their general solubility in lipids (lipophilic) and their limited solubility in water. Therefore, lipids, including triglycerides and cholesterol, require lipoproteins to transport them via blood to tissues of the body. Lipoproteins transport triglycerides and cholesterol in the blood to tissues where these molecules are needed. Following their digestion and absorption by cells in the intestine, triglycerides are incorporated into chylomicrons, a triglyceride-rich lipoprotein. From the cells of the small intestine, chylomicrons are transported to the lymph, then to the blood, and finally their remnants are taken up by hepatocytes after delivering most of their triglycerides to peripheral cells of the body. The proteins in each lipoprotein complex have special signaling mechanisms that initiate actions, such as enhancing enzymatic breakdown of triglycerides to fatty acids for cell uptake.

Peripheral tissues can remove the triglycerides from the chylomicrons and VLDL circulating in blood so the fatty acids can be used for energy or structures in muscle, fat cells, and other functional cells. Lipoprotein triglyceride degradation, also known as **lipolysis**, is accomplished by **lipoprotein lipase**. This enzyme breaks down triglycerides in lipoproteins for uptake by peripheral tissues, especially adipocytes and muscle cells. The quick removal of fatty acids and storage of resynthesized triglycerides from chylomicrons (and VLDL) by fat cells in adipose tissue means that the fats eaten at lunch are already being deposited in the adipose tissue before dinner! Chylomicrons distribute their contents quickly and typically disappear from blood within several hours after a meal. **Chylomicron remnants** (i.e., the remainder of the chylomicrons after passage through the body and removal of most of their triglycerides) are much smaller than chylomicrons, and they are promptly removed from circulation by the liver.

Triglycerides and cholesterol from the liver are also distributed to the periphery of the body by way of secreted VLDL. As with chylomicrons, VLDL complexes are delivered to the periphery and shrink in size after triglyceride breakdown and release of fatty acids to cells. The first of these smaller lipoproteins are known as intermediate density lipoproteins (IDLs). The smaller particles derived from VLDL are then called LDL, and they are returned via blood to be taken up slowly by the liver. If LDLs are not removed, they continue to circulate at elevated concentrations before they are removed, typically weeks later.

High LDL concentrations lead to fatty deposits in arteries that typically become more advanced deposits known as atherosclerosis. HDL acts primarily in reverse cholesterol transport by bringing cholesterol back to the liver from peripheral tissues and other particles for disposal. Each of these particles has a certain "lifetime" in the circulating blood; the average time that each type of particle resides in circulating blood is known as its **half-life**. LDL particles have the longest half-life and statin drugs are commonly prescribed to enhance liver uptake of these particles to shorten their half-life in the circulation. The removal of lipoproteins after their life cycle is referred to as clearance from the blood, and newly formed lipoproteins continue to replace the old disposed particles.

> " Triglycerides and cholesterol from the liver are distributed to the periphery by way of secreted VLDL. "

Dietary Fats and Energy Generation

A major function of dietary fats is to supply energy in their C-H bonds. Dietary fats are also needed to provide essential fatty acids for the synthesis of several molecules, including eicosanoids, and membrane structures. The energy in dietary fats can be stored as triglycerides in adipose tissue, muscle, and liver for later use. Just like carbohydrates, triglycerides can be degraded to generate cellular ATP in almost all cells of the body. Excessive accumulation of body fat, however, results from the overconsumption of energy (i.e., all the macronutrients, not just fat). Carbohydrates and proteins are typically oxidized for energy (ATP), and excess carbohydrates are also converted to triglycerides, which typically contribute to elevations of serum triglycerides. On the other hand, excess dietary fats and alcohol are largely converted to triglycerides that go into long-term storage until needed during periods of fasting. In times of fasting, the triglycerides are degraded in adipocytes by the process known as lipolysis, and the free fatty acids released to the blood are transported by albumin by the blood plasma, not by lipoprotein particles. These fatty acids are taken up from circulating blood by muscle cells and other metabolically active tissues, especially by the liver. The glycerol molecules released by triglyceride breakdown in fat cells directly enter blood plasma and are then transported back to the liver for re-use in metabolic reactions.

Any one of the energy-yielding macronutrients may be broken down and converted to fatty acids and then to triglycerides for long-term storage, especially during

lipolysis Fat (triglyceride) degradation in adipose tissue via hormone-sensitive lipase. Results in the release of free fatty acids and glycerol that then diffuse into the blood for distribution to other body tissues.

lipoprotein lipase Enzyme found in the capillary beds that degrades triglycerides in lipoproteins during their passage through the circulation.

chylomicron remnant The residual and smaller part of the chylomicron left after partial degradation of triglycerides by lipoprotein lipase and release of other lipids in the peripheral capillary beds. The remnants are taken up by the liver and degraded. They are not found in the circulating blood of healthy fasting individuals.

half-life The amount of time it takes for half of a particular molecule to disappear from the blood. For example, the half-life of insulin is 5 to 10 minutes.

> **"** A central understanding of energy metabolism is that sugars can be converted into fatty acids, but fatty acids cannot be converted back into sugars. **"**

lipogenesis The synthesis of a new fatty acid in the liver through the combining of two acetyl CoA molecules and the successive addition of acetyl CoA molecules. The fatty acids produced by the liver are fully saturated. The acid or carboxyl end of each fatty acid can be linked to glycerol phosphate to produce a triglyceride or phospholipid.

ketone Molecule produced from the accumulation of excess acetic acid molecules. The three most common ketones are acetone (a true ketone) and the organic acids acetoacetic acid and hydroxybutyric acid. Ketones are typically elevated in uncontrolled diabetes mellitus (type 1) and, to a lesser extent, during conditions of fasting or starvation.

ketogenesis The pathway through which ketones are formed in the mitochondria of the liver due to insufficient amounts of oxaloacetate or excessive generation of acetate from fatty acid oxidation or alcohol degradation.

fatty liver Accumulation of fat stores in hepatocytes following excessive calorie and/or alcohol consumption that serves as an indicator of abnormal metabolism.

periods of excessive caloric intake. The amino acids must undergo deamination (removal of nitrogen) before their carbon backbones enter the common metabolic pathway for triglyceride synthesis. When in excess, glucose molecules are enzymatically degraded to two-carbon fragments, known as acetyl CoA, prior to conversion to fatty acids and triglycerides. The hepatic synthesis of new fatty acids with 16 carbons, also known as **lipogenesis**, results from the initial combination of two acetyl CoA molecules and the successive addition of acetyl CoA molecules. The fatty acids made by human tissues are fully saturated. The acid or carboxyl ends of each fatty acid can be linked to glycerol phosphate to produce a triglyceride or phospholipid.

A central understanding of energy metabolism is that although sugars can be converted into fatty acids, fatty acids cannot be converted back into sugars because the pathway from glucose to fat has one key enzymatic reaction that is irreversible (acetyl CoA cannot be converted to a three-carbon carbohydrate or triose). For most cells of the body this is not a problem because they can use both fats and glucose as sources of energy. However, some tissues, mainly brain neurons and red blood cells, operate almost exclusively on glucose, and the liver must keep providing glucose at minimal levels during fasting periods as fuel for these tissues. As the body runs low on glucose from the previous meal, it must turn to other sources to maintain the blood glucose level. Amino acids from proteins can, rather inefficiently, be converted into glucose via gluconeogenesis.

As fasting continues, the body turns to yet another energy source. The liver generates and secretes into the blood a family of small ketone-containing molecules, which are characterized by an oxygen atom attached to carbon by double bonds. The **ketones** derived from fat and amino acid metabolism act as alternate energy sources for those tissues that require glucose, including the brain, by the process known as **ketogenesis**. In this process, ketones are generated at the expense of the body's other tissues. One of the ketones, acetone, is a volatile molecule that can be detected on the breath of those with low blood glucose, such as following the conversion of alcohol to ketones by alcoholics. This "ketotic breath" also may serve as a danger sign in a person with diabetes because it may indicate a severely low blood glucose concentration, such as following an insulin overdose or an oversecretion of insulin by an otherwise "healthy" person.

Storage of Fats in Extrahepatic or Peripheral Tissues

Fat cells (or adipocytes) located in almost all tissues, especially connective tissues, of the body store fats or triglycerides. The capacity for this storage is astoundingly large and allows a few people to weigh from over 300 pounds up to approximately 1,000 pounds! The liver cells themselves also store fat, even large amounts with chronic overnutrition. Excessive energy intake from macronutrients and alcohol over long periods typically results in a "fatty liver," a serious condition that reduces many of the critical liver functions.

Lipoproteins deliver triglycerides to fat cells and other cells. They also deliver cholesterol and phospholipids to cells in extrahepatic or peripheral tissues of the body. The synthesis of triglycerides in adipose tissue or other sites of the body requires fatty acids delivered via lipoproteins, glucose delivered in blood, and an enzyme for making new triglycerides. Fat cells require glucose for generation of glycerol phosphate, a key component in triglyceride synthesis. The triglycerides then become part of stored fat that can be used for energy at a later time.

Where the Macronutrients Go

On a piece of paper, draw a representation of a liver, adipose tissue, a brain, and the intestines. With three different color markers, show how the different macronutrients are absorbed, converted into triglycerides, stored, and released for energy. Keep in mind that each type of macronutrient may take several routes until it is finally metabolized in cells to carbon dioxide and water. ■

Metabolic Breakdown of Tissues for Energy

A man is marooned on a desert island with no food. He does have a case of bottled water. He is rescued after 2 weeks without consuming any food. Explain the sequence of energy sources that his body will use to survive. Consider the metabolic breakdown of storage molecules of energy (glycogen and fat) and muscle tissue (protein) for conversion to ATP. How will this metabolic breakdown affect his body weight, body composition, and appearance? How will these degradative processes affect the three components of his body composition: fat mass, lean body mass, and bone mass? ■

Fat Substitutes

The introduction of **fat substitutes** in the food supply has occurred because of our preference for fats in the diet—and for many, excessive fat intake! The types of substitutes being developed for fat are quite varied, but only a few have been approved for use by the FDA. When these molecules are hydrated, they form stabilized gels, which supply the needed lubricating and flow properties of fats. Most fat substitutes cannot be used in baking and frying at high temperatures. Because of their lack of flavor, fat substitutes are not widely accepted. Another negative factor is their relative solubility compared to true fats.

One popular fat substitute is Simplesse (NutraSweet Co.), which is derived from microparticulated protein (see **FIGURE 6.12**). Another fat-replacement product, olestra

> The introduction of fat substitutes in the food supply has occurred because of the preference for fats in the diet—and for many, excessive fat intake!

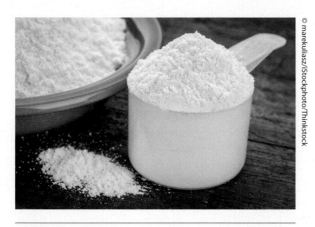

© marekuliasz/iStockphoto/Thinkstock

FIGURE 6.12 Simplesse. The fat substitute Simplesse is made from protein microparticles.

fat substitute Substances used to replace fats in foods in an effort to reduce fat intake. They have not found wide acceptance due to their lack of flavor, relative solubility compared to real fats, and the fact that most cannot be used in baking or frying.

(Olean from Procter & Gamble), is made by esterification of several fatty acids to sucrose. Olestra is largely resistant to digestive enzymes and passes through the entire gut unaffected. Olestra is not widely used, in part because of uncomfortable gastrointestinal effects such as indigestion and cramping in some consumers. This lipid-like molecule has similar sensory properties as fats, such as "mouth-feel," which makes it acceptable to consumers who do not mind the gastrointestinal side effects. Because of their lipid solubility, products containing olestra, such as potato chips, may interfere with the absorption of fat-soluble vitamins. Olestra has been approved by the FDA for use in chips and other snack foods, but fat-soluble vitamins must be added as fortificants to the food.

A prescription drug, orlistat (Xenical from Roche Laboratories, Inc.), inhibits the digestion of ingested fats in the intestine by about 30%. With less fat to absorb, caloric intake is decreased. This drug works best with people already consuming a low-fat diet. Like olestra, orlistat has similar adverse effects by interfering with fat-soluble vitamin absorption and causing undigested fats to pass through the digestive system intact.

PRACTICAL APPLICATIONS 6.4

Excess Energy Stored as Fat

Excessive caloric intake from a mix of the macronutrients that are not used to meet cellular metabolic needs must go to body tissues for storage as fats (triglycerides). This energy is not wasted. Which tissues of the body take up most of the excess energy as fats? Name three tissues that have been mentioned in this chapter, and think of another one or two tissues that may be involved in storage but of lesser amounts. ■

SUMMARY

Lipids are biological molecules that are soluble in organic solvents. They include fatty acids, triglycerides, phospholipids, cholesterol, steroid hormones, and eicosanoids. Fatty acids come in many forms based on the length of the hydrocarbon chain and the number and position of the double bond(s). The omega-6 (such as linoleic acid) and omega-3 fatty acids (such as alpha-linolenic acid) are essential fatty acids. They serve as precursors for the synthesis of eicosanoids, local factors, and hormones.

Fat-soluble molecules travel in blood as part of lipoproteins, small particles that contain triglycerides, cholesterol, phospholipids, and protein. The four types of lipoproteins are responsible for transporting the lipids to tissues. Except for the brain and red blood cells, all other tissues use fatty acids, in part, as sources of energy for ATP production. When consumed in excess, carbohydrates and proteins can be broken down into two carbon units that may go into the synthesis of new fatty acids and then triglycerides. The triglycerides, in turn, are stored for future use in adipose tissue.

Because of excessive fat consumption, triglyceride metabolism has become dominant in the lives of many adults. Lipoproteins deliver the extra triglycerides from the gut, and less so from the liver, after meals to peripheral storage sites. Once delivered, residual LDL particles increase their composition of cholesterol. High serum cholesterol concentrations result mainly from a high intake of total energy from all macronutrients, especially saturated fats rather than from dietary cholesterol, and high LDL-cholesterol concentrations are associated with increased risk of heart disease that results from atherosclerosis. The apolipoproteins carried in lipoproteins have important signaling roles in peripheral tissues for triglyceride degradation and other metabolic steps.

STUDENT ACTIVITIES

1. List the major classes of lipid molecules.

2. What are the general structural components of a triglyceride and how does phosphatidyl choline differ from a triglyceride? You may wish to draw the two structures on paper.

3. How do saturated fatty acids, monounsaturated fatty acids, and polyunsaturated fatty acids differ in general structure and length (number of carbons)? What is the difference between polyunsaturated fatty acids regarding the place of the last (omega) double bond?

4. Which foods are high in fat content?

5. Define hydrogenation and state how it is used in the industrial formation of trans fats.

6. List the four major lipoproteins and their tissues of origin and state the major molecular components.

7. Name a common fat substitute. Why might consumers seek out products with fat substitutes?

8. Explain what happens to fat cells when excessive energy is consumed over a long period of time.

9. Explain how triglycerides are broken down in fat cells and name the products released to blood. What are dietary fats used for in the body?

10. Which two lipoproteins deliver triglycerides to peripheral tissues?

11. Which two lipoproteins return cholesterol from peripheral tissue to the liver?

12. Which lipoprotein delivers cholesterol from the liver to peripheral tissues?

13. Name the precursor molecule used to synthesize bile acids (salts), steroid hormones, and vitamin D (skin).

14. Explain how the metabolism of cholesterol differs from that of phytosterol in the synthesis of cell membranes.

15. State what an eicosanoid is and explain how different types of polyunsaturated fatty acids contribute to the synthesis of eicosanoids.

16. Why can carbohydrates be degraded to acetyl CoA (2 C unit) and then into fatty acid synthesis, but acetyl CoA *cannot* be converted back to a carbohydrate? Hint: Think about enzymes.

17. Explain what an atheroma is. Then state how atheromas contribute to atherosclerosis. Why do saturated fats (and trans fats) contribute more readily than unsaturated fats (in the cis form) to the formation of atheromas?

WEBSITES FOR FURTHER STUDY

Dietary Fats
www.nlm.nih.gov/medlineplus/dietaryfats.html
Dietary Fats: Know Which Types to Choose
www.mayoclinic.com/health/fat/NU00262
Fat Substitutes
http://vm.cfsan.fda.gov/~lrd/fats.html

National Cholesterol Education Program
www.nhlbi.nih.gov/about/ncep/index.htm
U.S. Department of Agriculture
www.usda.gov

REFERENCES

Committee on Dietary Reference Intakes, Institute of Medicine. *Dietary Reference Intakes for Energy, Carbohydrate, Fiber, Fat, Fatty Acids, Cholesterol, Protein, and Amino Acids (Macronutrients).* Washington, D.C.: National Academies Press; 2002.

Jones PJH, Papamandjaris AA. Lipids: cellular metabolism. In: Erdman JW Jr, MacDonald IA, Zeisel SH (eds.), *Present*

Knowledge in Nutrition. 10th ed. Ames, IA: John Wiley & Sons: 2012; 233–259.

Lichtenstein AH, Jones PJH. Lipids: absorption and transport. In: Erdman JW Jr, MacDonald IA, Zeisel SH (eds.), *Present Knowledge in Nutrition.* 10th ed. Ames, IA: John Wiley & Sons: 2012; 213–232.

Reflection on Cardiovascular Disease

Cardiovascular disease (CVD) is a collection of diseases that strike different parts of the circulatory system through a similar mechanism involving damage to and clogging of the arteries. Two of the most common and deadly of these diseases are **coronary heart disease (CHD)**, including myocardial infarction (heart attack), and cerebral damage, or **stroke**.

The incidence of CVD increased in the first half of the 20th century, declined during World War II, and then increased again during the post-war period until early in the 21st century when food became more plentiful. Death rates, have traditionally paralleled morbidity rates, but with better medical care, CVD death rates have dropped about 60% since World War II. Deaths from heart disease have declined much faster than those from other diseases and disorders, such as cancer (see **FIGURE 1**). Declines in deaths from CVD are the result of both better prevention and better treatment. Today, fewer people smoke and cholesterol levels are lower than they were 50 years ago because of changes in the American diet and the widespread use of statin drugs. However, the recent epidemic of obesity has the potential to reverse these healthy CVD trends.

Coronary Heart Disease, Atherosclerosis, and Arteriosclerosis

CHD occurs when the blood flow via coronary arteries to the heart is diminished or blocked. Ischemia, or low supply of oxygenated blood, is the basic problem that leads to a **myocardial infarction (MI)**, also known as a heart attack. A decline in blood flow to the heart muscle typically occurs over decades as an artery narrows and even closes off, as in a heart attack or stroke, because of mineral deposits in the arterial vessel's intimal layer. In addition, some individuals can experience **angina pectoris** or chest pain without a heart attack. They also can have some muscle death when vessels narrow from

cardiovascular disease (CVD) A disease that develops from atherosclerosis in the arteries and arterioles of the general circulatory system; includes coronary heart disease, peripheral artery disease, and stroke.

coronary heart disease (CHD) Disease resulting from narrowing of the small blood vessels that supply blood and oxygen to the heart.

stroke A blockage of an artery of the brain (ischemic stroke) or a bursting of a vessel in the brain (hemorrhagic stroke).

myocardial infarction (MI) Also called a heart attack. Death of myocardial tissue in an area of the heart because of total occlusion of a coronary artery or arteriole by a blood clot. Tissue death occurs because the heart muscle does not get any blood supply and thereby delivery of oxygen and nutrients. Preceded by atherosclerosis, which causes a narrowing of the artery or arteriole. Often leads to death.

angina pectoris A myocardial condition in which the heart muscle does not get adequate oxygen delivery because of a partial, but not total, occlusion (blockage) of a coronary artery or arteriole.

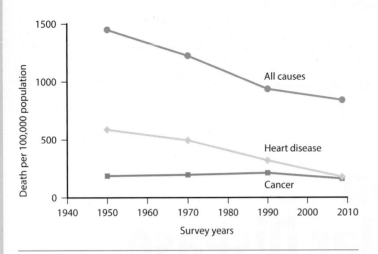

FIGURE 1 Declines in Mortality Rates. Mortality rates from CVD have dropped much more rapidly than mortality rates for other diseases.

Data from Centers for Disease Control and Prevention. *Health, United States, 2011: With Special Feature on Socioeconomic Status and Health.* Washington, DC: National Center for Health Statistics; 2012. Available at: www.cdc.gov/nchs/data/hus/hus11.pdf

fatty deposits, though they do not completely close. **Atherosclerosis** is the progressive process by which fat deposits are laid down in the walls of major arteries throughout the body, especially the coronary arteries that supply the heart muscle and the cerebral arteries that supply the brain (see **FIGURE 2**). The fatty deposits, known as fatty plaques, are potentially reversible in the early stages, but when calcification occurs in the adjacent medial layer of the artery by the process of **arteriosclerosis**, the damage can no longer be reversed. The deposit of fatty plaques can start quite early in life. Autopsies on children who have died from accidents or other causes often show the beginnings of these fatty deposits. As young adults and adults, practically everyone has some evidence of these deposits. How fast the deposits grow and become a problem for blood flow is largely based on a person's genetic makeup and lifestyle choices, especially diet and activity levels.

Atherosclerotic plaque is composed mainly of fat, cholesterol, and material from cell breakdown. As it enlarges, it forms patches in the arteries, which alter the rate of blood flow. As a plaque expands, it partially blocks a portion of an artery so that blood flows unevenly at the site of the plaque. The irregular blood flow in the artery contributes to clots, which may totally block blood flow or contribute to advancing CVD by affecting the medial or smooth muscle cells of an arterial wall. Some of the muscle cells of the medial layer of the arterial walls may convert to bone cells, causing minerals to precipitate on the organic bone matrix at these unusual sites by a process called calcification. Ultimately, this leads to arteriosclerosis as the vessels become calcified and less flexible.

atherosclerosis An early form of arteriosclerosis characterized by plaques or lipid accumulations (atheromas) in the arterial wall; any such lesion can become sufficiently extensive to interfere with or even block blood flow through the vessel, causing a clot (thrombus) to form at the site of obstruction. Plaques contain cholesterol, triglycerides, other fatty molecules, and tissue debris, including mineralizations.

arteriosclerosis Cardiovascular disease of the arteries with advanced pathology that is preceded by atherosclerosis.

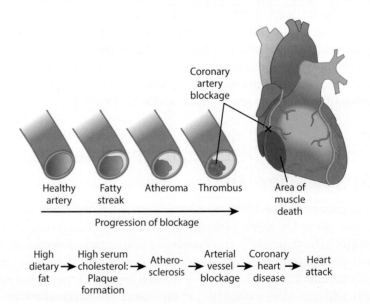

FIGURE 2 Progression of Atherosclerosis. The formation of arterial plaques contributes to the development of atherosclerosis, whereby the artery walls thicken or become blocked.

Reproduced from Anderson JJB. *Nutrition and Health: An Introduction.* Durham, NC: Carolina Academic Press; 2005.

Arteriosclerosis often occurs in later life. The hard lesions on the arterial walls produced by mineralization (calcification) and hardening are not reversible. Rigid arteries lose their elasticity, which can cause adverse effects. For example, if the aorta that leaves the left side of the heart becomes calcified, it loses much of its contractility, reducing back blood perfusion of the heart via the coronary arteries.

Thrombosis is the process leading to the formation of a blood clot, usually from an existing plaque. A small piece, or **thrombus**, breaks away from the larger clot and can lead to a heart attack or stroke. Sometimes a clot will get stuck in a capillary bed in the body, often the lungs, and contribute to the development of serious tissue complications.

Although mortality rates have dropped in recent years, CHD remains the number one cause of death in the United States, Canada, and many other nations. Once blood flow through a coronary artery (i.e., one directly supplying the heart) is reduced by 70% or more, the limited blood flow to the heart causes a person to begin to have difficulty with daily activities such as climbing stairs. Some people will have chest pain, called angina pectoris, which is a serious problem that reflects that the heart is not getting enough oxygenated blood. A person may experience a myocardial infarction, or heart attack, when the blood flow to a portion of the heart muscle is completely blocked and a segment of heart muscle dies from lack of oxygen and nutrients.

Other conditions that contribute to heart disease include damage to the aortic and mitral **valves in the heart**, damage to the heart chambers, "electrical" irregularities in the timing of heart contractions, and infectious diseases that weaken the heart. In late life the aorta may become stiffened due to arteriosclerotic calcification, which reduces blood flow to the heart muscle and may increase the risk of death.

Other serious, even deadly, forms of CVD include pathologic changes to peripheral vascular tissues, which result from blockage of an artery in the periphery, and deep vein thrombosis (DVT). Both of these conditions are common in the legs. These blockages are painful and cause serious damage. Thromboses typically generate clots.

Stroke

Cerebral vascular disease is a condition whereby blood vessels in the brain narrow or become blocked, resulting in stroke; these are similar to the events leading to a heart attack or angina. The two major types of stroke are ischemic or hemorrhagic. If an artery of the brain becomes blocked, depriving the brain and its neurons of oxygen and nutrients, ischemic stroke results. A hemorrhagic stroke occurs when a blocked or narrowed blood vessel bursts when subjected to high blood pressure. Hemorrhagic strokes typically result in instant death. In Western countries, about 80% of strokes are ischemic and 20% are hemorrhagic. The opposite is true in Asian countries, such as for Japan, Korea, and China, where high salt intake contributes to very high **blood pressure** and levels of **hypertension**. Blood pressure depends on the ability of the heart to pump and the backpressure from the capillary beds of the body. When these functions are compromised, it results in hypertension. Another condition arises when only a small temporary blockage of a cerebral (brain) artery occurs. This is a **transient ischemic attack (TIA)**, or ministroke. TIAs are generally serious precursors of future danger, including a full stroke.

Risk Factors for Cardiovascular Diseases

Two broad classes of risk factors contribute to CVD: dietary and nondietary. The discussion here emphasizes dietary or nutritional risk factors, but nondietary risk factors also are briefly noted.

thrombosis The formation of a clot within an artery or arteriole, which leads to total blockage of blood flow at that specific site. Can lead to a myocardial infarction or stroke.

thrombus The plug that is formed in the arteries due to thrombosis.

valves (heart) The heart has four valves that open to let blood flow through or out of the heart and then shut to keep blood from flowing backward.

blood pressure Arterial pressure measured at peripheral sites such as in the upper arm (brachial artery). It is the amount of pressure required to push blood throughout the body. Blood pressure depends on both cardiac output (the ability of the heart to pump) and peripheral resistance (the back pressure from the capillary beds of the body).

hypertension Also called high blood pressure. Abnormally elevated blood pressure resulting from either an increase in cardiac output, peripheral resistance, or both; a risk factor for cardiovascular disease.

transient ischemic attack (TIA) A ministroke that may result in only a brief blockage of an artery in the brain. May cause a blackout or temporary loss of function of the brain. A risk factor for stroke.

> **"** Investigators of the Framingham Heart Study and other prospective studies have identified several risk factors that account for a large proportion of the preventable causes of the disease (CVD), including hypertension, cigarette smoking, high LDL-cholesterol, and low HDL-cholesterol. **"**

Nondietary Risk Factors

Epidemiologic studies indicate that the causes of CVD are complex. The term *risk factors* has been used to help describe the many possible contributors to CVD. Of the more than 30 potential risk factors involved in the development of CHD, investigators of the **Framingham Heart Study** and other prospective studies have identified several that account for a large proportion of the preventable causes of the disease, including hypertension, cigarette smoking, high LDL-cholesterol, and low HDL-cholesterol. Two additional major risk factors discovered later by Framingham investigators are obesity and impaired glucose tolerance (including type 2 diabetes). Nutrition is a contributor to several of these risk factors. Other risk factors for CHD and stroke include age, gender (men), family history, personality type (aggressive and time-driven behavior), and physical inactivity.

FOCUS 1   Framingham Heart Study

Framingham, Massachusetts is a small city west of Boston. The Framingham Heart Study was initiated in 1948 when this small suburb had only about 5,000 residents, and the study was designed to determine the risk factors for heart disease in adults. However, because of population increases in the city, what was once a small epidemiologic study has turned into a multigenerational investigation of many other chronic diseases beside CVD. One of the study's earliest findings was the relationship between heart disease and elevated blood lipids, especially LDL-cholesterol, which has been instrumental in advancing both dietary and drug strategies to prevent CVD and other chronic diseases. ●

A recently discovered factor contributing to CVD is systemic inflammation. The **inflammatory response** in the arteries is a type of self-defense mechanism related to the swelling at injury sites and local fever. Increased levels of systemic inflammation that contribute to cardiovascular diseases are common in obese individuals and cigarette smokers, but they also may affect others. Genetic factors contribute to CVD risk, which are currently being investigated by researchers.

FOCUS 2   Role of Micronutrients and Phytochemicals in Improving Cardiovascular Health

Micronutrients and a wide variety of other molecules from plant foods have recently been shown to provide benefits to health, and to cardiovascular tissues specifically. For example, foods containing antioxidants may act to protect the endothelium (lining) of arteries from oxidative damage. Some phytochemicals, such as those found in garlic, red wine, olive oil, and other plant sources, may act to slow or reverse the clotting process. Recent reports also have shown that inflammation can be reduced by weight loss, smoking cessation, and exercise. ●

risk factor A contributor to disease, such as genetic predisposition, lifestyle, or an environmental factor. Also called a determinant.

Framingham Heart Study A study that was started in 1948 to investigate heart disease. Over time, it has been used to study practically all chronic diseases. Many of the epidemiologic and clinical findings of this study have had broad implications for the entire U.S. population.

inflammatory response A physiologic response to environmental and physical insults, such as infection, injury, burn, arthritis, surgery, and smoking; involves a rise in body temperature, changes in blood variables, and an enhanced immune response.

TABLE 1
Foods That Can Help to Lower Blood Cholesterol Concentrations

Vegetables	Fruits	Grains	Meat/Poultry/Fish	Legumes	Nuts	Other
• Asparagus • Broccoli • Eggplant • Garlic • Onion • Tomatoes • Spinach	• Apples • Blueberries • Citrus fruits • Grapes • Strawberries	• Barley • Oats • Wheat • Wild rice	• Lean meats • Lean poultry • Salmon and other fish	• Garbanzos • Peanuts • Lentils	• Walnuts • Other nuts	• Green tea • Red wine

Vegetable oils (e.g., canola, soy, olive, safflower) are recommended for cooking rather than animal-based fats and vegetable shortening.
Data from Lichtenstein, AH et al. Diet and lifestyle recommendations revision 2006: A statement from the American Heart Association Nutrition Committee. *Circulation* 2006;114:82–96.

Dietary Risk Factors

Major nutritional factors associated with high blood cholesterol concentrations include excessive energy intake from macronutrients and alcohol; high saturated fat intake; and too little consumption of micronutrients, fiber, and phytochemicals from plant foods. Saturated fats from animal sources are considered a major contributor to the elevation of serum total cholesterol, a major factor in the development of CHD, but the role of saturated fats remains controversial. Whereas some foods contribute to elevations in serum total cholesterol, others can help to improve cholesterol levels (see **Table 1**). CVDs are highly associated with serum cholesterol.

Dietary cholesterol had long been considered to contribute to high levels of serum cholesterol, but recent findings suggest that saturated fats from animal foods, rather than dietary cholesterol in the presence of excessive total energy intake, are a major determinant of high serum cholesterol concentration. Reducing intake of saturated fats typically has a substantial positive impact on blood cholesterol levels but less so on serum triglycerides.

Consider the impact of switching to margarine from butter. **Margarine** is made from vegetable oils, so it contains no cholesterol. In addition, margarine is also higher in "good" fats—polyunsaturated and monounsaturated fatty acids—than butter is. **Butter**, like many animal-based foods, is high in saturated fats. **Table 2** shows the serum lipid changes in a study where subjects were placed on low-fat diets containing either butter or margarine, with the type of fat being the only distinguishing feature. The polyunsaturated fats in the margarine lowered serum total cholesterol and LDL-cholesterol levels compared with equivalent amounts of saturated fatty acids in the butter-based diet.

Lipoproteins, Triglycerides, and Cardiovascular Diseases

Low-density lipoprotein (LDL) particles carry most of the cholesterol in the serum. Of the components of cholesterol in the blood, LDL-cholesterol (LDL-C) is most responsible for the damage leading to CVD. Although elevated plasma triglycerides, primarily in VLDL particles, may also be implicated in atherosclerotic disease, the evidence is less clear for the role of triglycerides than for the cholesterol fraction in LDL, especially

> *Dietary cholesterol had long been considered to contribute to high levels of serum cholesterol, but recent findings suggest that saturated fats from animal foods, rather than dietary cholesterol in the presence of excessive total energy intake, are a major determinant of high serum cholesterol concentration.*

margarine (oleomargarine) Imitation spread developed as a replacement for butter that is composed of modified fats, often hydrogenated vegetable oils. Recent modifications have greatly reduced the amount of trans fats in margarines.

butter A dairy product made by churning fresh or fermented cream or milk. It is generally used as a spread and a condiment, as well as in cooking, such as baking and frying. Like many animal-based foods, it is high in saturated fat.

TABLE 2
Plasma Cholesterol Levels for Diets with Butter Versus Margarine

Cholesterol Fraction	Butter Diet		Margarine Diet	
	Before	After	Before	After
Total cholesterol (mg/dL)	254	242*	251	228*
LDL-cholesterol (mg/dL)	172	163*	169	148*
HDL-cholesterol (mg/dL)	49	49	49	48

* Statistically significant difference between the butter and margarine diets.
Data from Chisholm A, Mann J, Sutherland W, et al. Effects on lipoprotein profile of replacing butter with margarine in a low fat diet: randomised crossover study with hypercholesterolaemic subjects. *BMJ.* 1996;312:931–934.

> Of the components of cholesterol in the blood, LDL-cholesterol (LDL-C) is most responsible for the damage leading to CVD.

oxidized LDL. High-density lipoprotein cholesterol (HDL-C) is protective against heart disease, and thus an elevated serum HDL-C concentration is beneficial for health. The role of HDL is the reverse transport of cholesterol (i.e., from the periphery back to the liver). This step removes cholesterol from other lipoproteins and tissues. A high HDL level favors good heart and vascular health.

The relationship between serum cholesterol and death from CHD is shown in **FIGURE 3**. Adult men and women have similar average blood concentrations of LDL-C, but men do not receive the same protective benefit of HDL-C that women do. Premenopausal women in particular are protected from the effects of high cholesterol because of their much higher level of estrogen and HDL-C concentration than similarly aged men. Therefore, high blood cholesterol is fairly common in adult men under 50 but not in women. LDL-C levels increase abruptly in women following menopause and the loss of ovarian estrogens at approximately age 50. **FIGURE 4** compares LDL-C and HDL-C levels of men and women. Accordingly, heart attacks and other CVD events in women also rise after age 55 (i.e., early postmenopause). Therefore, a two-to-three decade delay in significant CVD rates typically occurs in women in comparison with men. This delay is attributed to the loss of the protective effects of estrogens. Older postmenopausal women have essentially the same risk factors for CVDs as men at the same age. Men, however, usually have other CVD risk factors, such as poor eating habits, cigarette smoking, and greater iron stores compared with women. Thus the different CVD rates between *older* men and women are not solely attributable to estrogen.

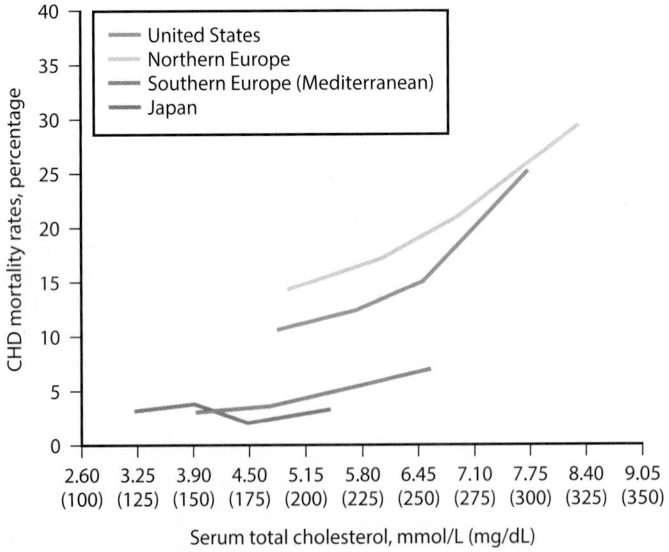

FIGURE 3 Relationship Between Total Serum Cholesterol and CHD Mortality.

Data from Verschuren WMM, Jacobs DR, Bloemberg BPM, et al. Serum total cholesterol and long-term coronary heart disease mortality in different cultures: Twenty-five-year follow-up of the seven countries study. *JAMA.* 1995;274:131–136.

Serum Cholesterol Measurements

How is serum cholesterol measured? In most cases, blood is drawn at a physician's office or lab. Most of the cholesterol components in the blood can be directly measured with instrumentation; from these measurements, serum LDL-cholesterol is calculated from the other subfraction measurements of total cholesterol. (Chylomicron cholesterol is absent during fasting in healthy individuals.) Total cholesterol (TC) is measured directly, and in adults it is usually in the range of 150 to 250 milligrams per deciliter. Values above 200 milligrams per deciliter are cause for concern. HDL-C is measured in blood after a precipitation step, and in Americans it usually ranges between 30 and 80 milligrams per deciliter. It is usually 10 mg/dL higher in women than men. Triglycerides are measured in fasting blood samples (usually 4 to 8 hours after the last meal). Because triglycerides are carried predominantly by VLDL, a simple ratio (1 to 5) has been determined that converts triglyceride concentrations into VLDL-cholesterol (VLDL-C) concentrations. The **Friedewald equation** is used to approximate LDL-C levels, as follows:

$$\text{LDL-C} = \text{TC} - \text{HDL} - \text{VLDL-C, where VLDL-C} = \text{TGs}/5$$

Thus, the LDL-C of a typical male with a total cholesterol of 220, HDL of 45, and triglycerides of 100 would be:

$$\text{LDL-C} = 220 - 45 - 100/5 = 155 \text{ mg/dL (too high a value—not heart healthy!)}$$

Significant associations between lipid risk factors with CHD and other CVDs have been supported by clinical trials. Treatment recommendations for blood lipids have been developed and updated over time by the **National Cholesterol Education Program (NCEP)**, whose goal it is to lower the incidence of illness and death from coronary heart

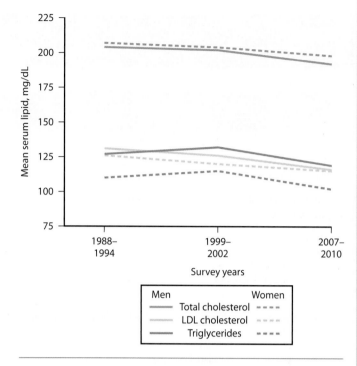

FIGURE 4 Serum Lipids Over Time.

Data from Carroll MD, Kit BK, Lacher DA, Shero ST, Mussolino ME. Trends in lipids and lipoproteins in US adults, 1988–2010. *JAMA.* 2012;308(15):1545–1554.

> The optimal level of < 100 mg/dL LDL-C, possibly even lower, is recommended for all adults, not just high-risk people who have CHD or type 2 diabetes.

Friedewald equation An equation used to calculate LDL-cholesterol based on known values of triglycerides, HDL-cholesterol, and total cholesterol.

National Cholesterol Education Program (NCEP) The National Heart, Lung, and Blood Institute (NHLBI) launched the NCEP in November 1985. The goal of the NCEP is to lower the incidence of illness and death from coronary heart disease (CHD) in the United States by reducing the percentage of Americans with high blood cholesterol.

PRACTICAL APPLICATION **1**

Your Own LDL-Cholesterol Level and Heart Disease Risk

If you know your total cholesterol, HDL-C, and triglyceride levels, then you can calculate your own LDL-C level. You may have a report of these at your doctor's office or a local hospital, or even in your own health records. If not, then use the following somewhat average values: total cholesterol = 206 mg/dL, HDL-C = 45 mg/dL for a male or 55 mg/dL for a female, and serum triglycerides = 85 mg/dL. Calculate, in either case, the LDL-C value using the Friedewald equation. Now compare your personal lipid values with the ATP III goals in Table 3. ∎

TABLE 3
Guidelines for Drug Treatment of High Blood LDL-Cholesterol

Risk Category	LDL-C Goal	Initiate Therapeutic Lifestyle Changes[1]	Consider Drug Therapy
High risk: CHD or CHD risk equivalents[2] (10-year risk > 20%)[3]	< 100 mg/dL (optional goal: < 70 mg/dL)	≥ 100 mg/dL	≥ 100 mg/dL (< 100 mg/dL: consider optional drug options)
Moderately high risk: 2+ risk factors[4] (10-year risk 10%–20%)	< 130 mg/dL	≥ 130 mg/dL	≥ 130 mg/dL (100–129 mg/dL: consider optional drug options)
Moderate risk: 2+ risk factors (10-year risk < 10%)	< 130 mg/dL	≥ 130 mg/dL	≥ 160 mg/dL
Low risk: 0–1 risk factor	< 160 mg/dL	≥ 160 mg/dL	≥ 190 mg/dL (160–189 mg/dL: LDL-lowering drug optional)

[1] Therapeutic lifestyle changes include: (1) reduced intake of saturated fat to < 7% of total calories; (2) consumption of plant stanols/phytosterols and increased viscous (soluble) fiber; (3) weight reduction; and (4) increased physical activity.
[2] CHD equivalents include other cardiovascular diseases and type 2 diabetes.
[3] Heart disease risk is calculated using a table specifically designed to assess multiple risk factors (not given here).
[4] The additional risk factors are smoking, hypertension, HDL < 40 mg/dL, family history of premature CHD (father or brother before age 55 or mother or sister before age 65), age (men ≥ age 45 or women ≥ age 55).
Modified from Third Report of the National Cholesterol Education Program (NCEP) Expert Panel on Detection, Evaluation, and Treatment of High Blood Cholesterol in Adults (Adult Treatment Panel III).

disease. The latest guidelines are the third version of the **Adult Treatment Panel (ATP III)**. The classifications of blood lipids are listed in **Table 3**. An optimal LDL-C level of 100 milligrams per deciliter, even lower if possible, is recommended for all adults and not just high-risk people who have CHD or type 2 diabetes. Whereas lower concentrations of LDL-C and triglycerides are healthier, higher concentrations of HDL-C are difficult to attain during a lifetime, even from excessive running.

Diet and Prevention of Cardiovascular Diseases

The **American Heart Association** is a nonprofit organization in the United States that advocates a lifestyle of healthy diet and exercise to prevent cardiovascular disease and stroke. The dietary changes recommended by the American Heart Association represent the latest advice of health experts in the use of diet to prevent CVD[1]:

- Balance calorie intake and physical activity to achieve or maintain a healthy body weight (BMI between 18.5 and 25).
- Consume a diet rich in vegetables and fruits.
- Choose whole-grain, high-fiber foods.
- Consume fish, especially oily fish, at least twice a week.
- Limit intake of saturated and trans fat and cholesterol.
- Minimize intake of beverages and processed foods with added sugar.
- Choose and prepare foods with little or no salt.

Adult Treatment Panel (ATP III) Guidelines based on extensive research that have been developed by the National Cholesterol Education Program (NCEP) on the detection, evaluation, and treatment of high blood cholesterol.

American Heart Association A nonprofit organization in the United States that fosters appropriate cardiac care in an effort to reduce disability and deaths caused by cardiovascular disease and stroke. Advocates the use of physical activity and diet to reduce the risk of developing cardiovascular disease.

[1] Reproduced from Lichtenstein AH, et al. Diet and lifestyle recommendations revision 2006: A statement from the American Heart Association Nutrition Committee. *Circulation*. 2006;114:82–96.

- If you consume alcohol, do so in moderation.
- When you eat food that is prepared outside of the home, follow the AHA 2006 Diet and Lifestyle Recommendations.

Animal protein sources typically increase blood cholesterol concentrations. Total protein intake should be kept at approximately 15% of total calories or less. Furthermore, most meat consumers should increase their consumption of protein from legumes and grains while reducing protein from animal sources.

In addition to the above guidelines, the National Cholesterol Education Program of the National Institutes of Health (NIH) has recommended therapeutic lifestyle changes (TLC) that include physical activity and are similar to AHA guidelines. Regular physical activity helps to lower LDL-C, but in most people who exercise these activities have no effect on HDL-C. Because of these modest changes in people who exercise regularly, the ratio of LDL-C to HDL-C or of TC to HDL-C is improved. Another benefit of regular physical activity is a possible decrease in body weight with an improvement in the ratio of lean body mass to fat. A decrease in body weight is usually also accompanied by a decline in blood pressure and an improvement in blood glucose regulation. Thus, exercise has several positive outcomes that reduce risks of chronic diseases.

> *Regular physical activity helps to lower LDL-C, but in most people who exercise these activities have no effect on HDL-C.*

Statin Drugs

Dietary modification alone can sometimes be effective in decreasing cholesterol levels, but it is often complemented by drug therapy. Cholesterol-lowering drugs can lower serum cholesterol much more quickly than diet therapy alone. One class of cholesterol-lowering drugs, the **statins**, has proved to be highly effective in reducing total cholesterol and LDL-C. The statins have been so successful that most physicians have stopped providing patient education emphasizing dietary modifications to achieve healthier diets that lower LDL-C levels.

Statins act in two ways. First, they partially inhibit a key enzyme (HMG CoA reductase) in the cholesterol synthesis pathway in the liver and then they increase the activity of liver membrane receptors for taking up LDL particles from blood. Reductions in LDL-C of 20% to 30% often occur early in treatment. Research has demonstrated that statins significantly reduce both CVD and death rates. Unfortunately, statins need to be taken for life, and these drugs do have potentially adverse side effects. Taking a statin does not, however, eliminate the benefits of a healthy diet that is low in saturated fat and high in fruits and vegetables. The two types of therapy together—diet and a statin—are effective in reducing the risk of CVDs.

statins Class of cholesterol-lowering drugs that have proven to be highly effective in reducing total cholesterol and LDL-C.

SUMMARY

The risk factors implicated in cardiovascular disease have been identified from epidemiologic studies throughout the world. Dietary links have been established for hypertension, atherosclerosis, arteriosclerosis, stroke, coronary heart disease, and other CVDs. Three of the major risk factors for CVD—namely, obesity, hypertension, and high serum cholesterol—have significant dietary contributions. CVD risk reduction through a healthy diet and regular physical activity is important for children, young adults, mid-life adults, and even the elderly. A major goal is to keep LDL-C at less than 100 milligrams per deciliter.

Today, Americans eat less fat and are less likely to smoke than in the past, which has contributed to the impressive recent declines in mortality from CHD, stroke, and related CVDs. Further CVD control is still needed in North America and other nations. In addition to type 2 diabetes, CVDs are the most preventable diseases through changes in diet, lifestyle (smoking cessation, increasing exercise), and drug therapy. The growing epidemic of obesity and the metabolic syndrome, however, may reduce recent beneficial trends of lowered heart disease rates. The traditional interventions of diet and exercise, delivered in a culturally palatable manner, remain needed to improve CVD mortality rates.

STUDENT ACTIVITIES

1. Distinguish the differences among atherosclerosis, arteriosclerosis, and thrombosis.

2. List the four original Framingham risk factors for CHD and then list two more recently identified risk factors.

3. Which lipoprotein is considered most atherogenic? Explain.

4. Explain why chylomicrons and VLDL particles are similar in their composition and roles.

5. What types of foods are recommended for lowering blood cholesterol concentration?

6. Explain how the Friedewald equation is used to estimate VLDL and LDL cholesterol. Calculate the LDL-C level for a man with total cholesterol of 205, HDL-C of 54, and triglycerides of 95.

7. Why is the cholesterol content of chylomicrons not generally measured when a blood sample is drawn for determining total cholesterol and its subfractions?

8. List five recommendations of the American Heart Association for reducing the risk of CHD and stroke.

9. Explain how statin drugs act in lowering total cholesterol concentration.

10. Why do women have an increased risk of heart disease after menopause, even though their HDL-cholesterol concentration may remain high and unchanged from pre-menopause?

WEBSITES FOR FURTHER STUDY

American Heart Association
www.americanheart.org
Dietary Fats: Know Which Types to Choose
www.mayoclinic.com/health/fat/NU00262
Dietary Fats, NIH
www.nlm.nih.gov/medlineplus/dietaryfats.html
Mayo Clinic Heart Health
www.mayoclinic.com
National Heart, Lung, and Blood Institute
www.nhlbi.nih.gov

National Cholesterol Education Program
www.nhlbi.nih.gov/about/ncep/index.htm
Risk Assessment Tool for Estimating Your 10-Year Risk of Having a Heart Attack
http://cvdrisk.nhlbi.nih.gov/calculator.asp
WebMD, Heart Disease
www.webmd.com/heart

REFERENCES

American Heart Association Nutrition Committee, Lichtenstein AH, Appel LJ, Brands M, et al. Diet and lifestyle recommendations revision 2006: a statement from the American Heart Association Nutrition Committee. *Circulation.* 2006;114:82–96.

Barzi F, Woodward M, Marfisi RM, Tavazzi L, Valagussa F, Marchioli R; GISSI-Prevenzione Investigators. Mediterranean diet and all-cause mortality after myocardial infarction: results from the GISSI-Prevenzione trial. *Eur Jour Clin Nutr.* 2003;57:604–611.

Cheng TO. Effect of rising serum cholesterol on risks of cardiovascular disease in northern China. *Int J Cardiol.* 2007;119:1–2.

de Lorgeril, M, Salen P, Martin JL, Monjaud I, Delaye J, Mamelle N. Mediterranean diet, traditional risk factors, and the rate of cardiovascular complications after myocardial infarction: Final report of the Lyon Diet Heart Study. *Circulation.* 1999;99:779–785.

Expert Panel on Detection, Evaluation, and Treatment of High Blood Cholesterol in Adults. Executive Summary of the Third Report of the National Cholesterol Education Program (NCEP) Expert Panel on Detection, Evaluation, and Treatment of High Blood Cholesterol in Adults (Adult Treatment Panel III). *JAMA.* 2001;285:2486–2496.

Friedewald WT, Levy RI, Frederickson DS. Estimation of the concentration of low-density lipoprotein cholesterol in plasma, without use of preparative ultracentrifuge. *Clin Chem.* 1972;18:499–502.

Holligan SD, Berryman CE, Wang L, Flock MR, Harris KA, Kris-Etherton PM. Atherosclerotic cardiovascular disease. In: Erdman JW Jr, MacDonald IA, Zeisel SH (eds.), *Present Knowledge in Nutrition.* 10th ed. Ames, IA: John Wiley & Sons; 2012;1186–1277.

Menotti A, Lanti M, Nedeljkovic S, Nissinen A, Kafatos A, Kromhout D. The relationship of age, blood pressure, serum cholesterol and smoking habits with the risk of typical and atypical coronary heart disease death in the European cohorts of the Seven Countries Study. *Int J Cardiol.* 2006;106:157–163.

Ridker, PM. C-reactive protein and the prediction of cardiovascular events among those at intermediate risk: moving an inflammatory hypothesis toward consensus. *J Am Coll Cardiol.* 2007;49:2129–2138.

Root M, Anderson JJB. Dietary effects of non-traditional risk factors of heart disease. *Nutr Res.* 2004;24:827–838.

ADDITIONAL READING

Levy D, Brink S. *A Change of Heart: How the Framingham Heart Study Helped Unravel the Mysteries of Cardiovascular Disease.* New York: Knopf; 2005.

Proteins

The proteins in foods supply the amino acids required for the synthesis of proteins in the body as well as the nitrogen (N) needed for the production of other biomolecules. **Proteins** are unique among the macronutrients because they alone supply nitrogen. In the normal course of metabolism, the body turns over and excretes nitrogen each day. Therefore, essential amino acids and nitrogen must be provided daily in order to maintain the body's everyday processes and, in children and pregnant women, to sustain growth. Unlike carbohydrates and fats, the body does not keep a long-term store of extra protein. Protein obtained from the diet is used to synthesize new cellular and extracellular proteins and to provide energy.

Proteins serve as the structural units of tissues and as functional components of cell membranes. Proteins also are important components of hormones; antibodies; enzymes; blood constituents, including albumin and clotting factors; collagen and elastin in connective tissues; hair fibers; apolipoproteins; and many other biomolecules. Proteins are found in all tissues inside and outside of cells throughout the body because they are highly variable and useful. No wonder protein is referred to as the "first" nutrient!

Today, dietary protein represents about 15% of the total energy in U.S. diets. (Note that only the hydrocarbon portion, not the nitrogen part, is converted into usable energy in our cells.) This percentage translates to approximately 75 to 80 grams of protein per day for women and 100 to 125 grams per day for men, exceeding the adult RDAs by about 100%. Affluent populations typically consume much more protein than needed to meet their age- and sex-specific RDAs. Dietary sources of protein include dairy, meat (red meat, poultry, and fish), eggs, cereal grains, vegetables, and beans and other legumes (see **FIGURE 7.1**).

This chapter examines the chemical structure of amino acids and proteins, food sources of dietary proteins, life cycle requirements and RDAs for proteins, functions of proteins in tissues, amino acid metabolism, and protein nutrition in special populations, including vegetarians and athletes. An estimated 1% to 3% of the adult U.S. population is vegan (i.e., no animal proteins are consumed). Much of the world's population does

> *Protein obtained from the diet is used to synthesize new cellular and extracellular proteins and to provide energy.*

protein Macronutrient composed of chains of amino acids. Contributes nitrogen (N) for synthesis of biological molecules and energy for ATP production.

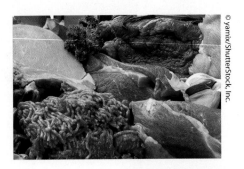
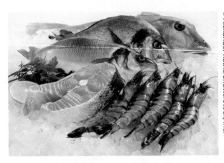
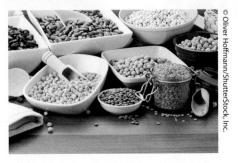

> Dietary sources of protein include dairy, meat (red meat, poultry, and fish), eggs, cereal grains, vegetables, and beans and other legumes.

FIGURE 7.1 Sources of Protein. Proteins are obtained from a variety of plant- and animal-based foods.

protein synthesis A complex system that involves the ribosome, enzymes, and messenger RNA derived from nuclear DNA (genetic information) to assemble amino acids into proteins.

amino acid An organic molecule with a central carbon atom with four groups: COOH, NH₂, H, and R. The R-group is unique to each amino acid; amino acids are the structural units of peptides and proteins.

amino (NH₂) group A side group found in every amino acid that can combine with a carboxyl group to form a peptide bond, be transferred to an organic keto acid to form a new amino acid via transamination, or be removed via deamination in the liver and used to make urea. Also called an amine group.

peptide bond An organic bond formed between two amino acids, the organic acid group of one and the amine group of the other; formation of the peptide bond involves the removal of a water (H₂O) molecule.

carboxyl group (carboxylate group, COOH) Functional group that is added or removed in metabolic reactions; also known as an organic acid.

polypeptide A polymer of many amino acids (i.e., 20 or so in human proteins) that includes numerous peptide bonds.

not consume adequate amounts of protein because of poverty or a lack of available plant and animal protein sources.

Structure of Amino Acids and Proteins

Proteins synthesis in living cells uses basic molecular components called **amino acids**. Twenty different amino acids may be used in making the linear array (polymer) of a protein, one amino acid after another. Each amino acid has different properties. The specific amino acids used and their precise order in the linear chain during protein synthesis dictate the properties of the resulting protein, and hence its function. Each type of protein is synthesized according to specific instructions in the DNA genetic blueprint, also known as the genetic code. In addition, each protein is synthesized only to meet a specific need of a cell. The synthetic molecular machinery (in ribosomes) is then activated and copies of that protein, with all of the amino acids in the correct order, are made. As shown in **FIGURE 7.2**, the amino group (also known as an amine group) of one amino acid binds to the acid group of the next amino acid, forming a carbon–nitrogen (C-N) bond. This linkage is known as a **peptide bond**, and these bonds are responsible for the linear structure of proteins.

In addition to their **amino (NH₂) group** and **carboxyl** or **acid (COOH) group** that make the peptide linkage, amino acids have side groups (R) that influence their ultimate three-dimensional shape, which dictates the role that a specific protein plays in cells or body fluids. Depending on the side group, the amino acid may be more or less water soluble. Some amino acids contain sulfur side groups that can form sulfur–sulfur cross links between amino acid strands within the same protein. Such links can hold the protein in a folded shape that is critical to its function. The side groups of amino acids are integral to the ultimate structure and role of the resulting protein.

Long chains of amino acids linked by peptide bonds are called **polypeptides**; they can be many hundreds of amino acids long. Once polypeptides are more than about 100 amino acids in length they are usually referred to as proteins, with the shorter polymers

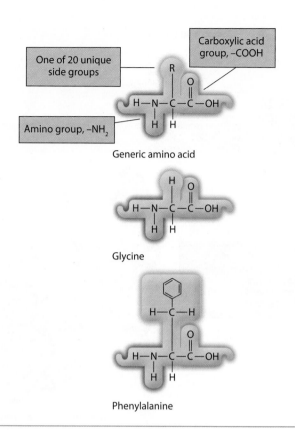

One of 20 unique side groups

Carboxylic acid group, –COOH

Amino group, –NH₂

Generic amino acid

Glycine

Phenylalanine

FIGURE 7.2 Amino Acids. All amino acids have an amino (NH₂) group, an acid (carboxyl or COOH) group, and a side group. The carbon–nitrogen bonds between adjacent amino acids are called peptide bonds. A protein is generated when multiple amino acids are joined together, one after another. The side group, R, is the residual structure of an amino acid.

> The shape and structure of a protein are intimately tied to the protein's function.

retaining the name polypeptide. Shorter polypeptides of 10 or fewer amino acids often are referred to simply as peptides.

The diversity of protein structures is great, partly because of the number and order of the amino acids in the protein but also partly because the bending and folding resulting from the side groups of amino acids of the polypeptide permit additional conformations. After synthesis, some proteins become globular, looking like a loose ball of string, such as the globin portion of hemoglobin molecules, which only function when they are in a particular three-dimensional configuration. Other proteins are fibrous or web-like, such as muscle proteins. The shape and structure of a protein are intimately tied to the protein's function (see **FIGURE 7.3**).

Nine **essential (or indispensable) amino acids** are required by the body; 11 other nonessential amino acids are also utilized (see **Table 7.1**). The essential amino acids cannot be synthesized by human cellular pathways and must be consumed in the diet. **Nonessential amino acids** can be synthesized in human tissues from other amino acids and from the byproducts of carbohydrate and fat metabolism. **Incomplete proteins** are deficient or lacking in one or more essential amino acids. The required amount of dietary essential amino acids decreases from infancy to adulthood. In infancy, the essential amino acids need to make up a much larger percentage of the dietary protein than in adulthood because of the limited ability to make metabolic conversions of amino acids early in life. The growth rate in infancy is so rapid that proteins are made and cells divide at a very rapid rate. When growth has stopped in adulthood, only small amounts of the essential amino acids are needed to replace proteins that are slowly turning over.

essential (indispensable) amino acid Amino acid that must be supplied in the human diet because humans do not have enzymes that can synthesize them, as opposed to nonessential amino acids, which can be synthesized by the body. Animal products generally contain greater amounts of the essential amino acids than plants.

nonessential amino acid An amino acid whose structure can be synthesized by usual pathways in the body and therefore does not need to be consumed in the diet.

incomplete protein A protein that is deficient or lacking in one or more essential amino acids. Examples include corn protein and collagen.

Amino acid sequence

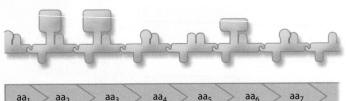

A simple illustration of a protein just shows the sequence of amino acids that form one or more polypeptide chains.

| aa₁ | aa₂ | aa₃ | aa₄ | aa₅ | aa₆ | aa₇ |

A more complex illustration of a protein shows its three-dimensional structure. This molecule of hemoglobin is composed of four polypeptide chains. The square plates represent nonprotein portions of the molecule (heme) that carry oxygen.

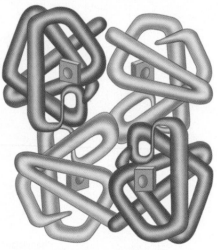

Three-dimensional structure

FIGURE 7.3 Three-Dimensional Structure of Proteins. Proteins come in a variety of shapes and sizes. The structure of a particular protein determines its ultimate role in the body. The terms aa₁, aa₂, etc. designate the first, second, and subsequent amino acids in order of use in protein synthesis.

> Nine essential, or indispensable, amino acids are required by the body; 11 other nonessential amino acids are also utilized.

TABLE 7.1
Essential and Nonessential Amino Acids

Essential	Nonessential
Histidine*	Alanine
Isoleucine*	Arginine
Leucine*	Asparagine
Lysine	Aspartic acid
Methionine	Cysteine
Phenylalanine	Glutamic acid
Threonine	Glutamine
Tryptophan	Glycine
Valine	Proline
	Serine
	Tyrosine

In certain conditions, nonessential amino acids, including cysteine, arginine, and tyrosine, may become essential.
* Branched chain amino acids.

Functions of Protein in the Body

Proteins serve an incredibly diverse array of functions in the human body (see Table 7.2). Fibrous and elastic proteins make up the outer layers of the skin and form the first defensive barrier against pathogens. Proteins also make up the antibodies in the human immune system that recognize and attack foreign microbial intruders.

TABLE 7.2
Examples of Proteins and Their Functions in the Human Body

Protein	Structure	Function	Action
Immunoglobulin	Small folded protein with highly variable portions at two ends	Immunity	The variable portion of the antibody molecules binds to invading pathogens.
Hemoglobin	Globular protein with four heme groups holding iron atoms	Transporter	Binds to oxygen in the lungs and transports it to tissues.
Collagen	Long twisted fibrils, triple helix	Connective tissue, bone	Overlapping fibrils form strong attachments to hold muscles, bones, and cells in place.
Actin and myosin	Long overlapping fibrils	Muscle fibers	Interaction between actin and myosin fibers moves muscles.
Insulin	Small folded protein	Hormone	Secreted by pancreas, binds to cells to facilitate movement of glucose from blood into cells.
Superoxide dismutase	Large folded protein with copper and zinc atoms at the center	Enzyme	Degrades the dangerous superoxide to the less dangerous hydrogen peroxide.
Albumin	Large globular cross-linked protein	Fluid balance	Maintains fluid balance by holding water in the blood.
Apolipoprotein B	Very large protein integrated into small fat droplets	Lipoprotein	Holds lipoprotein together, improves water solubility, and directs binding to receptors.

The most abundant protein in our bodies is collagen, which consists of three tightly knit polypeptides (triple helix). These polypeptides form coiled fibrous strands that comprise the ligaments and tendons that hold the bones and muscles in place. **Collagen**, the most abundant protein in the body, also is a predominant protein in connective tissues, including the organic matrix of bone. At the microscopic scale, the strong collagen fibers hold our cells and tissues in place.

Two additional proteins, actin and myosin, interact in the three types of muscle (skeletal, heart, and smooth) to cause contractions. **Hemoglobin** is a globular protein with four binding sites for oxygen that gives the red color to our blood and brings oxygen to our muscles and organs.

All of the enzymes that speed up the synthetic pathways in the body are proteins. Every cell has hundreds, if not thousands, of specific enzymes for every function, including the very reactions that make the enzymes. In addition, many of the body's messenger molecules—hormones—are also polypeptides or small proteins. For example, insulin, a polypeptide with two chains of amino acids linked by disulfide bonds, is considered a small protein because of its low molecular weight. Because of their large size and

collagen A protein molecule found in connective tissues that consists of a triple helix of polypeptide coils. It provides strength to connective tissues in tendons and ligaments. It is part of the organic matrix (osteoid) of skeletal tissues, where collagen fibers are arranged in an orderly array.

hemoglobin The oxygen-carrying molecule in red blood cells that utilizes iron in the heme portion to hold oxygen atoms being delivered from the lungs to other tissues.

> Although DNA contains the code of life, the proteins do the work of life, including the dramatic orchestration of cell division with its myriad interlocking steps and the sequential steps of the clotting process. Proteins are, indeed, the protean material of life.

solubility, blood proteins, such as albumin, help control fluid balance and acid-base balance. Other proteins act as transporters for less water-soluble materials such as lipids, lipid-soluble vitamins, and hormones. Still other proteins attach to the surface of cells and act as identifiers, address labels, or mailboxes for incoming bloodborne messages.

Although DNA contains the code of life, the proteins do the work of life, including the dramatic orchestration of cell division with its myriad interlocking steps and the sequential steps of the clotting process. Proteins are, indeed, the protean material of life.

Protein Quality and Food Sources

The protein content of foods varies considerably, but **protein quality** refers to the presence of all essential amino acids in amounts that support growth. Ratios of the protein content relative to energy (kilocalories) of select foods used around the world are provided in **Table 7.3**. The approximate **protein-to-energy ratio** needed to support reasonable growth and development, assuming a reasonable mixing of protein sources, is about 4 grams of protein per 100 kilocalories of food energy. This translates to

protein quality An index of the amount of all essential amino acids in a single food protein; protein quality of animal and plant foods varies considerably, with animal proteins generally having higher values. Milk and egg proteins have the highest quality for humans.

protein-to-energy ratio Ratio of protein content relative to energy (kilocalories). A good source of protein has about 4 grams of protein per 100 kilocalories of food energy.

TABLE 7.3
Protein-to-Energy Ratios of Common Foods

Food Item	Protein Content (grams per 100 kilocalories)
Fish (tuna)	18.0
Chicken (breast)	14.0
Soybeans, boiled	9.6
Beef (steak)	8.0
Egg (whole)	8.0
Cow's milk, (3.3% fat)	8.0
Broccoli, cooked	6.8
Green beans (snap)	6.0
Peanuts	4.0
Wheat (whole, hard)	4.0
Corn	3.0
Rice	2.5
White potato	2.5
Sweet potato	1.5
Banana	1.0
Cassava	0.5

A value of 4.0 grams per 100 kilocalories is considered minimal for supporting health.
Reproduced from Anderson JJB. *Nutrition and Health: An Introduction*. Durham, NC: Carolina Academic Press; 2005.

60 grams of protein per 1,500 kilocalories of food energy, which is in the neighborhood of the RDA for protein of adult women.

The quality of a dietary protein is based on its amino acid content, particularly the quantity of essential amino acids, and how well it is digested and absorbed. The proteins in animal products are generally of higher quality than those found in plant foods because they contain sufficient quantities of the essential amino acids and are more easily digested and absorbed. This makes them **complete proteins**. Plant proteins are generally of lower quality because they are low in one or more of the essential amino acids and because they are digested and absorbed less efficiently due to their fiber content. Note that protein from soy and from a few other legumes (e.g., peas, beans) is of high quality but generally provides less of the sulfur-containing amino acids.

An index called the Protein Digestibility-Corrected Amino Acid Score (PDCAAS) is used to score protein quality. It is used on nutrient labels of foods to equalize protein content when determining the %DV of protein of the food. **Table 7.4** provides some protein digestibility values of common foods used in calculating the PDCAAS and the %BV for protein used on food labels. Biological value (BV) is the proportion of the protein absorbed from a food that becomes part of the proteins of the person's body. In effect then, digestibility is how available to the body the protein is, and biological value is how efficiently the body uses the protein, once absorbed. Both values are needed to determine a food protein's true value.

The highest quality proteins are found in egg white and milk protein. The protein collagen, found in animal connective tissues, is of poor quality because it is totally deficient in tryptophan and low in a few other essential amino acids. Grain proteins, such

> *The quality of a dietary protein is based on its amino acid content, particularly the quantity of essential amino acids, and how well it is digested and absorbed.*

TABLE 7.4
Protein Digestibility Values or Quality Indices of Common Foods

Protein Source	Digestibility Value (%)	Biological Value (%)
Corn (whole)	89	59
Crisped rice cereal	77	64
Bread (whole wheat)	92	65
Milk (whole)	94	85
Eggs (scrambled)	96	94
Lima beans	78	66
Peanut butter	95	—
Soybeans	91	73
Beef	95	74
Tuna (canned)	90	76
Chicken	100	74

Maximum quality = 100; decreasing quality < 100.
Data from *Federal Register*, 58(3), January 6, 1993; 2079–2195. Food labeling: Mandatory status of nutrition labeling and nutrient content revision, format for nutrition label; and Hegsted, DM. *Improvement of Protein Nutriture*. National Academy of Sciences, Washington, DC, 1974, p. 70.

complete protein A high-quality protein that contains all the essential amino acids in reasonable quantities.

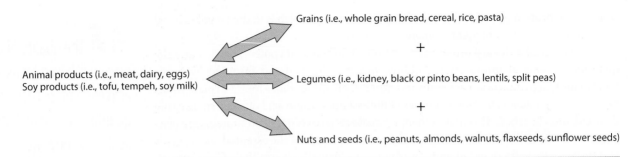

Grains (i.e., whole grain bread, cereal, rice, pasta)

+

Animal products (i.e., meat, dairy, eggs)
Soy products (i.e., tofu, tempeh, soy milk)

Legumes (i.e., kidney, black or pinto beans, lentils, split peas)

+

Nuts and seeds (i.e., peanuts, almonds, walnuts, flaxseeds, sunflower seeds)

FIGURE 7.4 Complementary Proteins. Foods that are low in one essential amino acid but high in another can be combined in a meal such that reasonable amounts of the essential amino acids are obtained. One particularly common pairing is rice and beans, a staple meal in many parts of the world.

> In the diets of infants and young children, protein quality is of greater importance because of higher requirements for essential amino acids used in growth and development.

as those in corn and wheat, tend to be low in lysine and tryptophan, whereas those in legumes such as beans and soybeans contain more of these essential amino acids and less of the sulfur-containing amino acids, such as methionine. Combining various plant proteins with differing missing essential amino acids in the same meal provides adequate amounts of all the essential amino acids. Foods like rice and legumes or corn and beans, when combined, offer good overall protein quality (see **FIGURE 7.4**). The mixing of different plant proteins in the same meal (or over 24 hours) is referred to as **complementation of proteins** and has been practiced by vegans and other vegetarians for centuries to meet their protein needs long before RDAs were established. Inadequate protein intakes are rare among practicing vegetarians because they consume complementary proteins each day. In the diets of infants and young children, protein quality is of greater importance because of higher requirements for essential amino acids used in growth and development.

Some diets that are low in protein quality have limited amounts of one or more essential amino acids, such that one or more of these amino acids are considered to be limiting in the diet. Typically, amino acids that contain sulfur and benzene (phenyl group) are limited in plant proteins. Diets that are low in one or more essential amino acids can restrict growth and place individuals at increased risk of disease because fewer key proteins can be synthesized.

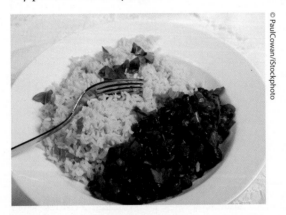

© PaulCowan/iStockphoto

complementation (complementarity) of proteins The combining of two or more plant proteins in the same meal to provide adequate amounts of all essential amino acids for the synthesis of proteins; for example, the use of corn and beans or other legumes together in a meal.

Protein Intake and Turnover

Proteins are digested within the gastrointestinal tract and yield amino acids. The amino acids are then absorbed by the enterocytes lining the small intestine. Absorbed amino acids are transported from the gut cells to the liver via the hepatic portal vein. Only about half of the amino acids are extracted for the hepatic synthesis of various proteins, both for export and for internal use as enzymes and in cell membranes. Proteins made in the liver and secreted to the rest of the body include the lipoproteins, which transport lipids, and other serum proteins, including albumin, which transports calcium and other ions, and transferrin, which transports iron in blood. The remaining 50% of absorbed amino acids pass through the liver and continue in the circulation to supply all other body tissues and organs. The brain, in particular, has a large need for amino acids, especially for the synthesis of neurotransmitters that are derived from a few specific amino acids.

The proteins in the body are always in a dynamic state of being degraded and synthesized (i.e., turned over). This constant activity of **protein turnover** of a specific protein throughout the day (24 hours) is thought to replace degraded proteins and to minimize the level of damaged proteins remaining in the body. About 50% of the free amino acids in the circulation, including alanine, have just come from proteins that were degraded and will soon be taken up by cells for the synthesis of new proteins. Some of the nitrogen from degraded amino acids in cells is recycled for the synthesis of new molecules, including nonessential amino acids made by transamination and other nitrogen-containing molecules. The turnover of the body's pool of amino acids is illustrated in **FIGURE 7.5**.

Protein turnover represents the sum of the synthesis and degradation of proteins by body tissues during the course of normal metabolism. The overall body turnover of protein is about three to four times larger than the total intake from food or the excretory losses of nitrogen from amino acids used in urea synthesis. This high turnover rate is based on healthy nonexcessive dietary intake of proteins and other macronutrients. Therefore, amino acids, both essential and nonessential, are always circulating in blood, though in lower concentrations when dietary protein intake is not sufficient. The metabolic steps involved in protein turnover constitute a significant share of the energy expended as part of the basal metabolic rate.

> *The overall body turnover of protein is about three to four times larger than the total intake from food or the excretory losses of nitrogen from amino acids used in urea synthesis.*

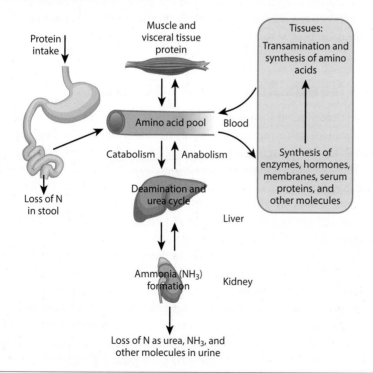

FIGURE 7.5 Amino Acid Pools in the Body. The overall daily turnover of proteins through protein synthesis and protein degradation of amino acids is about fourfold greater than the absorption of amino acids from the diet.

Reproduced from Anderson JJB. *Nutrition and Health: An Introduction.* Durham, NC: Carolina Academic Press; 2005.

protein turnover The dynamic synthesis and breakdown of proteins by the body.

Only about 33% of the amino acids used in protein synthesis come initially from the diet. Where do the remaining 67% of the amino acids come from? Most people consume approximately 70-100 grams of protein each day. The turnover of existing proteins in the body provides a pool of about 200 grams of amino acids a day from recycling. The protein requirement for a 70-kilogram person, at 0.8 grams of protein per kilogram of body weight per day, would be 56 grams per day. Indispensable (essential) amino acids account for about 0.1 grams per kilogram body weight per day, or about 10% to 12% of the protein requirement for adults.

The amino acids available to the body from both protein recycling and dietary sources end up in one of four places: (1) resynthesis into new proteins; (2) use of the hydrocarbon backbone for energy; and conversion of amino groups into other nitrogen-containing constituents that are lost in (3) feces and (4) urine. Of the 300 grams of amino acids available each day after protein digestion, about 200 grams go to new protein, about 75 grams go to energy needs, and about 25 grams are lost to feces and urine. ●

In times of short supply of dietary protein but adequate energy intake, the body adapts by conserving its amino acid pools. Under these conditions, the loss of total urinary nitrogen decreases to obligatory low levels and protein turnover decreases substantially. Thus, several dietary conditions contribute to the dynamic processes of protein turnover, both synthetic and degradative. With excessive protein intake, as in the standard American diet, extra amino acids not needed for protein synthesis or other molecules have their amino groups removed, a process known as **deamination**. The hydrocarbon part of the amino acid is then used for ATP production for cellular energy or for triglycerides synthesis and fat storage. The amino groups removed from amino acids are used mainly in urea synthesis and its excretion. Nitrogen balance, a measure of the balance between the nitrogen intake from protein and the excretion of nitrogenous products, like urea, is used to assess overall health.

Protein Needs Across the Life Cycle

In the United States, most people do not have any trouble meeting the RDA for protein. In fact, protein consumption by the vast majority of the U.S. population is close to twice the RDA. Most Americans consume 15% to 17% of their total energy intake as protein. Thus, an adult female who consumes 2,000 kilocalories per day will be getting approximately 75 grams of protein daily, which is equivalent to 300 kilocalories of energy intake. Compare this value with the protein RDA of 46 grams per day for females 19 years of age and older. For men, the comparable RDA is 52 grams per day, but intakes typically exceed 100 grams per day.

All protein allowances include a safety factor above the Estimated Average Requirement (EAR) to ensure adequate intakes for specific populations. During pregnancy and lactation, an additional 25 grams per day is needed. For the growth of infants and children, protein is recommended at higher levels on a per kilogram body weight basis. During the first year of life, the RDA is 1.52 grams of protein per kilogram body weight. Late in childhood, it decreases to about 0.85 grams per kilogram body weight per day. Children in their adolescent growth spurt require about 0.95 grams per kilogram per day. In adulthood, the protein allowance decreases to 0.8 grams per kilogram per day for both sexes.

In order to estimate the EAR for protein, balance studies of different protein intakes have been conducted, typically in young adults, for periods of 3 to 4 weeks. An EAR of

> **"** In the United States, most people do not have any trouble meeting the RDA for protein. **"**

deamination The enzymatic removal of an amine group; in the liver these amine groups enter the urea cycle for elimination from the body.

FOCUS 7.2 High-Protein Diets

High-protein diets, such as those recommended by the Atkins Diet, the South Beach Diet, and the Zone Diet, emphasize a dietary regimen that greatly reduces intake of carbohydrate-containing foods such as potatoes, breads, and beans. These diets tend to have early success with weight loss and, if maintained, can lead to considerable weight loss. However, they are not generally recommended by nutritionists because they put the body under metabolic stress for the duration of the diet. Without some carbohydrates in the diet the body must go to extreme lengths metabolically to keep up the blood glucose levels required for fueling the brain, nerves, and red blood cells. When all else fails, the body turns fats into ketone bodies, the small acidic molecules that can substitute for glucose as a fuel in some tissues. Unhealthy side effects of these metabolic shifts include low blood glucose, loss of appetite, lethargy, and acidic blood. These

acid compounds can lower the pH of the blood, altering many basic physiological processes of the body. These diets put individuals in a metabolic fasting state while they are still eating meals rich in meat and cheese. Diets balanced in healthy, low-fat foods consumed in smaller amounts will lead to progressive weight loss without the metabolic stress of a high-protein diet. ●

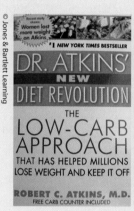
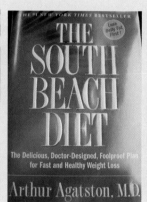
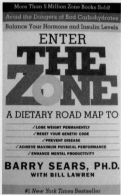

© Jones & Bartlett Learning

0.66 grams per kilogram per day has been established for healthy adults. The RDA, which includes a built-in safety factor of 25%, has been raised to 0.8 grams per kilogram per day to account for human variation. This RDA applies to both sexes, and it should meet the needs of 97.5% of the healthy adult population because of the safety factor. Heavily muscled individuals who work out regularly need slightly higher protein intakes than the RDAs to meet their needs. In addition, some nutritionists advocate even higher levels of dietary proteins as a way to lose weight; however, this practice is controversial.

Protein allowances for the various age and sex groups are provided in **Table 7.5**. This table of RDAs takes into consideration the typical pattern of U.S. dietary protein intake; that is, a diet with high quality protein (amino acid scoring pattern) and high digestibility (approximately 75%) of all food proteins typically consumed.

PRACTICAL APPLICATIONS 7.1

Protein Intake Compared with Protein Allowance

A 31-year-old man has a breakfast of two large eggs over easy with two pieces of white bread toast and 8 ounces of 1% milk. Lunch is 3 ounces of lean ham and 2 ounces of Swiss cheese with 1 tablespoon mayonnaise on a large Kaiser roll, together with half a cup of frozen yogurt. For dinner, he has a broiled 6-ounce lean pork loin, 1 cup of broccoli, and a baked potato with 2 ounces

of American cheese spread. For dessert he has half a cup of chocolate ice cream. Use food composition tables or Nutrition Panel labels to determine the protein content of these meals. How much protein did he consume? What is his protein RDA? What percentage of his RDA for protein did he consume from all his meals? ■

> Although it is probably true that vegans, on average, consume less protein than their omnivorous counterparts, this lower level is probably still above their RDA and poses little concern nutritionally. Several servings of legumes provide sufficient amounts of protein for vegans. "

TABLE 7.5
Estimated Average Requirement and Recommended Dietary Allowance for Protein

Age	EAR (g/kg/day) for Both Genders		RDA (g/kg/day) for Both Genders	
0–6 months	—		1.52*	
7–12 months	1.0		1.20	
1–3 years	0.87		1.05	
4–8 years	0.76		0.95	
9–13 years	0.76		0.95	
	Males	**Females**	**Males**	**Females**
14–18 years	0.73	0.71	0.85	0.85
			52 g/d	46 g/d
≥ 19 years	0.66	0.66	0.80	0.80
			56 g/d	46 g/d
Pregnancy		1.05		25 g/d†
Lactation		1.05		25 g/d†

* Adequate Intake (AI), rather than RDA, in g/kg/day; † EAR in g/kg/day = 71g/kg/d.
Data from Institute of Medicine, Food and Nutrition Board. *Dietary Reference Intakes for Energy, Carbohydrate, Fiber, Fat, Fatty Acids, Cholesterol, Protein, and Amino Acids.* Washington, DC: National Academies Press; 2002.

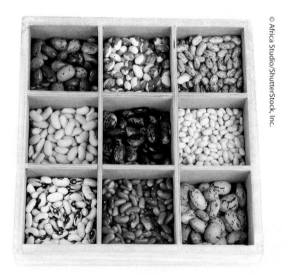

© Africa Studio/ShutterStock, Inc.

FIGURE 7.6 Vegan Protein Needs. Vegans can meet their protein needs by eating complementary proteins such as legumes and cereal grains.

Protein Needs of Vegetarians

Vegetarians have the same protein requirements as omnivores. The challenge for vegetarians is in ensuring that their protein requirements are met. Vegetarians, particularly vegans, usually consume complementary proteins from legumes and grains. In most cases, the total amount of protein consumed from these sources compensates for the lower quality (limited essential amino acids and lower digestibility) of vegetable and grain proteins sources.

Vegans may need to eat more legumes because of their higher intake of fiber, which decreases the digestibility of proteins. Table 7.3 shows that a number of foods consumed in a vegan diet—such as soy, green beans, other legumes, and broccoli—are fairly high in protein in terms of their protein–energy ratio. Although it is probably true that vegans, on average, consume less protein than their omnivorous counterparts, this lower level is probably still above their RDA and poses little concern nutritionally. Several servings of legumes provide sufficient amounts of protein for vegans (see **FIGURE 7.6**).

Most of the world subsists primarily on grain staples, such as wheat, rice, and corn, and root crops. Most of these foods contain low, but appreciable, levels of protein. Referring back to Table 7.3, note that the staple energy sources consumed in poorer nations of the world are essentially low-protein foods. For example, cassava has only 0.5 grams of protein per 100 kilocalories.

Protein Use by Tissues

Proteins play a major role in human nutrition. Dietary proteins—actually the amino acids derived from them—have several metabolic uses. As discussed earlier, proteins provide the essential amino acids required for the synthesis of tissue proteins, as well as enzymes and other molecules. The amino (NH_2) groups of amino acids also provide the nitrogen used in the synthesis of nonessential amino acids in cells as well as the synthesis of other nitrogen-containing molecules, such as the **nucleic acids— deoxyribonucleic acid (DNA)** and **ribonucleic acid (RNA)**—that govern protein synthesis. In addition, the hydrocarbon backbone of amino acids can be completely oxidized to carbon dioxide and water to generate cellular ATP. Under certain conditions, such as fasting or inadequate dietary protein intake, a larger fraction than normal of the diet-derived amino acids can be converted in the liver via gluconeogenesis to glucose for release to the blood and potential use by all other cells of the body. Lastly, amino acids are used for the synthesis of other essential molecules, such as neurotransmitters and hormones.

Protein Synthesis

Protein synthesis requires not only each amino acid programmed in the genetic code (DNA) for each specific protein, but it also needs messenger RNA (mRNA) and transfer RNA (tRNA). mRNA and tRNA govern the assembly of each protein in the ribosome attached to the cellular endoplasmic reticulum (organelle). The key enzyme in protein synthesis is protein synthase. The amino acids required for the synthesis of proteins are obtained from dietary proteins (~33%) and from the amino acid pool (~67%).

Protein Degradation

During times of extended fasting (greater than 24 hours) or chronic insufficient intake of energy and protein, the body degrades proteins in its own tissues (i.e., lean body mass) for gluconeogenesis to replenish glucose levels in the blood. These conditions of undernutrition are defined according to the degrees of deprivation of protein and energy. Marasmus or starvation, one form of undernutrition, results from too little of all macronutrients. Another form of **protein–energy malnutrition (PEM)** is known as kwashiorkor, which results from too little protein but nearly sufficient energy intake.

In these conditions, tissue proteins of skeletal muscle and visceral organs (even the heart muscle), are degraded by peptidase enzymes, a process called **proteolysis**. The amino acids are then carried in the blood to the liver for new glucose production. As a consequence of either extended fasting or a poor diet with inadequate energy, the protein in body tissues becomes further depleted. An example of a change in tissue proteins in semistarvation or severe undernutrition is the decline in serum albumin.

> During times of extended fasting (greater than 24 hours) or chronic insufficient intake of energy and protein, the body degrades proteins in its own tissues (i.e., lean body mass) for gluconeogenesis to replenish glucose levels in the blood.

nucleic acids Deoxyribonucleic acid (DNA) and ribonucleic acid (RNA). These molecules, which consist of nucleotides in long polymer chains, govern protein synthesis.

deoxyribonucleic acid (DNA) A complex molecule that has a double-helix structure. Portions of DNA comprise genes. Long DNA strands are linked to nucleoproteins in chromosomes in the nucleus of cells; these molecules comprise the genetic code, regulating all cellular activities at the most fundamental level through the synthesis of specific functional proteins.

ribonucleic acid (RNA) Nucleic acid polymer that controls protein synthesis in ribosomes by transferring the genetic code for a specific protein from the DNA to the ribosome; also the genetic material of many viruses.

protein–energy malnutrition (PEM) Balanced or unbalanced undernutrition with respect to calorie and protein intake. Can be a severe life-threatening nutritional disorder that requires medical attention. PEM is often coupled with infection as part of a malnutrition–infection cycle.

proteolysis The degradation (catabolism) of protein molecules to their constituent amino acids by proteolytic enzymes (peptidases) that hydrolyze peptide bonds. Occurs both within the GI tract and within cells.

Monitoring Protein Malnutrition

You are a World Health Organization (WHO) nutritionist newly assigned to an area with known high levels of general undernutrition. You will want to be able to detect adults and children with malnutrition (i.e., kwashiorkor and marasmus) so you can help them to overcome these conditions. You also want to detect villages and regions where PEM is likely to exist. What diagnostic tests would you consider using for detecting PEM among the adults and children? Consider the usefulness of the blood test for serum albumin and other circulating liver proteins, which is a standard approach for monitoring protein status. What clinical indicators of undernutrition would you look for in these children? In examining a village or region, what environmental and social factors would you consider in their diet, agricultural practices, culture, and current political and social state? ■

Protein Metabolism in Starvation, Dieting, and Excessive Intake

Protein in our diet and in our tissues, given the right stimuli, can be metabolized and then converted into other proteins, carbohydrates, or triglycerides. Given this interchangeability, it is not surprising to find that protein plays a key role in both dietary deprivation and excess. When a person is starving, usually all nutrients and calories are deficient. In this dire situation, the body is left to its own adaptive mechanisms. In the course of the millennia of evolution, those who have endured starvation have mostly survived.

Finely tuned mechanisms have evolved to conserve resources when undernutrition begins. For example, body temperature drops slightly, the basal metabolic rate decreases, protein recycling slows, and people generally become less physically active to conserve energy. The body draws upon both functional lean tissues and fat stores for energy. Although no reserves of spare amino acids exist in the body, the large amounts of functional proteins in tissues, such as muscle, can be degraded to provide proteins and amino acids for other uses. (**Protein-sparing modified fast** diets provide overall low energy consumption but a good amount of high-quality protein.) Muscle proteins are slowly degraded for needed blood glucose via gluconeogenesis and for amino acids needed for the minimum amount of new protein synthesis. The removal of amino groups from amino acids (i.e., deamination) leaves the hydrocarbon backbone (C-H) available for further degradation and entry into the metabolic pathways that generate ATP. Ketone bodies, such as acetone, are also synthesized during fat degradation to spare some protein conversion into glucose. Eventually, critical systems such as the immune system become compromised, such that infectious diseases may become much more serious. Similarly, heart muscle function declines. These conditions are usually made even more serious by a limited intake of required vitamins and minerals in the diet.

FIGURE 7.7 shows patterns of protein metabolism during intermeal periods, short-term fasting, and starvation. Protein degradation (i.e., proteolysis) is low during fasting and high during long-term starvation. Under starvation conditions most amino acids in muscle and other tissues are converted via **transamination** to alanine, which then enters blood. In this process, an amine group transfers from an amino acid to an organic keto acid to form a new amino acid. Once in the liver, alanine may be converted to glucose via the gluconeogenesis pathway. This glucose is then secreted by the liver for transport to the brain and red blood cells, which have high glucose requirements. The alanine–glucose cycle is illustrated in **FIGURE 7.8**.

protein-sparing modified fast A severe dietary approach to weight loss involving low-energy, high-protein intake.

transamination The transfer of an amine group from an amino acid to an organic keto acid to form a new amino acid.

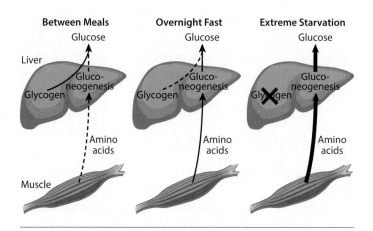

FIGURE 7.7 Patterns of Protein Metabolism. Different scenarios of protein synthesis and degradation occur under different conditions, such as between meals during the day, after an overnight fast, and during extended and extreme starvation.

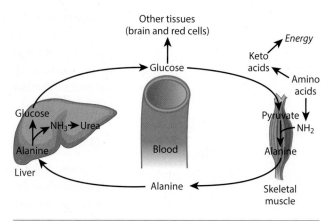

FIGURE 7.8 Alanine–Glucose Cycle. The alanine–glucose cycle involves liver utilization of alanine from skeletal muscle tissue and other tissues for the generation of new glucose molecules (i.e., gluconeogenesis). Glucose is secreted into the blood from the liver for use by all other cells of the body.

Reproduced from Anderson JJB. *Nutrition and Health: An Introduction*. Durham, NC: Carolina Academic Press; 2005.

The key to successful dieting is to lose weight while avoiding the severe effects of long-term fasting or semistarvation that lead to tissue protein (LBM) losses. In particular, a successful diet should maintain muscle mass and lower blood glucose to within the normal range (and provide feelings of fullness or satiety), while keeping the total calories consumed in a day low. Well-balanced diets, such as Weight Watchers, accomplish this by a mix of low-fat meats and cheeses, together with moderate amounts of carbohydrates, in small portion or serving sizes (see **FIGURE 7.9**). Emphasis is placed on careful calorie counting and on tasteful food preparation. Protein in the diet gives a long-term feeling of satiety, the carbohydrates keep blood glucose levels up, and small serving sizes keep calorie intake low.

As energy intake becomes chronically excessive, the body adapts by modifying its use of proteins. Instead of being converted into carbohydrate (glucose or glycogen) in the liver, the carbon backbones of amino acids (i.e., after deamination) are largely converted to fatty acids and then into triglycerides before being transported by VLDL particles to

> *A successful diet should maintain muscle mass and lower blood glucose to within the normal range (and provide feelings of fullness or satiety), while keeping the total calories consumed in a day low.*

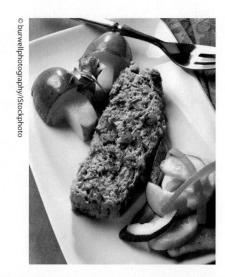

FIGURE 7.9 Managing Portion Sizes. Modest portion sizes for all meals, including during holiday periods, keep the caloric intake within the normal range and help prevent weight gain.

storage sites in the body. Of course, excess carbohydrates may also be converted to fat. During both starvation and protein breakdown, a large amount of urea is synthesized from the amino groups by the liver, coupled with CO_2 production, and then excreted by the kidneys. The amount of urea nitrogen in urine can provide information about the protein content of one's diet.

Special Protein Needs of Athletes

Adequate intake of protein is necessary for optimal growth and development of all tissues, including skeletal muscles and the skeleton. In the United States, typical protein intakes are more than adequate to meet these requirements, even during the adolescent growth spurt and with muscle development through exercise. Protein requirements for muscle building increase only minimally. Many athletes believe they need much higher intakes of protein each day to build muscle, but this has no basis in fact. Protein powders are not needed; meals with an extra serving of protein should be sufficient (see **FIGURE 7.10**). Vegetarian athletes typically do very well with only plant proteins from at least one legume per meal and one or more other sources if they are consumed in adequate amounts.

Competitive body builders and other athletes who "bulk up" may be the exception because they may need almost twice the RDA for protein to support muscle growth under these training conditions. However, this requirement can be easily met through a balanced diet that meets the increased energy and additional protein needs of their sports. (Protein-rich powders are not recommended.) The male hormones, mainly testosterone, and the weight-bearing strains of intense exercise significantly contribute to the increased muscle mass of strength athletes. Furthermore, the most efficient dietary energy source for athletes and power lifters is complex carbohydrates, not proteins. The use of protein is really an inefficient way to provide energy to meet tissue needs once protein requirements are met. In addition, the nitrogen waste products from excess protein intake can exert additional stress on the kidneys.

Protein supplements are increasingly being used by body builders and others to improve muscle mass or general health. Many nutritional formulations contain protein supplements with the promise to consumers that these supplements will prolong life, optimize health, or prevent disease. Much of this additional protein enters the pathways leading to fat synthesis.

Creatine is an amino acid that has been used by athletes as a supplement to generate creatine phosphate, a storage energy molecule in muscle cells. This is believed to enhance athletic performance. The scientific evidence suggests that creatine also increases muscle mass (lean body mass) slightly when combined with resistance exercise. Creatine is especially effective for short-duration activities requiring muscle bursts of energy from creatine phosphate made in tissues. However, **creatine phosphate** as a supplement (more than plain creatine) is not considered healthy because the excessive phosphate consumed may have adverse effects, such as soft tissue calcification.

> Many athletes believe they need much higher intakes of protein each day to build muscle, but this has no basis in fact.

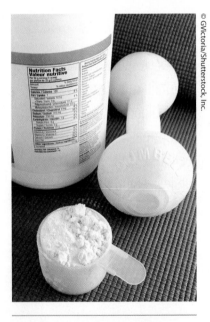

© GVictoria/Shutterstock, Inc.

FIGURE 7.10 Commercial Protein Powders. Most, if not all, protein consumed in protein supplements is degraded to generate ATP or to promote fat synthesis. Little or none is used for protein synthesis in muscle and other tissues.

creatine phosphate The high-energy molecule in skeletal muscle that serves as a readily available store of energy for muscle contractility and the events associated with movement.

SUMMARY

Protein plays a major role in human nutrition. Most Americans exceed the recommended intake. Proteins are made up of combinations of the 20 amino acids common to all of life. Humans require nine essential amino acids in a diet comprising about 0.8 grams of protein per kilogram body weight per day for adults. The nonessential amino acids can be synthesized by the body. Amino acids and proteins are needed for growth and development as well as numerous cellular functions, for the synthesis of extracellular proteins in blood (e.g., albumin), and for the supporting structures (e.g., collagen) of the body. Proteins also undergo degradation at different rates in different tissues; this is especially rapid when protein and energy intakes are not adequate. The diet must supply these amino acids and the nitrogen needed for the renewal of these proteins and other nitrogen-containing molecules, such as nucleic acids. Protein requirements vary according to the stage of the life cycle. Protein–energy deficiency diseases, such as kwashiorkor and marasmus, affect many children in the developing parts of the world. Vegetarians can easily obtain sufficient dietary protein through the careful choice of complementing proteins in plant foods, namely legumes and other grains. Athletes may need additional protein above their RDA, but almost certainly not so much as many are consuming.

STUDENT ACTIVITIES

1. Define the following: essential amino acid, nonessential amino acid, protein quality.

2. In infancy, essential amino acids from dietary proteins need to make up a larger percentage of the diet than during adulthood. What is the reason for this decline in the need for essential amino acids beyond infancy?

3. List some of the highest quality proteins. List some of the lowest. What makes a protein a "high-quality" protein?

4. It could be said that half of all proteins in our bodies are made from recycled amino acids. Explain.

5. Distinguish between marasmus and kwashiorkor.

6. What are complementary proteins? Why are they so important in vegetarian eating plans?

7. Being on the Atkins (high-protein) diet is like "starving" while eating a steak. Explain.

8. Should strength athletes consume more than their RDA of protein? Explain.

9. Name the three major waste products of proteins following complete metabolism.

10. In contrast to carbohydrates (glycogen) and fats (triglycerides), proteins are not stored for later use. Because of the need for tissue protein degradation during fasting and starvation, explain why this statement is not as simple as it sounds.

WEBSITES FOR FURTHER STUDY

The Doctor Will See You Now
www.thedoctorwillseeyounow.com/content/nutrition/art2059.html

Food and Agriculture Organization (FAO)
www.fao.org

Food Navigator
www.foodnavigator.com/news/ng.asp?n=77016-solanic-avebe-potato-protein

Harvard School of Public Health
www.hsph.harvard.edu/nutritionsource/what-should-you-eat/protein

Vegetarian Resource Group
www.vrg.org/nutrition/protein.htm

Do You Need Protein Powders?
www.webmd.com/vitamins-and-supplements/lifestyle-guide-11/protein-powder

REFERENCES

Aoi W, Naito Y, Yoshikawa T. Exercise and functional foods. *Nutr J.* 2006;5:15.

Das SK, Roberts SB. Energy metabolism in fasting, fed, exercise, and re-feeding states. In: Erdman JW Jr, MacDonald IA, Zeisel SH (eds.). *Present Knowledge in Nutrition.* 10th ed. Ames, IA: John Wiley & Sons; 2012: 117–133.

Evans WJ. Protein nutrition, exercise, and aging. *J Am Coll Nutr.* 2004;23:601S–609S.

Food and Nutrition Board, Institute of Medicine. *Dietary Reference Intakes for Energy, Carbohydrate, Fiber, Fat, Fatty Acids, Cholesterol, Protein and Amino Acids (Macronutrients).* Washington, DC: National Academies Press; 2005.

Morais JA, Chevalier S, and Gougeon R. Protein turnover and requirements in the healthy and frail elderly. *J Nutr Healthy Aging.* 2006;10:272–283.

Pencharz PB. Protein and amino acids. In: Erdman JW Jr, MacDonald IA, Zeisel SH (eds.). *Present Knowledge in Nutrition.* 10th ed. Ames, IA: John Wiley & Sons; 2012;134–155.

Pencharz PB, Ball RO. Different approaches to define individual amino acid requirements. *Annu Rev Nutr.* 2003;23:101–116.

Reeds PJ. Dispensable and indispensable amino acids for humans. *J Nutr.* 2000;130;1835S–1840S.

Tomè D, Bos C. Dietary protein and nitrogen utilization. *J Nutr.* 2000;130:1868S–1873S.

8

Vitamins

Vitamins serve a variety of functions in the body, both within cells and in extracellular fluids, which makes it difficult to generalize about them. Vitamins are classified based on whether they are **water-soluble** or **lipid-soluble (fat-soluble)**. Following intestinal absorption, water-soluble vitamins typically dissolve readily in blood for transfer throughout the body. The fat-soluble vitamins, however, require special protein carriers in the blood because of their poor water solubility. Two fat-soluble vitamins, vitamins A and E, are stored primarily in liver and fat tissues for relatively long periods of time. To a limited extent, vitamin D is stored in fat tissue, but vitamin K is not. Most of the water-soluble vitamins have limited storage capacity and thus need to be consumed in the diet almost every day. Daily intakes of vitamins D and K also are needed.

Consuming a variety of foods ensures adequate daily intake of most vitamins. Many of these essential vitamins are also provided in fortified foods. Vitamin supplements can provide an additional safety net for those whose diets do not provide adequate amounts. However, foods, rather than supplements, should serve as the basis of a healthy diet because they provide macronutrients and phytochemicals in addition to vitamins that aid in promoting health. National surveys of nutritional status have found that significant percentages of U.S. adolescents and adults have marginal intakes of several vitamins, especially those provided by dark green, leafy vegetables. Many have low or even deficient vitamin D measurements.

This chapter provides information on the water-soluble and the fat-soluble vitamins. For each class of vitamins, dietary sources, functions in the body, effects of deficiencies and toxicities, and the Recommended Dietary Allowances (RDAs) are described.

> " Vitamins are classified based on whether they are water-soluble or lipid-soluble. "

Water-Soluble Vitamins

Diversity characterizes the chemical structures and functions of the **water-soluble vitamins**. The water-soluble vitamins that are essential for human health are listed in

water soluble A substance that dissolves in water. Organic molecules with hydroxyl (OH), aldehyde (CHO), keto (=O), or carboxylic acid (COOH) groups tend to be water soluble.

lipid soluble (fat-soluble) A substance that dissolves in fats, oils, lipids, and organic solvents. Also known as being fat soluble.

water-soluble vitamin Vitamins that are soluble in water. Includes the B complex vitamins and vitamin C.

TABLE 8.1
Water-Soluble Vitamins Essential for Human Health

Vitamin	Function	Disease or Condition Caused by Dietary Deficiency
Thiamin	Coenzyme in metabolism (pyruvate dehydrogenase)	Beriberi
Riboflavin	Hydrogen (H) transfer as FAD	Ariboflavinosis
Niacin, nicotinic acid, nicotinamide	Hydrogen (H) transfer as NAD and NADP	Pellagra
Pyridoxine (B_6), pyridoxal, pyridoxamine	Amino (NH_2) group transfer; other functions in amino acid metabolism	Convulsions in infants
Folacin, folic acid, folate	Transfer of carbon atom (nucleic acid metabolism)	Megaloblastic anemia, neural tube defects
Cobalamin (B_{12})	Isomerization, methylation (nucleic acid metabolism)	Megaloblastic anemia, nerve damage
Pantothenic acid	Acyl transfer as part of coenzyme A	None reported
Biotin	Carboxyl (COOH) transfer	Rare
Ascorbic acid (C)	Collagen synthesis, oxidation-reduction (redox system) as an antioxidant	Scurvy

Reproduced from Anderson JJB. *Nutrition and Health: An Introduction*. Durham, NC: Carolina Academic Press; 2005.

> Diversity characterizes the chemical structures and functions of the water-soluble vitamins.

> Most of the water-soluble vitamins have limited storage capacity and thus need to be consumed in the diet practically every day.

vitamin C (ascorbic acid) An essential water-soluble vitamin that functions as an oxidation-reduction system in tissues and in the gut. It is also responsible for the hydroxylation of collagen and is a powerful antioxidant. If intake is inadequate, the deficiency disease scurvy will develop.

B vitamins A group of water-soluble vitamins that includes thiamin, riboflavin, niacin, pyridoxine, folic acid, cobalamin, pantothenic acid, and biotin. These vitamins play important roles in the body's metabolic pathways and in the synthesis of RNA and DNA.

Table 8.1. **Vitamin C**, which is also known as ascorbic acid, has one of the simplest chemical structures of the vitamins and is a powerful antioxidant. The eight **B vitamins** listed in Table 8.1 can be divided into two groups: (1) six vitamins involved in the pathways that extract cellular energy (ATP) from carbohydrates, fats, and amino acids and (2) two vitamins required for the synthesis of DNA and RNA. The B vitamins are found in a diverse array of foods, but are particularly plentiful in plant foods. Supplements of the water-soluble vitamins may be needed during pregnancy and lactation, under conditions of weight loss when using low-calorie diets, and when undergoing regular periods of vigorous physical activity. Most of the water-soluble vitamins have limited storage capacity and thus need to be consumed in the diet practically every day. All have RDAs and upper tolerance levels (ULs) established for the different stages of the life cycle.

Food Sources

Water-soluble vitamins are provided in both plant and animal foods. Relatively rich sources of vitamin C are provided in **Table 8.2**; sources of the various B vitamins are provided in **Table 8.3**. All of the water-soluble vitamins can be found in plant foods, with the exception of cobalamin, which is found only in animal products. Thus, consuming

TABLE 8.2
Vitamin C Content of Foods

Food	Serving Size	Ascorbic Acid (mg)
Fruits		
Orange juice	½ cup	62
Frozen (diluted)	½ cup	48
Canned	½ cup	43
Orange (peeled)	1 small	51
Grapefruit juice	½ cup	47
Grapefruit	½ small	34
Strawberries	10 large	106
Cantaloupe	¼ medium	51
Honeydew melon	⅛ large	29
Vegetables		
Potato		
Baked in skin	1 medium	17
Mashed	½ cup	1
French fried	medium serving	16
Chips	4 oz	35
Tomato		
Raw	1 medium	16
Canned	½ cup	11
Ketchup	1 tbsp	2
Juice	½ cup	22
Cabbage		
Raw	½ cup	15
Coleslaw	½ cup	20
Cooked	½ cup	15
Asparagus (cooked)	½ cup	44
Beet greens (cooked)	½ cup	36
Broccoli (cooked)	½ cup	51
Brussels sprouts (cooked)	½ cup	48
Cauliflower (cooked)	½ cup	27
Collards (cooked)	½ cup	17
Kale (cooked)	½ cup	27
Spinach (cooked)	½ cup	9
Turnip greens (cooked)	½ cup	20
Green pepper	½ cup	60

Data from U.S. Department of Agriculture, Agricultural Research Service. USDA National Nutrient Database for Standard Reference, available at: www.nal.usda.gov/fnic/foodcomp/search.

TABLE 8.3

Good Food Sources of the B Vitamins

Thiamin	Riboflavin	Niacin	B₆	B₁₂	Folate	Biotin
Grains, fortificant	Grains, fortificant	Grains, fortificant	Whole grains, wheat, and rice	Fortified cereals	Fortificant	Whole grains
Vegetables		Mushrooms, green peas	Leafy green vegetables*		Mushrooms, asparagus, leafy green vegetables*	Swiss chard, carrots
Sunflower seeds, pistachios, pecans	Paprika, almonds	Seeds	Chili powder, pistachios, garlic	Fortified tofu	Oranges, melons, strawberries, sunflower seeds	Almonds, walnuts, strawberries, raspberries
Legumes	Soybeans, legumes†	Peanuts, legumes	Legumes		Peanuts, legumes	Legumes
Pork, fish	Meats, salmon	Chicken, turkey, fish	Liver, fish	Clams, liver, crab, fish, beef	Liver	Halibut, liver
Dairy and eggs	Dairy, eggs			Swiss cheese, eggs	Dairy, eggs	Dairy

Note that vitamin B₁₂ (cobalamin) is found only in animal foods.

* Leafy green vegetables, especially dark greens; corn (folate); and a few others.

† Most legumes but not all.

Reproduced from Anderson JJB. *Nutrition and Health: An Introduction.* Durham, NC: Carolina Academic Press; 2005.

> **"** Consuming a variety of meats, dairy products, eggs, cereal grains, legumes, vegetables, and fruits will adequately supply all of the water-soluble vitamins. **"**

a variety of meats, dairy products, eggs, cereal grains, legumes, vegetables, and fruits will adequately supply all of the water-soluble vitamins (see **FIGURE 8.1**).

Fruits tend to be low in the B vitamins, but rich in vitamin C. Citrus fruits, whether fresh or frozen, are especially high in vitamin C. Other foods, such as tomatoes, peppers, potatoes, and leafy vegetables, also provide good amounts of ascorbic acid. Cereal grains, liver and meats, vegetables, and some fruits are good sources of the B vitamins. Some foods are especially good sources of specific B vitamins, such as riboflavin in milk products, and thiamin, riboflavin, niacin, and folate in enriched (fortified) baked goods.

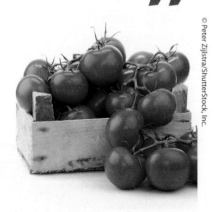 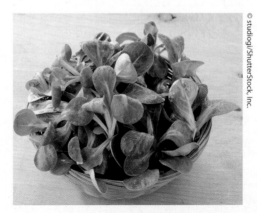 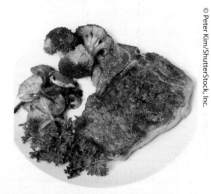

© Peter Zijlstra/ShutterStock, Inc.   © studiogi/ShutterStock, Inc.   © Peter Kim/ShutterStock, Inc.

FIGURE 8.1 Foods Rich in Water-Soluble Vitamins. The water-soluble vitamins are plentiful in a variety of foods from both plant and animal sources.

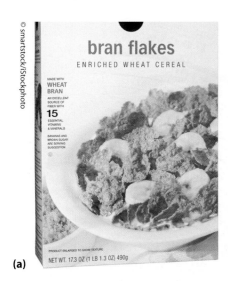

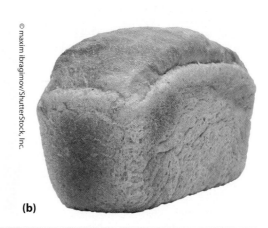

FIGURE 8.2 Fortified Foods. A variety of processed foods, such as breakfast cereals (a), are fortified with water-soluble vitamins, particularly folate. Bread (b) often is fortified with B vitamins.

Although a wide distribution of the B vitamins exists in foods, dark green, leafy vegetables, which supply folate and several other vitamins, are not consumed in adequate amounts by most of the U.S. and Canadian populations. Therefore, people who consume few fruits and vegetables may benefit from fortified foods or supplements to help them meet their vitamin needs. Fortified foods, especially breakfast cereals, provide both vitamin C and the B vitamins (see **FIGURE 8.2**). Foods has been fortified with folate in the United States for almost 20 years, and fetal defects caused from folate deficiencies have fallen as a result. However, some recent evidence of adverse effects suggests that the level of folate supplementation may be too high.

> People who consume few fruits and vegetables may benefit from fortified foods or supplements to help them meet their vitamin needs.

Supplements

Supplements of vitamins are increasingly being recommended because of perceived poor eating habits and low micronutrient intake. Many Americans do not follow the recommendation of eating a regularly balanced diet with a selection of foods from each of the food groups. Daily micronutrient supplements, which contain most of the essential vitamins, can be taken to ensure adequate micronutrient intake as long as the amounts do not exceed the recommended intakes (RDAs or AIs) (see **FIGURE 8.3**). At most, individuals taking such supplements would only be consuming levels of roughly twice the RDAs each day from the combination of foods and supplements. Amounts

PRACTICAL APPLICATIONS **8.1**

Folate Sources in the Diet

Use the USDA Food Composition Tables to identify several foods, including dark green, leafy vegetables and other sources that are good sources of folic acid or folate. Determine the amount of folic acid in micrograms per serving. Create a simple table with the food in the first column, the serving size in the next column, and the amount of folate in each serving in the third column. How could you change your diet to include more of these folate-rich foods? If you do not already eat any of these foods on a weekly basis, how else might you be able to obtain enough folate to support your cell and tissue needs? ■

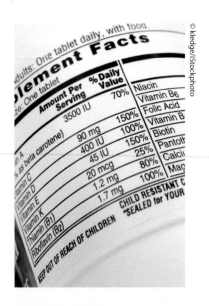

FIGURE 8.3 Vitamin Supplements. The content of multivitamin supplements varies based on the specific product. When choosing a multivitamin, look carefully at the Percent Daily Value (%DV) for each vitamin.

> ❝ Daily micronutrient supplements, which contain most of the essential vitamins, can be taken to ensure adequate micronutrient intake as long as the amounts do not exceed the recommended intakes (RDAs or AIs). ❞

of water-soluble vitamins exceeding the body's needs typically are excreted in the urine either as the unchanged vitamin or as a metabolite of the vitamin. An estimated 40% to 50% of adult Americans are currently taking vitamin (or vitamin/mineral) supplements (see **Table 8.4**).

Megadose supplementation (i.e., doses at many times the RDAs) of water-soluble vitamins is not recommended because of the potential for exceeding the upper limit of safety (UL) of the vitamin. Although water-soluble vitamins are generally less toxic than vitamins A and D, they nevertheless may exert adverse effects if consumed at excessive intake levels. Megadose supplementation is risky behavior except when prescribed by a physician.

megadose Excessive consumption of a particular nutrient, typically as a supplement in pill form. For water-soluble vitamins, a megadose is greater than 5 times the RDA; for fat-soluble vitamins, it is greater than 10 times the RDA. For the more toxic minerals, the ratios of megadose intakes to the RDAs are much lower.

TABLE 8.4
Supplement Intake by U.S. Adults: 2003–2006

Characteristic	Any Dietary Supplement (%)	Multivitamin/ Multimineral (%)	Botanicals (%)
Gender			
Male	44	31	13
Female	53	36	15
Age (years)			
19–30	39	27	13
31–50	49	35	18
51–70	65	44	20
≥ 71	71	46	17
Total	**49**	**33**	**14**

Data from Bailey RL, Gahche JJ, Lentino CV, et al. Dietary supplement use in the United States, 2003–2006. *J Nutr.* 2011;141:261–266.

Women tend to use vitamin supplements slightly more often than men, and both sexes prefer to take vitamins and minerals together. Households with higher annual incomes are more likely to take such supplements than families with lower incomes, who may have a greater need for them. An interesting fact about supplement users is that a large percentage of them are also on some type of special diet, presumably diets for weight reduction. This use of supplements is appropriate because dieters who reduce their usual caloric intakes substantially are not likely to obtain foods with sufficient amounts of the water-soluble vitamins, as well as of other micronutrients, without a supplement.

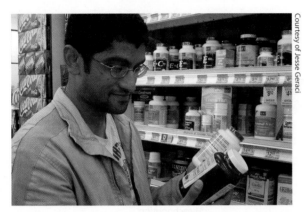

Courtesy of Jesse Geraci

A recent survey found that only a small percentage of the U.S. population has marginal or insufficient intakes of the water-soluble vitamins. Marginal deficiencies of folate, especially among adult women, were reported, despite recent food fortification with folate. Specific subpopulations identified as needing vitamin supplements are the poor, especially ethnic minorities; pregnant and lactating women; and older adults. Many older adults do not have adequate nutrient intake. However, these subpopulations do not typically use nutrient supplements.

Functions

The water-soluble vitamins serve a variety of roles in the human body. Adequate intake of these essential vitamins is critical to maintaining a healthy body.

Functions of Vitamin C

The primary role of vitamin C (ascorbic acid) in the body is as an antioxidant within the water compartments of cells, keeping highly reactive oxygen species (free radicals) from attacking macromolecules. This essential vitamin neutralizes these potentially harmful free radicals. Vitamin C also functions in the small intestine to convert dietary nonheme iron into a more readily absorbable form.

Another important function of ascorbic acid is to enhance the synthesis of collagen that is used in connective tissues, such as bones, ligaments, and tendons. Collagen in connective tissues is turned over regularly as old, ineffective molecules are replaced by new ones. As such, vitamin C also serves in wound healing, which involves considerable formation of new collagen.

B Vitamins: Energy Extraction from Macronutrients

Six of the B vitamins—thiamin, riboflavin, niacin, pyridoxine, biotin, and pantothenic acid—are coenzymes (molecules that assist the enzymes in catalyzing specific reactions) in the pathways that generate cellular energy (ATP) from the basic organic macronutrients. Thus, the B vitamins are critical to energy metabolism in the body (see **FIGURE 8.4**).

> The primary role of vitamin C (ascorbic acid) in the body is as an antioxidant within the water compartments of cells, keeping highly reactive oxygen species (free radicals) from attacking macromolecules.

> Thiamin and pantothenic acid, among other B vitamins, are required for the key step in initiating the citric acid cycle, which generates ATP.

thiamin An essential B vitamin found in pork and whole grains and fortified cereals. Plays a critical role in the body's energy-producing pathways. The deficiency disease is beriberi. It was the first vitamin discovered.

pantothenic acid (pantothenate) An essential B vitamin that is widely available in foods. It contributes to the structure of coenzyme A (CoA).

niacin An essential B vitamin found in meats, whole grains, and legumes. It is converted into two key cofactors—NAD and NADP—that are used in many energy pathways. Its deficiency disease is pellagra.

riboflavin An essential B vitamin that is a component of flavonoid proteins, flavin adenine dinucleotide (FAD), and other coenzymes that play key roles in the body's energy pathways. Good sources include liver, dairy products, and fortified cereal products.

biotin A B vitamin that is involved in multiple pathways that interconvert nutrients and energy-providing molecules throughout the body.

pyridoxin(e) (vitamin B$_6$) An essential B vitamin that plays a role in amino acid metabolism by transferring amino groups to other keto acids or to intermediate molecules in the urea cycle.

folic acid (folate, folacin) A B vitamin that is essential for the renewal of tissues that are turned over because of its role in facilitating cell division (mitosis) and nucleic acid synthesis. If not present in adequate amounts during pregnancy, neural tube defects may occur in the fetus.

cobalamin (vitamin B$_{12}$) A B vitamin with a complex structure containing a cobalt atom. It is found only in animal foods and is produced by a few specific intestinal microorganisms. It requires binding by intrinsic factor (IF) before it can be absorbed and participates in the transfer of methyl groups. Humans have a large storage capacity in the liver for cobalamin. It is essential for cell division and nucleic acid synthesis.

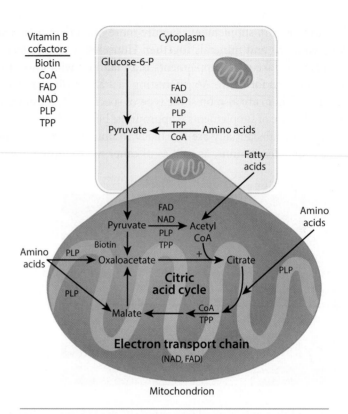

FIGURE 8.4 Integration of Pathways Requiring the B Vitamins Involved in Energy Extraction. This diagram shows the major steps in which B vitamins are involved in the modification of food-derived organic molecules for the production of energy (ATP) in cells. Note that the reaction of pyruvate to acetyl CoA involves four different B vitamins as coenzymes. Also note that the electron transport chain utilizes nicotinamide adenine dinucleotide (NAD) and flavin adenine dinucleotide (FAD). Pyridoxal phosphate (PLP) serves as a coenzyme in amino acid metabolism in at least five steps in the pathways shown. TPP = thiamin pyrophosphate.

Reproduced from Anderson JJB. *Nutrition and Health: An Introduction.* Durham, NC: Carolina Academic Press; 2005.

Thiamin and **pantothenic acid**, among other B vitamins, are required for the key step in initiating the citric acid cycle, which generates ATP. **Niacin** is converted into two key cofactors called NAD and NADP that are used in many energy pathways. Likewise, **riboflavin** is converted into FAD, which is used in the citric acid cycle and in many other metabolic reactions. NAD and FAD are key cofactors in the electron transport chain in mitochondria that generates most of the body's ATP. **Biotin** and **pyridoxin(e) (vitamin B$_6$)** are involved in multiple pathways that interconvert nutrients such as amino acids and energy-providing molecules throughout the body.

B Vitamins: Purine and Pyrimidine Metabolism

The B vitamins **folic acid (folate)** and **cobalamin** are essential for the renewal of tissues that are turned over because they facilitate cell division (mitosis). They are also required for nucleic acid (DNA and RNA) synthesis. Cells cannot multiply and divide properly without the formation of new DNA. Rapidly dividing cells include the red bone marrow, where erythrocytes (red blood cells) and leukocytes (white blood cells) are produced, and epithelial tissues of the lining of the intestine and the skin.

In early embryonic and fetal growth, development of the brain and spinal cord require massive numbers of cell divisions that depend on the availability of folate. If this critical vitamin is not available in sufficient amounts in prepregnancy and early pregnancy, neural tube defects may result. Folate is also required for the conversion of homocysteine to methionine. If dietary folate remains too low, the elevated serum homocysteine concentration that results is considered a risk factor for heart disease.

Older adults are at risk for cobalamin deficiency. Older adults have decreased function of the gastric mucosa (cells of the stomach lining). This decreased function, especially the reduced secretion of **intrinsic factor (IF)**, which is a glycoprotein secreted by the stomach, results in poor cobalamin absorption (see **FOCUS BOX 8.1**). Neuronal cells of the body and brain may be compromised by insufficient intake. Supplements or injections may be required. Deficiencies of cobalamin also may occur in vegans because plant foods are totally deficient in this vitamin.

Choline: A Conditionally Essential Vitamin

Choline has been established by the Institute of Medicine as a **conditionally essential vitamin** because it cannot be synthesized in human tissues. Large amounts of choline are typically consumed from animal foods each day. Choline is needed in the brain and other tissues for the synthesis of **phosphatidylcholine, or lecithin**, a phospholipid, as well as for acetylcholine, a neurotransmitter, and other molecules. Choline also serves as a source of methyl groups needed for DNA methylation and for regulation of gene expression.

> If folate is not available in sufficient amounts during prepregnancy and early pregnancy, neural tube defects may result.

> Deficiencies of cobalamin also may occur in vegans because plant foods are totally deficient in this vitamin.

FOCUS 8.1 Intestinal Absorption of Cobalamin

Dietary cobalamin (vitamin B_{12}) must combine with intrinsic factor (IF), which is made by cells in the epithelial lining of the stomach, before intestinal absorption of this vitamin can occur. The complex formed between vitamin B_{12} and IF (IF-B_{12}) is then absorbed in the lower part of the small intestine, the ileum, where specific receptors exist for the IF-B_{12} complex. When IF is completely lacking, pernicious anemia develops. **Pernicious anemia** does not result from a dietary deficiency of vitamin B_{12}, but rather from a metabolic defect in the production of IF in the stomach (usually the destruction of the IF-producing cells). **FIGURE A** illustrates the steps of digestion and absorption of vitamin B_{12}. ●

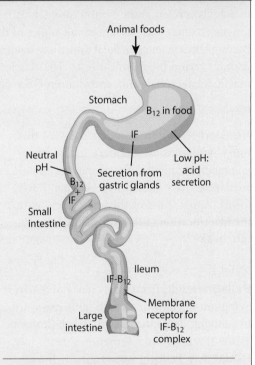

FIGURE A Vitamin B_{12} Absorption. Intrinsic factor (IF), which is produced and secreted by gastric glands, combines with vitamin B_{12} in the duodenum of the small intestine. The complex, IF-B_{12}, then travels down the GI tract to the ileum, where epithelial cells (enterocytes) have special receptors for absorbing this complex.

Reproduced from Anderson JJB. *Nutrition and Health: An Introduction.* Durham, NC: Carolina Academic Press; 2005.

intrinsic factor (IF) A glycoprotein secreted by the stomach that binds vitamin B_{12} in the upper small intestine prior to absorption of the vitamin in the lower ileum of the small intestine.

choline An organic base used in the synthesis of phosphatidylcholine and other organic molecules. It is a source of methyl groups for the body.

conditionally essential vitamin A vitamin that is essential in the diet because it cannot be synthesized in human tissue. Choline is considered to be a conditionally essential vitamin.

phosphatidylcholine (PC, or lecithin) A phosphatide found in membranes that has a role in signaling information from hormones and other molecules that influence membrane receptors.

pernicious anemia A classic form of macrocytic anemia resulting from a deficiency of intrinsic factor (IF) or some defect in its linkage with cobalamin or in the IF–cobalamin receptor in the lower ileum, but not from a deficiency of cobalamin in the diet.

> The classic deficiency diseases of the water-soluble vitamins are extremely rare today in North America and when they do occur, they exist predominantly among infants, the poor, the elderly, or may be caused by other extreme medical or social conditions.

deficiency disease A disease that results from a severe deficiency of a particular macronutrient or micronutrient.

beriberi A classic deficiency disease resulting from severe deficiency of thiamin; "wet" beriberi results from concurrent very low protein intake and the development of edema. May develop in people who eat large amounts of white rice.

pellagra A classic deficiency disease resulting from chronically low intakes of niacin that manifests as a skin disorder. Alcoholic pellagra results from the combination of low dietary niacin and excessive alcohol consumption.

macrocytic, megaloblastic anemia A type of anemia characterized by large immature red blood cells that typically results from a deficiency of either folic acid or cobalamin. Oxygen insufficiency results because of an inadequate number of red blood cells with too little hemoglobin within them.

Deficiencies

Living organisms have gained the ability to synthesize a great variety of molecules in the process of evolution. Because the capacity of humans to synthesize water-soluble vitamins has been lost, nearly all vitamins must be obtained from food sources (i.e., plants and animals) that manufacture them. A net loss of the water-soluble vitamins occurs because of the rapid turnover and limited storage capacity of the water-soluble vitamins, except for cobalamin, which means that these vitamins need to be consumed in the diet almost every day. With extended inadequate intakes, moderate deficiency symptoms (insufficiency) appear; if the deficiency is not resolved, more serious signs of severe deficiency follow.

Diagnosis of a severe deficiency requires prompt medical attention; however, marginal (subclinical) deficiencies or insufficiencies are difficult to determine without extensive biochemical tests. The classic **deficiency diseases** of the water-soluble vitamins are extremely rare today in North America and when they do occur, they exist predominantly among infants, the poor, the elderly, or may be caused by other extreme medical or social conditions. Marginal deficiencies are more common, and they remain an issue in U.S. and Canadian populations. Specific biochemical tests of blood or other tissues for water-soluble vitamin deficiencies, which are not routinely performed at most hospitals, are needed to detect deficiencies. Vitamin supplements may help to prevent a deficiency or correct a deficiency that already exists. Medical care for a deficiency may involve an initial treatment period with massive doses that are followed with tapering doses as tissue concentrations return toward normal. Consideration also must be taken of the underlying dietary, medical, or social causes.

Individuals with deficiencies of one or more of the B vitamins associated with energy metabolism often show symptoms such as lassitude and signs such as skin, lip, and tongue changes and fissures at the angles of the mouth. These nonspecific effects of a B-complex deficiency make it difficult to determine which specific B vitamin is deficient without serum biochemical tests. The classic vitamin deficiencies involving thiamin, niacin, folate, cobalamin, and vitamin C are described in the following sections.

Beriberi

Beriberi results from a deficiency of thiamin. Symptoms of beriberi include heart enlargement, mental deterioration, muscle weakness ("dry" form), or edema ("wet" form). Appearance of this deficiency led to the identification of thiamin as the first vitamin in 1897.

Pellagra

Pellagra results from a deficiency of niacin. Symptoms include dermatitis upon exposure to sunlight, dementia, and diarrhea (known as the three Ds) and sometimes death (see **FIGURE 8.5**). Pellagra was originally thought to be caused by an infectious agent (virus or bacterium) before careful studies showed that it resulted from a niacin deficiency.

Macrocytic, Megaloblastic Anemia

A deficiency of folate or cobalamin can result in **macrocytic, megaloblastic anemia**. This type of anemia is characterized by large

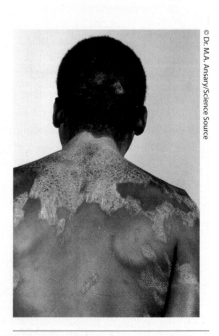

FIGURE 8.5 Pellagra with Dermatitis. In people with niacin deficiency, skin lesions occur upon exposure to sunlight.

© Dr. M.A. Ansary/Science Source

FOCUS 8.2   Niacin Deficiency, Pellagra, and the Appalachian South

Much of the niacin in our diets is supplied by meats and poultry. People whose diets are limited in these animal products, and especially those subsisting on corn-based diets, are at particular risk for niacin deficiency, which can result in pellagra. Historically, pellagra was prevalent in the South, especially the Appalachian region, and in Central and South America. In the 1920s up until the 1940s, large numbers of young men in the South had moderate to severe pellagra resulting from niacin deficiencies, which led to the rejection of many military enlistees from southern states prior to World War II. It was thought that pellagra was caused by a bacterium until Dr. Joseph Goldberger (see **FIGURE A**) identified it as a nutritional deficiency in the 1920s when he worked for the U.S. Hygiene Institute, a predecessor of the National Institutes of Health. He conducted a famous experiment on prisoners in which he fed them only cornmeal. Within 3 weeks his subjects showed clear signs of pellagra. By increasing the protein intake and overall diversity of their diets, he was able to cure the disease. Others were later able to identify the active agent as niacin. Goldberger, a physician, was able to determine that pellagra was a micronutrient deficiency. Because of his work and that of others, wheat flour fortification with niacin

(and also thiamin, riboflavin, and iron) was instituted in the United States in the early 1940s, resulting in sharp decreases in the incidence of pellagra. ●

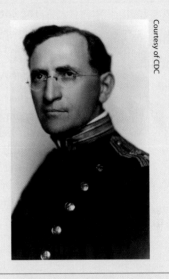

Courtesy of CDC

FIGURE A   Joseph Goldberger, MD. Dr. Goldberger of the U.S. Hygiene Institute conducted studies that determined that the causative agent of pellagra was not a bacterium or virus but rather a micronutrient deficiency.

immature red blood cells. Oxygen insufficiency results because of an inadequate number of red blood cells with too little hemoglobin within them.

Neural Tube Defects

Folate deficiency during early pregnancy contributes to **neural tube defects (NTDs)** in the developing fetus, including spina bifida (see **FIGURE 8.6**). Thus, folate

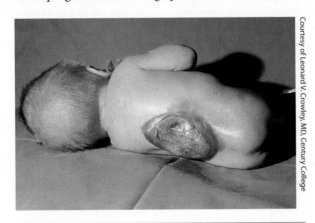

Courtesy of Leonard V. Crowley, MD, Century College

FIGURE 8.6   Spina Bifida. In this infant, a bone in the vertebral column did not close around the spinal cord in the lumbar region (lower back). Other cases of spina bifida have involved nonclosure up to the neck as far as the brain case (skull).

neural tube defect (NTD) Birth defect resulting from incomplete closure of the neural tube during fetal development. Results, in part, from insufficient folate intake during prepregnancy and early gestation (first 2 months). Defects may be severe, resulting in spina bifida.

> **"** Folate deficiency during early pregnancy contributes to neural tube defects (NTDs) in the developing fetus, including spina bifida. Thus, folate supplementation has a protective role against NTDs. **"**

supplementation has a protective role against NTDs. Prepregnancy supplemental folate generates higher blood concentrations of folate, which greatly reduces the risk of these birth defects during pregnancy. Substantial increases in the folate allowance have been recommended by the Institute of Medicine for preventing NTDs. The role of folate in protecting against one or more chronic diseases, however, has not been sufficiently supported as a general preventive recommendation by scientific evidence.

Neurological Effects

The consequences of cobalamin deficiency are much greater than that of just anemia. Cobalamin deficiency can result in serious and permanent neurologic effects that often are not detected in time to reverse the damaged peripheral nerves.

Scurvy

A classic example of a water-soluble vitamin that the body needs almost daily is ascorbic acid. If dietary intake is absent for 1 to 2 weeks, bleeding of the gums and small skin hemorrhages (petechiae) may occur. If dietary intake continues to be deficient, the full-blown deficiency disease, known as scurvy, may follow. **Scurvy** was common among British sailors before the use of lemons (called "limes"), which contain ascorbic acid, became standard fare on long voyages. British sailors were nicknamed "limies" after that.

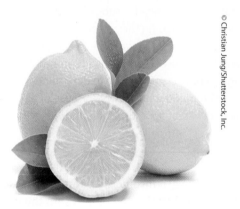
© Christian Jung/Shutterstock, Inc.

Toxicities

Large amounts of water-soluble vitamins generally are not toxic, largely because the water-soluble nature of these vitamins permits their rapid excretion or metabolism to waste products. Toxicities of water-soluble vitamins from food consumption alone are extremely rare, but **nutrient toxicities** from supplemental excesses of a few vitamins have been reported.

Megadoses of vitamin C may have potential toxic or adverse effects. The kidney excretes most of the excess ascorbic acid, but the liver can modify some of the ascorbic acid molecules to oxalic acid, which may eventually lead to kidney stones. The main adverse effect of excessive vitamin C consumption is generally diarrhea. Reported cases of metabolic abnormalities or toxicities of vitamin C have been rare.

Niacin, especially in the form of nicotinic acid used to treat patients with hypercholesterolemia and low HDL-cholesterol, has toxic side effects (flushing) that limit the usefulness of this form of therapy.

Recommended Dietary Allowances (RDAs)

RDAs or Adequate Intakes (AIs) have been set for all the water-soluble vitamins. In the United States and Canada, ingestion of key water-soluble vitamins at levels equal to or

scurvy A classic deficiency disease of ascorbic acid (vitamin C) characterized by bleeding gums, skin hemorrhages, and developmental defects in infants and children.

nutrient toxicity Adverse effects resulting from megadoses of nutrient supplements. Does not usually occur from high intakes of nutrients in foods consumed in excess. Most commonly observed with vitamins A and D.

greater than the RDAs has recently been achieved because of the consumption of so many foods that are fortified with select water-soluble vitamins. Federal food programs may have had a role in improving vitamin intakes of low-income families on food stamps (SNAP) and participating in supplementary food programs such as Women, Infants, and Children (WIC). The use of vitamin supplements usually puts total intake of these vitamins above the recommended allowances. **Table 8.5** lists the RDAs for most of the water-soluble B vitamins; pantothenic acid, biotin, and choline have AIs.

Fat-Soluble Vitamins

The **fat-soluble vitamins** are vitamins A, D, E, and K (see **Table 8.6**). A distinguishing characteristic of these vitamins is that they are soluble in lipid or organic solvents, rather than in water. They are obtained from the fat components of foods, such as oils, fat, liver, egg yolks, nuts, seeds, and wheat germ (see **FIGURE 8.7**). Carotenoids, plant precursors of vitamin A, are also often considered fat-soluble vitamins, but they are classified as **provitamins**.

Basic information on the metabolism, food sources, typical intakes, RDAs, deficiencies, and toxicities of the fat-soluble vitamins is provided in this section. In addition, some background on the digestion, absorption, and metabolism of these molecules, especially of vitamins A and D, is provided. These two vitamins are the ones most likely to be deficient in the diet or to be consumed in excess from supplement overdoses. Widespread fortification of these vitamins in foods increases the risk of toxicity.

> The fat-soluble vitamins are vitamins A, D, E, and K. A distinguishing characteristic of these vitamins is that they are soluble in lipid or organic solvents, rather than in water.

TABLE 8.5
Adult Recommended Dietary Allowances (RDAs) of the B Vitamins (1998)

Vitamin	RDA Units/Day		
	Males Ages 19–50	**Females Ages 19–50**	**Pregnant Women**
Thiamin	1.2 mg	1.1 mg	1.4 mg
Riboflavin	1.3 mg	1.1 mg	1.4 mg
Niacin	16 mg NE	14 mg NE	18 mg NE
Vitamin B_6	1.3 mg	1.3 mg	1.9 mg
Folic acid	400 µg DFE	400 µg DFE	600 µg DFE
Vitamin B_{12}	2.4 µg	2.4 µg	2.6 µg
Biotin*	30 µg	30 µg	30 µg
Pantothenic acid*	5 mg	5 mg	6 mg
Choline*	550 mg	425 mg	425 mg

NE = niacin equivalent; DFE = dietary folate equivalent.
* Adequate Intake (AI), not RDA.
Data from Food and Nutrition Board, Institute of Medicine. *Dietary Reference Intakes.* Washington, DC: National Academies Press; 1998.

fat-soluble vitamin Vitamins that are soluble in fats, oils, lipids, or organic solvents. Includes vitamins A, D, E, and K; beta-carotene is also considered a fat-soluble provitamin.

provitamin A precursor molecule of a vitamin. For example, carotenoids such as beta-carotene are provitamins of vitamin A and can be converted into vitamin A (retinol) in the GI tract.

TABLE 8.6
Fat-Soluble Vitamins: Functions, Deficiencies, and Toxicities

Vitamin	RDA/AI	Functions	Deficiency Diseases	Toxicities
A (retinol and beta-carotene)	RDA	Rod vision, cone vision, epithelial integrity, growth	Eye disorders, xerophthalmia, night blindness	Hypervitaminosis A
D (calciferol)	RDA	Intestinal calcium and phosphate absorption, skeletal metabolism, kidney function, calcium homeostasis, pleiotropism	Rickets, osteomalacia	Hypervitaminosis D, including soft-tissue calcification or calcinosis associated with renal failure
E (tocopherol)	RDA	Antioxidant, particularly for lipids	Anemia in premature infants and newborns	None
K (menadione)	AI	Formation of certain clotting factors	Impaired blood coagulation	Hemolytic anemia in infants receiving synthetic vitamin K (menaquinone)

Reproduced from Anderson JJB. *Nutrition and Health: An Introduction.* Durham, NC: Carolina Academic Press; 2005.

Fat-soluble vitamins must have protein carriers to transport them in aqueous solutions, such as blood. After digestion or separation from foods, the fat-soluble vitamins enter the intestinal epithelial cells in micelles along with the products of fat digestion. Following absorption, the fat-soluble vitamins are incorporated within the epithelial

> Following absorption, the fat-soluble vitamins are incorporated within the epithelial cells into newly formed chylomicrons.

> Regular consumption of the few nutritious foods containing vitamins D and K is critical for maintaining health.

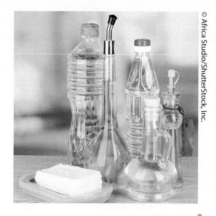

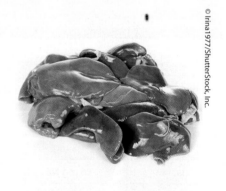

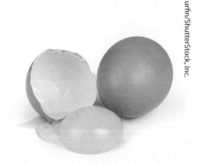

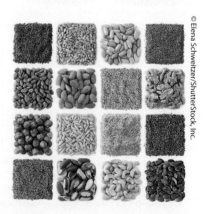

FIGURE 8.7 Foods Rich in Fat-Soluble Vitamins. A variety of foods are good sources of fat-soluble vitamins.

cells into newly formed chylomicrons that are released to the lymphatic vessels for distribution to the body. The chylomicrons travel to the peripheral tissues and then, via the chylomicron remnants, to the liver. When these molecules are released from storage sites in the liver, they are transported in the blood by special carrier proteins (i.e., binding proteins) to cells where they are needed. Fat-soluble vitamins cannot be distributed to tissues via blood without being bound to the special water-soluble protein carriers. Waste metabolites of the fat-soluble vitamins are generally excreted in the bile, but some are excreted in urine.

In reasonably well-nourished adults, liver stores of **vitamin A** increase with each decade of life because of continuing adequate intakes of both vitamin A and carotenoids. Thus, vitamin A supplements are not likely to be needed by adults. The three forms of vitamin A are important for the eyes and epithelial integrity. For elderly shut-ins and adults who get little exposure to sunlight in summer months, **vitamin D** supplements may be recommended in order to enhance calcium absorption for the maintenance of bone health. A large percentage of older adults in North America have vitamin D insufficiency, rather than true deficiency, as determined by measurement of serum 25-hydroxyvitamin D. **Vitamin K** consumption may also be low in many adults because they consume too few dark green vegetables. Vitamin K is important for blood clotting and the formation of bone matrix proteins. Therefore, regular consumption of the few nutritious foods containing vitamins D and K is critical for maintaining health. Adult deficiency of **vitamin E** is very rare.

Food Sources

The fat-soluble vitamins remain reasonably stable in stored foods. At usual cooking temperatures, some destruction of vitamins A and E occurs. Losses are greater at higher temperatures, such as with deep-frying. Vitamin E also is light sensitive, and both vitamin A and beta-carotene are readily oxidized when exposed to oxygen. However, the fat-soluble vitamins are generally not as sensitive to heat or light as the water-soluble vitamins, which are more readily destroyed when exposed to these conditions.

Dietary sources of vitamin A are split between plant pigments (the provitamin carotenoids) and the animal preformed vitamin, retinol. Animal sources of retinol include red meats, liver, and dairy products. Good plant sources of beta-carotene include yellow and orange vegetables (carrots, squash, sweet potatoes), green vegetables (broccoli, spinach, green beans), and yellow fruits (peaches, apricots, mangoes). In addition to beta-carotene, several other carotenoids in plant foods may provide vitamin A, although the enzymatic conversion is typically not efficient. In the typical Western diet, about 75% of vitamin A is derived from animal sources, whereas in most developing nations as little as 5% to 10% comes from animal sources, with the vast majority coming from carotenoids in plants.

Vitamin D is primarily obtained from skin biosynthesis following exposure to ultraviolet B (UVB) rays from the sun and secondarily from dietary sources, such as fatty fish and fortified milk. A few foods, such as mushrooms, provide vitamin D_2 (ergocalciferol), whereas animal sources contain predominantly vitamin D_3 (cholecalciferol).

Usual dietary sources of vitamin E include soy and corn oils, such as found in salad dressings and cooking oils, and in whole grains. Nuts and seeds, such as sunflower seeds and almonds, also are good sources of vitamin E.

Food sources of vitamin K are limited to the dark green, leafy vegetables, which contain appreciable amounts. Soybeans, cauliflower, cabbage, spinach, and a few other foods contain modest amounts of vitamin K. In the United States and Canada, vitamin K intake in older adults often is lower than the AI because many do not consume dark green, leafy vegetables. Another source of small amounts of vitamin K is intestinal bacteria. These bacteria release vitamin K into the lumen of the lower small intestine and

> Dietary sources of vitamin A are split between plant pigments (the provitamin carotenoids) and the animal preformed vitamin, retinol.

> Vitamin D is primarily obtained from skin biosynthesis following exposure to ultraviolet B (UVB) rays from the sun and secondarily from dietary sources, such as fatty fish and fortified milk.

vitamin A An essential fat-soluble vitamin with three distinct forms: retinol (an alcohol), retinal (an aldehyde), and retinoic acid (an organic acid). Retinol is a storage form found in the liver; it is carried by retinol-binding protein (RBP) to the eye and other tissues for use. Retinal participates in the visual cycle; retinoic acid functions like a steroid hormone in cells and is responsible for growth and epithelial integrity.

vitamin D Fat-soluble vitamin made in the skin under the influence of ultraviolet light. Dietary sources include dairy products and other fortified foods. Vitamin D plays a critical role in calcium absorption and homeostasis. Children who are deficient in vitamin D develop the deficiency disease rickets.

vitamin K A fat-soluble vitamin essential for blood clotting and formation of bone matrix proteins, including osteocalcin. Gut bacteria synthesize some vitamin K that is then absorbed by the GI tract.

vitamin E A fat-soluble antioxidant vitamin that operates in the highly lipophilic portion of cell membranes to protect polyunsaturated fatty acids (PFAs) and monounsaturated fatty acids (MFAs) from oxidation.

TABLE 8.7
Common Foods Containing Good Amounts of Fat-Soluble Vitamins

Vitamin	Vitamin-Rich Foods	Fortified Foods
A	Liver, carrots, sweet potatoes, broccoli	Dairy, cereals (ready to eat)
D	Egg yolks, fish, fish oils, liver	Dairy, orange juice
E	Vegetable oils, fats, nuts	Cereals (ready to eat)
K	Dark greens, legumes (peas, soybeans)	None

the large intestine where they are then absorbed. **Table 8.7** lists common foods with good amounts of fat-soluble vitamins.

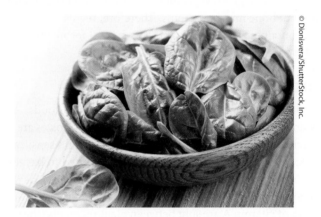

© Dionisvera/ShutterStock, Inc.

Supplements

All the fat-soluble vitamins can be obtained in supplement form. Because vitamins A and D are more commonly insufficient, supplements are more frequently recommended for these vitamins. Vitamin E has been recommended as an antioxidant supplement in the past, but results of recent population-based studies have not supported benefits of vitamin E supplements in preventing disease. Recommendations of vitamin K supplementation are rare.

Both vitamin A and vitamin D may be toxic if taken daily in sufficiently high doses. These two vitamins are metabolized, in part, to hormonal forms that act on nuclear DNA. High intakes may result in excessive protein synthesis and serious, negative consequences. The plant carotenoid forms that may be converted to vitamin A are considered safe because their enzymatic conversion to vitamin A is governed (i.e., feedback inhibited) by the amount or concentration of vitamin A.

A newly recognized exception to the rule about the general safety of vitamin supplements at RDA levels exists primarily for vitamin A consumption by the elderly. The amounts of vitamin A in supplements consumed by the elderly may push them into the UL or toxic range (upper limit of safe intake) because of the narrow window of safe intakes of this vitamin. Beta-carotene supplements are considered safe for all but cigarette smokers, as reported from a study of supplemented Finnish men who smoked for many years and then developed cancers at a high rate after taking a beta-carotene supplement for a few years.

Functions

The fat-soluble vitamins play a number of critical roles in the human body. The following discussion details the functions of these essential vitamins.

Functions of Vitamin A

Vitamin A has important roles in several biological pathways. It is essential for vision and for growth through the synthesis of nucleic acids and proteins. It also plays a role in immune system function and in maintaining the integrity of epithelial tissues, including gut tissue and skin. The growth-promoting activities of vitamin A result from the hormonal form of this vitamin, known as retinoic acid. Beta-carotene and many related carotenoid molecules found in plant foods have antioxidant roles in inhibiting free radical damage in cells. The two circulating forms of vitamin A, retinol and retinoic acid, act by distinctly different mechanisms within cells. Retinal is the aldehyde derivative of vitamin A that participates in the visual cycle.

Beta-carotene, also known as provitamin A, is a symmetrical long-chain hydrocarbon molecule. About 50% of dietary beta-carotene molecules are cleaved at the middle C-C bond to produce two retinol molecules in the enterocytes. The other 50% of dietary beta-carotene molecules are absorbed intact by the body directly, without being split in the gut cells to retinols; they are stored as intact carotenoids in fat tissue.

Liver cells store vitamin A in lipid droplets. Therefore, vitamin A can be retrieved from liver stores for use by other cells of the body to meet their needs. Once retinol is released by hepatic cells, it is immediately picked up in the blood by its specific carrier, **retinol-binding protein (RBP)**, which is a serum protein produced by the liver. An assessment of vitamin A nutritional status can be made by measuring the serum concentration of retinol. Values below a specified threshold indicate deficiency.

The role of vitamin A in the black–white visual cycle of the rod cells has been well established. **Retinol** is converted to 11-cis-**retinal**, which combines with opsin (a protein) to form the light-sensitive **rhodopsin** (see **FIGURE 8.8**). When a light photon hits a

> Beta-carotene, also known as provitamin A, is a symmetrical long-chain hydrocarbon molecule. About 50% of dietary beta-carotene molecules are cleaved at the middle C-C bond to produce two retinol molecules in the enterocytes.

> Liver cells store vitamin A in lipid droplets. Therefore, vitamin A can be retrieved from liver stores for use by other cells of the body to meet their needs.

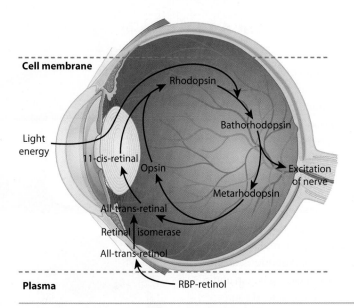

FIGURE 8.8 The Black-White Visual Cycle in the Rod Cells of the Eye. Retinol-binding protein (RBP) supplies the all-trans-retinol that is required by this cycle. Also, the protein, opsin, must be synthesized in the rods for this cycle to operate. Note the critical enzyme that converts all-trans-retinol to all-trans-retinal.

Reproduced from Anderson JJB. *Nutrition and Health: An Introduction.* Durham, NC: Carolina Academic Press; 2005.

retinol-binding protein (RBP) A serum protein made by the liver that circulates in the blood with transthyretin. Transports retinol from liver stores to extrahepatic tissues. RBP has a short half-life in the blood circulation.

retinol The hydroxyl (alcohol) form of vitamin A.

retinal The aldehyde form of vitamin A.

rhodopsin A color pigment in the rods of the retina (eye) that participates in the black-and-white visual cycle. The pigment requires retinal.

TABLE 8.8
Functions of Vitamin A in the Body

Vitamin A Molecule	Functions
Retinol	Precursor molecule for retinal and retinoic acid
Retinyl fatty acid ester	Transport form and storage molecule of retinol
Retinal	Participates in visual cycle as all-trans-retinal and 11-cis-retinal after conversion from retinol
Retinoic acid (hormone)	Cell differentiation and growth, epithelial cell function, glycoprotein synthesis (e.g., in gastric mucosa), activates DNA in most cells; immune role

Reproduced from Anderson JJB. *Nutrition and Health: An Introduction.* Durham, NC: Carolina Academic Press; 2005.

> Retinoic acid is the hormone form of vitamin A that influences gene expression.

rhodopsin molecule, it falls apart, releasing the retinal and sending a signal to the brain that a photon has been received at that point in the retina.

Retinoic acid is a hormonal form of vitamin A that influences gene expression. Vitamin A molecules also may be essential in the immune system and in preventing the growth and development of some cancers. **Table 8.8** lists the known functions of vitamin A.

PRACTICAL APPLICATIONS 8.2

Sources of Vitamin A in the Diet

Vitamin A is found only in animal foods, whereas beta-carotene, a precursor of vitamin A, is found only in plant foods. Use the USDA Food Composition Tables to identify five animal foods that are rich in vitamin A (typically listed as retinol or retinol equivalents). Create a table with the foods in the first column, the serving size in the next column, and the amount of vitamin A in a serving in the third column. Do you think your intake of vitamin A meets your age- and gender-specific RDA? Explain. If you were a vegan and consumed none of the animal sources of vitamin A, how would you be able to meet your recommended intake (RDA) for vitamin A? ■

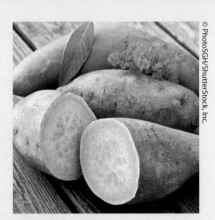

© PhotosGH/ShutterStock, Inc.

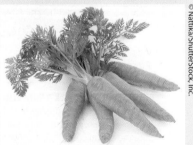

© Nattika/ShutterStock, Inc.

retinoic acid The acid (organic) form of vitamin A that influences gene expression as a hormone.

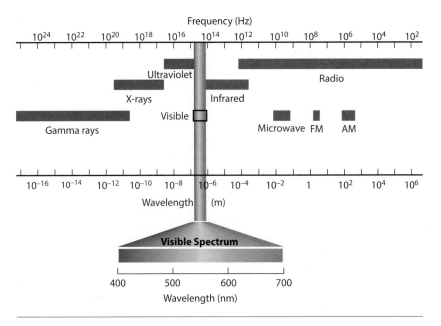

FIGURE 8.9 Biosynthesis of Vitamin D. Vitamin D can be synthesized by the skin in the presence of UV light. UVB must be able to penetrate the atmosphere before skin production of vitamin D occurs.

Functions of Vitamin D

Vitamin D, also called cholecalciferol or simply calciferol, can only be obtained from a few whole foods, select fortified foods, and from biosynthesis upon exposure of skin to ultraviolet light, exclusively the narrow range of UVB light (see **FIGURE 8.9**). Cholecalciferol is transformed in the liver to **25-hydroxyvitamin D, or calcidiol**, through the addition of a second hydroxyl (OH) group. Calcidiol is the major circulating form of vitamin D, and it serves as the "storage" molecule in circulating blood. Blood concentrations of calcidiol are measured to evaluate vitamin D status. A second transformation in the kidneys generates the active hormonal form of vitamin D, called **1,25-dihydroxyvitamin D or calcitriol**, with a third OH group added. Calcitriol acts as a hormone after it leaves the kidney and travels in the circulation to peripheral tissue targets, especially the skeleton, gut, and kidneys, for its actions. All three forms of vitamin D circulate in blood bound to **D-binding protein (DBP)**, which is made by the liver.

Calcitriol production in the kidney is stimulated by two major factors: low serum calcium concentration and elevated parathyroid hormone (PTH) levels. Calcitriol has three major functions. In the small intestine, calcitriol stimulates intestinal calcium absorption. In bone, calcitriol aids in the formation of new organic matrix of bone that helps calcium uptake occur in the mineral phase of bone tissue. Finally, calcitriol positively activates practically all cells of the body to improve general cellular activities and ward off diseases, such as a few specific cancers, or prevent adverse immune conditions. This last function is currently receiving considerable research attention.

The metabolic conversions of vitamin D in the body, whether the molecule is derived from the diet or the skin, are summarized in **FIGURE 8.10**. This figure also illustrates the actions of the hormone form of this vitamin, calcitriol, at its target sites.

Functions of Vitamin E

Vitamin E, a general name for the tocopherols and related tocotrienols, is found in fats of plant foods. The only known function of vitamin E is to prevent the oxidation of unsaturated fatty acids, which serve as constituents of human cellular membranes. Thus, it serves as an antioxidant within the membranes of cells.

> *Calcitriol acts as a hormone after it leaves the kidney and travels in the circulation to peripheral tissues targets, especially the skeleton, gut, and kidneys, for its actions.*

> *In the small intestine, calcitriol stimulates intestinal calcium absorption.*

> *The only known function of vitamin E is to prevent the oxidation of unsaturated fatty acids, which serve as constituents of human cellular membranes.*

25-hydroxyvitamin D (calcidiol) A vitamin D metabolite made in the liver via a hydroxylation at the 25-carbon position. This is the major circulating and storage form of vitamin D. Serves as an indicator of vitamin D status.

1,25-dihydroxyvitamin D (calcitriol) The hormonal form of vitamin D that is made in the kidneys from 25-hydroxyvitamin D. It acts on cells in the small intestine to increase calcium absorption. Also known as 1,25-dihydroxycholecalciferol.

D-binding protein (DBP) A protein synthesized and secreted by the liver that has the capacity to bind all vitamin D molecules and metabolites in the blood.

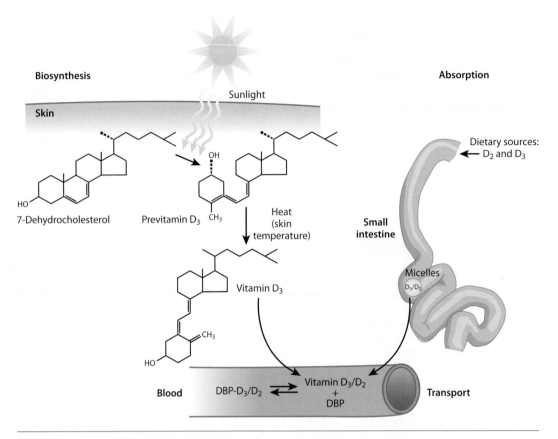

FIGURE 8.10 Metabolic Conversions of Vitamin D.

Reproduced from Anderson JJB. *Nutrition and Health: An Introduction.* Durham, NC: Carolina Academic Press; 2005.

PRACTICAL APPLICATIONS 8.3

Vitamin D and a Vegan Diet

If a person's diet contains no animal products (i.e., no eggs, liver, fish, or fish oils), no foods fortified with vitamin D, and no vitamin D supplements, how can a person obtain enough vitamin D to meet the body's needs? What if this person lives in an area of North America that has long, cloudy winters? Will he or she be able to manufacture enough vitamin D from sunlight? What might a vegan need to do to support bone health throughout the year? ■

Despite relatively low intakes of vitamin E by many in North America, severe deficiency is a rarity. As with several other vitamins, fortification of breakfast cereals and other foods has made a difference in the adequate nutritional status of vitamin E.

Functions of Vitamin K

Vitamin K, which is also called the antihemorrhagic factor, is essential in several steps of the **clotting, or coagulation**, system, where blood proteins bind with calcium ions in the blood to result in a fibrin clot or plug of an artery/arteriole. It also is essential in the organic matrix of bone. Vitamin K is required for the conversion of prothrombin and at least three other blood-clotting factors to their active forms in the normal

clotting (coagulation) The process whereby specific blood proteins combine with calcium ions in the blood, starting a cascade of reactions that results in a fibrin clot or plug of an artery or arteriole at the site of an atheroma dissection or break or other damage to a vessel.

clotting scheme. A true dietary deficiency of vitamin K is rare except in newborn and premature infants, who have not yet established sufficient intestinal colonies of bacteria to synthesize this essential vitamin. A common practice in many countries is to administer a small dose of vitamin K to all newborns. Coumadin (warfarin), a blood thinner taken by those with atrial fibrillation to prevent clotting, interferes with the action of vitamin K in the clotting or coagulation cascade.

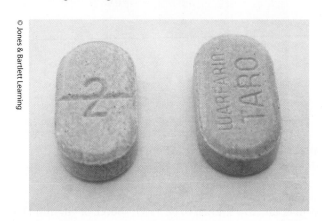

> Vitamin K, also called the antihemorrhagic factor, is essential in several steps of the blood-clotting system and in the organic matrix of the bone.

It has recently been discovered that vitamin K plays a role in bone health. Vitamin K enhances carboxylation of glutamic acid amino acids in **osteocalcin**, a common protein in bone, and promotes good bone health.

Deficiencies

Deficiencies of fat-soluble vitamins occur when dietary intake of one or more of these micronutrients is not adequate or when maldigestion of dietary fats or malabsorption of products of digestion occurs. In cases of steatorrhea (fatty stools) resulting from abnormalities of fat digestion or absorption, deficiencies of several fat-soluble vitamins invariably are present. Other potential causes of poor fat absorption, and hence poor absorption of fat-soluble vitamins, are drugs and dietary components such as olestra that interfere with the digestion and absorption of fats.

Vitamin A Deficiency

The first signs of vitamin A deficiency are **night-blindness** followed by drying of the conjunctiva (white tissue of the eye surface) and the cornea (**xerophthalmia**). If the cornea collapses, then total blindness follows. Blindness from vitamin A deficiency is common on the Indian subcontinent because few vitamin A–containing foods are consumed there. In many areas, dietary sources of either provitamin A or preformed vitamin A, including vitamin A–fortified milks, are very limited. Poorly nourished children in impoverished countries are the most likely to suffer from deficiency. Such a severe deficiency is extremely rare in North American infants because nearly all infant formulas and dairy products are fortified with vitamin A. Breast milk is also a good source of vitamin A. After infancy, a variety of vegetable sources is readily available, and most children in the United States and the rest of the developed world consume fortified dairy products. In India, a national program of vitamin A supplementation of young children has considerably reduced the incidence of blindness.

Vitamin D Deficiency

A prolonged deficiency of vitamin D in infants and young children results in **rickets,** a classic disorder characterized by abnormally shaped, or rachitic (rickety), bones. This disease occurs because of deficits of *both* vitamin D and calcium. It is especially prevalent in northern latitudes that have little exposure to sunlight in the winter months. A

osteocalcin A vitamin K–dependent matrix protein in bone that may be involved in the mineralization process. It serves as a marker of bone turnover.

night-blindness An early condition of vitamin A deficiency resulting from insufficient retinal. Rhodopsin (opsin–retinal combination) is needed to detect black-and-white patterns of light.

xerophthalmia An eye disease resulting in the drying of the cornea that occurs from a dietary deficiency of vitamin A.

rickets A classic deficiency disease that results from vitamin D and calcium deficiency in infants and children. Characterized by misshapen bones, especially of the tibia (bowed) and pectoral (chest) region.

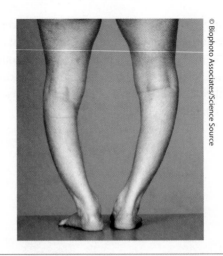

© Biophoto Associates/Science Source

FIGURE 8.11 Rickets. In children with rickets, the bones of the lower legs, pelvic girdle, and chest become malformed.

> A prolonged deficiency of vitamin D in infants and young children results in rickets, a classic disorder characterized by abnormally shaped, or rachitic (rickety), bones.

> Osteomalacia is the milder, adult form of rickets.

osteomalacia An adult form of rickets resulting from deficiency of both vitamin D and calcium. This classic deficiency disease is characterized by widened osteoid seams that fail to mineralize; however, there is no distortion of the skeleton, as in rickets.

daily dose of cod-liver oil, now known to be a rich source of vitamin D, was used in the late 19th century in industrial England to prevent or treat rickets, and this practice was continued in northern cities in the United States and Canada where winter exposure to UVB in sunlight is zero.

The classic rachitic signs in children are bowed legs, a "pigeon" breast cage with rachitic "rosary" beads where the ribs bend inwards, and a narrowed and pinched pelvic girdle (see **FIGURE 8.11**). In the United States, several cases of rickets of breast-fed children who have dark pigmented skin have recently been reported; dark skin reduces the efficiency of skin synthesis of vitamin D. Treatment for rickets generally consists of high daily doses of vitamin D for weeks to months, plus adequate dietary calcium and phosphorus intakes. The severe developmental defects of rachitic children, if not corrected medically, usually last a lifetime.

Osteomalacia is the milder, adult form of rickets. In adults, the weight-bearing bones have achieved maturity, so they do not bow or bend as in young children. Although osteomalacic adult bones are softer and more flexible than normal, they are more likely to fracture than are the soft, flexible bones of rachitic infants. The blood biochemical changes, such as low serum 25-hydroxyvitamin D and changes in bone markers, also are similar to those seen with rickets. Osteomalacia is treated with high doses (5,000 to 10,000 IU) of vitamin D each day until blood calcium levels return to normal. Lower amounts of vitamin D are given to osteomalacic adults than are provided to rachitic children.

A recent concern has arisen about vitamin D deficiency among the elderly, especially shut-ins who get little exposure to sunlight on a daily basis. Older adults over age 65 may benefit from a supplement of vitamin D at 800 IU (20 micrograms) per day in addition to any vitamin D provided by the diet in an attempt to improve the serum 25-OH vitamin D concentration.

Vitamin E Deficiency

Deficiency of vitamin E has only been clearly demonstrated in premature infants and early postnatal infants. Adult deficiency has not been produced except as a secondary result of fat malabsorption syndrome and of cystic fibrosis, a genetic disorder.

Vitamin K Deficiency

If the diet is poor in plant foods, the low vitamin K intake may remain sufficient for blood clotting but not enough for osteocalcin production and optimal long-term bone health. This "differential" insufficiency of vitamin K probably affects older adults the most, but further research is needed for better understandings of specific vitamin K requirements for clotting and bone proteins.

Toxicities

Toxicities of both vitamins A and D are well known though rare, and each can be corrected readily by cessation of vitamin intake. Vitamin D toxicity is less common than toxicity of vitamin A, but it is more severe and life-threatening. Toxicities of vitamins A and D, also known as **hypervitaminoses**, may be severe. Retinoic acid (vitamin A) and calcitriol (vitamin D) have nuclear receptors that continue to respond when high doses are given over a period of time. These toxicities have only been observed in individuals taking excess supplements of vitamin A or D for a few months or longer. They have not been observed from food consumption, with one exception. Milk that was accidentally fortified with excessive amounts of vitamin D by a dairy in the Boston area resulted in severe toxicities and a death.

Excessive carotene consumption is not toxic, but it can result in hypercarotenemia, a high plasma concentration of carotene. Hypercarotenemia is characterized by a yellowish cast or hue of the palms and other normally light surfaces, and it readily disappears when dietary sources containing carotene are reduced or eliminated. Toxicities from vitamin E or vitamin K are extremely rare because these molecules do not have nuclear DNA receptors. **Table 8.9** lists the relative toxicity of the fat-soluble vitamins.

Dietary Reference Intakes

The RDAs and AIs for the fat-soluble vitamins A, D, E, and K are listed in **Table 8.10**. Note that an RDA has not been established for beta-carotene or other carotenoids.

The RDA for vitamin A for young females (9 to 13 years) is 600 micrograms per day; for adult women it is 700 micrograms per day. The RDA for young males (9 to 13 years) is 600 micrograms per day; for adult men it is 900 micrograms per day. These RDAs are based on estimated intakes of both carotenoids and vitamin A.

The RDAs for vitamin D for both males and females are set at 15 micrograms per day from early childhood to 70 years of age, when it increases to 20 micrograms per day. Older adults need more vitamin D each day to enhance calcium absorption and to retain calcium in the mineral phase of bone because of the reduced efficiency of

> Toxicities of vitamins A and D, also known as hypervitaminoses, may be severe.

TABLE 8.9
Ratios of UL to RDA for the Fat-Soluble Vitamins as an Index of Potential Toxicity from Excessive Intake in Adults

Vitamin	Ratios of UL to RDA	
	Adult Males	**Adult Females**
A	3.3	4.2
D	6.7	6.7
E	66.7	66.7
K	No UL for toxicity established	

Note: Ratios for the elderly are the same as for adults.
Data from Food and Nutrition Board, Institute of Medicine. *Dietary Reference Intakes.* Washington, DC: National Academies Press; 2011.

hypervitaminoses Toxicities of vitamins A and D.

TABLE 8.10
Recommended Adult Dietary Reference Intakes of Fat-Soluble Vitamins

Vitamin and Unit	RDA/AI	Ages 19–30		Ages 31–50		Ages 51–70	
		Males	Females	Males	Females	Males	Females
A (µg RE)*	RDA	900	700	900	700	900	700
D (µg)†	RDA	15	15	15	15	15;20**	15;20**
E (mg)	RDA	15	15	15	15	15	15
K (µg)	AI	120	90	120	90	120	90

* RE = retinol equivalent. † 10 micrograms of cholecalciferol = 400 IU of vitamin D. ** Vitamin D recommendation (RDA) for those over 70 years is 20 micrograms (800 IU).
Data from Food and Nutrition Board, Institute of Medicine. *Dietary Reference Intakes.* Washington, DC: National Academies Press; 1997, 2000, 2004, and 2011.

vitamin D biosynthesis that occurs with aged skin. (For conversion to common labeling, 1 microgram of vitamin D or cholecalciferol is equivalent to 40 IU.) For many shut-ins, especially those living in northern latitudes, ultraviolet exposure is too limited for substantial biosynthesis. Thus, good dietary sources and supplements of vitamin D need to be consumed by such individuals to prevent the combination disorders of osteomalacia and osteoporosis.

The RDA for vitamin E for adults is the same for both genders: 15 milligrams per day. RDAs across the life cycle are chosen to match the fat intake in the United States at about 30% of total energy. If daily fat consumption is greater than 30% and is very high in polyunsaturated fatty acids (PFAs), dietary vitamin E intakes may need to be increased because of the vitamin's role in protecting against the oxidation of membrane PFA.

Most segments of the U.S. population fall somewhat short in meeting the RDA for vitamin E intake, and thus modest insufficiencies are common. Supplements of vitamin E are often recommended for individuals at high risk of chronic diseases such as coronary heart disease, certain cancers, diabetes, Alzheimer's, and possibly other diseases of the brain. However, no clear-cut evidence exists to support the use of supplements by the general adult population. High doses of vitamin E, perhaps 1,000 milligrams per day, may be potentially toxic, but observed toxicity is very rare.

The AI values for vitamin K are based on conservative estimates of the needs of the body. Because the contribution of bacterial biosynthesis of vitamin K in the intestine is difficult to assess, the AI values are merely best guesses. The AIs may be set too low to support adequate formation of osteocalcin and other vitamin K–dependent matrix proteins in bone tissue of older adults.

❞ Supplements of vitamin E are often recommended for individuals at high risk of chronic diseases such as coronary heart disease, certain cancers, diabetes, Alzheimer's, and possibly other diseases of the brain. ❞

SUMMARY

Water-soluble vitamins are present in a wide variety of foods. Thus, regular well-balanced diets should ensure reasonable intakes at the recommended levels. Low intakes of plant foods may contribute to suboptimal status of several water-soluble and fat-soluble vitamins. Thiamin, riboflavin, niacin, and folate are fortified in practically all breads and ready-to-eat cereals, and milk contains naturally good amounts of riboflavin and cobalamin (and is fortified with vitamins A and D). Many fruit drinks are fortified with vitamin C. Supplements of water-soluble vitamins are not normally recommended for healthy adults or those who eat balanced meals on a regular basis. Exceptions to this rule of thumb would be individuals on low-calorie diets for the purpose of weight reduction, those who have poor dietary habits, those under extreme stress, the elderly, and pregnant and lactating women. Because of a limited storage capacity, food sources rich in the water-soluble vitamins should be consumed each day at the DRI level.

In general, the water-soluble vitamins function as coenzymes in biological reactions. Also, each vitamin is often involved in several different reactions, and for some reactions more than one vitamin may be involved. Deficiencies for most B vitamins have been well characterized. The classic deficiency diseases of scurvy, beriberi, and pellagra are not usually seen today in North America except among alcoholics, severely deprived infants and children, and the very old. Vitamin C deficiency also is extremely rare today because of the wide availability of good sources of this vitamin. If the recommended nine daily servings of fruits and vegetables are consumed, plenty of vitamin C is obtained. Excessive intakes of the water-soluble vitamins, from foods or supplements, rarely result in metabolic dependencies or toxicities.

Food sources of fat-soluble vitamins are varied. Consumption of a wide variety of plant and animal foods is needed in order to meet RDA or AI levels. Vitamin D is an unusual nutrient because it can be provided by both foods and skin biosynthesis from the sun, under appropriate conditions. The fat-soluble vitamins have diverse roles in body functions. They serve as structural components (retinal in the rods and cones of the visual tissue); (2) hormones (calcitriol and retinoic acid); (3) enzyme cofactors in reactions (vitamin K actions on clotting and bone proteins); and as (4) nonenzymatic antioxidants (vitamin E actions to protect PFA).

Deficiencies of the fat-soluble vitamins have become less common in recent decades because of widespread fortification. Vitamin D insufficiency, however, has become prevalent in adults, especially among elderly shut-ins and institutionalized residents because of too little exposure to sunlight. Supplements of vitamin D may be recommended for the elderly in conjunction with calcium in order to prevent osteomalacia and skeletal fractures resulting from low bone mineral content (i.e., osteoporotic fractures). Low vitamin K and vitamin E intakes appear to be of little concern, except among the elderly. Vitamin A (and carotene) intakes tend to be better than those of fat-soluble vitamins D and K. Vitamin A deficiencies, however, are common in much of the developing world, especially in India and many other Asian nations.

Toxicities of vitamin A in the elderly, though rare, are almost always related to excessive intake of supplemental vitamin A (but not carotene). Toxicity of vitamin D also is rare, but with increasing vitamin D supplement use, more toxicity may be expected.

STUDENT ACTIVITIES

1. State the major difference between the two broad classes of vitamins.

2. Name one food rich in each of the following (do *not* use fortified foods): vitamin C, thiamin, riboflavin, niacin, pyridoxine, folic acid, cobalamin.

3. Name the deficiency disease or condition associated with each of the following vitamins: vitamin C, niacin, folate, cobalamin, thiamin.

4. How does vitamin C act within cells to protect macromolecules against damage? Explain.

5. Name two water-soluble vitamins for which toxic or adverse effects may occur when high supplemental doses are consumed.

6. Identify one function (reaction or other role) for each of the following B vitamins: thiamin, riboflavin, niacin, biotin, pantothenic acid, pyridoxine, folate, cobalamin.

7. Describe the absorption of cobalamin. Start in the stomach with gastric secretion and end with ileal receptor-mediated absorption by mucosal cells (enterocytes).

8. Describe the role of folate in converting homocysteine to methionine and the potential beneficial metabolic changes in cells. If serum homocysteine concentration increases, what are the potential adverse effects?

9. Identify one food each that is rich in the following (do *not* use fortified foods): vitamin A, vitamin D, vitamin E, vitamin K.

10. State one function of each of the following molecules: retinol/retinal, retinoic acid, 1,25-dihydroxycholecalciferol, vitamin E, vitamin K.

11. Speculate how beta-carotene may act within cells in the prevention of cancer.

12. Explain why vitamins A and D are toxic at high doses (i.e., hypervitaminoses) but vitamins E and K are not.

13. State the biochemical transformations of vitamin D synthesis in skin, starting with cholesterol (or 7-dehydrocholesterol).

14. Identify the deficiency diseases or conditions that occur when prolonged deficits of each the following occur: vitamin A, vitamin D, vitamin E, vitamin K.

15. Explain why vitamin D deficiency or insufficiency is more common in North America compared to countries nearer the equator.

16. Explain why dietary carotenoids can substitute for dietary vitamin A in body functions that require one form or another derived from vitamin A.

WEBSITES FOR FURTHER STUDY

NIH Office of Dietary Supplements
http://ods.od.nih.gov/factsheets/DietarySupplements.asp
Folic acid—CDC
www.cdc.gov/ncbddd/folicacid/index.htm
Vitamins and minerals—USDA
http://fnic.nal.usda.gov/food-composition/individual-macronutrients-phytonutrients-vitamins-minerals/vitamins-minerals

Dr. Joseph Goldberger, NIH
http://history.nih.gov/exhibits/Goldberger/index.html
The history of vitamins—Wellness Directory of Minnesota
www.mnwelldir.org/docs/history/vitamins.htm

REFERENCES

Bailey LB, Caudill MA. Folate. In: Erdman JW Jr, MacDonald IA, Zeisel SH (eds.), *Present Knowledge in Nutrition*. 10th ed. Ames, IA: John Wiley & Sons; 2012: 529–562.

Ballew C, Bowman BA, Sowell AL, Gillespie C. Serum retinol distributions in residents of the United States: Third National Health and Nutrition Examination Survey, 1988–1994. *Am J Clin Nutr*. 2001;73:586–593.

Bettendorff L. Thiamin. In: Erdman JW Jr, MacDonald IA, Zeisel SH (eds.), *Present Knowledge in Nutrition*. 10th ed. Ames, IA: John Wiley & Sons; 2012: 435–465.

Botto LD, Moore CA, Khoury MJ, et al. Neural-tube defects. *New Engl J Med*. 1999;341:1509–1519.

Committee on Dietary Reference Intakes, Institute of Medicine. *Dietary Reference Intakes for Calcium, Phosphorus, Magnesium, Vitamin D, and Fluoride*. Washington, DC: National Academies Press: 1997.

Committee on Dietary Reference Intakes, Institute of Medicine. *Dietary Reference Intakes for Thiamin, Riboflavin, Niacin, Vitamin B6, Folate, Vitamin B12, Pantothenic Acid, Biotin, and Choline*. Washington, DC: National Academies Press: 1998.

Committee on Dietary Reference Intakes, Institute of Medicine. *Dietary Reference Intakes for Vitamin C, Vitamin E, Selenium, and Carotenoids*. Washington, DC: National Academies Press: 2000.

Committee on Dietary Reference Intakes, Institute of Medicine. *Dietary Reference Intakes for Calcium and Vitamin D*. Washington, DC: National Academies Press: 2011.

Da Silva VR, Russell KA, Gregory JF. Vitamin B6. In: Erdman JW Jr., MacDonald IA, Zeisel SH (eds.), *Present Knowledge in Nutrition*. 10th ed. Ames, IA: John Wiley & Sons; 2012: 509–528.

Ervin RB, Wright JD, Wang C-Y, Kennedy-Stephenson J. Dietary intakes of selected vitamins for the United States population: 1999–2000. *Adv Data*. 2004 Mar 12(339):1–4.

Ferland G. Vitamin K. In: Erdman JW Jr., MacDonald IA, Zeisel SH (eds.), *Present Knowledge in Nutrition*. Ames, IA: John Wiley & Sons; 2012: 384–411.

Holick MF. Resurrection of vitamin D deficiency and rickets. *J Clin Invest*. 2006;116:2062–2072.

Holick MF. Vitamin D deficiency. *New Engl J Med*. 2007;357: 266–281.

Holick MF. Vitamin D: a D-lightful health perspective. *Nutr Rev*. 2008;66(suppl 2):182S–194S.

Jialal I, Traber M, Devaraj S. Is there a vitamin E paradox? *Curr Opin Lipidol.* 2001;12:49–53.

Johnston CS. Vitamin C. In: Erdman JW Jr, MacDonald IA, Zeisel SH (eds.), *Present Knowledge in Nutrition.* 10th ed. Ames, IA: John Wiley & Sons; 2012: 412–434.

Lindshield BL. Carotenoids. In: Erdman JW Jr, MacDonald IA, Zeisel SH (eds.), *Present Knowledge in Nutrition.* Ames, IA: John Wiley & Sons; 2012: 321–339.

Mayo-Wilson E, Imdad A, Herzer K, Yakoob MY, Bhutta ZA. Vitamin A supplements for preventing mortality, illness, and blindness in children aged under 5: systematic review and meta-analysis. *BMJ.* 2011;343:d5094. doi: 10.1136/bmj.d5094.

McCormick DB. Riboflavin. In: Erdman JW Jr, MacDonald IA, Zeisel SH (eds.), *Present Knowledge in Nutrition.* 10th ed. Ames, IA: John Wiley & Sons; 2012: 466–486.

Miller JW, Rucker RB. Pantothenic acid. In: Erdman JW Jr, MacDonald IA, Zeisel SH (eds.), *Present Knowledge in Nutrition.* 10th ed. Ames, IA: John Wiley & Sons; 2012: 611–636.

Norman AW, Henry HL. Vitamin D. In: Erdman JW Jr, MacDonald IA, Zeisel SH (eds.), *Present Knowledge in Nutrition.* Ames, IA: John Wiley & Sons; 2012: 340–360.

Penberthy WT. Niacin. In: Erdman JW Jr, MacDonald IA, Zeisel SH (eds.), *Present Knowledge in Nutrition.* 10th ed. Ames, IA: John Wiley & Sons; 2012: 487–508.

Rebouche CJ, L-Carnitine. In: Erdman JW Jr, MacDonald IA, Zeisel SH (eds.), *Present Knowledge in Nutrition.* 10th ed. Ames, IA: John Wiley & Sons; 2012: 637–658.

Rogovik AL, Vohra S, Goldman RD. Safety considerations and potential interactions of vitamins: should vitamins be considered drugs? *Ann Pharmacother.* 2010;44:311–324.

Solomons NW. Vitamin A. In: Erdman JW Jr, MacDonald IA, Zeisel SH (eds.), *Present Knowledge in Nutrition.* Ames, IA: John Wiley & Sons; 2012: 259–320.

Stabler SP. Vitamin B_{12}. In: Erdman JW Jr, MacDonald IA, Zeisel SH (eds.), *Present Knowledge in Nutrition.* 10th ed. Ames, IA: John Wiley & Sons; 2012: 563–586.

Tanumihardjo SA, Palacios N, Pixley KV. Provitamin A carotenoid bioavailability: what really matters? *Int J Vitam Nutr Res.* 2010;80:336–350.

Traber MG. Vitamin E. In: Erdman JW Jr, MacDonald IA, Zeisel SH (eds.), *Present Knowledge in Nutrition.* Ames, IA: John Wiley & Sons; 2012: 361–383.

Vieth R, Chan PC, MacFarlane GD. Efficacy and safety of vitamin D_3 intake exceeding the lowest observed adverse effect level. *Am J Clin Nutr.* 2001;73:288–294.

Yang QH, Carter HK, Mulinare J, Berry RJ, Friedman JM, Erickson JD. Race-ethnicity differences in folic acid intake in women of childbearing age in the United States after folic acid fortification: findings from the National Health and Nutrition Examination Survey, 2001–2002. *Am J Clin Nutr.* 2007;85:1409–1416.

Zeisel SH. Choline: critical role during fetal development and dietary requirements in adults. *Ann Rev Nutr.* 2006;26:229–250.

Zeisel SH, Corbin KD. Choline. In: Erdman JW Jr, MacDonald IA, Zeisel SH (eds.), *Present Knowledge in Nutrition.* 10th ed. Ames, IA: John Wiley & Sons; 2012: 659–681.

Zempleni J, Wijeratne SSK, Kuroishi T. Biotin. In: Erdman JW Jr, MacDonald IA, Zeisel SH (eds.), *Present Knowledge in Nutrition.* 10th ed. Ames, IA: John Wiley & Sons; 2012: 587–610.

ADDITIONAL READING

Combs GF. *The Vitamins*, 4th ed. London: Academic Press; 2012.

Presman AH, Buff S. *The Complete Idiot's Guide to Vitamins and Minerals.* 3rd ed. Indianapolis, IN: Alpha; 2007.

Shils M, Shike M, Ross AC, Caballero B, Cousins RJ (eds.). *Modern Nutrition in Health and Disease.* 10th ed. Baltimore: Lippincott Williams & Wilkins; 2005.

CHAPTER 9

Water and Minerals

Several minerals, both macrominerals and microminerals, are essential for human health. Most of the essential macrominerals are found in Groups I and II of the periodic table of chemical elements. These macrominerals have relatively low atomic numbers and are generally quite abundant in the earth's surface. A few other essential elements are from other groups of the periodic table. The macrominerals, or bulk elements, are those minerals that are needed in large amounts each day; the microminerals, or trace elements, are those needed only in small, or "trace," quantities each day. These essential minerals are found in plants and animals that are consumed as food. They function as structural components in the body as well as enzyme cofactors and protein stabilizers within cells.

Of the essential macrominerals, several operate in the intracellular fluid compartment of cells as well as in the fluid outside of the cells. Calcium, for example, has well-known intracellular roles in the contraction of muscle cells and in the functioning of nerve cells. It also plays important extracellular structural roles in the crystals of bones and teeth and in blood clotting. Phosphate anions are needed for bone minerals and for the synthesis of many intracellular molecules. Sodium and potassium serve as electrolytes with positive charges in body fluids, whereas chloride ions are negatively charged electrolytes. Microminerals also have diverse functions, but most act intracellularly as enzyme cofactors. Iodine is an exception because it is a required component of thyroid hormones. **FIGURE 9.1** highlights the position of the essential minerals in the periodic table. Other minerals found in the periodic table may be found in the human body, but their essentiality has not been established.

The **macrominerals** required by the body each day include calcium (Ca), phosphorus (P), magnesium (Mg), sodium (Na), potassium (K), and chloride (Cl) (see Figure 9.1). Sulfur (S) is also considered an essential element, but because sulfur metabolism is linked primarily with the sulfur-containing amino acids, little coverage of this element is given in this chapter. The essential **microminerals**, or **trace elements**, that have established RDAs or AIs are iron (Fe), zinc (Zn), iodine (I), selenium (Se), manganese

> *Most of the essential macrominerals are found in Groups I and II of the periodic table of chemical elements. These macrominerals have relatively low atomic numbers and are generally quite abundant in the earth's surface.*

macromineral Mineral elements needed in large amounts in the diet each day. Calcium, phosphorus, magnesium, sodium, potassium, and chloride are the macrominerals needed by the body each day.

micromineral (trace element) An essential mineral needed in small quantities in the diet. At present, RDAs or AIs have been set for the following trace elements: iron, zinc, iodine, selenium, manganese, copper, chromium, and fluoride.

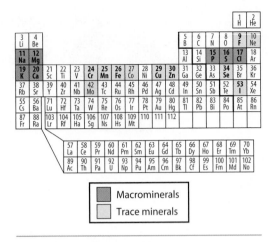

FIGURE 9.1 Position of the Nutritionally Essential Minerals in the Periodic Table.

Data from Gropper SS. Smith JL, Groff JL. *Advanced Nutrition and Human Metabolism*. 5th ed. Belmont, CA: Wadsworth/Cengage Learning; 2009; and Stipanuk MH. *Biochemical and Physiological Aspects of Human Nutrition*. 2nd ed. Philadelphia: WB Saunders; 2006.

> ❞ Each day the body loses water through urine, feces, exhaled breath moisture, and sweat; this water must be replaced. The goal is to replace daily losses of fluids and thereby maintain water balance. ❞

water A molecule consisting of two hydrogens and one oxygen (H_2O) that normally exists as a liquid at room temperature. The human body requires water to function.

water balance The maintenance of the body's water compartments, both extra- and intracellular, through the consumption of water and the generation of metabolic water to equal the losses in urine, feces, sweat, and evaporation via the lungs and skin.

(Mn), copper (Cu), chromium (Cr), and fluoride (F) (see Figure 9.1). The essentiality and functions in humans of other microelements, the ultratrace elements, remain uncertain; thus, the description of the role of these elements in this chapter is brief.

Water is essential to life. The body can survive much longer without food than it can without water. Water can be obtained from almost any type of food or fluid beverage, including tap water. It is especially important in the optimal functioning of the kidneys. This chapter focuses on water, the macrominerals, and the microminerals.

Water

Some consider water to be the most overlooked of all the nutrients. Water is extremely important to the human body, making up 60% of a person's body weight! (**FIGURE 9.2**) The water content of the body is somewhat greater in males because, in general, they have greater muscle mass (LBM) than females. Each day the body loses water through urine, feces, exhaled breath moisture, and sweat; this water must be replaced. The goal is to replace daily losses of fluids and thereby maintain **water balance**. In most cases this balance is maintained because of the thirst mechanism that stimulates one to consume fluids. Water intake is imperfectly regulated by thirst, a basic mechanism originating in the brain that leads us to drink.

Although experts recommend eight or more glasses of water or other fluids, such as juices, nephrologists (physicians who specialize in the kidneys) state that no physiologic basis for this recommendation exists for healthy people. This recommendation is made primarily to emphasize the importance of drinking enough water. In particular, pregnant and lactating women need to ensure adequate fluid intakes to remove toxic agents and to avoid complications. The kidneys have the capability of making either a concentrated or a dilute urine in response to a wide range of fluid intake (volume), ranging from 0.5 to 10 liters per day. It is important to ensure adequate water intake, especially if the thirst mechanism is not operating precisely.

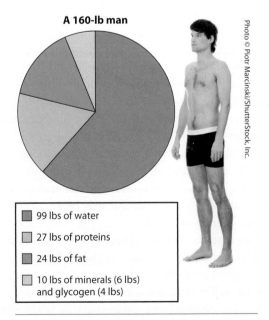

A 160-lb man

■ 99 lbs of water
■ 27 lbs of proteins
■ 24 lbs of fat
■ 10 lbs of minerals (6 lbs) and glycogen (4 lbs)

Photo © Piotr Marcinski/ShutterStock, Inc.

FIGURE 9.2 Water Content of the Body. Males have slightly more body water than females, mainly because mature males have more muscle mass than females.

Both foods and beverages supply water. Water is also produced as a byproduct of metabolic pathways, especially the citric acid cycle. This metabolic water, also called water of oxidation, amounts to approximately 250 milliliters per day. The amount of water obtained from beverages typically ranges between 850 milliliters in less active individuals and 1,500 milliliters in very active individuals. Food supplies only about 100 to 200 milliliters of water in an adult diet.

On the loss side (output) of the water balance equation, water lost through **urine** and **sweat**, including evaporation or insensible water loss, accounts for approximately 1,000 to 1,200 milliliters each per day; fecal losses are only 100 milliliters per day or so. These values are fair approximations for most adults. Additional losses occur in lung exhalations.

Water balance is maintained when the input equals the output. The best biomarker for adequate water hydration is the osmolality of blood (osmolality is the mass of solutes in a liter of fluid). Urine osmolality may also be helpful. The **kidney** may adapt and decrease fluid output when inadequate amounts of water are ingested, but a minimal water loss (urine and sweat losses) of approximately 200 milliliters occurs per day, mostly as urine. Adult males typically excrete more fluid than adult females.

Water has several roles in human tissues. It serves as an essential component of molecules synthesized by cells in oxidation reactions, as a solvent for carrying molecules and ions, as a vehicle for chemical reactions, as a thermoregulator, and as a pH **buffer**. Because of its high heat capacity, water is resistant to rapid temperature changes. Water also provides mechanical benefits as a cushion or shock absorber and as a lubricant. Finally, water in saliva bathes the teeth 24 hours a day, which, together with the minerals in saliva, helps to prevent dental caries.

Mineral salts dissolve in water to form ions that contain electrical charges (i.e., **electrolytes**). These charged ions, whether positive (cations) or negative (anions), typically exist in body fluids within limited ranges of concentrations. The clinically significant serum electrolytes include sodium, potassium, and chloride ions.

Water balance exists when input equals output. Hormones help to regulate water balance, but insufficient water intake remains the major factor contributing to water imbalance and dehydration. Problems in water balance arise because the thirst mechanism that governs fluid intake is an imperfect gauge of body needs when excessive water loss or dehydration occurs. Dehydration may occur relatively easily; thus, daily fluid replacement from water, juices, and other beverages is recommended. Deficits must be made up within a few hours following losses. Hot, humid days and excessive physical activity are two situations that contribute to large water losses as well as to electrolyte losses.

Although alcohol is a dehydrating agent that induces modest diuresis (water loss in urine), most alcoholic beverages provide some water that can go toward daily intake needs. The same may be said for beverages containing caffeine and for several medications that induce water loss. However, coffee, cola drinks, and alcoholic beverages are not recommended for water replacement because they act as mild diuretics and increase water losses in urine.

The consumption of almost any fluid is beneficial for maintaining blood volume and other body fluid compartments and for dilution of molecules that may contribute to kidney stone formation, especially in people who are predisposed to forming kidney stones. Although the causes of kidney stones are not well understood, it is thought that insoluble materials or precipitates act as microscopic seeds in initiating the growth of crystals that become renal stones. Thus, the consumption of adequate amounts of fluids on an everyday basis reduces the risk of stones.

Water losses can be especially high for those involved in outdoor activities on hot days as well as on cold, windy days. On cold, windy days, sweat losses are not noticed (i.e., they are insensible), but water losses may be great. Any form of water—tap, filtered,

> Water is also produced as a byproduct of metabolic pathways, especially the citric acid cycle. This metabolic water, also called water of oxidation, amounts to approximately 250 milliliters per day.

> Problems in water balance arise because the thirst mechanism that governs fluid intake is an insensitive gauge of body needs when excessive water loss or dehydration occurs.

urine The fluid made by the kidneys that contains nitrogenous waste products (urea, creatinine, ammonia, uric acid, and hydroxyproline), various chromes (colored products), water-soluble metabolites of vitamins, and minerals, such as potassium, calcium, sodium, and many others. Does not usually contain sugar (glucose) or proteins.

sweat Salty fluid produced by the sweat glands that helps the body to dissipate heat through evaporation.

kidney Organ that helps maintain homeostasis of the blood and other body fluids. Reabsorbs much of the filtered load of blood of sodium, calcium, glucose, and other important nutrient molecules and ions, keeping these substances in the body. Removes and eliminates waste products such as urea, uric acid, and creatinine.

buffer A molecule in solution that can neutralize the effects of both acids (H^+) and bases (OH^-) and thereby help to maintain acid–base balance within a narrow range. Also a class of food additives used to maintain a specific pH in order to prevent deterioration.

electrolyte A charged ion in solution. The three major mineral ions found in serum (and also in cells) are sodium (Na^+), potassium (K^+), and chloride (Cl^-) ions.

> *The consumption of almost any fluid is beneficial for maintaining blood volume and other body fluid compartments and for dilution of molecules that may contribute to kidney stone formation, especially in people who are predisposed to forming kidney stones.*

bottled, or other—supplies this needed nutrient. Although the need to drink eight glasses of water a day has not been confirmed by research, individuals do need to consume sufficient amounts of water each day. The recommended intakes of water are now given as AIs. For adult males (19 years and over), the AI is 3.7 liters per day; for adult women it is 2.7 liters per day. If a person does not like to drink plain water, fruit juices, soups, milk, or other noncaffeinated drinks work as well as plain water for replacing lost fluids.

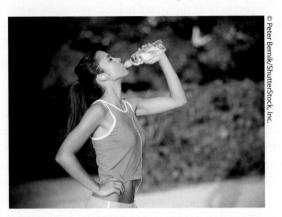

© Peter Bernik/ShutterStock, Inc.

Rapid and excessive water loss may result in serious medical complications, including fatigue, dry mouth and membranes, and headaches. Dehydration commonly occurs in individuals with elevated temperatures. If as much as 20% of total body fluids are lost, coma and death may follow. Vomiting or diarrhea may also lead to rapid dehydration. Infants with intestinal infections are especially vulnerable to dehydration because they do not have large amounts of body water. Although a rare condition, excessive water intake may also compromise body functions and health because of excessive dilution of body fluids and disordered regulation of electrolytes.

Macrominerals

The macrominerals, also known as the bulk elements, are needed each day in considerably greater amounts than the microminerals. This section on macrominerals discusses the electrolytes first, and then provides information on magnesium, calcium, and phosphorus.

Electrolytes: Sodium, Potassium, and Chloride

Electrolytes are charged ions that conduct electrical current in water or body fluids. Electrolytes exist in both foods and body fluids. The serum concentrations of the two cations—**sodium** (Na^+) and **potassium** (K^+)—are normally maintained within narrow ranges. The sodium–potassium (Na^+-K^+) pump in cell membranes helps maintain these concentrations within cells. Mechanisms in the kidney work to maintain constant electrolyte concentrations in blood serum and other extracellular fluids. Serum electrolytes are clinically monitored to assess the degree of change in response to illness or disease, especially diarrhea and vomiting and diseases of the kidneys.

Sodium ions are the primary extracellular electrolytes, whereas potassium ions are the primary intracellular electrolytes (intracellular fluid compartment). Within cells, potassium ions act as enzyme cofactors in several important reactions and have roles in other cellular functions. Sodium ions help to maintain the fluid volume of the body and, along with proteins, aid in the regulation of the osmotic concentration of these fluids. Sodium and potassium ions are transferred across cell membranes (sodium out of and potassium into cells) in order to maintain an electrical charge differential; this

sodium A monovalent mineral cation (Na^+) found predominantly in blood and extracellular fluids. Excess sodium consumption can lead to hypertension.

potassium A major intracellular cation (K^+) that is essential for the function of neurons and muscle cells and for growth of muscle tissue. Also serves as an enzyme activator in several reactions involving energy production. The body's total potassium content is directly related to lean body mass (LBM), especially muscle mass.

differential is essential for cell functions. Considerable amounts of energy (ATP) are used by the **sodium-potassium (Na⁺-K⁺) pump** to maintain the differential across cell membranes. Membrane charge gradients are an essential characteristic of living cells, and hence living organisms. The energy required by the Na⁺-K⁺ pump is a major portion of the basal metabolic rate.

The negatively charged **chloride** (Cl⁻) ions (i.e., anions) have higher extracellular than intracellular concentrations. The chloride anions serve to balance the cations in solution, mainly sodium, potassium, and positively charged proteins in fluids.

Food Sources

Sodium consumption by Americans and Canadians is generally higher than recommended, but a few decades ago it was even higher. In the United States, salt (sodium chloride, or NaCl) intake averages more than 6 grams per day. (Table salt is 40% sodium by weight.) In many Asian countries, sodium intake is even higher. However, only 115 to 230 milligrams of sodium per day is required for health. In general, the human body can adapt to a wide range of sodium intakes, at least for limited periods.

Changing the U.S. population's pattern of high salt intake has been aided by major modifications in the processing methods used by the food industry. Processed foods that have added salt are the major contributor to sodium intake in the United States, even though food processors have reduced the amount of salt added. Another contributor to salt intake (less than 25%) is salt from table salt shakers, and many people are cutting down on salting their foods. Low-salt foods are becoming increasingly available in the marketplace because of consumer pressure on food manufacturers to reduce the salt content of foods. However, many popular snack foods, such as various types of chips, remain high in salt. Foods high in salt should be reduced or eliminated because of the increased risk of developing hypertension from excess sodium intake. At present, soups, salt-cured meats, snacks, and other salt-fortified foods remain the largest sources of dietary sodium (see **FIGURE 9.3**).

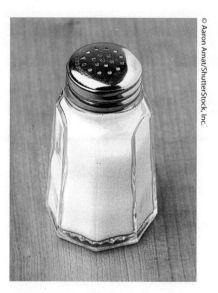

© Aaron Amat/ShutterStock, Inc.

Very few natural, whole foods contain much sodium; it is the processing of foods that adds the sodium. Salt historically was a scarce commodity until the advent of deep mining for salt. Thus, the "salt appetite" is a learned behavior that may be difficult to reverse. Because sodium is used as an additive or taste amplifier in so many foods, most people get enough sodium to meet their nutritional requirements, even without adding salt at the table. **Table 9.1** lists several common processed foods that contain added sodium. Compare these amounts with the AI for sodium, which is 1,500 milligrams. Consider the

> **❝** Sodium ions are the primary extracellular electrolytes, whereas potassium ions are the primary intracellular electrolytes. **❞**

> **❝** Considerable amounts of energy (ATP) are used by the Na⁺-K⁺ pump to maintain the differential across cell membranes. Membrane charge gradients are an essential characteristic of living cells, and hence living organisms. **❞**

> **❝** At present, soups, salt-cured meats, snacks, and other salt-fortified foods remain the largest sources of dietary sodium. **❞**

sodium–potassium (Na⁺-K⁺) pump The pump that transfers sodium out of and potassium into cells in order to maintain the electrical charge differential across cell membranes. The energy required by the Na⁺-K⁺ pump is a major portion of the basal metabolic rate.

chloride Macromineral required by the body. Exists as an anion (Cl⁻) in the body's fluids, balancing the charge of cations in solution. Extracellular concentrations are higher than intracellular concentrations.

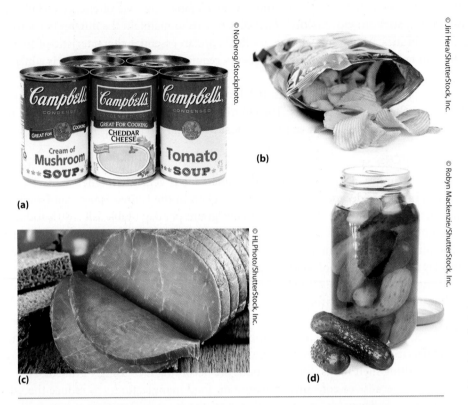

FIGURE 9.3 Foods High in Salt. Most of the salt in our diets comes from processed foods and foods from restaurants. (a) Canned soups, (b) potato chips, (c) ham, and (d) pickles. Only about a quarter of our salt intake comes from the salt shaker.

TABLE 9.1
Sodium Content of Commonly Consumed Processed Food Items

Food Item	Serving Size	Sodium (mg)
Dill pickle	1 large	1,181
Pork and beans	½ can	1,145
Turkey dinner	Frozen meal	1,051
Soy sauce	1 tbsp	1,003
Spaghetti and meatballs (canned)	1 cup	925
Chicken noodle soup (canned)	5 oz	655
Beef hotdog	1	513
French fries	Small order	337
American cheese	1 slice	282
Potato chips	1 oz	149

Data from U.S. Department of Agriculture, Agricultural Research Service. USDA National Nutrient Database for Standard Reference. Available at: www.nal.usda.gov/fnic/foodcomp/search

changes in sodium content from the raw state of potatoes to the processed state of this common food in French fries with salt additions. Salted fries represent a major source of sodium intake by fast-food consumers.

Dietary sodium from table salt and processed food sources has been directly linked to the development of hypertension and cardiovascular disease (CVD). Excess salt consumption requires an increase in fluid consumption to maintain normal serum electrolyte concentrations.

Potassium is present in good amounts in fruits and vegetables (see **FIGURE 9.4**). Potassium is not used as a food additive or as a supplement. **Table 9.2** lists common foods that are rich in potassium. Dietary potassium is well supplied by a variety of foods, especially citrus fruits and other fruits, most vegetables, and meats and dairy foods. However, these foods must be consumed in the amount recommended by MyPlate to supply the required amounts of potassium. Many North Americans actually consume inadequate amounts of potassium because they do not eat enough servings in these critical groups of foods, especially plant foods, each day. A comparison of the content of sodium and potassium in selected foods, mostly raw or unprocessed, can be appreciated by examining the amounts of each electrolyte in fruits and vegetables (see **Table 9.3**).

Chloride ions accompany both sodium and potassium to maintain electrical charge neutrality in all foods that contain the other two electrolytes (cations). No deficiencies of this mineral exist when foods are consumed naturally. Specific dietary recommendations for chloride have little meaning except for the formulation of baby foods and foods for older adults.

> Excess salt consumption requires an increase in fluid consumption to maintain normal serum electrolyte concentrations.

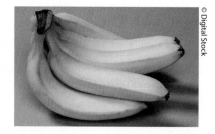

© Digital Stock

FIGURE 9.4 Food Sources of Potassium.

TABLE 9.2
Good Sources of Potassium

- Raisins
- Oranges
- Bananas
- Orange Juice
- Cantaloupe
- Potatoes
- Avocado
- Tomatoes
- Dried Dates
- Tomato Juice
- Dried Prunes
- Beans
- Peaches
- Milk
- Meat, Fish, Poultry (lean)

Reproduced from Anderson JJB. *Nutrition and Health: An Introduction*. Durham, NC: Carolina Academic Press; 2005.

TABLE 9.3
Sodium and Potassium Content of Selected Fruits and Vegetables Per Serving

Food	Serving Size	Sodium (mg)	Potassium (mg)
Fruits			
Apple	1 medium	1	148
Blueberries	1 cup	1	114
Grapes	10	1	94
Cantaloupe	1/4	22	368
Orange	1 medium	3	312
Dried prunes	5	1	348
Vegetables			
Broccoli (raw)	1 cup	30	286
Mushrooms (raw)	1 cup	4	223
Peas (cooked)	1 cup	6	384
Potato with skin (baked)	1 medium	17	926
Sweet potato (baked)	1 medium	41	542
Tomato (raw)	1 cup	6	292

Data from U.S. Department of Agriculture, Agricultural Research Service. USDA National Nutrient Database for Standard Reference, Available at: www.nal.usda.gov /fnic/foodcomp/search

TABLE 9.4
AIs for Sodium and Potassium Across the Life Cycle

Age	Sodium (mg/day)	Potassium (mg/day)	Chloride (mg/day)
9–13 years	1,500	4,500	2,300
14–18 years	1,500	4,700	2,300
19–50 years	1,500	4,700	2,300
51–70 years	1,300	4,700	2,000
≥ 71 years	1,200	4,700	1,800

Data from Food and Nutrition Board, Institute of Medicine. *Dietary Reference Intakes for Water, Potassium, Sodium, Chloride, and Sulfate.* Washington, DC: National Academies Press; 1997, 2004, 2011.

TABLE 9.5
Median Intakes of Sodium and Potassium

Age	Sodium (mg/day)	Potassium (mg/day)
12–19 years (males and females)	3,563	2,362
20–39 years		
Males	4,453	3,069
Females	3,116	2,322
40–59 years		
Males	4,421	3,429
Females	3,002	2,491
≥ 60 years		
Males	3,597	3,006
Females	2,742	2,441

Data from U.S. Department of Agriculture, Agricultural Research Service. 2012. Total Nutrient Intakes: Percent Reporting and Mean Amounts of Selected Vitamins and Minerals from Food and Dietary Supplements, by Gender and Age. What We Eat in America. NHANES 2009–2010. Available at: www.ars.usda.gov/ba/bhnrc/fsrg

Supplementation

Potassium may be prescribed for some individuals with high blood pressure who are taking antihypertensive drugs. Otherwise, no general recommendation for potassium supplementation exists. Too much potassium may have adverse effects on heart muscle, including death. Because adequate amounts of sodium and chloride are obtained from the diet, supplementation is not recommended.

Dietary Reference Intakes

AIs have been established for sodium, potassium, and chloride (see **Table 9.4**). The AIs for sodium are intended to help consumers lower their salt intake and decrease the risk of developing hypertension. AIs for sodium are 1.5 grams per day for both men and women ages 19 to 50 years and 1.3 grams per day for those ages 50 to 70 years. The allowances for sodium have been substantially reduced over recent years.

Because consumers generally do not get enough potassium, the AIs for potassium can help consumers focus on obtaining this mineral by consuming more servings of fruits and vegetables. The AI for potassium is 4.7 grams per day for adults, both men and women, older than 18 years.

Actual intakes of sodium and potassium as estimated by NHANES survey data are summarized in **Table 9.5**. Note that compared with the age-specific AIs, deficits typically occur beyond 11 years for potassium, especially in females. Sodium intakes are too high compared with their AIs. In fact, average sodium intakes are well above the UL of safe intake of 2,300 milligrams per day. Healthy intake ratios of Na:K range between 1:3 and 1:4!

Functions

The narrow ranges of blood concentrations of sodium and potassium are continuously maintained by regulatory mechanisms in order to sustain life. The range of serum potassium is about 3.5 to 5.0 milliequivalents per liter (mEq/L, or mmol/L), and it is critical for the function of heart muscle and other cells. The range of sodium in the blood is even narrower, about 135 to 145 mEq/L (or mmol/L). If concentrations of these two ions go outside these ranges, the health of an individual may be seriously compromised and medical care may be required immediately. For example, vomiting or diarrhea may seriously affect the normal concentrations of both sodium and potassium, which, if severe enough, may require replacement fluids, especially saline solution, a weak salt solution at a physiologic concentration (i.e., similar in sodium concentration to body fluids).

FOCUS 9.1 Dietary Sodium and Hypertension

Hypertension (i.e., high blood pressure) is a common problem among Americans, affecting approximately 50% of the U.S. adult population. Those who are inactive and overweight or obese are at increased risk for developing hypertension. It is also more common among older adults. Because there are few overt symptoms, many people do not realize they have high blood pressure. Hypertension is a major risk factor for cardiovascular disease (CVD), especially heart attack and stroke. It also typically accompanies obesity and type 2 diabetes and its complications. Thus, hypertension has taken an enormous toll in both disability (morbidity) and death (mortality) in the United States and in other affluent nations.

Hypertension is common in countries where the populations consume excessive sodium and food energy. Other common dietary risk factors contributing to hypertension are diets high in saturated fat, alcohol, and limited intakes of fruits and vegetables. Because hypertension and related chronic conditions are mainly the result of poor food choices and inactivity, they can be prevented by increasing healthy lifestyle behaviors. ●

Electrolytes function in blood and other body fluids. Sodium ions exist primarily in extracellular fluids with a gradient of about 140 mEq/L outside the cell to 10 mEq/L inside the cell. The sodium–potassium pump that sends sodium ions out of cells and potassium ions into cells requires energy as ATP, which may be as high as 50% of the total energy expenditure of the cells, a significant portion of our basal metabolic rate.

Potassium ions exist primarily inside cells and their concentrations in cells and in blood are also governed by the sodium–potassium pump. Life cannot exist if the cells cannot maintain their high intracellular potassium concentration of approximately 100 mEq/L. The potassium (K^+) gradient from outside to inside cells is opposite that of sodium; that is, about 5 mEq/L outside to 100 mEq/L inside.

Chloride ions accompany sodium and potassium in body fluids and tissues to help maintain charge neutrality, their major role. Other anions also help in maintaining electrical balance within fluids.

Deficiencies

The only electrolyte that is likely to be deficient due to inadequate dietary intake is potassium. Poor food selection (i.e., very few servings of fruits and vegetables) is the primary reason for deficiency. Processed foods usually have sufficient chloride and, without processing, sufficient sodium. A serious deficiency of sodium is very rare, except among athletes who sweat profusely and lose excessive amounts of sodium. Both sodium and potassium may be low in highly active athletes without increased intakes of foods and beverages, in addition to plain water, despite the presence of minimal amounts of these electrolytes in some water sources.

Toxicities

Although foods contain typically harmless amounts of potassium, supplements of potassium may have toxic effects on the heart and, if too high, could even cause the heart to stop beating. Individuals who need to take additional potassium because of heart problems must be cautious and under the close care of a physician. Sodium has adverse effects when consumed in excess because it may lead to hypertension. Excessive sodium intakes are associated with excessive fluid intake and sodium retention in body fluids.

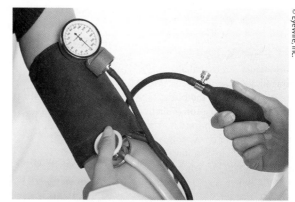

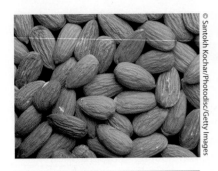

FIGURE 9.5 Good Food Sources of Magnesium.

© Santokh Kochar/Photodisc/Getty Images

> In the United States, magnesium intake is typically below the RDAs for both men and women. In general, insufficient intakes result from low consumption of dark green vegetables, which are the richest food sources of this mineral.

> Magnesium functions mainly as an intracellular cofactor for approximately 300 different enzymes.

magnesium An essential intracellular divalent cation (Mg^{2+}) that is abundant in the body, particularly the skeleton. Functions mainly within cells where it acts as an enzyme cofactor or enzyme activator. Most magnesium-requiring enzymes are involved in ATP synthesis or degradation.

Magnesium

Magnesium (Mg^{2+}) is an essential intracellular divalent cation (an ion with two positive charges). Magnesium is quite abundant in the body, especially in the skeleton, with 60% to 70% of the body's magnesium being stored in the bones. However, it has no known role in bone tissue except as a storage site. Like potassium, magnesium functions mainly within cells, where it acts as an enzyme cofactor or activator of different cellular enzymes. Most of the magnesium-requiring enzymes involve ATP synthesis and degradation. Other magnesium-dependent enzymes are involved in nucleic acid metabolism and other pathways.

Food Sources

Magnesium is found in good amounts in the chlorophyll of dark green vegetables and other plant foods (see **FIGURE 9.5**). Fairly good amounts are also provided by meats (muscle) and a few other foods. **Table 9.6** lists the magnesium content of common foods, especially dark green, leafy vegetables.

Supplementation

Small amounts of magnesium are included in daily vitamin-mineral supplement formulations. It is supplied in amounts to reduce the risk of deficiency.

Recommended Dietary Allowances

The adult RDAs for magnesium are 420 milligrams per day for men and 320 milligrams per day for women. A value of 6 milligrams per kilogram of body weight is frequently recommended for adults. During pregnancy, females need 40 milligrams more magnesium each day and only a little more is needed during early lactation. The UL is 350 milligrams per day for both genders and only comes into consideration when ingesting supplements and foods that are high in magnesium.

In the United States, magnesium intake is typically below the RDAs for both men and women. In general, insufficient intakes result from low consumption of dark green vegetables, which are the richest food sources of this mineral. Intestinal absorption of this divalent cation ranges between 25% and 60%, depending on the amount of magnesium in the diet.

Functions

Magnesium functions mainly as an intracellular cofactor for approximately 300 different enzymes. Magnesium is also found in blood serum, both as a free ion and bound to proteins or other molecules. Magnesium also has important roles in heart muscle function and nerve activity. Adequate intakes of magnesium may help prevent strokes. It may also have a protective role against the onset of type 2 diabetes.

Deficiency

National surveys of magnesium intakes have shown that over 70% of the adult population, and especially older adults, consume less than the gender-specific RDAs for magnesium. Although subclinical or marginal deficiency of magnesium may be prevalent in the United States, as suggested by low dietary intakes, adverse effects are not common. Excessive alcohol consumption and the use of diuretics and other drugs may lead to magnesium deficiency. Adequate intakes of magnesium as well as potassium may reduce hypertension, improve brain function, and reduce the risk of type 2 diabetes.

Toxicity

Excessive magnesium intake from foods is highly unlikely, but it may occur as a result of excessive use of magnesium supplements. Magnesium excesses from food consumption alone are highly unlikely.

TABLE 9.6
Magnesium Content of Commonly Consumed Foods

Food by Group	Serving Size	Magnesium (mg)
Dark Green Vegetables		
Green peas (cooked)	1/2 cup	21
Spinach (raw)	1 cup raw	156
Other Vegetables		
Potato with skin, baked	1 medium	48
Legumes		
Pinto beans (boiled)	1 cup	86
Soy tofu, nigari (Mg-set)*	1/5 block	48
Cereals and Grains		
Whole wheat bread	1 slice	12
White bread	1 slice	6
Cheerios	1 oz	39
Raisin Bran	1 oz	48
Meat, Poultry, Fish		
Ground beef, 90% lean (broiled)	3 oz	36
Chicken breast (baked)	3 oz	16
Halibut (baked)	3 oz	91
Dairy		
Milk, 1%	1 cup	27
Fruits		
Apple (raw)	1 medium	7
Nuts		
Cashews	1/4 cup	89
Peanuts	1/4 cup	67
Chocolate		
Cocoa powder	2 tbsp	51

* Processed magnesium-set tofu differs from calcium-set tofu; one of these two divalent cations is used in the preparation of any type of soy tofu.
Data from U.S. Department of Agriculture, Agricultural Research Service. USDA National Nutrient Database for Standard Reference, Available at: www.nal.usda.gov/fnic/foodcomp/search

Calcium and Phosphorus

Calcium exists in the body's fluids as a divalent cation (Ca^{2+}). Phosphorus is present in the body primarily as a divalent phosphate anion (HPO_4^{2-}). These two minerals are closely associated in the metabolism of the mineral phase of bone and their linked regulation via calcium-regulating hormones.

Calcium and **phosphate ions** also are essential in the formation of the hydroxyapatite crystals in bones and teeth. In addition to its role in bone formation and maintenance, calcium is essential for many other of the body's functions, including muscle contraction, nerve conduction, and blood clotting. Phosphate has many intracellular functions and is required for the synthesis of high-energy molecules, such as ATP and creatine phosphate. It also plays a critical role in DNA and RNA synthesis (see **FIGURE 9.6**).

Food Sources

Calcium and phosphorus are found in different amounts in a variety of foods, but both minerals are provided in good amounts by dairy foods. Because of the wide

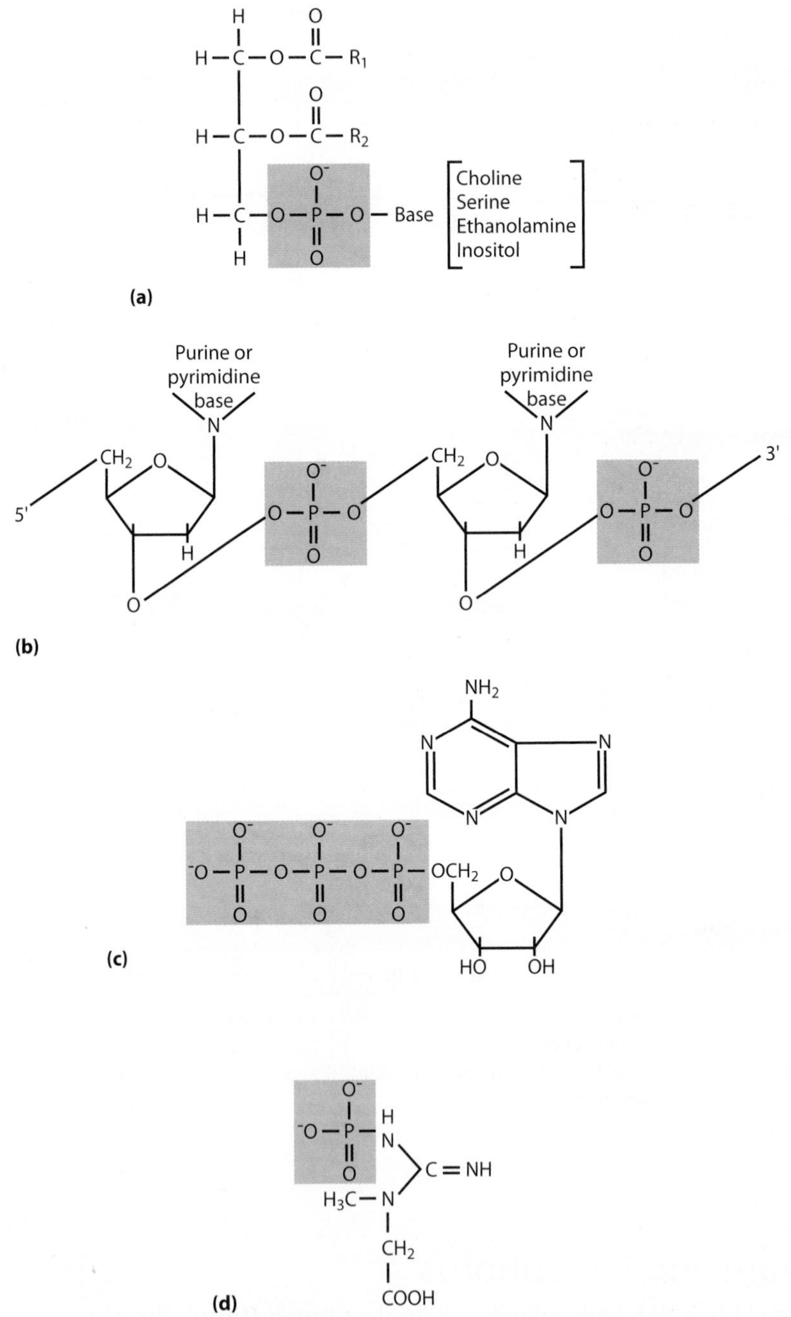

(a)

(b)

(c)

(d)

calcium A macromineral necessary for the mineralization of the skeleton and for many other functions, including extracellular blood clotting and intracellular regulation.

phosphate ion Inorganic phosphate ions (i.e., PO_4^{2-}) are present in the body's intracellular fluids, blood, other extracellular fluids, and secretions into the gut lumen. Phosphate is essential for the formation of hydroxyapatite in bone and teeth. Its most important role is in the formation of high-energy molecules, such as ATP and creatine phosphate. It also is a critical component of RNA and DNA.

FIGURE 9.6 Phosphate-Containing Molecules. The diversity of the important molecules containing phosphorus (as phosphate) shows how critical this element is for life. (a) Phospholipids, (b) deoxyribonucleic acid (DNA), (c) adenosine triphosphate (ATP), and (d) creatine phosphate.

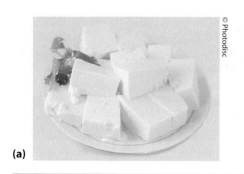
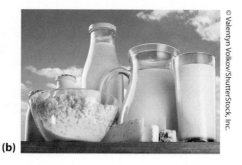

FIGURE 9.7 Foods Rich in Calcium. (a) Tofu and (b) dairy products.

availability of phosphorus in foods, ingestion of large amounts of phosphorus is common. However, the reverse is true for calcium because of the limited distribution of calcium among the food groups (see **FIGURE 9.7**). Based on food consumption surveys, approximately 60% of the calcium consumed by adults in North America and most Western nations is from dairy foods. The remainder of calcium is obtained from baked goods; dark green, leafy vegetables; and only a few other foods. Adults who consume little or no dairy products obtain most of their calcium from breads and baked goods, which provide a significant amount of this mineral, but not enough to meet the RDAs. In Asian countries, people obtain calcium from small fish, greens, and other sources, but typically they do not consume enough calcium to meet dietary recommendations.

One cup (8 oz) of milk of any kind, including skim milk, provides approximately 300 milligrams of calcium. This value is the standard to which other foods are compared. **Table 9.7** lists the calcium content of selected food items from different food groups. **Calcium-to-phosphorus ratios** of breast milk, bone, and blood serum are shown in **FIGURE 9.8**, as examples of normal values.

> Based on food consumption surveys, approximately 60% of the calcium consumed by adults in North America and most Western nations is from dairy foods.

> Adults who consume little or no dairy products obtain most of their calcium from breads and baked goods, which provide a significant amount of this mineral, but not enough to meet the RDAs.

> One cup (8 oz) of milk of any kind, including skim milk, provides approximately 300 milligrams of calcium.

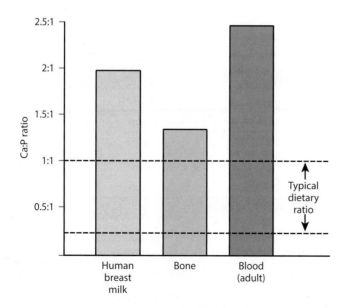

FIGURE 9.8 Calcium-to-Phosphorus Ratios of Breast Milk, Bone, and Blood. The ratios of these two macrominerals illustrate the importance of each ratio for specific functions in nursing infants, forming new bone mineral, and distributing the minerals to cells.

Ratios are based on mass amounts of each nutrient.

calcium-to-phosphorus (Ca:P) ratio The ratio of calcium to phosphorus in the diet or in a food.

TABLE 9.7
Calcium Content of Common Foods

Food Group	Serving Size	Calcium (mg)
Milk and Dairy Products		
Milk, whole	8 oz	276
Milk, skim	8 oz	299
Low-fat fruit yogurt	6 oz	258
Ice cream	½ cup	301
Ice milk	½ cup	258
Colby cheese	1 oz	92
American cheese	1 oz	107
Cheddar cheese	1 oz	194
Edam cheese	1 oz	159
Mozzarella cheese	1 oz	204
Ricotta cheese	½ cup	207
Muenster cheese	1 oz	143
Provolone cheese	1 oz	255
Cottage cheese	½ cup	203
Swiss cheese	1 oz	224
Colby cheese	1 oz	194
Protein Foods		
Tofu, firm, nigari	4 oz	198
Salmon with bones (canned)	3 oz	212
Sardines with bones	3 oz	325
Almonds	2 oz	141
Fruits and Vegetables		
Orange	1 medium	52
Kale	½ cup	90
Prunes	6	25
Green beans	½ cup	28
Winter squash	½ cup	23
Cereal Grains and Bakery Products		
White bread, enriched	1 slice	45
Whole wheat bread	1 slice	36
Cornbread, enriched	2½-inch square	88
Pancake, enriched	4-inch diameter	68
Corn tortilla, enriched	6-inch diameter	19

Data from U.S. Department of Agriculture, Agricultural Research Service. USDA National Nutrient Database for Standard Reference. Available at: www.nal.usda.gov/fnic/foodcomp/search

" Several processed foods, especially baked goods, highly processed cheeses, and luncheon meats, contain modest amounts of phosphate additives. "

Calcium intakes are plotted against age in **FIGURE 9.9** to illustrate the discrepancy between daily calcium intake and the RDAs for calcium. The median calcium intakes of females 11 years and older are much lower than their age-specific RDAs. Males do better, but still consume less calcium than recommended. Intakes of calcium by young females at median intakes suggest that peak bone mass (PBM) accrual may not be optimized in the lower 50% of consumers. Similar low calcium intakes are common in China and other Asian nations, although Japanese women have somewhat increased their calcium intakes in recent decades. Phosphorus intakes have been found to be considerably higher than calcium in almost all populations of the world.

Most foods (except fruits and vegetables) contain plentiful amounts of phosphorus. In addition, a 12-ounce can of cola contains approximately 30 to 60 milligrams of phosphorus. When soft drinks replace milk, the intake of calcium is reduced while the amount of phosphorus is typically increased, both of which contribute to a lowering of the Ca:P ratio. Several processed foods, especially baked goods, highly processed cheeses, and luncheon meats also contain significant amounts of phosphate additives. **FIGURE 9.10** shows the percentage of phosphate additives in the most commonly consumed processed foods. The extra phosphorus from additives just adds to the dietary imbalance between calcium and phosphorus (i.e., a less than 1:1 ratio, see **Table 9.8**).

Low-fat dairy products, such as live-culture yogurts, are excellent sources of calcium. One cup of yogurt contains about 30% to 50% more calcium than a cup of milk. Many consumers find yogurt appealing because it is low in dietary fat and has little or no effect on weight gain. Furthermore, one cup of yogurt provides enough calcium to meet about 33% of daily RDAs and at the same time avoids overconsumption of phosphorus (and fat). In contrast, a serving of cottage cheese, although still a dairy product and a good source of protein, contains much lower amounts of calcium compared with a serving of yogurt or milk.

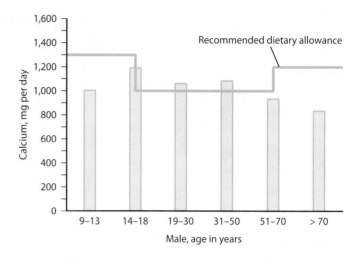

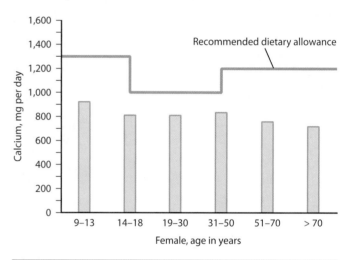

FIGURE 9.9 Median Calcium Intakes of Females Compared to the Recommended Dietary Allowances (RDAs). Plot based on data from USDA, 1994. After age 13, males did better than females, but they still did not achieve the RDAs at all ages.

Reproduced from Anderson JJB. *Nutrition and Health: An Introduction.* Durham, NC: Carolina Academic Press; 2005.

PRACTICAL APPLICATIONS **9.1**

Lactose Intolerance and Inadequate Calcium Intake

People who are lactose intolerant often reduce their consumption of milk and other dairy products. If milk consumption is totally stopped or greatly reduced, then both calcium intake and vitamin D intake may be reduced. Plan a dinner meal that does not contain milk, cheese, or yogurt, but does include a minimum of 300 milligrams of calcium from other foods. Create a table with three columns. In the first column, record the food item. Record the serving size in the second column, and then enter the amount of calcium per serving in the third column. Did you find it easy or difficult to incorporate nondairy calcium-containing foods into the meal? What milk-alternative products could you use to help a person with lactose intolerance meet his or her calcium needs? ■

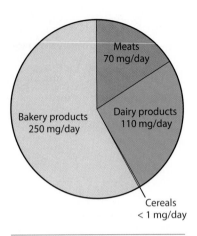

FIGURE 9.10 Phosphate Additives in Processed Foods (Percentage by Food Group).

* Estimated phosphorus intake per person. Data from Greger JL, Krystofiak M. Phosphorus intake of Americans. *Food Technol.* 1982;36(1):78–84.

TABLE 9.8
Phosphorus Content of Select Foods and Soft Drinks

Item (regular serving)	Phosphorus (mg)
Food Item	
Whole wheat bread	39
White bread	25
Oatmeal	96
Cheddar cheese	145
Skim milk	247
Egg	296
Banana	26
Orange juice	42
Apple	20
Tuna (water packed)	184
Ground beef	168
Turkey (roasted)	186
Broccoli (cooked)	51
Potato with skin (baked)	121
Tomato (fresh)	30
Corn, frozen	95
Coca-Cola Classic	41
Diet Coke	18

Data from U.S. Department of Agriculture, Agricultural Research Service. USDA National Nutrient Database for Standard Reference, Available at: www.nal .usda.gov/fnic/foodcomp/search; and Pennington JAT. *Bowes and Church's Food Values of Portions Commonly Used*. 17th ed. Philadelphia: J.B. Lippincott; 1998.

The Calcium–Phosphorus Ratio

The ratio of calcium to phosphorus is high in human breast milk (2:1), which supports bone mineralization and tooth formation in the developing infant. Cow's milk has a ratio of only 1.3:1. Later in childhood and during adolescence, the dietary Ca:P ratio often falls to less than 1:1 and the usual adult ratio typically falls between 0.5:1 and 0.8:1. This ratio depends greatly on the amount of milk or other dairy products an individual consumes each day. During the growth periods of the life cycle a sufficient supply of calcium (and phosphorus) and other nutrients is needed for optimal skeletal development; that is, to maximize the development of peak bone mass (PBM) by 20 years of age or so. An optimal Ca:P ratio during adolescence is approximately 1:1 for PBM development.

PRACTICAL APPLICATIONS 9.2

Phosphate Additives in Processed Foods

A comparison of the phosphorus content of three types of cheese products illustrates the significant increase in phosphates in a specific food after processing with phosphate salts as functional additives. The phosphorus values in each of the three types of cheese—cheddar, American, and Cheez-Whiz—show how adding phosphorus additives increases the total amount of phosphorus on a weight-for-weight basis. Using a food composition table, find the phosphorus content of one serving of each cheese type. Examine the ingredients label of each of the three cheese types for any phosphorus-containing ingredients that are added in processing.

Cheese Type	Serving Size	Phosphorus (mg)	Phosphorus-Containing Ingredient
Cheddar	1 oz	145	
American	1 slice	179	
Cheez-Whiz Squeeze	2 tbsp	266	Sodium phosphate

Does the use of phosphate additives appear to increase the total amount of phosphorus in the food item?

Can you explain why the food industry needs to add phosphate salts to processed foods? ■

Too much dietary phosphorus, as absorbed phosphate ions, may adversely affect the skeleton by drawing calcium from the bone to balance the high phosphorus in the blood (see **FIGURE 9.11**). This phenomenon occurs after a period of low calcium and high phosphate intakes because of the bone resorptive action of **parathyroid hormone (PTH)**. Bone may be compromised by such a diet with an unhealthy long-term low Ca:P ratio. An optimal dietary ratio of calcium to phosphorus for adults ranges between 1:1 and 0.5:1 (see Figure 9.8). Over a long period of time, low-calcium diets alter calcium

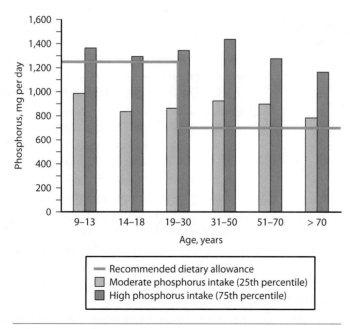

FIGURE 9.11 Phosphorus Intake in Adults Compared to the RDA.
Data from NHANES, 2005–2006.

parathyroid hormone (PTH) Hormone produced by the parathyroid glands that has a major role in regulating blood calcium concentration through its direct actions on bone and the kidneys and indirect actions on the small intestine via the hormonal form of vitamin D (1,25-dihydroxyvitamin D).

metabolism, resulting in excessive loss of bone mass and, possibly, osteopenia and later osteoporosis.

The reduced capacity to digest milk sugar, lactose, after infancy typically leads to the consumption of inadequate amounts of calcium in most affected individuals. Many African Americans, Asians, and even some Caucasians are lactose intolerant, and they have learned to avoid symptom-producing milk and other dairy products. People with lactose intolerance may eat other dairy products, such as calcium-rich yogurt (live culture preferably), in which lactose is broken down, or drink lactose-free cow's milk or soy milk. In recent years, additional alternative lactose-free milk products, some derived from almonds or coconut, have appeared on the market. People with lactose intolerance may also benefit from taking calcium supplements beginning as early in life as possible to try to optimize skeletal development and achieve **peak bone mass** and to maintain that bone mass during the adult decades.

> **"** In adults and older individuals, calcium supplements may have little or no impact in improving bone mineral density, and the additional calcium may actually contribute to arterial calcification. **"**

Supplementation

Supplementation of calcium in modest quantities may help maintain calcium balance and bone mass, especially in growing children and adolescents. In adults and older individuals, calcium supplements may have little or no impact in improving bone mineral density, and the additional calcium may actually contribute to arterial calcification. Thus, calcium supplementation in adults may improve overall calcium balance at the expense of calcification of arteries of the heart, the heart valves, the brain, and other organs. Note that supplementation with phosphorus is not recommended for healthy individuals.

Recommended Dietary Allowances

Recommended calcium and phosphorus intakes are almost the same for both sexes across the life cycle, despite the obvious differences in body size and bone mass between the genders. The RDA for calcium for ages 9 to 18 years is 1,300 milligrams per day. This amount may be more than enough for optimal skeletal development because although only small percentages of individuals in this age range consume calcium at or above the RDA, the majority of adolescents are still able to achieve reasonable bone development. The RDA for calcium is 1,000 mg per day for women 19 to 50 years of age and for men up to age 70. For women over age 50 and men over age 70, the RDA is increased to 1,200 milligrams per day.

The RDA for phosphorus is 700 milligrams per day for adults. However, phosphorus intakes for each age category greatly exceed recommended intakes. The desired adult Ca:P ratio, based on the RDAs, is a healthy 1.4:1 (from 1,000 milligrams of calcium and 700 milligrams of phosphorus per day), but rarely do adults have such ratios because of their high phosphorus intakes. Adult phosphorus intakes are too high compared with the RDAs. **Table 9.9** provides the DRIs for calcium and phosphorus for the different age groups. **Table 9.10** provides estimated calcium and phosphorus intakes.

In general, positive calcium balance is the rule from infancy through adolescence. Early adulthood (ages 20 to 40) is characterized by an equilibrium in calcium balance, with no net gains or losses. Negative calcium balance (steady bone loss) dominates during the resorptive postmenopausal phase of women and continues during the subsequent periods of life of both genders.

TABLE 9.9
RDAs of Calcium and Phosphorus

Age	Calcium (mg/day)	Phosphorus (mg/day)
9–13 years	1,300	1,250
14–18 years	1,300	1,250
19–50 years	1,000	700
51–70 years	1,000 M; 1,200 F*	700
> 71 years	1,200	700

* Male and female RDAs are different.
Data from Food and Nutrition Board, Institute of Medicine. *Dietary Reference Intakes for Calcium, Phosphorus, Magnesium, Vitamin D, and Fluoride (1997)* and *Dietary Reference Intakes for Vitamin D and Calcium (2011)*. Washington, DC: National Academies Press, 1997, 2011.

peak bone mass (PBM) The point at which greatest bone mass is attained. Typically occurs by 20 years of age or the decade thereafter.

TABLE 9.10

Median Intakes of Calcium and Phosphorus and Calcium:Phosphorus (Ca:P) Ratios

Age	Calcium (mg/day)*	Phosphorus (mg/day)	Ca:P Ratios
12–19 years (males and females)	1,124	1,408	0.8:1
20–39 years			
Males	1,260	1,726	0.73:1
Females	1,007	1,230	0.82:1
40–59 years			
Males	1,297	1,752	0.74:1
Females	1,143	1,196	0.96:1
≥ 60 years			
Males	1,153	1,413	0.82:1
Females	1,266	1,137	1.11:1

* Calcium values include supplements, which increases the Ca:P ratio. Phosphate values do not include phosphate additives to foods, which makes the ratio appear to be healthier.
Data from U.S. Department of Agriculture, Agricultural Research Service. 2012. Total Nutrient Intakes: Percent Reporting and Mean Amounts of Selected Vitamins and Minerals from Food and Dietary Supplements, by Gender and Age. What We Eat in America. NHANES 2009–2010. Available at: www.ars.usda.gov/ba/bhnrc/fsrg

Intestinal Absorption

Absorption of calcium and phosphate ions occurs in the absorbing epithelial cells (enterocytes). A major difference between these two mineral ions is that calcium cations are absorbed at a relatively low efficiency by adults compared with phosphate anions. When considering that almost all foods contain phosphorus and relatively few contain much calcium, the amount of phosphate ions typically absorbed exceeds that of calcium ions from a meal by a wide margin.

Dietary components such as **oxalic acid (oxalate)**, which is present in foods such as spinach, rhubarb, and beet greens, and phytic acid in cereals, bind with calcium ions within the small intestine, further reducing calcium absorption when both are consumed in the same meal (see **FIGURE 9.12**).

Under conditions of low calcium intake, calcium ions are more efficiently absorbed from approximately 25% to as high as 75%.

Excretion

The excretion of calcium in the urine is influenced by several nutrients in the usual diet. The average North American consumes protein from animal sources, such as meat, fish, poultry, milk, cheese, and eggs. When metabolized, animal proteins generate more urinary acid, especially sulfuric and phosphoric acids, than do vegetable sources of protein. The additional acids must be buffered by serum bicarbonate and bone calcium before being excreted by the kidneys. For consumers of low amounts of dietary calcium, high animal protein intakes may increase urinary calcium losses. However, this

> *Under conditions of low calcium intake, calcium ions are more efficiently absorbed from approximately 25% to as high as 75%.*

oxalic acid (oxalate) A short organic acid found in some plant foods, such as rhubarb, that binds calcium ions and to a lesser extent other divalent cations in the gut lumen, thereby reducing the intestinal absorption of calcium and other minerals. Also involved in renal tubular formation of oxalate stones (kidney stones).

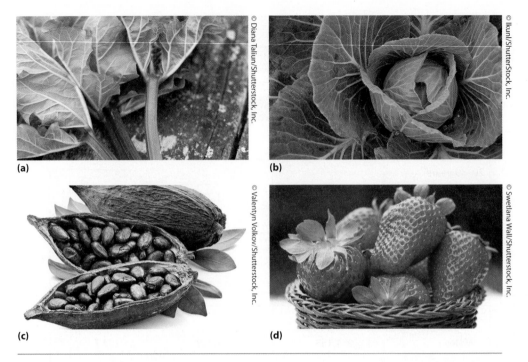

FIGURE 9.12 Foods Rich in Oxalic Acid. Oxalic acid inhibits the absorption of several minerals, especially calcium, iron, and zinc. (a) Rhubarb, (b) cabbage, (c) cacao beans, and (d) strawberries.

theory may be in doubt as newer data suggest that high protein intake may actually improve both calcium absorption and bone density. So, the concern about too much animal protein adversely affecting bone mass because of acid generation remains on hold, until new research findings appear.

A high-sodium diet also increases urinary calcium losses because urinary calcium excretion is tightly linked to urinary sodium excretion. These minerals are reabsorbed by a common mechanism in the renal tubules of the kidneys.

Deficiencies

Many people believe that a deficiency of dietary calcium, which is fairly common in the United States and other parts of the world, contributes to osteopenia or osteoporosis later in life, which can lead to an increased risk for bone fractures. However, newer

FOCUS 9.2 Interactions Between Calcium and Vitamin D

Calcium and vitamin D interact in two important ways. The first is in intestinal absorption and the other is in bone formation. In the intestine, the hormonal form of vitamin D (1,25-dihydroxyvitamin D) enhances the absorption of calcium ions. The vitamin D hormone, which is made by the kidneys, increases the efficiency of calcium absorption by stimulating the synthesis of calbindins by the gut absorbing cells. Each calbindin carries four calcium ions across the cytoplasm of the enterocyte to the basement membrane for absorption.

At sites of new bone formation in the skeleton, the hormonal form of vitamin D aids bone-building cells in taking up calcium ions that are used in making new bone mineral (i.e., hydroxyapatite, which is a complex phosphate of calcium).

When dietary calcium intakes are low, as in a young child who is no longer breastfeeding, the maintenance of calcium homeostasis and perhaps a positive calcium balance is aided by an increase in intestinal calcium absorption stimulated by serum 1,25-dihydroxyvitamin D (calcitriol). ●

research indicates that calcium intake in adults and elders has little impact on bone mineral density or the risk of fracture and that the calcium deficiency hypothesis of bone loss is incorrect. This research suggests that other risk factors, such as insufficient physical activity and other unhealthy behaviors, are major contributors to bone loss in older adults, in addition to high circulating levels of parathyroid hormone (PTH). In fact, it may be more important to maintain high calcium intake and regular physical activity early in life in order to accrue a higher peak bone mass, which may help prevent or delay fractures in later life.

Bone health programs at any age include the consumption of calcium at RDA amounts from foods and, if prescribed by a physician, supplements. Regular weight-bearing exercises, especially walking at a good pace, and strength exercises involving upper body muscle groups that help maintain the bone mass and quality of the proximal femur also are beneficial. At present, research suggests that consuming foods containing adequate amounts of calcium and vitamin D and engaging in physical activity at all phases of the life cycle can help to prevent or delay the onset of osteopenia, osteoporosis, and the fractures associated with osteoporosis.

> *At present, research suggests that consuming foods containing adequate amounts of calcium and vitamin D and engaging in physical activity at all phases of the life cycle can help to prevent or delay the onset of osteopenia, osteoporosis, and the fractures associated with osteoporosis.*

FOCUS 9.3   The Need for Calcium Supplements

The RDAs for calcium remain the best recommendations for the U.S. population, but many individuals have difficulty consuming these recommended amounts, especially the elderly, who have an RDA of 1,200 milligrams per day. As a general rule, adults and elders who obtain 800 milligrams or more of calcium per day from foods seem to be doing well. However, many adults, especially older adults, do not consume 800 milligrams of calcium per day, and thus may benefit from a calcium supplement (500 milligrams or less) as well as a vitamin D supplement (400 IU per day) to maintain bone mass and density.

The concern with calcium supplements is that excess calcium, once absorbed, may not go into bone but rather into arterial walls or other soft tissues. The UL for calcium is 2,500 milligrams per day for adults between 19 and 50 years but only 2,000 milligrams per day for those 51 years and older. Calcium intake at the upper range may impact cardiovascular health by increasing the risk of arterial calcification. This issue of excessive calcium supplement intakes by older adults needs to be closely monitored in the future. ●

Phosphorus deficiency is extremely rare, but it may exist in older adults who do not consume enough food energy, phosphorus, or other nutrients in their daily diet. Malnutrition is fairly common in shut-in and institutionalized elderly.

Toxicity

Calcium toxicity may occur with excessive intake, particularly in cases of overconsumption of calcium supplements. Calcium salts greatly limit the elasticity of the arteries, especially the aorta. The major adverse effect related to excessive calcium supplement use is constipation, especially in the elderly who usually consume too little water or other fluids. Two more severe conditions, renal stone formation and calcification of renal and other soft tissues, may result from causes other than excessive calcium intake, but dietary calcium is generally restricted in the treatment of individuals with these conditions.

Excessive additive phosphate intake, when combined with calcium deficiency, tends to decrease bone mass and density and may possibly lead to osteopenia and osteoporosis. Excessive phosphate induces the **calcium homeostatic** mechanisms to elevate

calcium homeostasis The regulation of blood calcium concentration (total) at about 10 milligrams per deciliter through the integrated actions of parathyroid hormone (PTH), the hormonal form of vitamin D (i.e., 1,25-dihydroxycholecalciferol), and other hormones working on the skeleton, gut, and kidneys.

parathyroid hormone secretion, increase bone resorption, and increase phosphate excretion. In addition, over decades arterial calcification may possibly result from calcium ions that are resorbed from bone.

Microminerals

The microminerals, also known as trace elements, include nine elements that are established as essential for human function: iron, zinc, iodine, selenium, copper, manganese, fluoride, chromium, and molybdenum. Possibly a dozen other trace elements may also be present in human tissues, but their requirements for human health remain unknown. As indicated by the term "trace elements," these nutrients are required in small amounts. All of the micronutrient recommendations are for less than 100 milligrams per day, and some are less than 1 milligram per day. Several minerals required in microgram amounts are referred to as ultratrace minerals.

Microminerals such as iron and zinc are abundant in meat and fish. Microminerals also are abundant in plant foods. Whole plant foods, such as vegetables, that are steamed or cooked briefly in small amounts of water retain their trace elements much better than when cooked in water for long periods of time. Fresh, uncooked vegetables, of course, retain these nutrients much more completely.

In recent years, concerns have been raised that because most Americans rely on highly processed foods many people may not be ingesting adequate amounts of some trace elements. Food processing, especially the conversion (milling) of cereal grains to flours, generally leads to reductions of between 25% and 75% of several trace elements.

North Americans who consume a **balanced diet** (i.e., adequate servings of a variety of iron-containing foods, including fortified cereals, each day) should be able to obtain reasonable intakes of all the trace elements. Individuals who do not consume meat, fish, or poultry (i.e., most vegetarians) will need to consume iron-rich legumes to avoid deficiencies of iron, zinc, and possibly chromium. Seafoods contain practically all the trace elements in good amounts. **Table 9.11** lists the food groups containing good amounts of different trace minerals.

> ❝ In recent years, concerns have been raised that because most Americans rely on highly processed foods many may not be ingesting adequate amounts of some trace elements. ❞

> ❝ North Americans who consume a balanced diet (i.e., adequate servings of a variety of iron-containing foods, including fortified cereals, each day) should be able to obtain reasonable intakes of all the trace elements. ❞

> ❝ Food fortification with selected trace elements, especially iodine and iron, has improved the intakes of North Americans, which some consider to be one of the great public health successes of the twentieth century. ❞

balanced diet A diet balanced with respect to macronutrients, micronutrients, and non-nutrients, providing all the essential nutrients and energy from foods to support the daily activities in a healthy individual. Energy intake is not excessive when maintaining energy balance. Such diets for healthy males and females contain nutrient intakes at approximately RDA levels.

TABLE 9.11
Food Groups Containing Good Quantities of the Trace Elements

Meats/ Poultry	Fish/Seafood	Dairy	Legumes	Cereals	Fruits/ Vegetables
Iron	Iron	Iodine	Iron	Iron	Iron*
Zinc	Zinc		Zinc	Zinc	Chromium†
Chromium	Selenium		Manganese	Manganese	Manganese
Copper	Chromium		Copper	Molybdenum	Molybdenum
Manganese	Copper				
Selenium	Iodine				
	Fluoride				

* Dark green, leafy vegetables; some dried fruits; † Especially broccoli.

Food fortification with selected trace elements, especially iodine and iron, has improved the intakes of North Americans, which some consider to be one of the great public health successes of the twentieth century. Other trace element fortificants include fluoride and zinc. The presence of many foods fortified with iron, especially flours of wheat and other cereal grains, and ready-to-eat breakfast cereals, has made it easier for consumers to obtain adequate amounts of this trace element. Many micronutrients are added to ready-to-eat breakfast cereals.

Once absorbed, trace elements generally become associated with proteins or other organic molecules and, typically, each trace element functions as part of a complex structure. For example, when a trace element becomes an integral part of a protein molecule, a metalloprotein results. The biological roles of some trace elements in these complex molecules, including several enzymes, are still unfolding. Research on trace elements represents one of the frontiers of nutrition that is being advanced with better chemical analytic methods and instruments for the detection of trace quantities of these elements in both tissues and foods.

This section of the chapter examines the essential micronutrients, including iron, zinc, iodine, selenium, copper, molybdenum, and others needed in ultra-low amounts. Each trace element is characterized by functions, food sources, and deficiencies or toxicities. **Iron** has a critical role in oxygen transport by red blood cells and it functions as an enzyme cofactor in all cells. Also, iron is the most commonly deficient nutrient in the diets of women throughout the world. Because of its importance, this section pays special attention to iron.

Iron

Iron is an essential micromineral. Free, or ionic, iron exists in two different forms in the body: the +2 (ferrous) state and the +3 (ferric) state. Oxidation or reduction (i.e., the loss or gain of an electron) readily occurs between the two states. Because iron binds so readily to protein, it is an essential constituent of several metalloprotein molecules, including **heme iron** in red blood cells.

Iron in plant-based foods is less readily available for intestinal absorption. In addition, one of the richest sources of iron, liver, is generally not consumed because of its high saturated fat and cholesterol content. Because low iron intake often is a problem in the human diet, iron fortification of foods is common throughout the world.

Of all the micronutrient deficiency diseases in the world, **iron deficiency** is the most common. Marginal or subclinical iron deficiency alone does not result in serious adverse health effects, and it is much more prevalent than the more severe form of iron deficiency that is associated with anemia. Mild (uncomplicated by anemia) to severe (accompanied by anemia, i.e., **iron deficiency anemia**) cases of iron deficiency have been identified in the U.S. population in recent nutritional assessments, such as the NHANES. For women, in particular menstruating females, and even for those who consume energy at the recommended level, it is difficult to ingest enough iron to meet the gender-specific RDAs.

Food Sources

Animal proteins, especially red meats, poultry, and fish, provide good supplies of iron in the form of heme iron. Certain metalloproteins, including hemoglobin, contain a central molecular cage, called a porphyrin, which holds an iron atom. This porphyrin and its iron are called heme iron. Liver contains large amounts of heme iron. Heme iron is absorbed more efficiently than nonheme iron. Nonheme forms of iron exist as ions (Fe^{2+} or Fe^{3+}) mostly in plant foods. Good sources of **nonheme iron** include dark green vegetables; soybeans; beans; peas; dried apricots and peaches; prunes; dates; figs; raisins; whole wheat breads and pastas; and iron-fortified breads, cereals,

> Once absorbed, trace elements generally become associated with proteins or other organic molecules and, typically, each trace element functions as part of a complex structure. For example, when a trace element becomes an integral part of a protein molecule, a metalloprotein results.

> Of all the micronutrient deficiency diseases in the world, iron deficiency is the most common.

iron A micronutrient that serves as a component of hemoglobin, myoglobin, cytochromes, and enzymes. It seldom exists in the free state. Present in foods in heme and nonheme forms.

heme iron Dietary iron derived from heme metalloproteins (e.g., hemoglobin, myoglobin).

iron deficiency A form of deficiency of iron resulting from inadequate consumption of iron-rich foods and characterized by low hematocrit and blood hemoglobin content; typically also characterized by low, but not exhausted, iron stores (ferritin).

iron deficiency anemia A severe form of iron deficiency characterized by low hemoglobin and depressed values of virtually all biochemical indices of iron status. Symptoms include tiredness and lack of energy.

nonheme iron Iron that is consumed in foods as ionic iron rather than as a component of heme (porphyrin plus iron). Nonheme iron is absorbed less efficiently than heme iron. Found primarily in plant foods.

TABLE 9.12
Common Food Sources Rich in Heme Iron and Nonheme Iron

Foods Rich in Heme Iron	Foods Rich in Nonheme Iron
Meats	Egg yolks
Fish	Dark green vegetables
Poultry	Soybeans
Liver	Beans and peas
Clams	Dried apricots
	Prunes
	Dates
	Figs
	Raisins
	Whole wheat bread
	Iron-fortified bread
	Iron-fortified baby foods

Reproduced from Anderson JJB. *Nutrition and Health: An Introduction*. Durham, NC: Carolina Academic Press; 2005.

and baby foods (see **Table 9.12**). Meats and other animal proteins contain nonheme iron in modest amounts (see **FIGURE 9.13**).

Functions

Iron has several important roles in the body. It is required for the formation of hemoglobin and myoglobin, and it acts as a cofactor for several different enzymes. Hemoglobin and myoglobin are required for the delivery of oxygen to the body's tissues. Heme iron is also a component of mitochondrial **cytochromes**, which are primarily mitochondrial enzymes involved in ATP generation. Nonheme iron is also a component of several enzymes.

Absorption

In general, iron is better absorbed from animal foods than from plant foods (see **FIGURE 9.14**). The absorption of nonheme iron is enhanced by the presence of vitamin C or a meat factor in the same meal, and it may be inhibited by tannins in tea and other components of some foods. The specific chemical structure of the so-called "meat factor" has not been identified. The intestinal absorption of both heme and nonheme iron is detailed in **FIGURE 9.15**.

cytochrome An enzyme in mitochondria that is part of the electron transport chain that captures energy from the C-H bonds of acetate molecules (and other molecules that convert to acetate) from the citric acid (Krebs) cycle. It enables the oxidation of the two hydrocarbons (C-H) of acetate to carbon dioxide and water (metabolic).

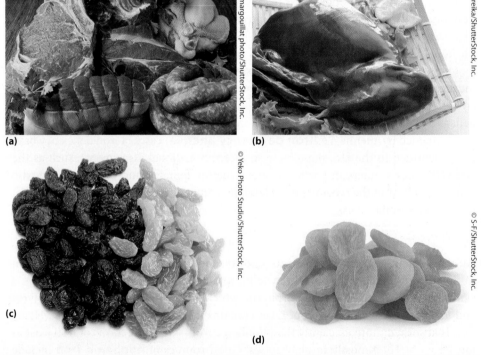

FIGURE 9.13 Foods Rich in Iron. Meats and other animal proteins are good sources of heme iron. Many plant-based foods are good sources of nonheme iron. (a) Red meat, (b) liver, (c) raisins, and (d) dried apricots.

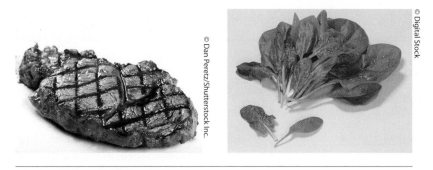

FIGURE 9.14 Absorption of Iron from Animal and Plant Foods. Iron is better absorbed from animal products than from plant foods.

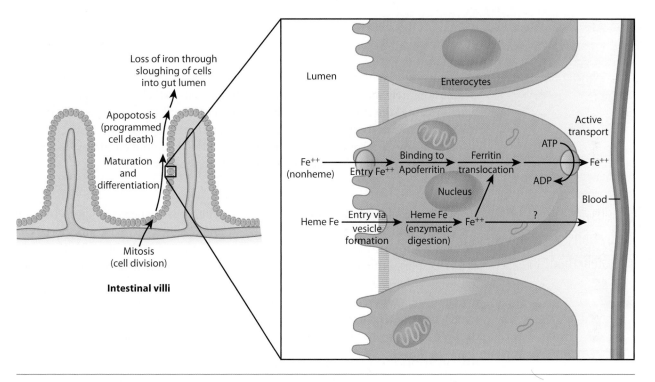

FIGURE 9.15 Intestinal Absorption of Iron. Iron absorption is complicated because of the two types of iron found in foods: ionic iron and heme iron. Each has a separate route of transcellular absorption beginning at the brush border of the surface of epithelial cells.

Reproduced from Anderson JJB. *Nutrition and Health: An Introduction.* Durham, NC: Carolina Academic Press; 2005.

For individuals with adequate iron intakes, heme iron is absorbed at 25% to 40% efficiency, whereas nonheme ionic (ferrous) iron is absorbed at 5% to 10% efficiency. Ferric iron (Fe^{3+}) is not well absorbed. Ascorbic acid and the so-called meat factor improve the efficiency of intestinal absorption of nonheme iron a few percentage points.

Iron balance is carefully regulated by the intestinal barrier, especially when iron intake is adequate. The efficiency of iron absorption depends on the body's need to produce red blood cells (e.g., during menses when blood losses are typically significant). The gut permits only so much iron to be absorbed. In a deficiency state, the efficiency of absorption is increased, whereas during periods of sufficient intake iron absorption may be reduced.

Unique among all minerals, iron is not normally excreted in the urine or secreted in bile or sweat. The body has no other major mechanism for controlling the elimination of iron, except for minor losses in skin desquamation (i.e., shedding of the outer skin layer). Menstruation, blood loss due to injury, or the presence of intestinal parasites

> For individuals with adequate iron intakes, heme iron is absorbed at 25% to 40% efficiency, whereas nonheme ionic (ferrous) iron is absorbed at 5% to 10% efficiency.

PRACTICAL APPLICATIONS **9.3**

Iron Content in Common Foods

Refer to a food composition table and determine the iron content (in milligrams) for the following foods:

- Green peas (1 cup, raw)
- Broccoli (1 cup, raw)
- Kale (1 cup, raw)
- Liver (3 oz, cooked)

- Beef patty (3 oz, cooked)
- Salmon (3 oz, cooked)

Which of these foods contain heme iron? Which contain only nonheme iron? In terms of the total amounts of iron, which foods typically provide the most total iron? Which provide the most heme iron? How would the type of iron consumed differ between omnivores and vegetarians? ■

> *Iron ions are carried in the blood by transferrin, a transport protein made in the liver.*

also can upset iron balance, especially when blood losses are heavy. Thus, iron balance is almost entirely maintained by the action of gut cells, which are thought to receive signals "telling" the small intestinal absorbing cells to increase or decrease absorption. High serum transferrin (with low percentage saturation) may be the key signal involved in intestinal iron absorption and, hence, iron regulation. This limit on elimination makes iron overload, or hemochromatosis, a potentially serious condition.

Metabolism

Heme, the metallo-organic molecule, is absorbed intact as the heme complex. The iron is removed from heme in the cells of the intestine and is then carried via the portal circulation to the liver (see **FIGURE 9.16**). Iron ions are carried in the blood by **transferrin**, a transport protein made in the liver. Iron is either stored in liver cells or transferred to the blood for distribution via transferrin to other tissues, especially to the red bone marrow for incorporation into heme that is needed by red blood cells for transporting oxygen to tissues. Iron is stored as the iron storage protein **ferritin**, which is present in the liver, red bone marrow, and other tissues, such as the spleen and lymphoid tissues.

Recommended Dietary Allowances

The RDAs for iron across the life cycle are provided in **Table 9.13**. Note the higher recommendation for pregnant women than for non-pregnant women in the childbearing years.

Deficiency

Iron deficiency is a generic name that includes both iron deficiency anemia and depleted (deficient) iron stores without the anemia, the less serious form of deficiency. In the United States and other developed countries in which iron-fortified foods are available, iron deficiency is less prevalent, but it is a much more common problem in the developing world where fortified foods and meat may not be available.

Iron nutritional status is assessed by simple measurements of hematocrit (the percentage by volume of red cells in a capillary tube of centrifuged and separated blood) and hemoglobin concentration. Red blood cells also can be examined microscopically. Perhaps the most sensitive measurement is of serum ferritin, the iron storage protein. Depletion of iron stores is indicated by low levels of serum ferritin and by low values of serum hemoglobin and **hematocrit** (see **FIGURE 9.17**).

In anemia, the more severe form of iron deficiency, functions that require iron are depressed, thus compromising oxygen delivery to muscle and other tissues, including the brain. Most people with iron deficiency function reasonably well until iron stores

transferrin A liver protein secreted into the blood to carry iron from the liver to tissues, especially the red bone marrow, where red blood cells are forming. A marker for acute disease because synthesis increases when the body is under stress.

ferritin Storage form of iron found primarily in liver but also measurable in blood serum. It is derived through the combining of iron with apoferritin, a protein synthesized in the liver that is capable of storing large quantities of iron.

hematocrit Packed cell volume of blood after centrifugation that is expressed as a percentage of cells to the total volume in the capillary tube.

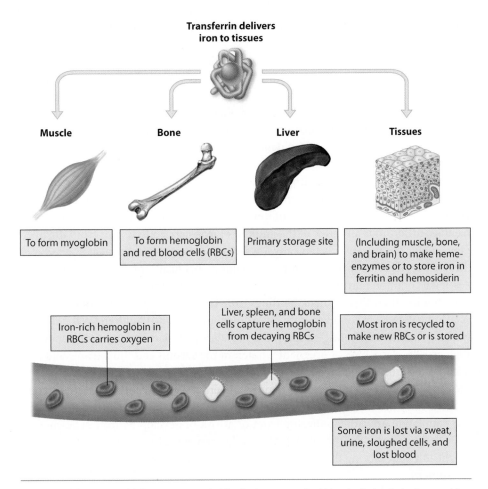

FIGURE 9.16 Iron Metabolism. Iron is needed for the formation of red blood cells, but it also is essential for the synthesis of several enzymes and skeletal muscle proteins.

TABLE 9.13
RDAs for Iron Across the Life Cycle

Life Stage	Male (mg/day)	Female (mg/day)
9–13 years	8	8
14–18 years	11	15
19–50 years	8	18
> 51 years	8	8
Pregnancy		27
Lactation		10 (9)*

* The RDA for lactating females 18 or younger is 10 mg of iron per day, whereas older women need only 9 mg per day until menstruation resumes.

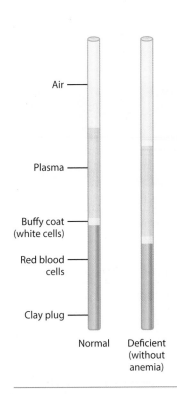

FIGURE 9.17 Low-Normal and Low Hematocrit Values.

become severely low, and excessive blood loss, such as from trauma, triggers acute blood losses that may lead to anemia.

Low hematocrit measurements mean that too little hemoglobin, i.e., iron, is present in the red blood cells. Clinical manifestations of the more severe form of iron deficiency with anemia include skin and nail changes; a pale, smooth tongue; tiredness; weakness; possibly faintness; pica (a craving for clay, starch, or ice); and general disinterest (lassitude). These symptoms result from poor oxygen delivery to tissues, such as the brain and muscle. The more severe form of iron deficiency does not occur until blood hemoglobin levels go well below 12 grams per deciliter and the hematocrit is less than 35%. Such values can be found in menstruating women and girls with iron-poor diets. **Table 9.14** shows the progressively worsening changes in iron indices as an individual moves from normal iron status through depletion of iron stores to anemia. The transferrin saturation percentage in serum is an index of the amount of iron carried to tissues from the liver; the percentage of saturation is typically low in iron-deficient individuals.

Severe iron deficiency with anemia is a major global health problem. In the United States, it is a common nutritional deficiency, affecting approximately 5% of menstruating females but less than 1% of others. Findings from the medical evaluation of the USDA's Special Supplementary Food Program for Women, Infants, and Children (WIC) showed that among infants and young children the prevalence of marginal iron deficiency was as high as 33%. Also, 25% of pregnant women in the second and third trimesters who had not taken iron supplements were found to be iron deficient. Other studies have suggested that a high percentage of U.S. preschoolers consume less than half the recommended dietary intake for iron. Hence, even in the United States, significant numbers of the population are either suffering from or at risk of developing iron deficiency. In the developing world, the prevalence of iron deficiency is even greater and is a major public health issue among those most at risk (i.e., toddlers and pregnant and menstruating women).

Conditions such as maternal iron deficiency, premature delivery, and low birth weight can lead to iron deficiency anemia in newborns. Infants experience a period of

TABLE 9.14
Changes in Blood Iron Indices from Normal to Iron Deficiency Anemia

Iron Parameter	Normal Erythropoiesis	Iron Depletion	Iron Deficiency Anemia
Iron stores	Good	Low	Depleted
Plasma ferritin	40–160 µg/mL	< 20 µg/mL	< 10 µg/mL
Iron absorption	5–10%	10–20%	10–20%
Transferrin (% saturation)	20–50%	< 15%	< 15%
Erythrocytes	Normal appearance	Normal	Microcytic and hypochromic
Hematocrit	> 35%	> 35%	< 35%
Hemoglobin	> 12 g/L	> 12 g/L	< 12 g/L

Data from Anderson JJB. *Nutrition and Health: An Introduction.* Carolina Academic Press, Durham, NC, Figure 17-04, p. 337 2005; and Herbert V. Recommended dietary intakes (RDIs) of iron in humans. *Am J Clin Nutr.* 1987;45:679–686.

very rapid growth at ages 6 to 18 months that increases the body's iron requirements, thus increasing the risk of deficiency in this group, especially those infants who are weaned to an iron-poor diet, as in many poor countries. Severe and persistent deficiency during infancy and early childhood may lead to permanent brain damage and delayed development.

Another period of rapid growth and increased need for iron is during adolescence. Adolescent girls, besides experiencing growth and maturation, also begin to lose iron in menstrual blood. Adolescent boys, generally between the ages of 13 and 18, experience an enlargement of muscle mass and expansion of blood volume, which also means an increased need for iron.

Supplementation

Some populations benefit from iron supplements. People following calorie-restricted diets to promote weight loss usually do not consume enough animal protein to provide the iron needed to meet their tissue requirements. Thus, people on weight-loss diets may require iron supplements. Endurance athletes, particularly women, lose iron at greater rates than normal, perhaps via cell loss throughout the small intestine, and they often require additional iron in the form of supplementation. And, as discussed earlier, iron supplementation by pregnant women can reduce the risk of iron deficiency.

Toxicity

Because the efficiency of intestinal iron absorption is low, iron overload and the toxic effects that may follow are highly unlikely. Iron overload, also known as **hemochromatosis**, occurs almost exclusively in individuals who have inherited a gene for more efficient iron absorption. Almost one in 100 to 200 people has inherited a gene for hemochromatosis, which increases the body's ability to absorb iron. The more common adverse effects of hemochromatosis, in addition to excessive iron stores that progress with age throughout the body, are heart damage and diabetes mellitus (the "bronze" form of hemochromatosis), which typically only presents in those older than 40 years. Iron overload can easily be detected by measuring transferrin (saturation values typically greater than 50% to 60%), and then treatment can begin.

Zinc

Zinc (Zn^{2+}), a trace element with an established RDA, is a component of many different enzyme systems. Because almost 100 enzyme systems require zinc, many aspects of metabolism are influenced by its nutritional status. Zinc as a component of enzymes has diverse roles in muscle, skeletal, and other tissues. Zinc interacts with vitamin A (retinol) in the liver and possibly in the eye. In addition to its roles in metalloenzymes and as an enzyme activator, zinc, in the form of zinc fingers, is also required for the hormonal regulation of DNA. Thus, zinc deficiency can diminish cell growth and repair and have a negative impact on many different biochemical pathways.

Food Sources

A variety of foods are good sources of zinc (see **Table 9.15**). Meat, poultry, and seafood are generally the best dietary sources of zinc. Wheat germ also is a good source of zinc. In order to meet the adult zinc RDAs (11 milligrams per day for men and 8 milligrams per day for women), a diet with reasonable amounts of protein, especially from animal sources, should be consumed. Zinc fortification of breakfast cereals began almost a decade ago to ensure that practically all adults consume sufficient zinc. Because the amount of zinc in processed infant foods has been shown to be low, these foods are now fortified with zinc additives, another example of fortification.

> Adolescent boys, generally between the ages of 13 and 18, experience an enlargement of muscle mass and expansion of blood volume, which also means an increased need for iron.

> In order to meet the adult zinc RDAs (11 milligrams per day for men and 8 milligrams per day for women), a diet with reasonable amounts of protein, especially from animal sources, should be consumed.

hemochromatosis Iron storage disease that results from increased intestinal absorption and excessive accumulation or overload of iron in the major storage organs (i.e., liver, spleen, bone marrow, heart). Complications resulting from this disorder have a severe negative impact on long-term health.

zinc An essential micromineral that exists in the body as a divalent cation (Zn^{2+}). Plays a role in more than 100 enzyme reactions and is a component of many other tissue proteins.

TABLE 9.15
Zinc Content of Common Foods

Foods Rich in Zinc	Foods Poor in Zinc
Oysters	Fruits
Wheat germ	Vegetables
Red meat	Milk
Poultry	White bread†
Fish	
Liver	
Nuts*	
Whole wheat bread	
Legumes*	
Fortified cereals	

* Zinc in plant sources, much of which is bound to phytic acid, has low bioavailability. † Processed sources generally are reduced in zinc by 33% or so. Reproduced from Anderson JJB. *Nutrition and Health: An Introduction.* Durham, NC: Carolina Academic Press; 2005.

> Absorption in the zinc-sufficient individual is about 20% to 30% efficient, but it is higher in deficient individuals.

iodine An essential trace mineral that exists as iodide (I⁻) in solution. Iodide is taken up by the thyroid gland so that the thyroid cells can synthesize the thyroid hormones thyroxin (T_4) and triiodothyronine (T_3).

thyroxin (T_4) A hormone produced by the thyroid gland that contains four atoms of iodine.

triiodothyronine (T_3) A hormone produced by the thyroid gland that contains three atoms of iodine.

Deficiency

Severe zinc deficiency in childhood contributes to poor growth (especially of the skeleton), skin abnormalities (dermatitis), poor taste acuity, reduced appetite, and hypogonadism (reduced functions of the ovaries or testes). Zinc supplementation of zinc-deficient young male Iranian dwarfs in the 1960s resulted in stimulation of growth as well as of gonadal development.

Severe zinc deficiency is rare in the United States. However, infants and young children are more likely to develop marginal zinc deficiency than adults. Marginal zinc deficiency has been reported in a study of preschool children living in Denver, Colorado, but zinc deficiency has not been observed in other locations. Deficiency of zinc in the developing world is much more prevalent, affecting as many as 2 billion people, according to the WHO. It contributes to many deaths because of zinc losses from diarrhea in infants. Zinc supplementation has been demonstrated to reduce infant mortality.

The relatively inadequate intake of zinc, averaging about two-thirds of the RDA by most North Americans, despite consuming a diet reasonably high in animal protein, suggests that marginal zinc deficiency is common. Daily servings from the protein food group, especially meat, poultry, fish, or other seafoods, provide most of the zinc required by tissues each day.

Absorption

The efficiency of zinc absorption largely depends on the zinc content of the diet. In general, zinc is better absorbed from animal products than from plant sources. In plants, zinc ions bind strongly to the phytic acid in whole grains and other plants, and, like other divalent cations, zinc may also bind to dietary fiber components. Absorption in the zinc-sufficient individual is about 20% to 30% efficient, but it is higher in deficient individuals.

Excretion

Zinc is lost primarily via pancreatic secretions of zinc-containing enzymes into the small intestine and is eventually eliminated in feces. Dermal zinc losses via sweat and sloughed skin are relatively high compared with other trace minerals. Urinary losses remain low but fairly constant. Athletes may need more zinc in their diets because of large losses of zinc in sweat.

Toxicity

When consumed in excessive amounts from supplements or cold lozenges, zinc may interfere with the absorption of copper ions because both zinc and copper ions are carried across the gut membranes by the same membrane carriers or porters. Thus, copper deficiency may result from excessive zinc intake.

Iodine

Iodine (I⁻) is another trace mineral that has an established RDA. Iodine is a component of the thyroid hormones. These hormones govern the basal metabolic rate (BMR), or energy-utilizing capacity of cells (and the body). Following absorption, iodide ions become trapped by the thyroid gland, and the ions are incorporated into the protein thyroglobulin by thyroid cells. From this molecule, the two thyroid hormones are split off: **thyroxin (T_4)**, which contains four atoms of iodine, and **triiodothyronine (T_3)**, which has three iodine atoms (see **FIGURE 9.18**). Iodine also is required for brain function, and deficiency during pregnancy increases the risk of cognitive deficit in infants.

Food sources of iodine include fish and seafood plus algae and other plants cultured in water. Most plant foods are low in iodine if the soil iodine content is low, which is the original reason for fortification of common table salt with iodine.

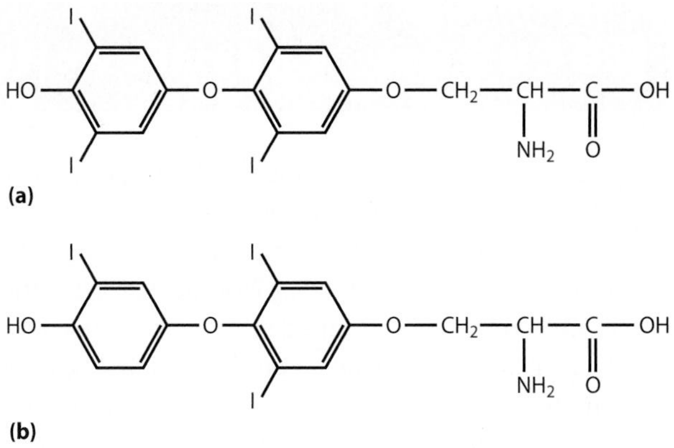

Deficiency

Severe dietary iodine deficiency is characterized by an enlarged thyroid gland, or goiter (see **FIGURE 9.19**). A goitrous thyroid gland contains cells that make too much **thyroglobulin** without enough iodine in an unsuccessful attempt to take up more and more iodide ions from blood. The blood of deficient individuals contains insufficient iodine to produce the iodinated hormones, and only small amounts of the fully iodinated thyroid hormones (T_4 and T_3) are then released to the blood. Individuals with iodine-deficiency **goiter** or simple goiter exhibit lowered BMR, lethargic behavior patterns, weight gain, and reduced mental function.

In some geographic areas of the world, soil deficiency contributes to widespread goiter in a population, which is referred to as endemic goiter. Endemic goiter can also result from the high consumption of iodide inhibitors, or goitrogens, such as cyanide and thiocyanates found in turnips and certain tropical plants, such as cassava. In tropical Africa, South America, and India, the carbohydrate-rich cassava (tapioca or manioc) is a significant source of iodine inhibitors, and, therefore, goiter is prevalent in these regions even today. Throughout the world, the use of iodized salt can help to ensure adequate iodine intake. Seafood consumption once or twice a week should also help to maintain normal serum concentrations of thyroid hormones.

Toxicity

Iodine toxicity is not a public health concern in the United States, even if there is excessive consumption of iodized salt. Excess iodine is easily excreted in the urine.

FIGURE 9.18 Thyroid Hormones. Structures of (a) thyroxin (T_4) and (b) triiodothyronine (T_3).

Severe dietary iodine deficiency is characterized by an enlarged thyroid gland, or goiter.

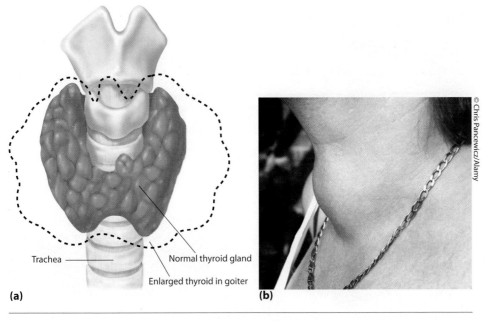

(a)

Trachea

Normal thyroid gland

Enlarged thyroid in goiter

(b)

© Chris Pancewicz/Alamy

FIGURE 9.19 Goiter. An enlarged thyroid gland resulting from consuming food deficient in iodine. Such goiters are now rare, but they may be found in those who live in mountainous or other types of terrain where the earth's surface iodine has been leached. A schematic diagram (a) illustrates the location of the thyroid gland in the neck and the photo of a person (b) illustrates the enlarged goiter.

thyroglobulin A protein found in the thyroid gland that is used to produce the hormones thyroxin (T_4) and triiodothyronine (T_3).

goiter (simple) A classic deficiency disease of iodine that results in simple enlargement of the thyroid gland. Endemic goiter refers to the prevalence of many individuals in a population with goiter because of iodine deficiency or consumption of goitrogens in the usual diet. Other types of goiter (i.e., metabolic) are not simple goiter.

FOCUS 9.4 Endemic Goiter and Iodized Salt

In the Great Lakes region of the United States, iodine has been greatly reduced in the topsoil because of widespread glaciations in the area approximately 10,000 years ago. Thus, as late as the 1930s, many individuals living in this region and eating foods raised in its soils developed goiter. The high prevalence of goiter prompted public health experts to try to fortify food with iodine in order to prevent the iodine deficiency disease. Common table salt was selected as the vehicle for iodine fortification.

The first trials using iodized salt (which was the first fortified food) were conducted in Akron, Ohio. These experiments proved how easy it was to correct iodine deficiency by using a common food as a vehicle for fortification. When iodized salt became widely accepted by consumers by the early 1940s, endemic goiter in the Great Lakes region and in other parts of the United States practically disappeared. However, goiter has not been so successfully eliminated in other parts of the world. ●

Selenium

Most North Americans consume 150 to 200 micrograms of **selenium (Se²⁻)** per day, which is more than enough to meet the body's needs. Selenium exists as part of a few enzymes, including glutathione peroxidase, which serves as an antioxidant in the cytoplasm of cells. In addition, several selenoproteins also function in the body. Whether intakes greater than recommended exert a protective effect against skin and other cancers, coronary heart disease, or other chronic diseases is not clear at this time.

Food Sources

Selenium intake closely parallels the consumption of meat, fish, and poultry (see **FIGURE 9.20**). People whose diets are high in animal proteins may ingest more than

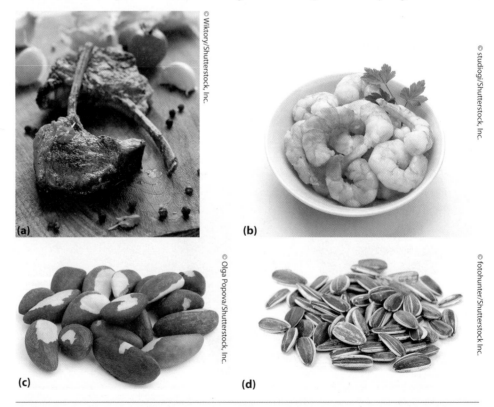

© Wiktory/Shutterstock, Inc.

© studiogi/Shutterstock, Inc.

© Olga Popova/Shutterstock, Inc.

© fotohunter/Shutterstock, Inc.

selenium An essential micromineral that exists as a divalent anion (Se²⁻). It activates the enzyme glutathione peroxidase, which protects fatty acids and other molecules against oxidative damage.

FIGURE 9.20 Foods Rich in Selenium. Animal foods such as (a) lamb chops and (b) shrimps are particularly rich in selenium. Some nuts, such as (c) Brazil nuts, and seeds, such as (d) sunflower seeds, also supply good amounts of selenium.

200 micrograms of selenium per day and may even approach the UL of 400 micrograms per day. Animal proteins are more likely to substitute selenium for sulfur in two amino acids, cysteine and methionine, which become part of several newly recognized functional selenoproteins. **Table 9.16** lists selected selenium-rich foods.

Deficiency

True selenium deficiency from inadequate dietary intake has only been documented in mainland China in the remote mountainous region of Keshan, where the soil content of selenium is the lowest in the world. The deficiency, called Keshan disease, is characterized by cardiomyopathy (enlarged heart). In China, it primarily affected women and children, who typically eat a lower quality diet than adult men do. Since supplementation of selenium in the Keshan region started in 1980, China has practically eliminated this deficiency disease.

Toxicity

Supplement users who consume amounts much greater than the recommended level are at risk of developing symptoms of toxicity, but no cases have been reported in the United States. Selenium intakes greater than 55 micrograms per day from foods are common in omnivores, but the UL for selenium (400 micrograms per day) and potential toxicity are probably not attainable by consuming only foods. Selenium toxicity has only been reported for miners and related workers who get excessive selenium from dust particles that get swallowed and absorbed.

Copper

Copper (Cu^+ and Cu^{2+}) is incorporated into a few enzyme systems, including ceruloplasmin in blood, and it is essential for the uptake of iron in the bone marrow for hemoglobin production during red blood cell formation. RDAs are established at 900 micrograms for both adult men and women. A varied diet should provide more than adequate amounts of this trace element.

Copper deficiency may occur in individuals who take zinc supplements because of a zinc–copper interaction. Zinc and copper are absorbed by the same membrane transport mechanism, and therefore excessive zinc reduces copper absorption. Copper deficiency is extremely rare, but when it occurs it is typically found in infants, in whom it may be life threatening.

Molybdenum

Molybdenum (Mo^{6+}), although essential in humans, is required in only one well-known enzyme system, xanthine oxidase. Both deficiencies and toxicities of molybdenum have long been known in animal nutrition, but no human deficiencies have been reported in the United States. The RDAs are set at 45 micrograms for adult males and females.

Other Essential Trace Elements

Three other essential trace elements have AIs: manganese (Mn), fluoride (F), and chromium (Cr). Not enough is known about the role of these elements in the body to establish an Estimated Average Requirement (EAR) for each (and the RDAs that are

TABLE 9.16
Selenium Content of Select Foods

Food Source	Amount per Serving (µg)
Ground beef (90% lean)	18
Chicken breast (baked)	23
Tuna (canned)	68
Shrimp (raw)	32
Beef liver (fried)	28
Whole wheat bread	7
Swiss cheese	15
Egg (large)	7
Soybeans (roasted)	16

Data from U.S. Department of Agriculture, Agricultural Research Service. USDA National Nutrient Database for Standard Reference, Available at: www.nal.usda.gov/fnic/foodcomp/search

> Most North Americans consume 150 to 200 micrograms of selenium (Se^{-2}) per day, which is more than enough to meet the body's needs.

> Copper (Cu^+ and Cu^{2+}) is incorporated into a few enzyme systems, including ceruloplasmin in blood, and it is essential for the uptake of iron in the bone marrow for hemoglobin production during red blood cell formation.

molybdenum An essential micronutrient that exists as a cation (Mo^{6+}) in the body. Is required only as a component of the xanthine oxidase system.

> Three other essential trace elements have AIs: manganese (Mn), fluoride (F), and chromium (Cr). Not enough is known about the role of these elements in the body to establish an Estimated Average Requirement (EAR) for each (and the RDAs that are based on the EARs).

> In bones and teeth, fluoride ions become part of hydroxyapatite, a mineral crystal, thereby making the mineral crystal harder.

manganese Essential micromineral that serves as an enzyme cofactor. Plays an important role in the body's energy-deriving pathways and in protein metabolism.

fluoride Ionic form of the trace mineral fluorine. Helps maintain healthy tooth enamel and surfaces in the oral cavity.

teeth Hard, mineralized tissue in the oral cavity that helps in the initial mechanical breakdown of food.

fluoridation Addition of fluoride ions to municipal drinking water for the purpose of preventing dental caries.

fluorosis Condition of excess fluoride accumulation in the hard tissue of teeth and bones. Teeth become discolored and, in extreme cases, flake off pieces, giving them an etched appearance. In bone, the quality of tissue is diminished and fractures (especially microfractures) are more likely to occur.

TABLE 9.17		
Essential Trace Elements with Recommended Intakes (AIs)		
Recommendation (AI)	**Males**	**Females**
Manganese	2.3 mg	1.8 mg
Fluoride	4.0 mg	3.0 mg
Chromium	35 µg	25 µg

Data from Food and Nutrition Board, Institute of Medicine. *Dietary Reference Intakes.* Washington, DC: National Academies Press; 1997–2001.

based on the EARs). **Table 9.17** provides the AIs for these three essential trace elements. Seafood is, in general, the best food source for all of the trace elements. Typical intakes of these elements in foods have been shown to be safe.

Manganese

Manganese serves as an enzyme cofactor and plays important roles in energy-deriving pathways and in protein metabolism. Food sources of manganese include animal meats and seafood. A manganese deficiency has not been reported for humans. This may mean that another mineral with similar properties, magnesium, can substitute for manganese in these enzyme-governed steps. No human toxicity of manganese from foods has been reported.

Fluoride

Fluoride exists naturally in water, foods, and the body primarily as fluoride (F^-) ions. In bones and **teeth**, fluoride ions become part of hydroxyapatite, a mineral crystal, thereby making the mineral crystal harder. Fluoride ions bind predominantly on the crystal surfaces rather than within the crystal structure after bone and tooth mineral have been developed. Whether these ions perform an essential function in human tissues is not entirely established, but fluoride is generally considered to be a "required" element because of its caries prevention. In the mouth, these ions may also inhibit bacterial activities, including acid production, and help reduce plaque formation on tooth surfaces, thus reducing dental caries.

Fluoridation of most U.S. municipal water supplies, instituted at 1 part fluoride per million (ppm) of water, has greatly decreased the incidence of dental caries (see **FIGURE 9.21**). (A recent recommendation to decrease this level to 0.75 ppm has been adopted by a few communities.) The routine consumption of too much fluoride (> 3 ppm) in the drinking water may lead to tooth mottling (discoloration), a condition known as **fluorosis**, and toxicity at the cellular level. An adverse cellular response to too much fluoride intake is poisoning of the mitochondrial ATP-producing steps that reduce availability of ATP molecules. So, the upper limits (ULs) of safety of fluoride are set for protecting the public health.

Fluoride is absorbed in the small intestine following food and beverage consumption. Much of the absorbed fluoride circulates in the blood to the salivary glands and the bones and, in infants and young children, to pre-erupted teeth. The developing teeth take up circulating fluoride ions in the dentin and enamel layers of teeth. The salivary glands secrete fluoride into the oral cavity, where the fluoride in the saliva bathes the enamel surfaces and exchanges with hydroxyl groups on the crystal surfaces. In this way, fluoride helps to maintain (with continuous salivary secretion) and preserve the hardness of the enamel surfaces. Fluoride mouth rinses benefit the health of teeth by binding of fluoride ions on the tooth surfaces.

Fluoride rinses and fluoridated community waters have clearly contributed to great reductions of dental caries in children, a major advance in public health dentistry. Nevertheless, children drinking fluoridated waters need to be periodically monitored by dentists and hygienists to assess for fluorosis of teeth and potential toxicity.

Chromium

Chromium is involved in glucose metabolism as well as in lipid metabolism. Research suggests that it may enhance the peripheral uptake of glucose by acting with insulin in some manner with the membrane receptor for insulin and, thus, permit more efficient entry of glucose into cells. A deficiency of chromium in humans leads to a diabetes-like condition and to elevations in blood cholesterol and triglycerides. In subjects with glucose intolerance, chromium supplementation may improve their condition. Much remains, however, to be learned about the metabolism of this trace element.

Many foods contain modest amounts of chromium, including most meats, poultry, fish and other seafoods, and fruits and vegetables. The losses of chromium in food processing are great: about 40% in high-extraction wheat flour and about 92% in processed sugar. Chromium tends to be in short supply in the diet, but a true deficiency is not common, although that might be expected from the relatively poor intake. The chromium content of blood and tissues declines with age, and it has been suggested that this decrement is linked to the aging process.

Concerns about the safety of chromium supplements, such as chromium picolinate, have been raised (see **FIGURE 9.22**). Because power lifters and other athletes often take this supplement, they need to be made aware of any potential adverse effects such as possible DNA damage. As far as is known, chromium has no established benefits as a dietary ergogenic aid for improving human performance in physical activities.

Trace Elements of Uncertain Significance

Several additional trace elements—aluminum, arsenic, boron, silicon, tin, vanadium, and a few others—may also be required by humans, but too little is known about the

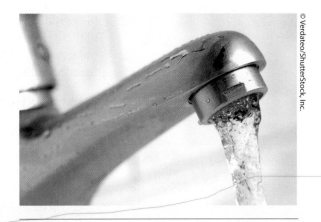

FIGURE 9.21 Fluoridation. Fluoridation of most municipal water supplies in the United States has greatly decreased the incidence of dental caries.

> Fluoride rinses and fluoridated community waters have clearly contributed to great reductions of dental caries in children, a major advance in public health dentistry.

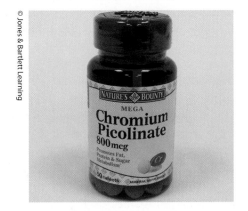

FIGURE 9.22 Chromium Picolinate. Chromium picolinate is sold as a nutritional supplement to prevent or treat chromium deficiency, despite the fact that no evidence of its benefits has been found.

chromium An essential trace mineral whose function has not been established. It is possibly involved with insulin regulation as a glucose tolerance factor.

biological effects of these trace elements at this time to classify them as essential. All of these elements are present in human tissues, but their functions in the body remain unknown or unclear. In general, supplements of these trace elements are not recommended. A high intake of arsenic, for example, has toxic effects on cells.

Dietary Reference Intakes of Trace Elements: RDAs or AIs

The adult DRIs and characteristics of trace elements are summarized in **Table 9.18**.

TABLE 9.18
Characteristics of Essential Trace Elements

Element	DRI	Function	Deficiency	Toxicity
Iron	RDA	Component of hemoglobin, myoglobin, enzymes	Iron-deficiency anemia	Hemochromatosis, perhaps coronary heart disease
Zinc	RDA	Component of enzymes, zinc fingers	Hypogonadism, poor growth, poor taste acuity	None known
Iodine	RDA	Component of thyroxin and triiodothyronine	Simple goiter	Toxic goiter
Selenium	RDA	Component of enzymes, selenoproteins	Keshan disease (cardiomyopathy)	Selenosis
Copper	RDA	Component of enzymes	Retarded infantile growth	Wilson's disease (genetic)
Manganese	AI	Component of enzymes	None known	None known
Fluoride	AI	Part of the mineral structure of bones and teeth	Poor crystal properties	Fluorosis
Chromium	AI	Glucose tolerance factor	Impaired glucose tolerance	None known
Molybdenum	RDA	Component of enzymes	Possible	Rare

Reproduced from Anderson JJB. *Nutrition and Health: An Introduction*. Durham, NC: Carolina Academic Press; 2005.

SUMMARY

Water is a critical nutrient that is lost through excretion, sweat, and other routes, and needs to be replaced by foods and fluids each day in order to maintain water balance and normal body functions. Water losses present special problems, especially for athletes.

Of the macrominerals, magnesium does not present any major problem because deficiency resulting from dietary inadequacies is exceedingly rare. Average magnesium consumption by Americans, however, is below the RDA, but symptoms of deficiency are typically not apparent. Calcium is moderately deficient in the diets of females and less so of males in North America. Rarely is the calcium RDA (1,300 milligrams per day for girls or 1,000 milligrams per day for women) achieved after 11 years of age. The importance of the calcium:phosphorus ratio of the diet cannot be minimized. Low calcium intake, coupled with high phosphorus consumption, especially from processed foods, may be one factor that contributes to the high prevalence rates of osteoporosis among older women. In general, a larger skeletal mass as a result of adequate calcium intakes and regular physical activity that develops by late adolescence continues into the adult years and the greater bone mass affords protection against osteoporosis in late life. If adequate amounts of calcium from foods are not consumed, modest supplements may be needed. Physician prescriptions of calcium, however, are recommended rather than self-medicating with calcium.

In addition to calcium, potassium is commonly low in the diets of U.S. children and adults because so few servings of fruits and vegetables are typically consumed each day by the vast majority of the population. Foods, not supplements, are recommended to increase the intakes of these macrominerals, but supplements also may be necessary. Excessive sodium intakes commonly exist and they may contribute to increased risk of heart disease because of sodium-induced hypertension.

The essential trace elements have diverse functions, and their deficiencies and toxicities have been fairly well characterized. Iron remains the micromineral most commonly deficient throughout the world. If individuals consume the variety of foods recommended by the USDA's MyPlate food guidance system, they should obtain sufficient amounts of all the trace elements. The major reason for insufficient intakes of most microminerals is the low intake of plant foods, which provide good amounts of so many of the trace elements. Also, the near total omission of seafoods that are rich in practically every trace element by many may also contribute to inadequate intake. Diet-related iron deficiency is more prevalent than for any other micromineral simply because of too little consumption of foods containing heme iron and iron-fortified foods. If the dietary intake of iron cannot be improved, iron supplementation is necessary.

STUDENT ACTIVITIES

1. In what ways is water released from the body?

2. List three functions of water in the body.

3. What AIs have been provided for water?

4. List the three minerals that are classified as electrolytes. Identify one function of each and state where it is concentrated in the body.

5. Identify one unprocessed food that has high sodium levels. List three foods in which sodium additives greatly increase the sodium content.

6. Which foods tend to be high in potassium? Explain why many people have low potassium intakes that are exacerbated by high sodium intakes.

7. What is the major role of magnesium ions in metabolism?

8. List three different foods that are fortified with calcium.

9. List three raw unprocessed foods, other than dairy, that contain high levels of phosphorus. List two foods that contain added phosphates.

10. What is an optimal dietary ratio of calcium to phosphorus (Ca:P) for adults and children? Explain.

11. Why is optimal bone development early in life so critical for girls and boys? Explain.

12. Intestinal calcium absorption efficiency declines after about 60 years of age. Explain why this decrease in efficiency may occur.

13. Explain in words (or use a diagram) the major components of calcium homeostasis.

14. When calcium intake is chronically low, which hormonal mechanism(s) help the body maintain calcium homeostasis? Explain.

15. How does vitamin C affect iron absorption?

16. Identify two animal foods and two plant foods that provide high levels of iron per serving.

17. Explain why adolescent girls (and some adult women) have such a high prevalence of iron deficiency and the more severe form of iron deficiency anemia.

18. What molecule carries (transports) iron from the intestinal absorbing cells through the blood to body tissues for uptake by cells? What molecule circulating in blood acts as an enzyme that aids the uptake of iron ions by forming red blood cells in the bone marrow?

19. Explain why excessive zinc intake may lead to copper deficiency.

20. List two molecules that require selenium for their function; then state how one of these molecules acts as an antioxidant.

21. Why is iodine needed by the body? Name two molecules that require iodine for their function. Explain the potential adverse effects of goitrogens on the utilization of iodine for its functional molecules.

22. Explain why fluoride has such a narrow window of safety.

23. What is the role of manganese in cell metabolism?

WEBSITES FOR FURTHER STUDY

Facts About Calcium, University of Florida IFAS Extension
http://edis.ifas.ufl.edu/pdffiles/FY/FY21600.pdf
Potassium, Micronutrient Information Center, Linus Pauling Institute
http://lpi.oregonstate.edu/infocenter/minerals/potassium/
Magnesium, Office of Dietary Supplements, NIH
http://ods.od.nih.gov/factsheets/magnesium.asp
Sodium, American Heart Association Recommendations
www.heart.org/HEARTORG/GettingHealthy/NutritionCenter/HealthyDietGoals/Sodium-Salt-or-Sodium-Chloride_UCM_303290_Article.jsp
Salt & Sodium, Nutrition.gov
www.nutrition.gov/nal_display/index.php?info_center=11&tax_level=2&tax_subject=388&level3_id=0&level4_id=0&level5_id=0&topic_id=1667&&placement_default=0

Iron Deficiency, Centers for Disease Control and Prevention
www.cdc.gov/nccdphp/dnpa/nutrition/nutrition_for_everyone/iron_deficiency/index.htm
Cassava's Link to Iodine Deficiency Requires Further Study
www.modernghana.com/news/198981/1/cassavas-link-to-iodine-deficiency-requires-furthe.html
International Zinc Consultative Group
www.izincg.org

REFERENCES

Aggett PJ. Iron. In: Erdman JW Jr, MacDonald IA, Zeisel SH (eds.). *Present Knowledge in Nutrition*. 10th ed. Ames, IA: John Wiley & Sons; 2012: 816–839.

Anderson JJB. Osteoporosis. In: Erdman JW Jr, MacDonald IA, Zeisel SH (eds.). *Present Knowledge in Nutrition*. 10th ed. Ames, IA: John Wiley & Sons; 2012: 833–842.

Anderson JJB, Garner SC, Klemmer PJ (eds.). *Diet, Nutrients, and Bone*. Boca Raton, FL, and London: Taylor & Francis; 2012.

Anderson JJB, Roggenkamp KJ, Suchindran CM. Calcium intakes and femoral and lumbar bone density of elderly U.S. men and women: National Health and Nutrition Examination Survey 2005–2006 analysis. *J Clin Endocrinol Metab*. 2012;97:4531–4539.

Dhingra R, Sullivan LM, Fox CS, et al. Relations of serum phosphorus and calcium levels to the incidence of cardiovascular disease in the community. *Arch Intern Med*. 2007;167:879–885.

Erdman JW Jr, MacDonald IA, Zeisel SH (eds.). *Present Knowledge in Nutrition*. 10th ed. Ames, IA: John Wiley & Sons; 2012.

Ervin RB, Wang C-Y, Wright JD, Kennedy-Steenson J. Dietary intake of selected minerals for the United States population: 1999–2000. *Advance Data* No. 341, April 27, 2004.

Finley JW. Bioavailability of selenium from foods. *Nutr Rev*. 2006;64:146–151.

Fleming RE, Sly WS. Mechanisms of iron accumulation in hereditary hemochromatosis. *Annu Rev Physiol*. 2002;64:663.

Food and Nutrition Board, Institute of Medicine. *Dietary Reference Intakes for Calcium, Phosphorus, Magnesium, Vitamin D, and Fluoride*. Washington, DC: National Academies Press; 1997.

Food and Nutrition Board, Institute of Medicine. *Dietary Reference Intakes for Vitamin A, Vitamin K, Arsenic, Boron, Chromium, Copper, Iodine, Iron, Manganese, Molybdenum, Nickel, Silicon, Vanadium, and Zinc*. Washington, DC: National Academies Press; 2001.

Food and Nutrition Board, Institute of Medicine. *Dietary Reference Intakes for Water, Potassium, Sodium, Chloride, and Sulfate.* Washington, DC: National Academies Press; 2004.

Food and Nutrition Board, Institute of Medicine. *Dietary Reference Intakes for Calcium and Vitamin D.* Washington, DC: National Academies Press; 2010.

Frassinetti S, Bronzetti G, Caltavuturo L, Cini M, Croce CD. The role of zinc in life: a review. *J Environ Pathol Toxicol Oncol.* 2006;25:597–610.

Goldhaber SB. Trace element risk assessment: essentiality vs. toxicity. *Regul Toxicol Pharmacol.* 2003;38:232–242.

Hambidge M. Biomarkers of trace mineral intake and status. *J Nutr.* 2003;133(suppl 3):948S–955S.

Heaney RP. Phosphorus. In: Erdman JW Jr, MacDonald IA, Zeisel SH (eds.). *Present Knowledge in Nutrition.* 10th ed. Ames, IA: John Wiley & Sons; 2012: 723–742.

Holt RH, Uriu-Adams JY, Keen CL. Zinc. In: Erdman JW Jr, MacDonald IA, Zeisel SH (eds.). *Present Knowledge in Nutrition.* 10th ed. Ames, IA: John Wiley & Sons; 2012: 840–872.

Jequier E, Constant F. Water as an essential nutrient: the physiological basis of hydration. *Eur J Clin Nutr.* 2010;64:115–123.

Karppanen H, Karppanen P, Mervaala E. Why and how to implement sodium, potassium, calcium, and magnesium changes in food items and diets? *J Hum Hypertens.* 2005;19(suppl 3):S10–9.

Kemi VE, Kärkkäinen MUM, Lamberg-Allardt CJE. High phosphorus intakes acutely and negatively affect calcium and bone metabolism in a dose-dependent manner in healthy young females. *Br J Nutr.* 2006;96:545–552.

Kemi VE, Kärkkäinen MU, Rita HJ, Laaksonen MM, Outila TA, Lamberg-Allardt CJ. Low calcium:phosphorus ratio in habitual diets affects serum parathyroid hormone concentration and calcium metabolism in healthy women with adequate calcium intake. *Br J Nutr.* 2010;103:561–568.

Kenefick RW, Cheuvront SN, Montain SJ, Carter R, Sawka MN. Human water and electrolyte balance. In: Erdman JW Jr, MacDonald IA, Zeisel SH (eds.). *Present Knowledge in Nutrition.* 10th ed. Ames, IA: John Wiley & Sons; 2012: 796–815.

Lopez MA, Martos FC. Iron availability: an updated review. *Int J Food Sci Nutr.* 2004;55:597–606.

Nielsen FH. Manganese, molybdenum, boron, chromium, and other trace elements. In: Erdman JW Jr, MacDonald IA, Zeisel SH (eds.). *Present Knowledge in Nutrition.* 10th ed. Ames, IA: John Wiley & Sons; 2012: 946–979.

Preuss HG, Clouatre DL. Sodium, chloride, and potassium. In: Erdman JW Jr, MacDonald IA, Zeisel SH (eds.). *Present Knowledge in Nutrition.* 10th ed. Ames, IA: John Wiley & Sons; 2012: 767–795.

Prohaska JR. Copper. In: Erdman JW Jr, MacDonald IA, Zeisel SH (eds.). *Present Knowledge in Nutrition.* 10th ed. Ames, IA: John Wiley & Sons; 2012: 873–896.

Terry EN, Diamond AM. Selenium. In: Erdman JW Jr, MacDonald IA, Zeisel SH (eds.). *Present Knowledge in Nutrition.* 10th ed. Ames, IA: John Wiley & Sons; 2012: 917–945.

Valtin H. "Drink at least eight glasses of water a day." Really? Is there scientific evidence for "8 × 8"? *Am J Physiol Regul Integr Comp Physiol.* 2002;283:R993–R998.

Volpe SL. Magnesium. In: Erdman JW Jr, MacDonald IA, Zeisel SH (eds.). *Present Knowledge in Nutrition.* 10th ed. Ames, IA: John Wiley & Sons; 2012: 743–766.

Weaver CM. Calcium. In: Erdman JW Jr, MacDonald IA, Zeisel SH (eds.). *Present Knowledge in Nutrition.* 10th ed. Ames, IA: John Wiley & Sons; 2012: 704–722.

Weaver CM, Proulx WR, Heaney R. Choices for achieving adequate dietary calcium with a vegetarian diet. *Am J Clin Nutr* 1999;70(suppl 3):543S–548S.

Weaver CM, Rothwell AP, Wood KV. Measuring calcium absorption and utilization in humans. *Curr Opin Clin Nutr Metab Care.* 2006;9:568–574.

Zimmermann MB. Iodine and iodine deficiency disorders. In: Erdman JW Jr, MacDonald IA, Zeisel SH (eds.). *Present Knowledge in Nutrition.* 10th ed. Ames, IA: John Wiley & Sons; 2012: 897–916.

CHAPTER 10

Nutrition During Pregnancy, Lactation, and Infancy

Optimal nutrition during a woman's pregnancy and subsequent lactation period helps to ensure proper fetal development and sustained growth of the resulting infant. The proper supply of nutrients and avoidance of harmful substances by the mother significantly influence the outcome of pregnancy. Breast milk is sufficient to support a baby's growth for the first 6 months; only after 6 months of age are supplementary solid foods recommended along with breast-feeding. After weaning, other environmental factors become more important for infant and child development, such as the amount of money available for purchasing quality foods, the wise selection and preparation of foods, the parents' educational level, the ability of parents to promote optimal child development and growth, proper housing, sanitation, and the availability of good health care. This chapter focuses on the physiologic changes and nutritional needs of pregnant and lactating women and the nutritional needs of infants during the first year of life.

Preconception Nutrition

The prepregnancy (preconception) nutritional status of women is very important. Many women who plan to become pregnant fail to consider their preconception nutritional needs. Women who are considering pregnancy need to ensure they are eating a healthy diet as well as consider their alcohol intake and cigarette smoking status. The reason for this admonition is that women who are healthy typically have healthy babies. Preconception nutritional status is very important because many women are not aware when they conceive; inadequate dietary folate, excessive alcohol use, and cigarette smoking negatively impact early fetal development.

Furthermore, good nutritional status between pregnancies is important, especially during the recovery period after the end of breast-feeding that allows appropriate spacing between pregnancies. It is generally recommended that a mother wait at least 1 year before planning for another baby. This time allows her body to recover from the prior pregnancy and lactation.

It is imperative that a woman who is planning a pregnancy, or in the early stages of pregnancy, begin prenatal care under the supervision of a healthcare provider. Nutritional research also indicates that it is important for women to take control of their own nutrition in the early adult years, during a pregnancy, and during lactation, and to take charge of the nutritional care of their infants both while breast-feeding and once they are weaned.

> **Women who are healthy also typically have healthy babies.**

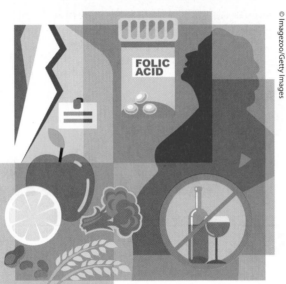

© Imagezoo/Getty Images

FOCUS 10.1 Folate and Birth Defects

In the United States, folic acid intakes tend to be low, even among otherwise healthy adolescent and young adult women. Women whose folate levels are low during the preconception period are likely to have low folate status during pregnancy, which may impact early fetal development of the central nervous system, including the spinal cord. Research has shown that women with low folate status are at increased risk of having a child with birth defects, especially damage to the brain and spinal cord; these birth defects are called neural tube defects. The most extreme of neural tube defects is spina bifida (see **FIGURE A**).

Folate supplements before and early during pregnancy can reduce the risk of these defects. The need for folate supplements is most critical during early gestation, often before a woman is even aware that she is pregnant. Women need to be aware that folate supplements can reduce the risk of birth defects. Fortunately, many women are aware of the link between folate supplements and fetal health. Unfortunately, women who are likely to have unplanned pregnancies, especially teens and others without birth control, are more likely to be poorly nourished and poorly informed about the need for folate supplements.

Nutrition experts agree that all young women should be consuming 400 micrograms of folate (the RDA) from foods on a daily basis. Foods rich in folic acid include dark green, leafy vegetables. In addition, nutrition experts also recommend that women of childbearing age take a daily supplement of 400 micrograms of folate.

Fortification of cereal products with folic acid was mandated by law in both the United States and Canada in the late 1990s primarily with the goal of reducing neural tube defects. Research indicates that this fortification has led to approximately a 30% to 40% decline in infants with neural tube defects. ●

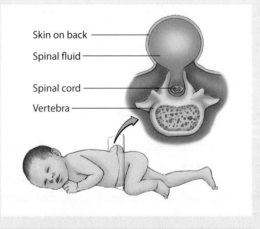

Skin on back
Spinal fluid
Spinal cord
Vertebra

FIGURE A Spina bifida. Spina bifida is a birth defect in which the bones of the spine (vertebrae) do not form properly around the spinal cord.

Physiologic Changes During Pregnancy and Lactation

A pregnant woman undergoes many physiologic changes that enable her body to nurture the **fetus** (developing human) during gestation and to support lactation after delivery. During **pregnancy**, a woman undergoes tremendous physiologic changes, especially with regards to the cardiovascular and reproductive systems. Hormones specific for reproduction increase and new tissue growth occurs. Tissue growth during pregnancy and lactation requires increases in nutrient intakes from foods. Many changes occur during **gestation**, which is the period of fetal development in the uterus.

The specific maternal physiologic adjustments made during the course of pregnancy include:

- Expansion of maternal blood volume, including both increased numbers of red blood cells and plasma volume.
- An increase in maternal extracellular fluid.
- An increase in maternal fat deposition.

> Tissue growth during pregnancy and lactation requires increases in nutrient intakes from foods.

FOCUS 10.2   Measurement of Hematocrit from a Blood Sample

To illustrate the change in hematocrit as a woman progresses through pregnancy, it may be helpful to explain how a hematocrit is determined in the laboratory. After a finger prick, a small capillary tube (about the size of a bobby pin) is used to collect the blood. The blood is drawn slowly up to the top of the tube, and one end of the tube is plugged with soft clay to hold the blood in place. The tube is then spun in a small centrifuge that has a special holder for the capillary tubes. After spinning for 5 minutes, the tubes are removed and, when held up to the light, the heavier blood cells, mostly red blood cells, can be seen to have collected at the bottom of the tube and the lighter plasma is at the top. Healthy young adults have roughly 40% packed cells at the bottom; the other 60% (that at the top) represents the plasma (fluid). This 40% packed red blood cells is called the hematocrit. The hematocrit decreases in pregnant women and may even go as low as 20% if a woman develops anemia during pregnancy. **Figure A** shows two sample hematocrits from the same woman, one from before pregnancy and the other from the third trimester. ●

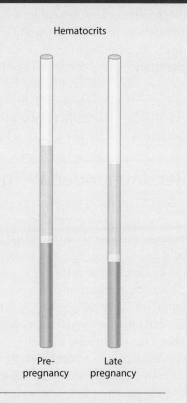

Hematocrits

Pre-pregnancy   Late pregnancy

FIGURE A Hematocrits. Two hematocrits are shown here: normal hematocrit (left) and normal hematocrit during pregnancy (right).

fetus The developing human in the uterus that receives its oxygen and nutrients from the mother via the placenta. The fetal nutritional supply depends on the mother's eating habits and other lifestyle practices, such as cigarette smoking, alcohol consumption, maternal weight gain, and health.

pregnancy The period of gestation (280 days) that consists of three terms (trimesters). Normally leads to a healthy baby and mother.

gestation Period of fetal development in the uterus from conception to birth; normally 280 days (or approximately 9 months) in humans.

- An increase in size of the uterus and the breasts.
- Formation and growth of the placenta.
- Production of amniotic fluid.

The uterus continues to enlarge during pregnancy in order to accommodate the growing fetus, and the mammary glands increase in size largely through the development of buds that will secrete milk after delivery. Cardiac output (volume of blood pumped per minute) also increases, as does the blood flow to the kidneys and the uterus. In general, the heart, kidneys, and most other organs increase their energy utilization. All of this means that the mother needs more nutrients in order to adapt to the demands of the developing fetus.

The increase in blood volume is reflected mainly in the serum (fluid) compartment, compared with the smaller increase in the number of new red blood cells produced. Therefore, the hematocrit (packed cell volume, or % of red blood cells in the total blood column in a capillary tube) actually decreases from approximately the end of the first trimester to term (delivery). This decline in hematocrit does not usually result from a deficiency of dietary iron (foods and supplements), but rather from the relatively greater increase in total blood volume than in red cell mass. The greater volume of blood is needed to deliver nutrients and oxygen to an expanded lean body mass (the mother's tissues and organs and the placenta and baby), resulting from both maternal and fetal growth.

Pregnancy

Pregnancy is characterized by weight gain, especially after the first trimester (i.e., first 3 months of pregnancy). During this critical period, it is essential that the mother's diet meets recommended intakes for energy, protein, and micronutrients. Furthermore, plants are needed for phytochemicals despite the absence of any specific recommendations. Major difficulties of a full-term gestation may occur when either too little or too much food is consumed during the 9-month period (i.e., status of underweight or overweight). The delivery of a baby also is known as **parturition**. The **pregnancy outcome** is hopefully a healthy baby within the normal weight range!

Recommended Weight Gain During Pregnancy

Adequate intake of both energy and nutrients by a prospective mother during pregnancy is essential for a good outcome; that is, a healthy baby of normal weight and length carried by the mother fully to term.

A normal, full-term pregnancy of 280 days (approximately 40 weeks, or 9 months) is divided into three equal terms called **trimesters**. During the first trimester, the fertilized egg develops into an **embryo**. By 4 weeks the embryo has implanted into the uterine wall and the placenta forms, marking the beginning of the fetus or fetal stage. The life-support system of the fetus is the highly vascularized **placenta** that supplies nutrients and oxygen to the developing fetus and that removes carbon dioxide and some wastes from the fetus (see **FIGURE 10.1**). Fetal development during

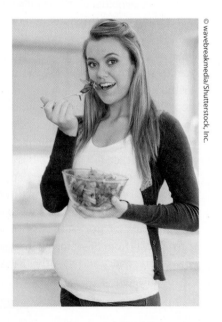

© wavebreakmedia/Shutterstock, Inc.

parturition The act of giving birth to a baby. Also referred to as delivery.

pregnancy outcome Ideally, the birth of a healthy, well-developed, full-term baby of weight greater than 5.5 pounds (2,500 grams) and of good length accompanied by good health of the mother.

trimester A term in the course of pregnancy. A normal full-term pregnancy contains three trimesters over approximately 9 months (280 days).

embryo An early stage of development of a fertilized egg prior to implantation in the uterus; the human embryo exists in utero for approximately 4 weeks, after which the circulation of the placenta supplies the nutrients and oxygen necessary for development as a fetus, the second stage of pregnancy.

placenta The organ formed within the uterus following the fertilization of an egg and implantation of the embryo that permits transfer of nutrients and oxygen from the mother to the growing fetus; some waste products from the fetus cross the placenta to the maternal circulation.

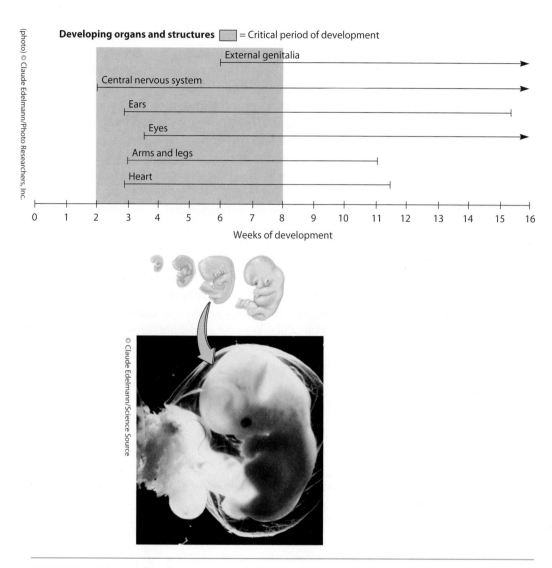

FIGURE 10.1 Embryonic Development. During the first 8 weeks of development all of the major systems are forming. The embryo is very vulnerable to nutrient deficiencies and toxins during this stage.

the last part of the first trimester involves limb budding, a period during which the fetus is especially sensitive to drugs and other toxic substances.

During the first trimester, many women have morning sickness (which may actually occur at any time during the day) and they do not, in general, have good appetites. Competition for nutrients among growing tissues and the lack of appetite may result in very little weight gain during the first trimester. Starting at approximately 9 to 12 weeks of gestation, maternal weight begins to increase slightly because of changes in several tissues, exclusive of the fetus itself. Weight gain results from increases in blood volume, fat tissue mass, gains of the uterus and breasts, as well as the development and growth of the placenta. A healthy woman gains only about 2 to 3 pounds during the first trimester of pregnancy.

During the second and third trimesters, the fetus draws on the maternal nutrients and nutrient stores for continued growth and development. Thus, fetal growth can be compromised by poor maternal intakes of nutrients. During the second and third trimesters, a healthy pregnant woman gains additional weight, particularly maternal fat stores. The maternal fat stores gained during pregnancy will be called upon during the lactation period for use as an energy source.

A healthy woman gains only about 2 to 3 pounds during the first trimester of pregnancy.

> By the time the pregnancy has come to term, a healthy pregnant woman will have typically gained 25 to 35 pounds.

Gradual weight gain is needed for healthy fetal development. The pregnant woman should gain approximately 1 pound per week from approximately the 10th to the 40th weeks of a healthy gestation (see **FIGURE 10.2**). This pattern of weight gain corresponds to the physiologic changes that occur in the woman's body as well as the developmental changes of the fetus. By the time the pregnancy has come to term, a healthy pregnant woman will have typically gained 25 to 35 pounds. The **prenatal development**, or growth of a fetus from conception to delivery, correlates with the weight gain pattern.

The recommended increase in weight during a full-term pregnancy should be based on a woman's prepregnancy weight. The most recent recommendations from the Institute of Medicine are presented in **Table 10.1**. These recommendations emphasize the importance for all women to gain weight during pregnancy, regardless of body size. A weight-reduction diet, therefore, is never warranted during pregnancy. **FIGURE 10.3** shows a pregnant woman near full term who has achieved the recommended weight gain of approximately 30 pounds.

Some experts are now suggesting that grids of gains in body mass index (BMI) during the course of pregnancy, rather than simply weight, may be more useful in monitoring the gestational health of women because BMI takes height into consideration. BMI grids have not yet replaced weight gain tables, but new guidelines for weight gain based on BMI are anticipated.

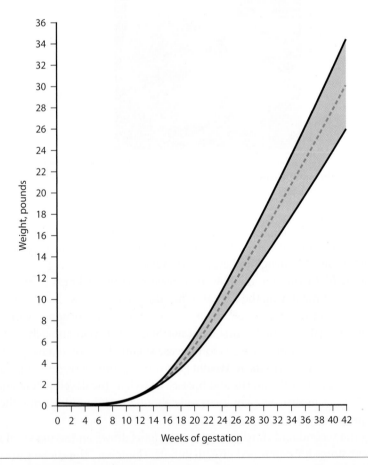

prenatal development Growth of the fetus from the fertilized egg and embryo up until parturition (delivery) of a baby, even if premature. Full-term development implies the delivery of a baby greater than 5.5 pounds (2,500 grams) at approximately 280 days of gestation.

FIGURE 10.2 Prenatal Weight Gain Grid. Note that the recommended gains in weight should fall within the limits of the curved lines. Too much gain or too little gain by the pregnant woman could signal a potential problem. Full-term gains should fall between 26 and 35 pounds for normal-weight women, but other recommendations exist for women who are overweight, obese, or underweight.

Reproduced from Anderson JJB. *Nutrition and Health: An Introduction.* Durham, NC: Carolina Academic Press; 2005.

TABLE 10.1
Pregnancy Weight Gain Recommendations

Prepregnancy Weight Status	Recommended Weight Gain (pounds)
Underweight (BMI < 18.5)	28–40
Normal weight (BMI 18.5–24.9)	25–35
Overweight (BMI 25.0–29.9)	15–25
Obese (BMI ≥ 30.0)	11–20

Data from *Weight Gain During Pregnancy*, The American College of Obstetricians and Gynecologists, 2013, http://www.acog.org/Resources_And_Publications/Committee_Opinions/Committee_on_Obstetric_Practice/Weight_Gain_During_Pregnancy.

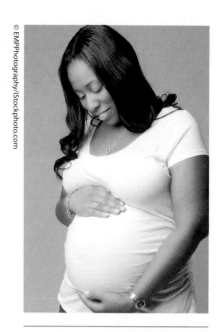

FIGURE 10.3 Pregnant Woman Late in Gestation. A well-nourished woman with a healthy prepregnancy weight will gain close to 30 pounds during full term. Most of this weight exists in the developing fetus, the uterus, placenta, and breasts. In addition, women accumulate additional fat tissue to aid with impending lactation.

Monitoring weight gain during the course of pregnancy has been useful in identifying maternal complications and anticipating adverse birth outcomes. For example, too rapid a weight gain—that is, more than 2 pounds per week during the second and third trimesters—along with edema or generalized swelling (hands, feet, and other sites) is indicative of pregnancy-induced hypertension. Poor weight gain in the first half of pregnancy (0 to 20 weeks) has been associated with intrauterine growth retardation, whereas inadequate weight gain during the second half of gestation (after 20 weeks) is predictive of a preterm birth (i.e., prior to completion of 37 weeks of gestation). **Low-birth-weight (small-for-term) babies** (i.e., those less than 5.5 pounds or 2,500 grams in weight) are far too common in the United States and may result from premature delivery or from poor nutritional status of the mother. Whether full-term or **premature** (born before eight months of gestation has occurred), babies may also be **small for gestational age (SGA)**, which is usually an indicator of improper uterine growth. SGA infants often result from factors such as maternal smoking or drug use, preeclampsia, diabetes mellitus (type 1 or type 2), or infection.

As mentioned earlier, weight reduction is never recommended for women who are pregnant. In fact, weight loss by overweight or obese women during the first trimester has been associated with birth defects. Early and routine prenatal care that tracks maternal weight gains can help to ensure the delivery of a healthy baby and prevent the development of unfavorable complications.

> ❝ Weight reduction is never recommended for women who are pregnant. ❞

Nutrient Requirements During Pregnancy

Energy requirements for pregnant women are higher than those for nonpregnant women. However, requirements for only some of the macronutrients and micronutrients are higher during pregnancy (see **Table 10.2**). Increased energy intake is required for the synthesis of new tissues (placenta, fetus, and mother's tissues) needed to support a healthy pregnancy and subsequent lactation. In addition to a requirement for increased intakes of energy, nutrients that generally need to be increased in pregnancy are protein, iron, folate, iodine, and vitamin B$_6$. Recent research suggests that cobalamin intake may also need to be increased during pregnancy in order to support the need for it during lactation.

Many physicians recommend supplements of these and other micronutrients for pregnant women. Supplements formulated to meet the micronutrient needs of women who are pregnant or who are considering becoming pregnant are often referred to as

low-birth-weight (small-for-term) baby A baby born at or near full term that is less than 5.5 pounds (2,500 grams) in weight. Low-birth-weight infants are at higher risk for poor nutrition and disease outcomes.

prematurity Preterm delivery of a baby, usually defined as occurring before 8 months of gestation or 250 days.

small-for-gestational-age (SGA) baby A baby who is low birth weight (i.e., less than 5.5 pounds or 2,500 grams) at term or a premature baby whose birth weight is lower than it should be for its gestational age.

TABLE 10.2

RDAs and Additional Amounts of Energy and Nutrients Recommended Following the First Trimester (Highest Value) Compared to Nonpregnant RDAs

Nutrient	RDA	Additional Amount per Day	Percent (%) Increase
Significant Increase Required			
Protein	71 g	25 g	~54
Iron	27 mg	9 mg	~50
Folate	600 μg	200 μg	~50
Vitamin B_6	1.9 mg	0.6 mg	~46
Iodine	220 μg	70 μg	~46
Zinc	11 mg	3 mg	~37
Thiamin	1.4 mg	0.3 mg	~27
Riboflavin	1.4 mg	0.3 mg	~27
Niacin	18 mg	4 mg	~29
Pantothenic acid	6 mg	1 mg	~20
Chromium	30 μg	5 mg	~20
Modest Increase Required			
Energy	~2,800 kcal	~400 kcal	~17
Water	3.0 L	0.3 L	~10
Fiber	28 g	3 g	~12
Vitamin A	770 μg	70 μg	~9
Vitamin C	85 mg	10 mg	~13
Vitamin B_{12}	2.6 μg	0.2 μg	~8
Choline	450 mg	25 mg	~6
Magnesium	350 mg	40 mg	~13
Selenium	60 μg	5 μg	~9
Copper	1,000 μg	100 μg	~11
Manganese	2.0 mg	0.2 mg	~11
Molybdenum	50 μg	5 μg	~11
No Extra Amounts Needed			
Vitamin D	15 μg	—	—
Vitamin E	15 mg	—	—
Vitamin K	90 μg	—	—
Biotin	30 μg	—	—
Calcium	1,000 mg	—	—
Phosphorus	700 mg	—	—
Fluoride	3 mg	—	—
Sodium	1.5 g	—	—
Potassium	4.7 g	—	—
Chloride	2.3 g	—	—

The percentage is based on calculation of the nutrient amount of the pregnant RDA (total) minus the additional amount for pregnancy (only) over the base of nonpregnant RDA. For protein: 71 − 25 = 46 and then 25 divided by 46 = 55%.

Data from Food and Nutrition Board, Institute of Medicine. *Dietary Reference Intakes.* Washington, DC: National Academies Press; 1997–2011.

"prenatal supplements" and include folate to prevent neural tube defects and iron to prevent anemia and to increase iron stores of both the mother and fetus. The additional amounts of specific nutrients (RDAs) recommended during pregnancy are given in Table 10.2.

Because of the widespread use of prenatal supplements, anemias of pregnancy resulting from deficiencies of iron and B vitamins have been reduced in the United States. However, iron deficiency anemia still occurs in 9% of women in the first trimester and up to 25% in the third trimester. The CDC estimates that almost one-third of low-income women are anemic during the third trimester. In nations where iron intake is low or deficient, iron deficiency anemia is much more frequent, becoming a significant risk factor for a poor outcome of pregnancy for both mother and child. In developing nations, the World Health Organization (WHO) estimates that the anemia rates of pregnant women range from 35% to 75%.

> In addition to a requirement for increased intakes of energy, nutrients that generally need to be increased in pregnancy are protein, iron, folate, iodine, and vitamin B$_6$.

Meeting Nutrient Requirements During Pregnancy

Pregnant women can meet the increased requirements for energy and nutrients by increasing the number of servings from MyPlate's five food groups, typically by one to two servings per day. Prenatal supplements also are recommended. Alcohol, along with cigarette smoking, should be eliminated (see **FIGURE 10.4**).

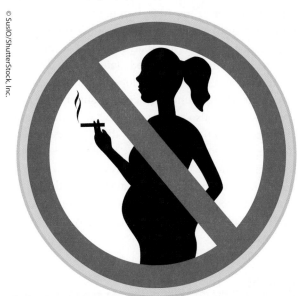

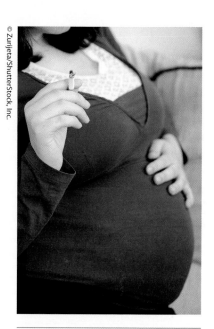

FIGURE 10.4 Smoking During Pregnancy. Both mother and child suffer from poor outcomes when the mother smokes while pregnant.

Recent emphasis has been placed on the increased intake of essential fatty acids, especially omega-3 fatty acids, by pregnant women. The fetus requires adequate amounts of essential polyunsaturated fatty acids to support the growth of the brain, the eyes, and other tissues. Because of the rapid development of the brain during the last two trimesters, the brains of newborns benefit from having large amounts of long-chain omega-3 fatty acids in the mother's milk or formula. Research findings of twins and multiple births have shown that the milk of many mothers of these infants may not have provided sufficient amounts of these essential fatty acids to support the rapid brain development of the fetuses. Although supplements of these fatty acids are not broadly recommended, foods that contain them are strongly recommended, particularly for women in their second and third trimesters. The current AI for alpha-linolenic acid, an omega-3 fatty acid, is about 25% higher for pregnant and lactating women than for other women. Considering that omega-3 fatty acids are typically low in the diets of women, some obstetricians may recommend intake of an omega-3 fatty acid supplement to ensure adequate development of the fetal brain and visual network.

> The fetus requires adequate amounts of essential polyunsaturated fatty acids to support the growth of the brain, the eyes, and other tissues.

Increases in intakes of calcium and vitamin D beyond the RDAs for nonpregnant women are not recommended for pregnant women. In fact, excessive intakes of several nutrients, including sodium, phosphate, and vitamin A (excluding carotenoids), may contribute to potential problems like hypertension and excessive urinary calcium losses.

Special Needs of Vegetarians During Pregnancy

Vegetarians, particularly vegans, who are pregnant should pay special attention to intakes of calcium, vitamin D, omega-3 fatty acids, protein, iron, and zinc. Consuming additional servings of milk or soy milk will help meet calcium, vitamin D, and protein requirements. Additional servings of legumes will help with protein, zinc, and iron needs. The increased need for vitamin B_{12} can be met by foods specifically fortified with vitamin B_{12} or through supplements. Vegetarians who do not consume fish may have difficulty meeting the requirements for the omega-3 fatty acids. Vegetarians should consume foods high in alpha-linolenic acid, such as flax seeds, walnuts, and canola oil to provide the raw material for the body to synthesize the necessary omega-3 fatty acids.

Nutritional and Other Risk Factors During Pregnancy

The health and nutritional status of a woman prior to conception is an important predictor of pregnancy outcome; that is, the health, weight, and length of her future baby! **Adolescent pregnancy** can be problematic for girls less than 18 years. Far too often, adolescent or teenage girls who become pregnant in the United States and in developing countries are not adequately nourished and not fully developed even though they are sufficiently mature to become pregnant. These young mothers may suffer from poor pregnancy outcomes. Good nutritional status is also critical for older women who are planning for a pregnancy later in their reproductive years. Other dietary, lifestyle, and disease risks are also of concern to pregnant women and public health professionals. The outcome of a healthy baby over a nine-month gestation always seems like a miracle, but good health behaviors greatly improve the chances of having a healthy baby.

A variety of risk factors can influence the course and the outcome of pregnancy by affecting either the nutritional status of the mother or the maternal supply of nutrients to the fetus. Some of these factors are as follows:

- *Maternal age:* Younger than 17 years or over 40 years.
- *Maternal weight:* Underweight (BMI < 18.5) or obese (BMI ≥ 30).
- *Maternal medical history:* Preexisting conditions such as renal disease, hypertension, or diabetes mellitus, which could lead to preeclampsia.
- *Poor maternal dietary habits:* Skipping meals, little variety of foods, poor quality foods, pica (abnormal eating of clay, starch, or ice).
- *Substance abuse:* Cigarette smoking, illicit drug use, and alcohol consumption.

Health Risks

Health risks that may adversely impact the outcome of a pregnancy include gestational diabetes, hypertension, edema, proteinuria (albumin and other proteins in the urine), and preeclampsia. **Gestational diabetes** is a form of type 2 diabetes that may develop late in pregnancy. The likely cause is an interference with maternal insulin receptors by a placental hormone. Gestational diabetes occurs in 3% to 10% of pregnancies. Having gestational diabetes also greatly increases the risk of developing type 2 diabetes after the pregnancy, especially among obese women.

Preeclampsia is characterized by a combination of hypertension and proteinuria. This serious, generally asymptomatic condition needs to be corrected promptly to

adolescent pregnancy Pregnancy in females younger than 18 years of age. Many teenagers are not fully developed and may not be adequately nourished to support a pregnancy, thus increasing the risk for adverse outcomes.

gestational diabetes A form of type 2 diabetes that may develop late in pregnancy. Occurs in 3% to 10% of pregnancies and may result in adverse outcomes for both the baby and mother. Development of gestational diabetes increases a woman's risk of type 2 diabetes after pregnancy.

preeclampsia A condition in pregnancy that includes high blood pressure, edema, and protein in the urine (proteinuria). It can cause further eclampsia and may result in fetal death.

prevent further complications of eclampsia, including risk of fetal death. The incidence rate is about 8% to 9% and the mortality rate is about 2% to 3%. Some women develop preeclampsia because their bodies have not fully recovered from the previous pregnancy before becoming pregnant again. Both gestational diabetes and preeclampsia are serious conditions that require monitoring by an obstetrician.

Maternal Age

Maternal age has also been found to influence pregnancy outcome. Women of young gynecologic age (based on years beyond menarche; that is, the first menstrual period) are at a higher risk of having preterm low-weight babies and complications. Adolescents typically have not completed their skeletal development, which may be revealed as limitations of the growth of the uterus and the placenta and of the expansion of the maternal blood volume. Girls younger than age 17 who become pregnant may not necessarily be at higher risk of poor pregnancy outcome if they are at least 2 years past menarche. Outcomes of adolescent pregnancies are commonly suboptimal in the United States because of low socioeconomic status (SES), poor dietary habits, poor prenatal weight gain, poor prenatal care, and other factors relating to the family environments rather than to the young age *per se.* In poorer countries the picture is much more dire, with more young pregnant mothers and poorer outcomes for babies and mothers (see **FIGURE 10.5**).

Older maternal age is also a risk factor, with older maternal age being linked with the increased incidence of preeclampsia and gestational diabetes. In addition, the risk of chromosomal problems is higher among older mothers, in particular in the incidence of Down syndrome in mothers older than 40 years. One possible explanation for this is that the primary ova (eggs) stored in the ovary from the time of birth are considerably older and have been subject to more environmental insults.

Maternal Weight

Several studies have shown that women with low prepregnancy weight are at increased risk of delivering low-birth-weight infants. Similarly, obese women who become pregnant may also suffer from potential complications and poor birth outcomes. Obesity puts the mother at risk for gestational diabetes, preeclampsia, and stroke. They are more likely to have problems with labor and require a C-section.

Iron Deficiency Anemia

In the United States, iron deficiency anemia occurs in 7% to 12% of pregnant women. Iron deficiency (depletion of stores as reflected by low serum ferritin) and the more severe iron deficiency anemia are global problems, occurring among pregnant women throughout the world who do not receive iron supplements.

Many pregnant women are anemic because they do not use prenatal nutrient supplements and they have little or no prenatal care. They become anemic because of inadequate dietary iron intake prior to conception and the virtual absence of iron stores in the body. The demands of pregnancy for increased red blood cell production and new tissue formation accelerate the onset of anemia. The iron demands of a pregnancy can rarely be met by diet alone.

Iron deficiency anemia has been associated with the delivery of premature infants and with increased maternal mortality. A less frequent but potentially serious cause of anemia and poor pregnancy outcome is folic acid (and much less commonly cobalamin) deficiency, which is characterized by macrocytic and megaloblastic

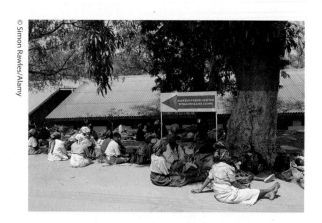

FIGURE 10.5 Maternal Care in Developing Countries. Maternal risks are very high in certain African countries where many villages lack electricity, running water, and paved roads, making it difficult for expectant mothers to obtain adequate health care.

> **The iron demands of a pregnancy can only rarely be met by diet alone.**

red blood cells. These two nutritional anemias (iron and folic acid) can be prevented or improved by additional intakes of micronutrients during pregnancy. Foods are the best sources of these additional amounts of nutrients. However, it is often difficult for a pregnant woman to consume an additional 9 milligrams of iron a day without taking a supplement. Because micronutrient-containing foods may not be consumed in sufficient amounts, most physicians recommend prenatal supplements containing iron and other micronutrients. Fortunately, the absorption efficiency for iron increases during pregnancy, thus making absorption of any dietary or supplemental iron more efficient.

Excessive Vitamin A and D Intake

Intakes of these two fat-soluble vitamins are needed at recommended intakes, but because excessive consumption may be possible from overzealous supplement usage, pregnant women need to be aware that these two vitamins may have potentially toxic effects on fetal skeletal development and contribute to calcifications of soft tissues of the developing fetus.

PRACTICAL APPLICATIONS 10.1

Prenatal Supplements

Doctors, midwives, and nutritionists all recommend prenatal supplements for pregnant women. These vitamin and mineral supplements are intended to supplement a healthy diet during pregnancy. The Academy of Nutrition and Dietetics and other organizations recommend that, in addition to a diet that meets the RDA of folate, pregnant women take a daily supplement of 400 micrograms per day of folic acid to reduce the risk of neural tube defects and other birth defects. A supplement of up to 30 milligrams of iron is recommended for pregnant women to reduce the risk of anemia. Women are encouraged to meet the RDA for calcium through dietary means. However, this is rarely accomplished, and the deficit can be met by supplementation. Other trace elements are occasionally recommended such as zinc and copper. Long-chain omega-3 fatty acids are recommended by some groups in the third trimester to enhance brain development. Although these supplements can be prescribed by a doctor, they are most commonly obtained over the counter at the pharmacy. In fact, many different prenatal supplements are available, with a bewildering array of additional ingredients and associated health claims.

Research prenatal supplements on the Internet and find at least five different formulations. How much folic acid, iron, and calcium do they contain? What additional micronutrients are supplied? Are omega-3 fatty acids added? What are the doses of vitamins A and D? Remember that these two vitamins are potential teratogens (poisonous to fetuses) when taken in large doses. If a woman is taking supplements, how do the vitamin and mineral doses compare with the RDAs? Are herbal non-nutrient supplements added? ■

fetal alcohol syndrome (FAS) A severe disorder in an offspring resulting from heavy alcohol consumption, frequently binge drinking, by the mother during pregnancy. Results in physical abnormalities in the development of the face, limbs, and internal organs, in addition to retarding brain development and severely affecting intelligence.

Alcohol Consumption

Chronic, heavy alcohol consumption during pregnancy—greater than two glasses of beer or wine or 5 ounces of whiskey a day—has been shown to be associated with retarded development of the fetus and physical and mental abnormalities in infants. Binge drinking (occasional but heavy drinking) also has been linked with these developmental abnormalities. Low birth weight and delayed postnatal growth are the most common findings of what is known as the fetal alcohol effects condition. This condition is far more common than the more severe **fetal alcohol syndrome (FAS)**, which is characterized by microencephaly (small brain), facial anomalies, cardiac defects, and limb deformities (see **FIGURE 10.6**). Children suffering from FAS may also later exhibit poor growth, mental retardation, learning difficulties, and aberrant behavioral patterns. Low birth weight, nervous system deficits, and even prematurity may result from regular intakes of even small amounts of alcohol.

In the developing fetus, alcohol use by the mother first causes biochemical abnormalities and then the anatomical defects. Although the biochemical abnormalities disappear after birth, the physical damage is already present in the infant and the effects remain. The nutrient supply from the mother to the fetus also is compromised by the presence of alcohol in the blood. In addition, the fetal liver is not able to efficiently metabolize ethanol that crosses the placenta. A high circulating ethanol concentration in fetal blood, therefore, will alter normal cellular pathways, adversely affecting cell division (proliferation) and differentiation in the developing fetus.

The difference between the more severe FAS and the milder **fetal alcohol effects (FAE)** is a matter of degree of alcohol consumption. Although it has not been fully established by research, some evidence suggests that even one drink a day by a pregnant woman may have adverse effects on fetal development. A safe level of alcohol consumption has not been determined for pregnant women. Therefore, the best rule for a woman who even thinks she may be pregnant is to avoid all alcoholic beverages until after lactation is completed; this is also the advice of the U.S. Surgeon General and the Academy of Nutrition and Dietetics.

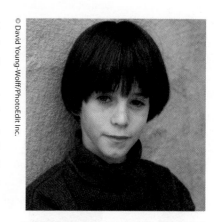

FIGURE 10.6 Characteristic Facial Changes of Infants and Small Children with the Fetal Alcohol Spectrum. Note the physical changes of the midline of the face, such as the absence of the philtrum (groove) running from the nose to the upper lip. These changes may be quite subtle as in this photograph, especially in cases of milder adverse effects of alcohol intake by pregnant mothers.

Drugs and Other Potentially Toxic Chemicals

Drugs and many other chemicals are risk factors during pregnancy and lactation. Any drug (prescription or over the counter) used during pregnancy and lactation should be approved by a physician prior to use. Many drugs, particularly those that are fat-soluble, readily transfer across the placenta and mammary glands. Thus, the developing fetus or breast-feeding infant is generally exposed to any drugs administered for the mother's benefit. Many drugs have potentially adverse effects at some stage of fetal or infant development.

Drug addiction of any kind, whether licit or illicit, is a potential hazard to fetal development or to the nursing infant. For example, babies born of mothers who are cocaine or heroin addicts are invariably of very low birth weight, and delivery is nearly always premature. These high-risk babies require special care and nurturing that their mothers generally cannot provide.

Oral contraceptive agents, or birth control pills, provide a good example of an unsuspected drug effect. These agents may reduce the blood concentrations of some of the water-soluble B vitamins. Because women may continue taking these agents without realizing they are pregnant, the fetus could then be directly affected by nutrient deficits.

Lastly, fetal complications resulting from excessive drug use may be complicated by the concurrent effects of maternal human immunodeficiency virus (HIV) in women with AIDS. The combined insults of drugs and HIV can have devastating consequences on the development of the newborn and the later life of the child.

Cigarette Smoking

Cigarette smoking by the mother also has deleterious effects on fetal development. Even reducing the number of cigarettes smoked a day from a full pack to just a few cigarettes is not enough to completely reduce the negative effects on fetal growth and size at delivery. Cigarette smoking reduces the delivery of oxygen and increases the delivery of carbon monoxide to fetal tissue as well as to maternal tissues. This behavior is especially detrimental if smoking is continuous throughout the waking hours. Smoking of any kind of tobacco is not recommended before or during pregnancy because it typically

fetal alcohol effects (FAE) A disorder observed in babies or young children of mothers who consumed excessive amounts of alcohol during pregnancy. Results in reduced intelligence test scores, but the overall effects on child development may be minor.

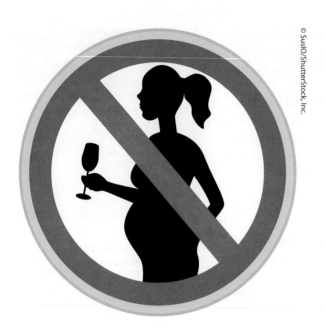

contributes to low birth weight. Smoking during breast-feeding will also deliver to the infant carcinogens from the cigarettes, in addition to the nicotine.

Tea, Coffee, and Herbals

When consumed in large quantities each day, caffeine-containing beverages such as coffee, tea, and cola-type drinks may modestly alter cell metabolism in both maternal and fetal tissues. Limiting these beverages to the equivalent of two servings of coffee a day (about 300 milligrams of caffeine) may be beneficial. Herbals, typically available as supplements, are not recommended during pregnancy because of potential adverse effects; however, more research is needed on the health effects of these supplements. The assumption cannot be made that these natural products are not harmful to a rapidly developing fetus. The wide variety of products available and the ranges of their efficacy and purity, in addition to their largely unknown effects, make caution advisable.

Potential Adverse Effects of Early Life Programming

Poor maternal nutrition status during pregnancy negatively influences birth weight and the infant's early development. Could adverse early life events contribute to the development of chronic diseases later in life? A growing literature supports an association between fetal growth and the development of chronic diseases later in life, revolving around the idea of **early life programming**. The "Barker hypothesis," named for David Barker, the original advocate of this hypothesis, suggests that delayed prenatal development of the fetus influences the development of chronic diseases later in life, especially cardiovascular diseases. Additional data now point to the effects of low birth weight and the development of hypertension, diabetes, cardiovascular diseases, and obesity later in life.

Although the public health implications of the Barker hypothesis are intriguing, the hypothesis and the data supporting it reinforce the importance of optimal nutrition of the woman during pregnancy because of the potential adverse effects on the late life development of nutrition-related chronic diseases.

Lactation

Lactation is the production and release of milk by the mammary glands for nourishing the infant and is commonly a time for the mother and infant to bond. Breast-fed infants generally grow well and thrive solely on breast milk for the first 6 months of life. Infants who are breast-fed typically have fewer infections and other complications (e.g., ear aches) than bottle-fed infants. Even twins can develop very well on breast milk, but the mother, who roughly doubles her production, may become more easily exhausted with two different feeding schedules. Maternal lactation is a wonderful opportunity for nurturing an infant. Thus, the mother's nutrition needs to be optimal. Unfortunately, many barriers such as career choices prevent women from being able to take full advantage of nursing.

Nutrient Allowances During Lactation

Lactating women require additional amounts of nutrients in order to have good **milk** production in both quantity and quality to meet the needs of their growing infant (see **Table 10.3**). The RDAs for lactating women go up by 330 kilocalories for energy

early life programming Theory that common chronic diseases in adult life originate during fetal life, such that low birth weight may be linked to later development of hypertension, diabetes, obesity, and cardiovascular disease. Also called the "Barker hypothesis."

lactation The production and release of milk by the mammary glands for nourishing the infant. Pediatricians currently recommended that mothers breast-feed their infants for a minimum of 6 months.

milk Secretion from the mammary glands of mammals. The composition of human breast milk differs considerably from cow's milk, especially in total energy, protein, and micromineral content.

TABLE 10.3

Nutrients Recommended (RDAs) During Lactation (Up to 6 Months) Compared to RDAs of NonPregnant and NonLactating Women*

Nutrient	RDA	Quantity	Percent Increase
Significant Increases Required			
Water	3.8 L	0.8 L	~27
Protein	71 g	25 g	~54
Vitamin A	1,300 µg	600 µg	~85
Vitamin E	19 mg	4 mg	~27
Vitamin C	120 mg	45 mg	~37
Vitamin B_6	2.0 mg	0.7 mg	~54
Thiamin	1.4 mg	0.3 mg	~27
Niacin	17 mg	3 mg	~21
Riboflavin	1.6 mg	0.5 mg	~45
Folate	500 µg	100 µg	~25
Pantothenic acid	7 mg	2 mg	~40
Choline	550 mg	125 mg	~29
Zinc	12 mg	4 mg	~50
Iodine	290 µg	140 µg	~93
Selenium	70 µg	15 µg	~27
Chromium	45 µg	20 µg	~80
Copper	1,300 µg	400 µg	~44
Manganese	2.6 mg	0.8 mg	~44
Modest Increase Required			
Energy	2,733 kcal	330 kcal	~14
Fiber	29 g	4 g	~16
Vitamin B_{12}	2.8 µg	0.4 µg	~17
Biotin	35 µg	5 µg	~17
Molybdenum	50 mg	5 mg	~11
Potassium	5.1 g	0.4 g	~9
No Extra Amounts Needed			
Vitamin D	15 µg	—	—
Vitamin K	90 µg	—	—
Calcium	1,000 mg	—	—
Phosphorus	700 mg	—	—
Magnesium	320 mg	—	—
Fluoride	3.0 mg	—	—
Sodium	1.5 g	—	—
Chloride	2.3 g	—	—
Iron	9 mg	—	—

* Increased amounts are needed for the first and second 6 months of lactation, but only the values for the first 6 months are provided here. See footnote in Table 10.2 for calculation of percentage.

Data from Food and Nutrition Board, Institute of Medicine. *Dietary Reference Intakes*. Washington, DC: National Academies Press; 1997–2011.

> Maternal milk also supplies immunoglobulins or antibodies that help the infant better fight infectious agents.

TABLE 10.4
Good Food Sources of Energy and Nutrients for Pregnant and Lactating Women

Energy Sources	Protein Sources	Micronutrient Sources
Cereals/breads	Meats	Dairy foods
Dairy foods	Legumes	Fruits
Eggs	Dairy foods	Vegetables
Fruits/juices	Eggs	Eggs
Vegetables	Whole-grain cereals	Nuts, seeds

Data from the USDA.

(a 14% increase) and by 25 grams per day for protein (a 54% increase). If the mother can nurse, breast milk is far superior to formula because it contains all the nutrients in the right proportions for the infant and the proteins it contains are not allergenic (i.e., allergy causing). Breast milk is also easier to digest and binds essential minerals to enhance their absorption by infants. Maternal milk also supplies immunoglobulins or **antibodies** that help the infant better fight infectious agents. Maintaining a healthy immune system is critical for the health of both the mother and her nursing infant.

Little or no increase in iron is recommended for women during lactation because menstruation does not typically resume until late in lactation. Breast milk contains little iron, but it is of high bioavailability so that little drain on maternal iron stores occurs in lactation. **Table 10.4** lists foods rich in nutrients needed by nursing mothers (i.e., energy, protein, micronutrients).

Breast Milk Versus Formulas

Nearly all types of **infant formulas** are extractions and modifications of milk obtained from cows. An exception is soy milk–based formula, which is extracted from soybeans (see **FIGURE 10.7**). Soy milk is considered nonallergenic and it contains less saturated fat than traditional formulas. Formulas based on cow's milk, like breast milk, contain lactose,

antibody An immunoglobulin made in response to antigenic stimulation by specific lymphocytes. Certain antibodies in the circulation exist because of a prior exposure to an antigen or other microorganisms (i.e., acquired immunity), whereas others are in the blood at birth (innate).

infant formulas Milk substitutes that contain nutrients in approximately the same concentrations as human breast milk. These formulas are typically modified cow's milk or soy milk. They are very important for infant growth for mothers who cannot produce their own milk or who choose not to breast-feed.

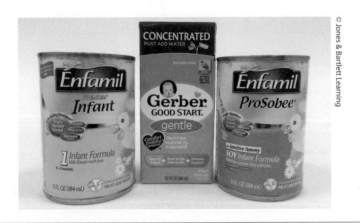

© Jones & Bartlett Learning

FIGURE 10.7 Infant Formulas. A variety of infant formulas is available. Many are based on cow's milk. Soy milk options are available for infants who have difficulty digesting cow's milk–based formulas. Many infant formulas are supplemented with omega-3 fatty acids, in addition to a variety of other nutrients, to meet the needs of the growing infant.

TABLE 10.5

Nutrient Content of Breast Milk Compared with Whole Cow's Milk and Generic Infant Formulas (per Liter)

Nutrient	Breast Milk	Whole Cow's Milk*	Generic Milk-Based Formula with Iron	Generic Soy Formula with Iron
Energy	728 kcal	629 kcal	578 kcal	578 kcal
Protein	11 g	34 g	13 g	17 g
Fat	46 g	34 g	37 g	32 g
Cholesterol	145 mg	144 mg	0 mg	0 mg
Lactose	72 g	48 g	—†	—†
Calcium	333 mg	1,227 mg	376 mg	542 mg
Phosphorus	145 mg	959 mg	257 mg	376 mg
Iron	0.3 mg	0.5 mg	11 mg	11 mg
Vitamin A	2,506 IU	1,299 IU	1,809 IU	2,268 IU
Vitamin D	42 IU	412 IU**	—**	—**
Vitamin C	52 mg	9 mg	51 mg	50 mg
Thiamin	0.14 mg	0.39 mg	0.64 mg	0.64 mg
Riboflavin	0.38 mg	1.7 mg	0.92 mg	0.92 mg
Niacin	1.8 mg	0.9 mg	4.5 mg	3.2 mg
Folic acid	52 µg	52 µg	46 µg	40 µg

* Vitamin D–fortified cow's milk. † Lactose values not given for generic formulas. ** Formula milks frequently are fortified with vitamin D. Data from Food and Nutrition Board, Institute of Medicine. *Dietary Reference Intakes.* Washington, DC: National Academies Press; 1997–2011.

a sugar that is used as a quick, readily available source of energy. The nutrient composition of breast milk is presented in **Table 10.5**, along with similar data for cow's milk and for generic infant formulas based on cow's milk and soy milk. Note that the amounts of the breast **milk proteins**, casein and lactalbumin, are much lower than in cow's milk!

FOCUS 10.3   Lactose Intolerance in Infants

Infants clearly need the energy and micronutrients provided by milk, either breast milk or milk-based formulas. Most infants will not suffer from lactose intolerance because the gut typically produces sufficient amounts of lactase in the first year of life. However, if an infant placed on a milk-based formula does develop intolerance to the lactose in the formula, a physician will often recommend soy-based products so the infant gets the needed micronutrient package (i.e., calcium, vitamin D, and riboflavin), along with the essential macronutrients. These nutrients are important for early infant development. ●

milk proteins The two major proteins found in milk are casein and lactalbumin (whey).

▌▌ Breast milk contains high amounts of saturated fat and cholesterol, both of which are needed for membrane synthesis, especially in the nervous tissue in the brain. **▐▐**

The mineral and vitamin mixtures of infant formulas are designed to duplicate or improve on mother's milk, but none of these formulas contain immunoglobulins and other molecules, such as bifidus factor, that are present in breast milk. Bifidus factor encourages the growth of the bacteria *Lactobacillus bifidus* in the baby's intestine. Such probiotic bacteria are beneficial to the health of the developing infant's digestive system. **Colostrum**, which is the milk produced in the first few days of lactation, is important for infants because it contains high concentrations of immunoglobulins that defend against bacteria and possibly viruses. These milkborne immunoglobulins help the infant's **immune system** for a few days until the baby can produce its own immunoglobulins. These immunoglobulins (proteins) are absorbed intact—without digestion—in the first few days of life, and thereby endow the infant with antibodies to fight harmful microorganisms. Many dietary proteins can be absorbed intact or practically whole because the infant's GI tract is so immature.

As shown in Table 10.5, the composition of breast milk differs considerably from cow's milk in the following nutrients: protein, lactose, fat, calcium, phosphorus, and cholesterol. Breast milk contains high amounts of saturated fat and cholesterol, both of which are needed for membrane synthesis, especially in the nervous tissue in the brain. Brain growth and development occur at a rapid pace during the first year of life. Infant formula milks may need to be fortified with omega-3 fatty acids to support the growth and development of the infant brain and nervous system.

The protein content of breast milk is much lower than that of cow's milk (see **FIGURE 10.8**). The major difference in protein composition—much lower in breast milk than cow's milk—is preferred for at least the first year of life because infant kidneys cannot process the

colostrum The first milk produced by a mother during the 2 to 3 days following the birth of an infant. Colostrum is rich in immunoglobulins that provide a short period of acquired immunity for the breast-feeding infant before the infant can adequately synthesize his or her own immunoglobulins.

immune system The network of cells, tissues, and organs that works to defend the body against attacks by "foreign" invaders, such as bacteria, viruses, parasites, and fungi, that can cause infections.

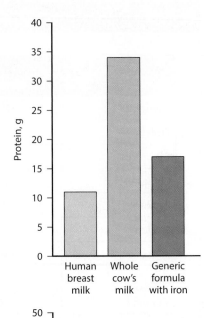
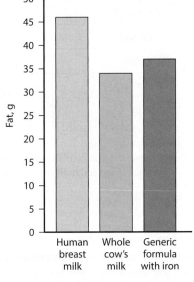
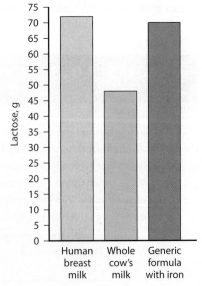

FIGURE 10.8 Macronutrient Distribution in Breast Milk, Cow's Milk, and Formula. Breast milk provides relatively more fat than cow's milk and soy milk. Fat is needed for the development of tissues, especially in the brain.

Data from Anderson JJB. *Nutrition and Health: An Introduction.* Durham, NC: Carolina Academic Press; 2005.

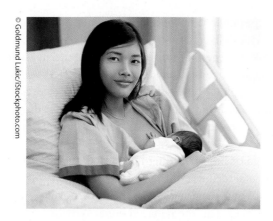

FIGURE 10.9 The Importance of Breast-Feeding. Breast milk is best for infants. Ideally, all mothers will breast-feed until their infants are at least 6 months of age in order to provide their child with needed immuno-globulins and fatty acids.

products of protein metabolism efficiently at this early stage. Note the large difference in protein of the types of milk in Figure 10.8. Formulas tend to be intermediate, but they still contain more protein than breast milk. Breast milk is considered the best food for infants for at least the first 6 months of life (see **FIGURE 10.9**).

Meeting Nutrient Requirements During Lactation

Lactating women should consume additional servings of nutrient-rich foods from each MyPlate food group to meet the increased energy, protein, and micronutrient demands of both her own body and that of the breast-fed infant. Cigarette smoking should be eliminated. Alcohol may be consumed in limited amounts if timed around feedings. An adequate diet remains the cornerstone of good health for lactating women.

Benefits of Lactation to Mothers

A major benefit to mothers who breast-feed for 6 months or longer is that they gradually lose the excess weight put on as adipose tissue stores during pregnancy in preparation for lactation. Weight-reduction diets are not recommended for lactating women, but physical activity is encouraged for both weight and fat loss following the gains during a full-term pregnancy.

In addition, many new mothers experience **lactational amenorrhea**, which is temporary postnatal infertility that occurs when a woman is not menstruating. Not all

> Breast milk is considered the best food for infants for at least the first 6 months of life.

> A major benefit to mothers who breast-feed for 6 months or longer is that they gradually lose the excess weight put on as adipose tissue stores during pregnancy in preparation for lactation.

lactational amenorrhea Temporary postnatal infertility that occurs when a woman is amenorrheic (not menstruating) and fully breast-feeding.

PRACTICAL APPLICATIONS 10.2

Soy-Based Formulas

Several soy-based formulas are now available on the market. These typically contain additional iron, vitamin D, and calcium plus a few other nutrients comparable with milk-based products. Refer to Table 10.5 and compare the nutrient composition of a generic soy-based formula with a cow's milk–based formula. What are the major differences between these two types of formulas? Do any differences appear so great that they might affect an infant's nutritional status? ■

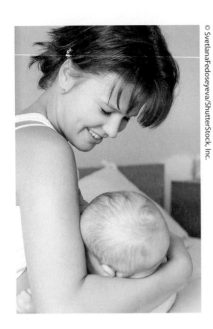

women, however, experience this, especially well-nourished mothers. Therefore, the several months following delivery is not guaranteed to be free from ovulation and potential conception. Another benefit of nursing is that the uterus shrinks more efficiently after birth. This happens once the baby initiates breast-feeding and the hormones are released that enhance milk let-down or release. Furthermore, nursing also nurtures a strong mother–infant bond that fosters healthy early infant development. Bonding is considered by many experts to confer a significant psychological benefit to both mother and infant.

Another advantage of breast-feeding is restored and improved bone mass of the mother. Maternal skeletal turnover during breast-feeding is substantial, perhaps as much as 35% of the total mineral mass (and matrix). This turnover results in the formation of new bone that is healthier than the replaced bone. Whether or not a net gain of bone mass can be achieved as a result of breast-feeding, coupled with a good calcium intake, has not been established. Breast-feeding also reduces the risk of breast cancer. In women with good nutrition, breast-feeding does not result in bone loss, but it may in those with poor nutrition or insufficient calcium.

One of the few problems with breast-feeding is that chemicals in the environment can enter the breast milk. Fat-soluble environmental chemicals, such as organic pesticides and heavy metals, can enter the mother's milk and then be passed on to the infant. The same is true of alcohol and many drugs, most of which are also fat-soluble. For example, alcohol will transfer into the milk a mother produces in direct proportion to the amount in her blood.

Teenage Mothers and Lactation

Teenage mothers (younger than 17 years) must be especially diligent in consuming extra servings of nutrient-rich foods each day in order to maintain their own growth and development as well as that of the breast-fed infant. Thus, the minimum numbers of servings recommended would be the same as for an adolescent female plus the additional servings needed during pregnancy or lactation. Lactation by adolescents is typically compromised by poor diets.

Unfortunately, teenagers who become pregnant usually are not prepared psychologically, even if they are ready physically, to have a baby. In general, their eating habits are not satisfactory, and many of these adolescents have not completed their skeletal development. Another problem is that pregnant adolescents typically delay too long in obtaining prenatal care and advice about diet and nutrient supplements.

The best approach to helping an adolescent who becomes pregnant is to arrange as early as possible for her to obtain prenatal care from an obstetrician or family physician so that her nutritional status can be improved and other aspects of prenatal health can be addressed.

Special Nutritional Needs of Vegetarians During Lactation

Sound vegetarian dietary practices should satisfy the nutrient needs of the fetus and breast-fed infant. High-quality protein is generally not a problem because of the mixing of several protein sources, including at least one type of legume. If several different plant proteins are consumed by a vegan mother, she should be able to satisfy both the nutritional requirements of fetal and early infant development as well as her own needs.

Nevertheless, four concerns about strict vegetarian (vegan) eating practices arise. First, these diets may be low in energy and a few micronutrients, especially vitamin B_{12}, that are provided in good quantities by animal products. Second, vegan diets are generally low in the omega-3 fatty acids typically found in fish and fish oils. Third, these diets may also be low in calcium and vitamin D. Fourth, pregnant or lactating vegan women may have difficulty consuming sufficient energy because strict vegetarian diets contain so much satiety-inducing dietary fiber.

One easy solution is sufficient consumption of soy milk, which is usually fortified with calcium and vitamin D and sometimes vitamin B_{12}. Substituting legumes and soy milk for meats and dairy foods during these critical phases of the life cycle should ensure that the fetus or infant will develop and grow. A vegan diet is considered safe if the mother practices sound nutrition with ample intake of legumes and possibly vitamin B_{12} and omega-3 fatty acid supplements.

Nutritional Supplements During Lactation

Some physicians recommend the use of nutritional supplements during lactation to ensure adequate micronutrient intakes. However, supplements should not take the place of balanced dietary intakes by lactating women.

Nutritional Intake by Nonlactating Post-parturient Mothers

The mother who does not lactate after delivery, of course, needs to reduce her energy intake and try to achieve normal body weight within a few months. If she has gained excess adipose tissue, it will take her longer to return to her normal body weight in the absence of lactation. Therefore, the nonlactating mother will have to be careful to obtain all the micronutrients needed during her recovery while at the same time reducing total caloric intake for weight control.

Infancy

Breast milk provides practically all the essential nutrients needed in **infancy**, which makes breast milk the preferred source of nutrition for infants in the first 6 months of life. Exclusive breast-feeding for the first 6 months is recommended by groups such as the American Academy of Pediatrics. Many organizations also recommend some continued breast-feeding until the infant is 1 year of age.

Infants who are not breast-fed should be fed human milk substitutes; that is, formulas that are based on the latest information about safe and healthy nutrient content in order to ensure optimal **growth** in hard and soft tissue mass. Small-for-gestational-age babies typically need specific nutritional care by pediatricians to get them into the normal range of weight and height. Information on the appropriate range of weight and height for age is available in growth charts, which are available from a number of different sources.

Nutritional Needs During the First Year

Macronutrient and micronutrient needs of infants during the first year of life are factored into the RDAs so infant foods should provide the recommended amounts of these nutrients. **Table 10.6** lists the nutrient RDAs over the first year of life broken down into the first 6 months and the second 6 months. Meeting the infant's needs during the first 6 months is easy if the infant is breast-fed, although micronutrient supplements such as omega-3 fatty acids may be recommended by a physician to ensure intake sufficiency.

After 6 months of age, solid foods are gradually introduced into the infant's diet. The quality of the child's diet remains important for continuing growth along healthy percentiles on the growth charts. Depending on the infant's rate of growth, parents may require additional guidance from healthcare professionals, including physicians and dietitians, regarding optimal nutrient intake.

> A vegan diet is considered safe if the mother practices sound nutrition with ample intake of legumes and possibly vitamin B_{12} and omega-3 fatty acid supplements.

infancy Period of life from birth to 1 year of age. Typically a period of rapid growth, with almost a doubling of birth weight and a significant enlargement of the head (and brain) relative to the rest of the body.

growth (general) The increase in tissue mass, especially soft tissues and hard (skeletal) tissues, through the formation of new cells (hyperplasia) and the enlargement of those cells (hypertrophy).

> The quality of the child's diet remains important for continuing growth along healthy percentiles on the growth charts.

TABLE 10.6
RDAs for the First Year of Life

Nutrient	Birth Through 6 Months of Age	6–12 Months of Age
Energy		
Female	520 kcal	676 kcal
Male	570 kcal	743 kcal
Protein	9.1 g	13.5 g
Calcium	210 mg	70 mg
Iron	0.27 mg	11 mg
Vitamin A	400 μg	500 μg
Vitamin C	40 mg	50 mg
Folate	65 μg	80 μg

Data from Food and Nutrition Board, Institute of Medicine. *Dietary Reference Intakes*. Washington, DC: National Academies Press; 1997–2011.

FOCUS 10.4   Fat Intake of Nursing Infants

Infants need a fairly high intake of fat (triglycerides) during the first 6 months of life and a little less during the second 6 months. Omega-3 fatty acids are particularly important to include in the diets of infants because of rapid brain growth for up to one year of age. Typically, fat should comprise 30% to 40% of total calorie intake. Breast milk has a high fat content and should fully meet the infant's fat requirements for the first 6 months. For formula-fed infants, the formula's fat content should closely parallel that of human milk (refer back to Table 10.5 for a comparison of breast milk and generic formulas). Infants have high fat requirements because they need large amounts of fat in order to support the growth of tissues such as those in the brain and nervous system.

In recent years, mothers with concerns about high-fat diets have been restricting the fat intake of their infants—to the detriment of their infants' health! The best rule for mothers is to let nature take its course by using breast milk as the major food source as long as possible (up to a year) and introducing solid foods starting at about 6 months. Healthcare providers should assure mothers about the appropriate amount of fat in the typical infant diet over the first year. Unless otherwise recommended, fat should not be reduced prior to 2 years of age, and then typically to about 30% of calories. ●

Weaning and Solid Food Introduction

Depending on the readiness of the child and mother, solid food is initially introduced at 6 months. Final weaning from breast-feeding typically occurs between 9 and 12 months postdelivery. Longer periods of breast-feeding are certainly acceptable, though less commonly practiced in the United States.

The first solid foods typically include iron-fortified rice or other cereals for babies and pureed vegetables and fruits. High-protein foods such as meats and eggs are introduced later. Adequate fluid intake is still needed to maintain water balance while the kidneys continue to mature. Regular full-fat cow's milk is generally not recommended until after

1 year of age because of its high protein content and the resulting stress it may place on the developing kidneys.

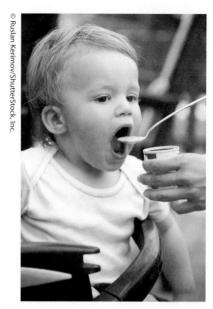

If iron-fortified cereals or other iron-containing foods are not provided after the first 6 months, infants may develop anemia. Even though the iron in breast milk is highly available, the overall level provided is low, and by 6 months of age the infant's iron stores may be depleted. Parents should also make sure that their infants are consuming adequate amounts of vitamin C and other vitamins from food sources if supplements are not used. It is important to check the food labels to determine if the foods provided have been fortified. The baby food industry has been active in ensuring optimal health of growing infants, and many infant foods are fortified with nutrients.

A few allergenic foods can be cautiously introduced into the diets of infants, one food at a time, every 2 to 3 days to identify any intolerances. Common allergies result from **allergens** (proteins) in foods, including peanut butter, eggs, cow's milk, and soy products. Such foods can be introduced carefully after 1 year of age, or after 2 years of age if there is a family history of allergies. Too much sugar and salt intake, especially from processed foods, also needs to be watched. Because of potential toxicity, honey should not be introduced until after 1 year.

Nutritional Supplements During Infancy

Most physicians recommend micronutrient supplements for infants. In particular, a vitamin D supplement (400 IU per day) is recommended for exclusively breastfed infants. Infants also receive an injection of vitamin K at birth to get them started before intestinal bacteria provide a source. In addition, for those without fluoridated water, a supplement of fluoride is recommended from birth through childhood.

Infants who are having difficulty breast-feeding or eating solid foods may also need additional macronutrients either in liquid form or in an easily consumable state. Many such formulations exist. If nutrient intake continues to be low, consultation with a physician or nutrition specialist may be necessary. Infant supplements may be recommended by a physician when an infant is not following an optimal growth pattern on the grid during the first year.

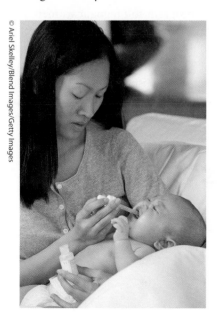

> Current recommendations are that infant milk formulas or milk substitutes, such as soy milk, should contain a minimum of 4% of energy from linoleic acid and 0.75% of energy from alpha-linolenic acid (ALA).

allergen A protein in food or other environmental material that induces an allergic response (i.e., excess production of antibodies and other immune defense molecules); a type of antigen.

Current recommendations are that infant milk formulas or milk substitutes, such as soy milk, should contain a minimum of 4% of energy from linoleic acid and 0.75% of energy from alpha-linolenic acid (ALA). ALA serves as the precursor for the essential long-chain omega-3 fatty acids. One omega-3 fatty acid, docosahexaenoic acid (DHA), is added to some formulas already. The balanced intake of omega-6 and omega-3 fatty acids seems important for healthy babies.

Federal Food Programs for Infants and Mothers

Several **federal food programs**, administered by the USDA, benefit low-income mothers and children. One of the most successful of these programs is the **Supplementary Food Program for Women, Infants, and Children (WIC)**. WIC serves pregnant women as well as mothers and their young children (up to 5 years of age). Foods offered by WIC, such as dairy, soy, eggs, cereals, fruits, and vegetables, are nutrient rich and are considered essential parts of a healthy diet (see **FIGURE 10.10**). WIC remains an outstanding program because the foods given to qualified mothers are limited to a few nutrient-dense, high-quality foods. Other USDA programs, such as the School Lunch Program, have had less of a measurable impact with regard to the health of children. The Supplemental Nutritional Assistance Program (SNAP) formerly called the Food Stamp Program provides food credits to low-income families, and infants may benefit from the food items purchased.

> WIC remains an outstanding program because the foods given to qualified mothers are limited to a few nutrient-dense, high-quality foods.

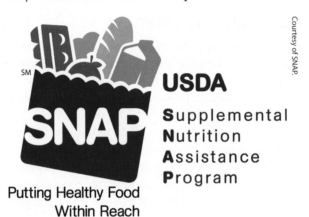

Courtesy of SNAP.

Despite the widespread availability of the WIC program to pregnant women and mothers and their infants and young children, infant mortality rates in the United States have remained steady at about 6.8 deaths per 1,000 live births since 2000, according to CDC reports. The highest rate, 13.6 deaths per 1,000 live births, occurs with African American infants, and the next highest rate is for non-white Hispanics. Also, teen mothers and mothers over 40 years have higher rates compared with those of mothers in their 20s and 30s.

federal food programs USDA programs that provide foods or food vouchers for needy individuals or families. These programs include the School Lunch Program, the Supplementary Food Program for Women, Infants, and Children (WIC), and the food stamp program (SNAP).

Supplementary Food Program for Women, Infants, and Children (WIC) A federal food-assistance program that provides nutrition education for medically qualified mothers and certain high-quality foods free for enrolled mothers and their children. Is considered the most cost-effective of the U.S. Department of Agriculture's food programs due to the strong gains in birth weights and growth of infants and children.

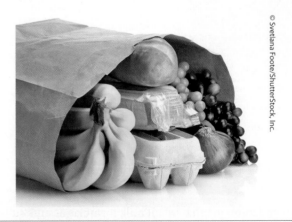

© Svetlana Foote/ShutterStock, Inc.

FIGURE 10.10 WIC-Approved Foods. The WIC program provides nutritious foods to women and their children to ensure optimal nutrition for at-risk populations.

SUMMARY

The nutritional status of a pregnant woman has a profound influence on the development and growth of her fetus, as well as on her own developing tissues (i.e., uterus, placenta, breasts). A good pregnancy outcome—a healthy baby in the normal weight range over nearly a full 40-week gestation—depends on sound eating habits both prior to and during pregnancy and good prenatal care by a physician. The DRIs for pregnant women are designed to optimize the intakes of energy, protein, and other nutrients during a full gestation. These intakes also help in accumulating the fat stores that are being laid down for use during the subsequent lactation period. Prenatal micronutrient supplements are typically recommended. Nevertheless, most authorities would prefer that pregnant women consume a diet that includes a broad variety of foods, such as fruits, vegetables, meats, dairy foods and eggs, plus micronutrient supplements, and even fish for omega-3 fatty acids. Vegan women have some difficulty getting adequate amounts of energy, omega-3 fatty acids, and vitamin B_{12}. Even though nutrient supplements are recommended during pregnancy, good diets containing a variety of foods remain the basic foundation for a healthy pregnancy outcome.

A healthy baby who grows at a steady rate within the normal weight range for his or her age depends greatly on sound eating habits of the mother for the length of her lactation period. Smoking, alcohol ingestion, and the use of drugs can have serious deleterious effects on both mother and baby during this critical period. An adequate volume of milk or infant formula should provide sustenance for the infant to grow normally for a period of up to 6 months. The DRIs for lactating women are designed to optimize the intakes of energy and nutrients during this demanding period of the life cycle. Lactating women need increased amounts of energy to maintain their own tissues as well as to support the production of milk, which contains energy primarily as lactose and fat. The immune system of breast-fed infants also benefits from mother's milk, which contains immunoglobulins (antibodies). Food guides are provided for lactating women to ensure adequate intakes of the most critical nutrients, namely, protein, calcium, macronutrients that provide energy, and other micronutrients. Good diets remain the basic foundation for high quality milk of a lactating mother that supports normal infant growth.

STUDENT ACTIVITIES

1. Why is it important for young women who might become pregnant to adopt habits that ensure a healthy baby (e.g., no smoking or drinking, start folic acid supplements, limit herbals) even before they are pregnant?

2. Explain why pregnant women, especially those in their second and third trimesters, have increased nutrient requirements.

3. Identify two micronutrients that pregnant women need in amounts 40% or greater (according to RDAs) than healthy nonpregnant women.

4. The incidence of neural tube defects declined in the United States and Canada by 30% to 40% in the late 1990s due to fortification of foods with folic acid. Developing countries that started requiring fortification have seen even larger decreases. Why do you think this might be?

5. What is the specific recommendation for folic acid (folate) for a pregnant woman?

6. Alcohol consumption, especially when excessive, is a risk factor for a healthy outcome (baby) of pregnancy. Explain why.

7. Name the USDA food program that provides high-quality foods for pregnant women. Why is this program so beneficial in terms of pregnancy outcomes?

8. The nutrient requirements (according to the RDAs) of a lactating woman increase substantially. List two micronutrients lactating women need in amounts 40% or greater than nonpregnant, nonlactating woman.

9. Identify three nutrients that have no increase in DRI during lactation. Why is there no increase?

10. State three major differences in macronutrient composition between breast milk and cow's milk.

11. Explain why pregnancy, breast-feeding, and infancy are so much more hazardous to mothers and babies in poorer countries around the world.

12. Explain why breast milk is so much higher in saturated fat and cholesterol than cow's milk.

13. Breast milk is considered to be beneficial for the infant's immune system, especially during the first 6 months of life. Explain why.

14. Infant nutritional requirements, especially of the macronutrients, are high for a specific purpose. Explain the reason for these high needs.

15. Why might nutrient supplements be recommended for infants? Explain.

WEBSITES FOR FURTHER STUDY

ChooseMyPlate
www.choosemyplate.gov/pregnancy-breastfeeding.html
Pregnancy and the Vegan Diet
www.vrg.org/nutrition/veganpregnancy.htm

Ask the Dietitian
www.dietitian.com/breastfeed.html

REFERENCES

Allen LH. Maternal nutrient metabolism and requirements in pregnancy and lactation. In: Erdman JW Jr, MacDonald IA, Zeisel SH (eds.). *Present Knowledge in Nutrition.* 10th ed. Ames, IA: John Wiley & Sons; 2012; 980–1002.

American Dietetic Association. Position of the American Dietetic Association and Dietitians of Canada: vegetarian diets. *J Am Diet Assoc.* 2003;103:748–765.

American Dietetic Association. Position of the American Dietetic Association and Dietitians of Canada: dietary fatty acids. *J Am Diet Assoc.* 2007;107:1599–1611.

Bhatia JJS, Greer FR. Clearing up confusion on the role of dairy in children's diets. *Am Acad Peds (AAP) News.* June 28, 2007.

De Wals P, Tairou F, Van Allen MI, et al. Reduction in neural-tube defects after folic acid fortification in Canada. *N Engl J Med.* 2007;357:135–142.

Food and Nutrition Board, Institute of Medicine. *Dietary Reference Intakes.* Washington, DC: National Academies Press; 1997–2011

Godfrey KM, Barker DJ. Fetal nutrition and adult diseases. *Am J Clin Nutr.* 2000;71(suppl):1344S–1352S.

Hannigan JH, Armant DR. Alcohol and pregnancy and neonatal outcome. *Semin Neonatol.* 2000;5:243–254.

Heird WC. Infant nutrition. In: Erdman JW Jr, MacDonald IA, Zeisel SH (eds.). *Present Knowledge in Nutrition.* 10th ed. Ames, IA: John Wiley & Sons; 2012; 1003–1020.

Kaiser L, Allen LH. Position of the American Dietetic Association: nutrition and lifestyle for a healthy pregnancy outcome. *J Am Diet Assoc.* 2008;108:553–561.

Kowaleski-Jones L, Duncan GJ. Effects of participants in the WIC Program on birthweight: Evidence from the National Longitudinal Survey of Youth. *Am J Pub Health.* 2002;92:799–804.

Lovelady C, Lonnerdal B, Dewey KG. Lactation performance of exercising women. *Am J Clin Nutr.* 1990;52:103–109.

Murphy MM, Molloy AM, Ueland PM, et al. Longitudinal study of the effect of pregnancy on maternal and fetal cobalamin status in healthy women and their offspring. *J Nutr.* 2007;137:1863–1867.

Penney DS, Miller KG. Nutritional counseling for vegetarians during pregnancy and lactation. *J Midwifery Womens Health.* 2008;53:37–44.

Stein Z, Susser M. The Dutch Famine, 1944–1945, and the reproductive process. I. Effects on six indices of birth. *Pediatr Res.* 1970;2:74–76.

ADDITIONAL READING

Delange FM, West KP (eds.). *Micronutrient Deficiencies in the First Six Months of Life.* Basel, Switzerland: Karger SG; 2003.

Johnson PK. Vegetarian diets in pregnancy and lactation. In: Sabate J (ed.). *Vegetarian Nutrition.* Boca Raton, FL: CRC Press; 2001: 195–219.

Klimis-Zacas D, Wolinsky E (eds.). *Nutritional Concerns of Women.* 2nd ed. Boca Raton, FL: CRC Press; 2003.

Messina MJ, Messina VL. *The Dietitian's Guide to Vegetarian Diets: Issues and Applications.* Gaithersburg, MD: Aspen; 1996.

Nutrition Across the Life Cycle

Healthy eating patterns are important during all phases of the life cycle, but they are particularly important early in life. Thus, healthy eating patterns need to be established during childhood and adolescence, and parents or caretakers have major roles in overseeing early eating behaviors. The second year of life begins the onset of childhood, a period with special energy and nutrient requirements to meet the demands of the growing body. This period of rapid growth requires adequate intake of energy and protein as well as micronutrients and phytochemicals.

Adults (21 to 65 years) continue to require nutrients, though typically at lower levels than during the growth phase. Thus, recommended intakes are based on the maintenance of body tissues and organs during the three or more decades after initial growth to adult height (age 20 or so). Regular physical activity helps govern energy intake and the consumption of protein in active individuals but not in those who are not active!

The nutritional requirements of older adults (older than 65 years) remain essentially the same as for adulthood, though they gradually decline over the later years. Gastrointestinal (GI) tract decrements in physiologic functions with age occur as a matter of course, but even more significant are the occasional pathologic changes of GI tissues that often affect the elderly. Despite declining physiologic requirements, intakes of some micronutrients may actually need to be increased later in life because of lowered efficiency of intestinal absorption. The uncertainties in establishing requirements for many nutrients because of widely varying declines in function late in life mean that the age-specific RDAs of older adults are considered less reliable than those for younger adults. During late-life **aging**, many organ systems undergo significant declines in function.

The nutrient allowances (RDAs) for all segments of the life cycle are set so the body obtains all of the nutrients and energy for growth as well as tissue maintenance after **skeletal growth** (height) has been completed. Healthy eating patterns should be accompanied by healthy lifestyle behaviors, including regular physical activity. Unfortunately, several nutrition-related problems arise at each stage of the life cycle, from early childhood (2 to 12 years) through adolescence (13 to 20 years), and into adulthood (beyond age 20).

aging The decline in biological functions that typically begins after age 50 years and leads to variable decrements in organ functions, reduced cell renewal, and losses of tissue in the lean body mass compartment, especially in muscle mass and bone mass.

skeletal growth The growth in height in childhood that is typically concluded by late adolescence; continuing accumulation of bone mass (mineral content) occurs during early adulthood (bone consolidation).

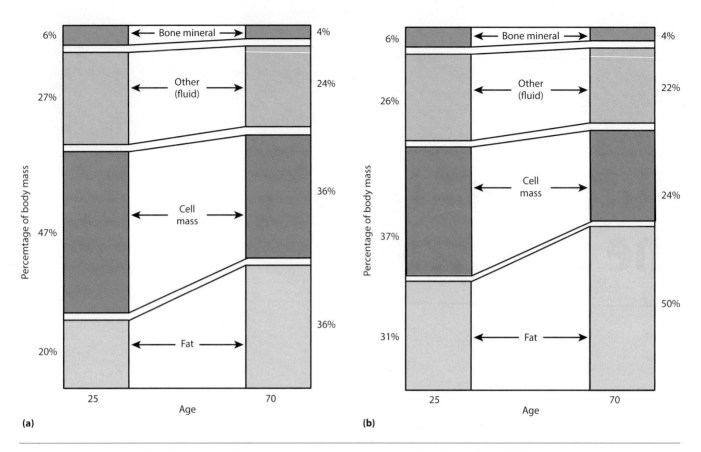

FIGURE 11.1 Body Composition Changes Over Time. Body composition changes over time for both (a) males and (b) females.

Reproduced from Anderson JJB. *Nutrition and Health: An Introduction.* Durham, NC: Carolina Academic Press; 2005.

This chapter begins with an overview of changes in body composition over the life cycle. It then presents nutrient requirements for healthy individuals during major stages of the life cycle—from 1 year of age to old age. The effects of nutritional deficits or excesses that may arise during these periods also are detailed.

Body Composition Changes Across the Life Cycle

The major compartments of the body—lean body mass (LBM), fat mass, and bone mass—undergo tremendous changes from early life to the elder years (see **FIGURE 11.1**).

Children and Adolescents

Childhood changes in body composition from 1 year to 20 years of age primarily involve growth and development of the skeleton and musculature. However, with adequate food intake, fat stores begin to accumulate in the preadolescent years. Fat mass remains fairly steady except for gains in girls around the time of **puberty**. The accumulation of fat tissue (especially by females) during the prepubertal period (approximately 9 to 12 years of age) is necessary for the development of reproductive function and the onset of **menarche** (first menses). The accumulation of muscle mass by adolescents, particularly males, in association with pubertal development, especially with the production of testosterone, is closely associated with the increase of bone mass. Suboptimal skeletal growth during childhood and adolescence may result from chronically low intakes of calcium.

childhood The period of life between infancy and adolescence; typically includes the onset of puberty. This period is marked by extensive growth (both general and skeletal) and extends from 1 year of age to 11 to 13 years in girls and 13 to 15 years in boys.

puberty The transitional period between late childhood and early adolescence that is marked by sexual development, including hormonal changes and increased physical development of the skeleton. In boys, it is also characterized by added muscle mass.

menarche The physiological/hormonal events surrounding the first menstruation (menses), which marks the pubertal transition of girls from late childhood (prepuberty) into adolescence.

Excessive gains of fat tissue or fat mass, however, may contribute to health-related problems of overnutrition and eventually lead to overweight and obesity. In recent decades, fat mass accumulation in children and adolescents has become much more significant in the United States and other developed countries, as reflected by increasing rates of obesity among these age groups.

Adults

The major changes in body composition occurring during **adulthood** are an upward shift in the percentage of body fat and a corresponding downward shift in LBM (see **Table 11.1**). The percentage changes in body composition across adulthood shown in **FIGURE 11.2.** are related to two physiologic events occurring at the same time: (1) a loss of LBM, principally as muscle, and (2) a gain in adipose tissue, or fat mass. During adulthood and the elderly period, individuals remain healthier if they are able to retain most of their LBM through exercise and physical activity, even if they gain some fat mass. Despite a relative decline in percentage of LBM, retention of the bulk of the LBM (in kilograms or pounds) to help support vital functions remains important (see discussion of sarcopenia below).

The most accurate method for measuring body composition is **dual-energy x-ray absorptiometry (DXA)**. DXA total-body measurements provide accurate data on an individual's fat mass, LBM, and bone mass. DXA is widely used to assess individual body composition, which is an indicator of health status. Although DXA is the most accurate measure of body composition, it is a relatively expensive test that requires special equipment. The body mass index (BMI) is a much easier and less expensive method of determining a person's body composition. In the United States, over the last several decades BMI has been used as a measure of weight status, with cutoff values determining whether a person is overweight or obese.

TABLE 11.1
Percent Body Fat Mass by Age and Ethnicity

| | Fat Mass (%) | | | | | |
| | Men | | | Women | | |
Age	White	Black	Hispanic	White	Black	Hispanic
20–39 years	26	24	27	37	40	40
40–59 years	29	26	29	41	42	42
≥ 60 years	21	29	31	43	42	43

Data from Li C, Ford ES, Zhao G, Balluz LS, Giles WH. Estimates of body composition with dual-energy x-ray absorptiometry in adults. *Am J Clin Nutr.* 2009;90(6):1457–1465.

> During adulthood and the elderly period, individuals remain healthier if they are able to retain most of their LBM through exercise and physical activity, even if they gain some fat mass.

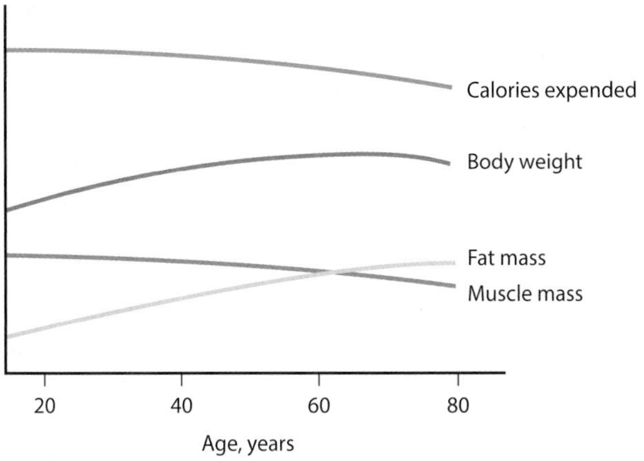

FIGURE 11.2 Percent (%) Change in Body Composition Over the Life Span.

Reproduced from Anderson JJB. *Nutrition and Health: An Introduction.* Durham, NC: Carolina Academic Press; 2005.

adulthood Period of life beginning after the conclusion of skeletal growth (height) (approximately age 18 to 20 years in females and 20 to 22 years in males). The main divisions are early adulthood from 20 to 30 years of age and later adulthood up to age 60.

dual-energy x-ray absorptiometry (DXA) A scan of bone and soft tissues of the body by a machine that uses two energy sources of x-rays to separate measurements of bone from soft tissues (i.e., adipose tissue). The total body scan permits estimations of mass of bone and fat, which enables the determination of lean body mass (primarily muscle). DXA is used to measure bone mineral content (BMC) and bone mineral density (BMD).

PRACTICAL APPLICATIONS 11.1

Body Composition Changes with Weight Gain

DXA measurements provide estimates of LBM, fat mass, and bone mass in metric units (i.e., kilograms). By subtracting the sum of the bone mass plus fat mass from total body mass (weight) of an individual, you obtain muscle mass (or LBM) by difference.

Changes in size (mass) of the three main body compartments reveal a great deal about a person's typical eating and exercise patterns over time, considering the various stages of the life cycle. The so-called ideal man weighs 70 kilograms, but most adult men in the United States today typically weigh well over 70 kilograms. Let's assume that a 22-year-old, 6-foot male graduate student, who spends much of his time at a computer, weighs 100 kilograms. He states that he has gained quite a bit of weight over the last few years because he has been less physically active. First, calculate his BMI and state the weight classification range (optimal BMI range is 18.5 to 25) he falls in. Then, based on his DXA-derived LBM of 65 kilograms, bone mass of 2 kilograms, and body fat mass of 33 kilograms, estimate his body fat mass as a percentage of total body mass. In late adolescence, this man weighed 70 kilograms, 10 kilograms of which was fat. Based on this information, which of the man's three main body compartments shows the greatest percentage increase? Briefly explain what happened to his body composition over the period from adolescence to early adulthood. ■

> *Sarcopenia and osteopenia, along with increased body fat, represent major changes in body composition in late life that are risk factors for chronic diseases and death.*

Excessive gains in fat mass lead to obesity. Obese adults are at increased risk for many chronic diseases, in particular type 2 diabetes and cardiovascular diseases. They are also at increased risk for breast cancer and a few other cancers. Obese individuals also generally have decreased respiratory function, which means oxygen delivery to tissues is reduced. Obese individuals are also at greater risk of developing sleep apnea and osteoarthritis.

The Elderly

All three major components of body composition change in the **elderly**. Continuing declines in LBM, which is reflected by **sarcopenia** (loss of muscle mass), and relatively greater fat mass are usually apparent among the elderly. In the old-old elderly (beyond age 80 years), however, body weight may decline even more, reflecting significant losses of the fat mass as well as continuing, but smaller, losses of LBM.

Loss in height typically occurs in this older segment of the population as vertebral bone mass declines and the vertebrae begin to crush against each other. Also, the bone mass of the appendicular (limbs) skeleton continues to decrease. Thus, sarcopenia and **osteopenia** (low bone mass), along with increased body fat, represent major changes in body composition in late life that are risk factors for chronic diseases and death.

In many elderly individuals, fat mass may represent more than 50% of total body weight. Bone mass continues to decline among the elderly and may be classified as either osteopenia or osteoporosis based on the degree of bone loss. Bone mass retention may be aided by increased intakes (or use of supplements) of both calcium and vitamin D when diets are deficient in these micronutrients and probably in most other nutrients as well (i.e., state of undernutrition). Bone mass and bone quality may be enhanced by increased physical activity, especially activities that stress the skeletal muscle groups (and bones) of the upper body through modest resistance exercises. Muscle strength has been improved immensely in old-old men (nonagenarians) by modest strength exercises. Aerobic activities, such as walking, improve both endurance and longevity. Therefore, both LBM and bone mass may be maintained and possibly improved in the elderly by regular strength activities.

elderly period The period after adulthood from about 60 years to the end of life. The young-old (early elderly) includes those ages 60 to 80 years; the old-old (late elderly) includes those from 80 to 100 years. Centenarians are those 100 years and older.

sarcopenia Age-related loss of muscle mass. It usually begins around age 45, when muscle mass begins to decline at a rate of about 1% per year.

osteopenia Low bone mass; a precursor to osteoporosis. Defined by the World Health Organization (WHO) as a bone mineral density (BMD) 1.0 to 2.5 standard deviations (SDs) below that of healthy 20 to 29 year olds.

Obesity continues to be highly prevalent among the elderly. Even if an elderly person eats reasonably well, the ratio of fat to lean mass typically continues to increase because of limited physical activity and exercise. Low LBM is associated with a reduction in the basal metabolic rate (BMR) at any stage of adult life. Because the elderly need to maintain their LBM for survival, dieting for weight loss is generally not recommended. Loss of LBM, as reflected by sarcopenia, is itself a risk factor for death during the later years of life.

> Because the elderly need to maintain their LBM for survival, dieting for weight loss is generally not recommended.

Nutritional Needs of Children and Adolescents

Energy and protein supply the building materials required by the hormone-driven growth rates early in life. Many micronutrients also support this growth. The RDAs for micronutrients are reasonable guidelines that will support growth during the first two decades of life.

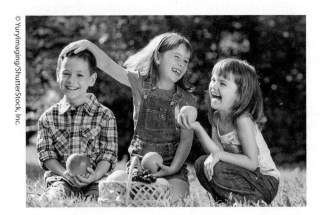

© YuryImaging/ShutterStock, Inc.

Growth Charts

The weight of children and adolescents should be monitored frequently in order to avoid underweight or overweight for height and age. The growth patterns of children between 1 and 3 years are represented by values of weight and height plotted on charts against age. Graphs of weight for height (with no age dimension) may also be useful in assessing the pattern of growth of young children. The growth patterns of older children and adolescents are also monitored by standardized charts that provide percentiles as guides. Regular checkups by a pediatrician or family physician should permit detection of abnormal growth patterns (curves on charts) and allow the institution of needed corrective steps. Adequate nutritional intakes are very important during the developmental period of life from birth to 18 to 20 years. See Appendix E.

Appetite and Eating Patterns

In general, **appetite** is the best guide for food consumption by children, especially during the years of rapid growth, but appropriate selection of foods and of modest food serving sizes remain important. Routine physical activity, of course, helps to stimulate appetite. Normal, active, growing children may eat almost anything in sight or they may be very selective about their food choices. The quantity of food intake and, hence, energy consumption, are controlled by mechanisms that generally serve to meet the body's needs, assuming adequate amounts of food energy are available. The diets of all children should be designed to provide adequate amounts of energy, protein and other macronutrients, and micronutrients. If intakes do not approach RDA levels, a

> In general, appetite is the best guide for food consumption by children, especially during the years of rapid growth, but appropriate selection of foods and of modest food serving sizes remain important.

appetite The desire to obtain and consume food. The appetite center in the brain, along with a satiety center, controls food intake. It is also influenced by external cues whether true hunger exists or not.

> ❝ Breakfast also is critical for growing children because intakes of foods at breakfast enable children to concentrate better on tasks and, in general, to learn better. ❞

> ❝ Affluence, which is often characterized by ample food availability, poor dietary habits, and too little physical activity, contributes to the overweight status and poor fitness of a large percentage of U.S. children. ❞

adolescence Period of life beginning at puberty (ending of childhood) and continuing until skeletal development is complete (i.e., approximately 11 to 18 years of age for females and 13 to 20 years for males).

TABLE 11.2
Food Guidelines for Children

- Include a variety of foods from each of the major foods groups.
- Minimize eating out at fast-food restaurants.
- Encourage selection of fresh fruits and vegetables as snacks.
- Provide adequate energy and nutrients, including fluids, to support normal growth.
- Reduce foods that contain large amounts of fat and cholesterol.
- Limit sugary drinks and snacks, salty foods, and processed foods.
- Model and encourage other healthy lifestyle habits, such as engaging in regular physical activity and abstaining from smoking and excessive alcohol.
- Monitor body weight to avoid overweight and prevent obesity.

---

nutritionist or physician should be consulted and a daily supplement of vitamins, iron, and other minerals at 100% of the RDAs may be recommended. Reasonable guidelines for food consumption (types of foods in servings) for children are listed in **Table 11.2**.

Preschoolers and young schoolchildren require a substantial breakfast to get an early start in meeting the daily growth requirements for energy, protein and other macronutrients, micronutrients, water, and phytochemicals. The breaking of the overnight fast is critical for children. Because most growth occurs while children sleep, by morning they have largely exhausted their glycogen stores. Breakfast also is critical for growing children because intakes of foods at breakfast enable children to concentrate better on tasks and, in general, to learn better. According to recent studies, adolescents also generally do better in school and other activities when they start the day with breakfast. Breakfast is less critical for adults because they are no longer growing and they typically obtain sufficient amounts of energy, if not more, during a day.

Some of the problems that U.S. parents face are the constant introduction of new food products for children in the supermarket, the conflicting nutritional messages in the media and advertising, and changing lifestyles that are so common in advanced societies. Therefore, dietary habits of children are continuously evolving. Affluence, which often is characterized by ample food availability, poor dietary habits, and too little physical activity, contributes to the overweight status and poor fitness of a large percentage of U.S. children.

Food habits during **adolescence** are frequently criticized. Adolescents often eat at irregular times, consume too much fast food, accept too many fad diets, and eat a limited variety of foods. Although many teens have poor food habits, their growth rates (height) often are not adversely affected. However, limited amounts of physical activity may negatively impact an adolescent's ability to achieve optimal skeletal growth.

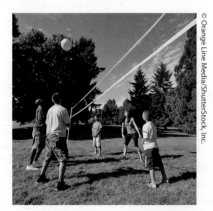

© Orange Line Media/ShutterStock, Inc.

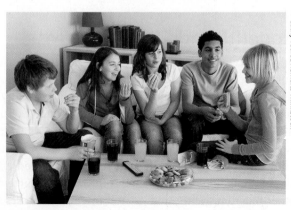

© Cathy Yeulet/Hemera/Thinkstock

Because adolescents are still growing, they tend to snack more often than other age groups in order to get enough calories. This increased snacking helps to meet adolescents' energy and protein needs to sustain growth. Today, American adolescents have achieved high growth standards, on average, compared with many other developed countries. Achievement of maximal height depends on an optimal supply of protein and energy, plus micronutrients, for sustaining the adolescent growth spurt. Thus, even though food habits may not be ideal, they are sufficiently good to meet the demands of growth. If energy intakes, however, are not coupled with energy expenditure, excessive weight accumulation will likely occur.

Energy and Protein Needs

The body's energy and protein requirements are met by the meals and snacks consumed during a 24-hour period. A regular pattern of eating on most days should provide all the nutrients and energy needed if sound food choices are made based on the USDA's MyPlate food guidance system. Energy (calorie) intakes by healthy weight and obese children and adolescents aged 1 to 17 years are shown in **FIGURE 11.3**. The mean energy intake of boys of healthy weight peaks at 15 to 16 years of age; it peaks earlier for girls at ages 10 to 11. Mean intake then declines with approaching adulthood. For energy, intakes closely approximate RDAs (kilocalories per kilogram body weight) for both sexes after adolescence.

The patterns of protein intake of boys and girls are similar to those of caloric intake, but actual mean protein intakes always exceed the sex-specific RDAs through age 19. This pattern of excessive protein intake continues across the adult years.

Energy and protein needs vary at different ages, and the RDAs are really "best guestimates" during the first two decades of life. The RDAs for energy and protein throughout the life cycle are provided in **Table 11.3**. Recommendations for energy and protein have been set to reflect gender differences in body size (weight and height) and developmental patterns (girls achieve their maximal height earlier than boys).

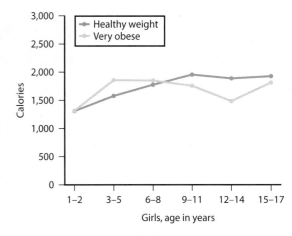

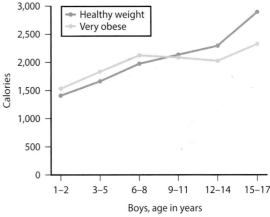

FIGURE 11.3 Energy Intakes by Children and Adolescents Ages 1 to 17 Years. Energy intakes increase from childhood through adolescence.

Data from Skinner AC, Steiner MJ, Perrin EM. Self-reported energy intake by age in overweight and healthy-weight children in NHANES 2001–2008. *Pediatrics*. 2012;130(4):e936–e942.

TABLE 11.3
RDAs for Energy and Protein for Children and Adolescents

Age	Energy (kcal per day)		Protein (grams per day)	
	Male	**Female**	**Male**	**Female**
1–2 years	1,046	992	13	13
3–8 years	1,742	1,642	19	19
9–13 years	2,279	2,071	34	34
14–18 years	3,152	2,368	52	46
> 18 years	3,067	2,403	56	46

Data from Food and Nutrition Board, Institute of Medicine. *Dietary Reference Intakes for Energy, Carbohydrate, Fiber, Fat, Fatty Acids, Cholesterol, Protein, and Amino Acids (Macronutrients) (2005)*. Washington, DC: National Academies Press; 2005.

> The mean energy intake of boys peaks at 15 to 16 years of age; it peaks earlier for girls at ages 10 to 11.

> Average intakes of calcium and iron of girls are much less than the RDAs after 11 years of age.

TABLE 11.4
RDAs for Calcium and Iron Across the Life Cycle

Age	Calcium (mg)		Iron (mg)	
	Male	Female	Male	Female
1–3 years	700	700	7	7
4–8 years	1,000	1,000	10	10
9–13 years	1,300	1,300	8	8
14–18 years	1,300	1,300	11	15
19–50 years	1,000	1,000	8	18
51–70 years	1,000	1,200	8	8
> 70 years	1,200	1,200	8	8

Data from Food and Nutrition Board, Institute of Medicine. *Dietary Reference Intakes.* Washington, DC: National Academies Press; 2001, 2011.

Micronutrient Intakes: Calcium and Iron

The recommended intakes of calcium and iron for children are provided in **Table 11.4**. Calcium needs are greatest during periods of rapid skeletal growth; that is, during childhood and adolescence. Iron needs are typically greater in menstruating girls and in boys who are building muscle.

Average intakes of calcium and iron by girls are much less than the RDAs after 11 years of age. For nearly all other micronutrients, girls' intakes meet or exceed the recommendations. The RDAs for calcium remain nearly the same for males and females across the life cycle despite the emergence of significant differences in body weight of the two genders beginning at age 11. The average intakes of most micronutrients of boys generally exceed the age-specific recommendations.

Nutritional Problems in Children and Adolescents

Energy imbalances and nutritional deficiencies can cause problems in growing and developing children and adolescents. In developed countries, an overabundance of high-calorie, low-nutrient foods is contributing to an increased incidence in overweight and obesity. At the same time, some adolescents are so concerned about their weight that they develop eating disorders in an effort to maintain what they perceive to be an ideal body weight. The situation in poor countries is much different. In poor, developing nations, children suffer from limited intakes of protein and energy, resulting in deficiency diseases that stunt growth and development.

Overweight and Obesity

Childhood obesity, like obesity among the adult population, is becoming more prevalent in the United States. Poor food habits and limited activity remain the major determinants. By adolescence, 15% to 20% of teens are estimated as being overweight or obese, according to the BMI cutoffs. This high estimate is an incredible figure!

Although the factors that contribute to childhood obesity have not been fully established, it seems to be rooted in family behavioral patterns, both in eating habits and in patterns of activity. Some snacking is acceptable, but large amounts of nutrient-poor foods can contribute to energy imbalance, and thus excess weight gain.

Low levels of physical activity, i.e., **sedentary lifestyle**, among children are prevalent. The evidence is mounting that sedentary activities such as watching television and playing computer games are a major factor in the development of obesity. In the United States, children, on average, watch almost 6 hours of television programming a day, and while watching they are often snacking, putting them on the path of becoming sedentary "couch potatoes." Sedentary lifestyle patterns are related to family and cultural habits, which schools and other social institutions cannot entirely counteract through physical education classes, sports programs, gymnastics schools, dance studios, scouting, and activities of other clubs and organizations.

> In the United States, children, on average, watch almost 6 hours of television programming a day, and while watching they are often snacking.

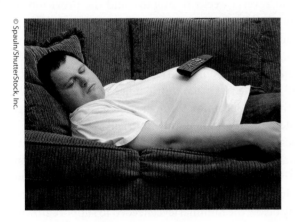

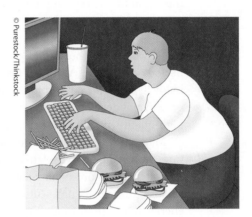

If both parents are obese, chances are high that their children will also become obese. The risk is lower if only one parent is obese, and it is very low if neither parent is obese. A family's eating and activity patterns greatly influence weight accumulation by children, whether the critical factors are hereditary or environmental. Environmental rather than genetic factors are likely the largest contributor to obesity in affluent societies. In 90% to 95% of obese American children the primary cause of obesity can be attributed to environmental factors.

Recommendations for reducing the risk of obesity in children emphasize more activity and fewer calories—that is, more foot and less fork. If a parent or caregiver recognizes that a child or adolescent is overweight or obese, professional help may be needed to improve the child's food habits, to adjust portion sizes, and to promote routine physical activity. Many specific changes are recommended, such as having less food available at the table for the child, reducing portion sizes, instituting a program of regular physical activity, and involving all household members in assisting the overweight child in efforts to control weight. The key step here is to modify eating and activity patterns that have contributed to the overweight or obesity. Early intervention for the purposes of weight reduction and increasing physical activity is strongly recommended for optimal long-term health benefits and for minimizing the possible risks of chronic diseases often associated with obesity during adulthood.

> In 90% to 95% of obese American children the primary cause of obesity can be attributed to environmental factors.

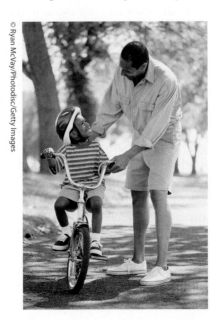

sedentary lifestyle Lifestyle characterized by low levels of physical actively. Believed to be a key factor in the development of obesity.

> The major clinical differences between these two disorders of undernutrition—marasmus and kwashiorkor—relate to the amount and quality of protein available in their diets as infants and young children.

> Undernourished children do not defend well against infectious diseases, which contribute greatly to the much higher morbidity and mortality rates in the developing world.

parenteral nutrition The delivery of nutrition to patients who cannot use their guts, typically by a venous catheter; also known as intravenous feeding or nutrition.

immune response The body's response to foreign agents, especially microorganisms (bacteria, viruses) and parasites, through the actions of lymphocytes and other cells, the production of immunoglobulins and cytokines, as well as the activation of diverse cells (lymphocytes and others) by antigens or foreign cells. The immune response is greatly blunted if nutrients are inadequate.

malnutrition–infection cycle The circular sequence starting with poor nutrition, especially among infants and young children, that leads to an infectious disease that, in turn, enhances malnutrition. This cycle may possibly even lead to death.

Deficiencies in Protein and Energy Intake

Undernutrition of a *severe* nature results in marasmus or kwashiorkor (or an intermediary form between these two forms). These two extreme forms of undernutrition are characterized by balanced undernutrition (marasmus) or unbalanced undernutrition (kwashiorkor). Marasmus is also known as protein–energy malnutrition, whereas kwashiorkor is the disorder that results from sufficient energy intake but lack of protein. Although these deficiency diseases remain quite rare among young children in North America, cases nevertheless do appear from time to time because of poverty, poor parental care, or for other reasons. The discovery of such cases should result in prompt medical intervention with the administration of intravenous nutrition or **parenteral nutrition** (bypass of the GI tract) in a hospital or clinic. Recovery from these conditions typically takes from several weeks to months, and the provision of nutrition education of the mother or caregiver is essential.

These disorders are far more common, even routine, in some developing nations of the world, and their numbers are greatly increased during war, drought, and other periods of disaster. Although protein is not the only nutrient deficient in the diets of many living in the developing world, it is the key macronutrient needed for reasonable growth and development from the time of conception through adolescence. (Note that high-quality protein foods also contain many essential micronutrients.)

Many developing nations are located on or near the equator. Because of their location, these nations have relatively limited amounts of land available for crop production and often have poor quality soils. The crops that can be easily produced by farmers in these countries are, unfortunately, low in protein but high in energy. The protein-to-energy ratio of these foods is typically below the minimal level needed to support growth early in life. Furthermore, animal livestock production is not generally practiced in most of these areas, and fish or seafood cultivation is limited or nonexistent.

Foods from equatorial countries, such as rice, cassava, yams, and plantains (see **FIGURE 11.4**), have low quantities of protein relative to their total caloric content. For this reason, many children of the developing world get too little dietary protein relative to energy, and they too often grow inadequately in height (i.e., become short and stunted). Children with inadequate protein often have short legs and arms relative to their trunk. Many develop clinically evident kwashiorkor or marasmus. The number of severe cases of these protein–energy disorders represents only the tip of the iceberg of the total number of children who suffer from moderate or mild subclinical forms of kwashiorkor and marasmus in the developing world. The major clinical differences between these two disorders of undernutrition relate to the amount and quality of protein available in their diets as infants and young children.

Undernutrition and Risk of Infectious Diseases

The presence of undernutrition in infants and children makes them far more vulnerable to the infectious diseases of childhood caused by bacteria and viruses. They have a poor **immune response** to infection. Undernourished children do not defend well against infectious diseases, which contribute greatly to the much higher childhood morbidity and mortality rates in the developing world. For example, measles, a viral disease of no great consequence among American children, has deadly consequences among undernourished children of developing nations in Africa because of nutritionally induced immune suppression. In equatorial Africa and South Asia, infectious diseases are more prevalent because of poor nutrient intakes, in particular vitamin A and zinc. Low intakes of vitamin A (or carotenoids), for example, have very adverse effects on the body's immune defenses against viruses and bacteria.

The relationship between undernutrition and depressed resistance to infection is often called the **malnutrition–infection cycle**. In this cycle, inadequate nutrition

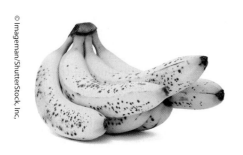
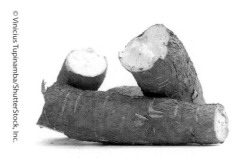

© Imageman/ShutterStock, Inc.

© Vinicius Tupinamba/ShutterStock, Inc.

FIGURE 11.4 Equatorial Food Crops. Many foods grown in equatorial regions are good sources of energy, but poor sources of protein. People who rely on bananas (left) rice, yams, cassava (right), and plantains as their primary food sources are at greater risk for developing a protein-deficiency disease.

depresses the response of the immune system to the invading organisms. The body, when sick, responds by lowering appetite, lowering the absorptive efficiency of ingested nutrients, decreasing the utilization of nutrients that are absorbed, and mobilizing and wasting the body's stored nutrients in tissues through an increase in excretion. These deficits, in turn, lower resistance. This cycle of depressed **immunity** coupled with poor diet can be represented as a reinforcing circle, with death as a potential end result (see **FIGURE 11.5**). Poor sanitation and poor diet drive the cycle around.

Diet and Dental Caries in Children and Adolescents

The process of tooth decay begins with the formation of bacterial colonies on the surface of teeth. These colonies are referred to as **dental plaque**. The bacteria in these plaques degrade the carbohydrates in food, especially retentive (sticky) sugars, to acids, which lowers the pH of the fluids in the oral cavity. The plaque enhances the tooth decay process by keeping the acid within the structure and adjacent to the tooth surface. First, the **enamel** is degraded or etched after many successive attacks by the acid and then the surface of the underlying mineral or apatite is dissolved. The result is caries, more commonly known as cavities. Caries directly result from bacterial infection of the oral cavity. They must be cleaned out and filled or teeth will be lost eventually from severe decay.

Diet has a major effect on the development of dental caries. The wise selection of tooth-healthy foods and beverages may have a large impact in reducing caries, whereas the choice of cariogenic foods enhances tooth surface defects. Sticky retentive sugars are the most cariogenic. Many sugar-based soft drinks also are cariogenic in principle, but the fluid resides so briefly in the oral cavity that they are only mildly cariogenic. Milk that remains in the mouth for long periods, such as in babies with bottles continuously

> The relation between undernutrition and depressed resistance to infection is often called the malnutrition–infection cycle.

immunity Innate and acquired immunity refers to antibodies (immunoglobulins) circulating in the blood either through natural production (innate) of nonspecific antibodies or through the stimulation by infecting organisms of the production of specific antibodies (acquired). Also includes temporary immunity or passive acquired immunity against infection obtained by giving preformed antibodies by injection, such as used in the prophylactic control of flu epidemics.

dental plaque Plaque formed by bacterial colonies on tooth surfaces.

enamel The hard outer layer of teeth that contains a highly ordered array of the mineral, hydroxyapatite. Can be strengthened by fluoride.

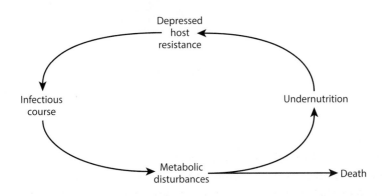

FIGURE 11.5 Undernutrition–Infection Cycle in Infants and Young Children.

in their mouths, is highly cariogenic. Any sweet fluids such as milk, juices, or soft drinks in baby bottles may contribute to caries. Fruits and vegetables rich in dietary fiber tend to be anticariogenic, but caution is needed about the sugars in many fruits. Finally, consistent dental hygiene—tooth cleaning, tooth brushing, flossing, fluoride treatment, and possibly other procedures—remain highly protective against the typical soft, highly processed diets consumed in North America, and other Western nations.

Periodontal disease, another problem related to diet and the oral tissues, refers to dysfunction of the gums and underlying tissues. In the case of poor oral hygiene and perhaps a poor diet, mineralized plaque or calculus resulting from bacterial activity collects on the teeth surfaces and penetrates the gums. Bacteria, then, also penetrate the gums or gingiva and lead to inflammation of the gums (gingivitis). If gingivitis persists, it can lead to a loosening of the tooth, loss of both hard tissue (bone) of the jaws (localized osteopenia) and soft oral tissue, and possibly the loss of one or more teeth.

Several factors contribute to caries. The prevention of further plaque formation, especially with topical fluorides, brushing, and flossing, will reduce or eliminate the recurrence of decay. Prevention of caries is best achieved by proper dental hygiene and a good diet. The dietary steps for the control of bacteria include: (1) eating a well-balanced diet containing all nutrients, which help maintain healthy gums (i.e., improved bacterial resistance); (2) decreasing the consumption of foods containing sugar, especially retentive sweet snacks, so the bacteria are denied their energy substrates; (3) using fluorides regularly to strengthen the tooth enamel; and (4) frequently consuming tooth-protective foods (i.e., firm foods that have a detergent effect on the teeth), such as raw vegetables and fruits. Plenty of fluids are also needed for rinsing the teeth and gums and, hence, for dental health.

Thus, good oral hygiene and proper eating habits (quantity, quality, and frequency or QQF) are important for healthy teeth and oral tissues, such as the gums and underlying connective tissue and bone. Some individuals may wish to keep a food diary of all consumption, particularly sweet snacks and foods with "hidden sugars" (read labels).

> **"** Prevention of caries is best carried out by proper dental hygiene and a good diet. **"**

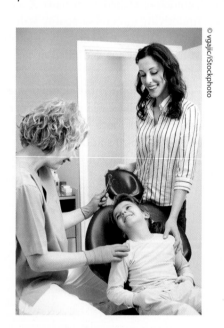

© vgajic/iStockphoto

periodontal disease Dysfunction of the gums and underlying tissues. Often related to poor diet.

Eating Disorders: Anorexia Nervosa and Bulimia Nervosa

Early adolescence (right around the time of puberty) is the period when eating disorders—primarily anorexia nervosa and bulimia—are most likely to develop. Adolescents' eating habits sometimes go astray, leading to poor intakes and other behaviors that counter the

FOCUS 11.1 The Vipeholm Study of Sugar-Related Dental Caries

A 5-year nutritional study of caries in over 400 adult patients at a mental institution (Vipeholm) in Sweden was undertaken to study the effects of frequency and retentiveness of sugar intake (or cariogenic diets) on the formation of dental caries. Both frequency and retentiveness were shown to increase the number of caries. **FIGURE A** shows the basic findings of this famous dental caries study. Some of the steps considered essential in the process of caries formation include bacterial culture or growth on the retentive nutrients (food-related or candy energy sources) and the generation of plaque, a polysaccharide, on the specific surface; the tough plaque serves as a protective shield for the bacterial colony. The colony of bacteria that adheres to the tooth surface is essential for this decay process. They stick to the surface because of the polysaccharide they secrete that becomes an umbrella-like plaque protecting the bacteria and the acid they secrete. ●

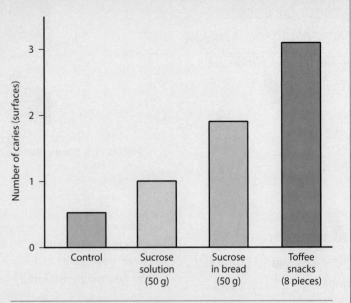

FIGURE A Vipeholm Study of Sugar-Related Dental Caries.

Reproduced from Anderson JJB. *Nutrition and Health: An Introduction.* Durham, NC: Carolina Academic Press; 2005.

---

benefits of the nutrients (i.e., vomiting or purging). Serious psychological problems and other behaviors contribute to the development of eating disorders; however, other factors also play important roles in the development of these disorders, including heredity.

Anorexia nervosa most commonly develops among postpubertal girls and may continue throughout adolescence and the remainder of life. **Anorexia** literally means loss of appetite. When girls gain weight, including new accumulation of fat, in association with reproductive development and the onset of regular menstrual cycles, they may skip meals to avoid gaining more weight and body fat. If they dislike their body's appearance, they may use drugs or induce vomiting to shed body fat. If this destructive pattern, which also may include not getting along with one or both parents, becomes so significant that they begin to lose too much weight and fat, anorexia nervosa will result—and it is accompanied by **amenorrhea**. The psychological effects of anorexia nervosa are said to last for the remainder of a person's life! Although much less common among males, they, too, can develop anorexia because of a strong dislike of their body image.

Those who are active in sports and activities that focus on body image, such as dance, gymnastics, cheerleading, and others, are at higher risk for developing anorexia nervosa. The causes are many and difficult to trace, but are thought to include family conditions, social environment, and issues of self-image. The incidence of anorexia nervosa varies significantly by ethnicity and country; the incidence is highest among middle-class white girls in affluent societies exposed to media images of very thin ideal women such as models and actresses.

Anorexia nervosa is not only a serious psychological problem, but it also has severe health effects because of the undernutrition that results. The dietary treatments for

anorexia nervosa A psychological disorder characterized by refusal to eat, extreme weight loss, loss of menstrual cycles, and depressed gonadotropin hormones.

anorexia A loss of appetite that is often, though not necessarily, associated with severe reduction in body weight for any reason, such as occurs in many cancer patients.

amenorrhea Never beginning menstrual cycles (primary amenorrhea) or absence of menstrual cycles for at least three consecutive months (secondary amenorrhea).

Anorexia nervosa is not only a serious psychological problem, but it also has severe health effects because of the undernutrition that results.

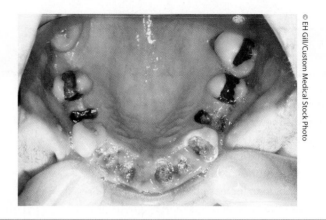

© EH Gill/Custom Medical Stock Photo

FIGURE 11.6 Effect of Bulimia on Dental Health. Bulimia can have devastating effects on dental health because of the corrosive actions of stomach acids on the tooth enamel.

Because bulimia nervosa is not so physically noticeable and typically occurs later in life, it is widely suspected that the condition is underreported and underestimated.

anorexia nervosa are secondary to the psychological and social causes and eventual primary psychological treatments. The usual treatment for anorexia nervosa is multifaceted and usually includes counseling, medications, and careful dietary regimens as well as counseling for family and friends. Recovery is slow and difficult. In extreme cases, anorexia nervosa may result in death.

Similarly, **bulimia nervosa** typically develops during the adolescent years, in both boys and girls, but it takes on a different pattern in girls because of their greater concern about body fat and therefore body image. Whereas anorexia nervosa is a condition of extreme undereating, bulimia is a condition of purging and vomiting. Bulimia is typically a cyclic condition. A person, usually a woman, will try to diet to keep her weight down and then during a period of stress or depression or some other trigger the dieter will give in and overindulge to an extreme extent. At this point, she will consume thousands of calories as fast as she can, often as cookies and cake or other soft, yummy foods. She will quickly regret this and force herself to throw up (vomit) her food or purge with **laxatives**. After recovering, she will go back on the diet, and the cycle starts again.

Obviously, this pattern is oversimplified, and no single person with this condition acts it out in the same manner. Several commonalities should be noted though. Most bulimics are near normal weight because this type of cycling balances out the dieting and purging. Many bulimics are discovered by their dentists because the corrosive stomach acids from repeated vomiting etch the teeth and may cause massive tooth decay (see **FIGURE 11.6**). As opposed to anorexics, many bulimics start these cycles later in life in their 20s and 30s and even later. Because bulimia nervosa is not so physically noticeable and typically occurs later in life than anorexia nervosa, it is widely suspected that the condition is underreported and underestimated. The usual treatment for this psychological problem is similar to that for anorexia: counseling, possible medication, and a very carefully guided dietary regimen.

Nutritional Needs of Adults

Sound dietary principles based on consuming a certain number of servings from each of the major food groups every day holds for adults as well as for all other age groups. Nutrient adequacy is met by eating a variety of foods in reasonably planned meals on a fairly regular basis. Coupled with regular physical activity, sound food habits promote good health and prevent the development of disease.

bulimia nervosa A psychological disorder characterized by bingeing and purging.

laxative Food components, such as dietary fiber, or over-the-counter formulations that enhance the flow of the contents of the large bowel (colon) toward elimination.

The Transition from Adolescence to Young Adulthood

Adolescent food habits tend to be replaced by healthier selections in early adult life because of changes in lifestyle and increased personal responsibilities, such as jobs and family considerations. During this early period of adulthood—that is, the childbearing years of 20 to 35 for women and a similar period for men—good food habits may improve one's health status. For women, pregnancy and lactation, of course, increase demands for energy, protein, and micronutrients as part of healthy eating patterns.

Similarly, late adolescent and young adult men benefit from improved food habits, but they typically become more sedentary and no longer participate in regular physical activities as they age. Because their "appetites" for foods usually remain the same as during their more active years, men commonly gain weight at a high rate during the period from about 25 to 34 years of age. Women usually follow this trend a decade or so later. The point is that early life food habits, especially during the teenage years, often turn into adult patterns of excessive food energy consumption relative to the body's physical expenditures of energy. Binge eating and consuming too much high-fat or high-sugar foods, often with alcohol, may become commonplace. A **binge-eating disorder** may emerge in some individuals who consume excessive amounts of food without any control. Intelligent food choices in modest servings can be learned and practiced by young adults as part of a healthy dietary pattern, especially when coupled with regular physical activities or workouts.

A variety of dietary patterns are available to consumers in North America, ranging from low-carbohydrate to high-carbohydrate diets, among others, but the diet that really counts is the one an individual can reasonably consume over a lifetime and stay healthy! Apart from the rare exceptions for genetic and familial factors, most people have considerable control over their own destinies with respect to the health and disease continuum by having good habits or by modifying bad habits. The locus of control, thus, resides to a great extent in each one of us. Beyond the availability of good health care, sound food habits, without the use of supplements, linked with regular physical activity and the practice of healthy behaviors should herald an adult life with minimal concerns about chronic diseases.

Energy and Protein Intake

Adults require energy and protein to maintain optimal health. Energy intake typically decreases with age because of declines in physical activity. This consequently leads to a decline in lean body mass (LBM). Protein intake, however, remains fairly high throughout adult life, providing essential amino acids needed by the immune system and for tissue replacement in organs and tissues, especially skeletal tissue and heart muscle.

Nutrient Intake Patterns

Macronutrient consumption percentages for U.S. adults are fairly consistent across the adult years. Carbohydrate intakes range between 49% and 53%, and fat intakes between 32% and 34% of calorie intake. The 15% to 17% of energy derived from protein during the adult years for both males and females is slightly higher than recommended. Alcohol consumption represents only 1% to 5% of energy intake, though a fraction of consumers may drink much more alcohol because so many adults consume no alcohol at all.

A recent analysis of American eating patterns over a 30-year period revealed that practically all socioeconomic and racial groups have been eating reasonably high-quality diets, as compared with recommended macronutrient guidelines, including more recent trends of decreased consumption of total fat and saturated fat. Nevertheless, data also show that practically all U.S. adults consume too few fruits and vegetables on a daily

> Late adolescent and young adult men benefit from improved food habits, but they typically become more sedentary and no longer participate in regular physical activities. Men commonly gain weight at a high rate during the period from about 25 to 34 years of age.

> The 15% to 17% of energy derived from protein during the adult years is slightly higher than recommended.

binge-eating disorder (BED) An eating disorder characterized by excessive eating without control.

PRACTICAL APPLICATIONS 11.2

Percentage Energy Composition of Macronutrients in a Sample Adult Diet

Consider a 50-year-old woman who consumes a diet that includes carbohydrates (180 grams), fats (80 grams), and proteins (40 grams) from plant sources only. Her vegan diet includes no alcoholic beverages. Using Atwater equivalents, calculate the percentages of total kilocalories of carbohydrate, fat, and protein in her diet. How do her percentages compare with the range of recommended percentages for the U.S. population? Explain. Can a plant-based diet provide a proper balance of the macronutrients? ■

basis. Despite the reasonable quality of the diet of the U.S. population over the last few decades, overweight and obesity have climbed steeply.

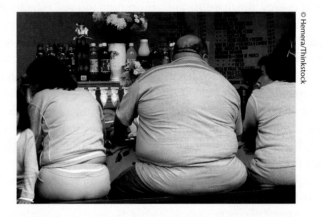

© Hemera/Thinkstock

> "Since the early twentieth century, the age of menopause has been delayed or extended by 5 to 7 years, presumably because of better nutrition."

Calcium intake for females typically falls to below the RDAs after age 11, but after age 20 calcium intakes have relatively little effect on bone mass. Starting in the perimenopausal years, women's needs for iron fall to approximately the same amounts recommended for men.

Nutrition and Menopause

A significant physiologic change that affects adult women is menopause. **Menopause** is the total cessation of menstrual cycling that occurs in a woman's late 40s or early 50s. This natural physiologic event represents the end of a woman's reproductive capability and period of ovarian secretion of **estrogens**. In the United States, the average age of menopause is currently 52 years. Since the early twentieth century, the age of menopause has been delayed or extended by 5 to 7 years, presumably because of better nutrition. Improved nutrient intakes, based largely on high-quality protein sources and micronutrient fortifications, support not only general health but also the functioning of the ovaries for 35 to 40 years in Western nations as part of the **hypothalamic-pituitary-ovarian (H-P-O) axis**. Diet has little or no influence on menopause itself—nutrition is only responsible for the delay of it.

The menopausal transition, which may last for several years, is typically characterized by increased body temperature accompanied by sweating (i.e., "hot flashes" or "night sweats"), insomnia, irritability, mood changes, and other effects. Weight gain also usually occurs at this time. All of these effects result from the loss of estrogens and possibly of progesterone.

Estrogen replacement therapy (ERT) alone may correct almost all of the adverse effects resulting from menopause, but endometrial tissue functions more normally when

menopause The cessation of menstruation and ovarian production of estrogens and progestins and the physiological changes in organ systems such that a woman can no longer become pregnant. Usually occurs in women of ages 45 to 55.

estrogens Female sex hormones. Natural estrogens are responsible for female sexual development and play an essential role in fertility, pregnancy, and lactation.

hypothalamic-pituitary-ovarian (H-P-O) axis The complex interactions among the hypothalamus, the pituitary, and the ovary that regulate the female reproductive cycle.

a progestin, a synthetic form of progesterone, is administered along with the estrogen. The combination form of treatment is called hormone replacement therapy (HRT). Estrogens have beneficial effects on bone mass and also lower blood cholesterol concentrations. However, because ERT may increase the risk for heart disease and for breast and other reproductive cancers in postmenopausal women, this therapy is no longer recommended. Estrogen alone may still be used to help early postmenopausal women overcome their heat regulatory disturbances, but only for a few years.

The explanation for the changes in functions during menopause is a direct outcome of a decline in ovarian function. The secretion of estrogen by the **ovaries** typically begins to fall in the late 30s or early 40s, but it decreases sharply in the period immediately preceding the menopause; amenorrhea then exists. The cells of the ovaries, therefore, have built into their genetic coding a rather fixed or finite life span (~35 to 40 years) that can only be slightly modified by good nutrition. Surgical removal of the ovaries (oophorectomy), of course, produces an early artificial menopause that results in virtually the same physiological changes that are associated with natural menopause. Earlier menopause, surgical or natural, increases the risks for osteoporosis as well as for heart disease and stroke.

The reduction of circulating estrogens from the ovaries leads to elevations of total blood cholesterol in women and to increased atherogenesis and plaque formation in major arteries. These changes place postmenopausal women at greatly increased risk of heart attack and stroke. The increased fat deposition in tissues, such as the breasts, of postmenopausal women may not result from lack of estrogen so much as from excessive food energy consumption because of the loss of the "braking" effect of estrogens on the brain center controlling appetite and food intake.

A major consequence of the loss of estrogens in postmenopausal women is a more rapid rate of bone loss, known as the early postmenopausal decline in bone mass. Increases in calcium intake alone have little effect in slowing the early postmenopausal bone loss, and this limited effect of calcium intake is also true in the late adult years. During the decade following the onset of menopause, it has been estimated that women can lose from 15% to 30% of their total skeletal mass.

Even in the years prior to the menopause, during which estrogen production begins to decline, women often increase their daily intake of food (i.e., energy, other nutrients). This pattern continues past menopause for almost a decade. During this decade or longer, nearly all women gain weight, mostly abdominal fat that contributes to significant changes in body composition. The chronic diseases of women, especially cardiovascular diseases and breast cancer, increase rather sharply during the first postmenopausal decade.

Men, of course, do not experience menopause, but some scientists use the term *andropause* to signal the onset of declining production of **androgens** and general male reproductive function. The timing of andropause is highly variable, and no easily measured variables mark its onset. Therefore, andropause is extremely difficult to pinpoint, in sharp contrast to the events associated with the menopause.

> " The explanation for the changes in functions during the menopause is a direct outcome of a decline in ovarian function. "

Nutritional Needs of the Elderly

In general, in the United States the elderly have a reasonably satisfactory nutritional status, but fair percentages of them are deficient in a few specific nutrients or are even undernourished. The reasons for this common suboptimal nutritional status are diverse and are related to social, psychological, and socioeconomic factors. One of the most devastating factors contributing to adverse changes in food habits is the loss of a spouse and subsequent loneliness, including eating alone. Older people who eat alone often consume monotonous diets that may lead to nutrient deficiencies because of the limited variety of foods selected. Another important factor contributing to nutritional imbalances of older adults is limited mobility caused by disease, limited activity, or

ovary Reproductive organ that produces eggs and estrogen hormones and progestins; part of the H-P-O axis.

androgens Male sex steroid hormones responsible for male secondary sex characteristics; also present in females at lower concentrations because of its production by the adrenal cortex in both sexes. Act as growth promoters.

depressive mood. Because of a gradual decline of LBM with age, and related gradual decrements of functions of the musculoskeletal, gastrointestinal, and other systems, the elderly tend to consume less than younger adults, even though they still require balanced meals providing all the essential nutrients on a regular basis.

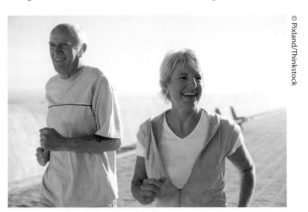

© Pixland/Thinkstock

Energy and Protein Intake

Food intake of the elderly, as represented by energy intake, is generally low and shows a significant decline in amounts over the decades from age 50 and beyond. The elderly tend to be low or deficient in total calories from the energy-providing macronutrients (except for protein) and deficient in several of the micronutrients in comparison with the RDAs. Intakes by females also tend to be generally lower relative to the sex-specific recommendations. Low energy intakes are common among many elderly. Protein intakes are typically above the RDAs for most North Americans.

Although the RDAs for energy intake for older adults are the same as for younger adults, the elderly tend to decrease their intake of food with increasing age. The decline in food consumption is related to the limited amount of daily physical activity. Body weight decreases and muscle mass tends to be replaced by fat mass in older adults.

Micronutrient Intake

Data on the nutritional status of the elderly have been collected by the USDA for many years. The mean intake of nutrients compared with the various recommended levels for men and women older than age 70 are summarized in **Table 11.5**. Actual intakes are compared with the recommended levels to yield a percentage of the recommended intake for each nutrient. Most nutrient intakes, including several not represented here, are in the adequate range, with values over 100%.

Fiber intake is inadequate in older adults. They can increase their fiber intake through increased consumption of complex carbohydrates and fruits and vegetables. Vitamin A intake is adequate and actually increases with age. Thiamin and the other B vitamins are well represented in the diets of the elderly. The one exception is folate, which is often consumed in low amounts, particularly by elderly women, and this deficit may seriously limit cellular DNA repair. Calcium intakes are also typically low, particularly compared with the latest RDA, but not as low as folate. Cobalamin intakes may also be low in some elders. Unfortunately, salt intake remains high for the elderly, as it is for other age groups. Because blood pressure tends to increase with age and taste acuity (number of taste buds) tends to decrease, limiting salt intake by the elderly is not so easy to accomplish. The elderly need adequate amounts of fluids each day, but thirst is usually the best guide.

Requirements for three micronutrients—calcium, vitamin D, and vitamin B_6 (pyridoxine)—are thought to be increased in the elderly according to their RDAs. Many older adults get little to no exposure to sunlight, especially in the winter months, which limits

Although the RDAs for energy intake for older adults are the same as for younger adults, the elderly tend to decrease their intake of food with increasing age.

Food intake of the elderly, as represented by energy intake, is generally low and shows a significant decline in amounts over the decades from age 50 and beyond.

TABLE 11.5
Intakes of Nutrients from Food as Mean Percentages of Dietary Recommendations for Adults 70 Years and Older

Nutrient	Recommended Dietary Allowance		Average Intake as a Percent (%) of Recommendation	
	Men	Women	Men	Women
Energy	3,000 kcal	2,400 kcal	64	64
Protein	56 g	46 g	133	131
Fiber	30 g	21 g	57	72
Vitamin A	625 µg	500 µg	118	122
Vitamin E	15 mg	15 mg	55	42
Vitamin C	90 mg	75 mg	100	106
Vitamin D	800 IU	800 IU	29	22
Thiamin	1.2 mg	1.1 mg	140	122
Folate (DFE)	400 µg	400 µg	142	113
Vitamin B_{12}	2 µg	2 µg	300	209
Calcium	1,200 mg	1,200 mg	75	68
Phosphorus	580 mg	580 mg	219	183
Iron	8 mg	8 mg	205	158
Sodium	1,200 mg	1,200 mg	267	216
Potassium	4,700 mg	4,700 mg	60	50

DFE = dietary folate equivalents.
Data from Food and Nutrition Board, Institute of Medicine. *Dietary Reference Intakes*. Washington, DC: National Academies Press; 1997–2011; and Moshfegh A, Goldman J, Cleveland L. (2005). *What We Eat in America, NHANES 2001–2002: Usual Nutrient Intakes from Food Compared to Dietary References Intakes*. Available at: www.ars.usda.gov/SP2UserFiles/Place/12355000/pdf/0102/usualintaketables2001-02.pdf

their skin's ability to produce vitamin D. Many elders also do not consume fortified dairy products. Therefore, during the winter months from about October to April in North America, almost all of the required vitamin D must come from foods, fortified foods, or supplements to replace the 60% or so of the RDA normally supplied by skin biosynthesis during the summer months. Vitamin K may also be underconsumed by many elderly. Vitamin K is found only in dark green, leafy vegetables that are poorly consumed by older adults. Many elderly may also need additional vitamin B_{12}, as requirements for this vitamin may be increased because of **hypochlorhydria**, reduced production of intrinsic factor, less storage in the liver, or increased degradation of the vitamin by hepatic enzymes. **Achlorhydria** also may occur in some elders. Older adults also benefit from greater intake of antioxidant nutrients from foods than currently are recommended in order to defend against free radicals.

hypochlorhydria Condition of too little production of hydrochloric acid (HCl) by the stomach.

achlorhydria Condition of essentially no production of hydrochloric acid (HCl) by the stomach.

Because of low total energy intakes, the consumption of many micronutrients by the elderly falls below RDA levels without supplementation. For this reason, many elderly have been recommended by their health providers to take a daily supplement containing nearly all the essential micronutrients at or near RDA levels, but not higher, as insurance against a poor diet. This practice, however, is under increasing attack.

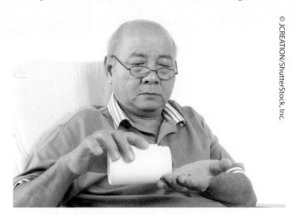

For two micronutrients, iron and vitamin A, the elderly clearly need lesser amounts than do younger adults. Too much iron can contribute to hemochromatosis among those genetically predisposed to this condition because of continuous storage. Many supplements marketed to older adults do not contain iron. Too much storage of vitamin A can lead to increased risk of hip fracture; thus, older adults should avoid taking supplements that contain vitamin A.

Recommended Dietary Allowances

Elder eating patterns need to provide sufficient nutrients to support all tissue functions. A reasonable set of nutrient guidelines for the elderly, based on the current RDAs, is given in **Table 11.6**. Note that energy and protein recommendations remain the same for the elderly as for younger adults.

The precise micronutrient requirements of the elderly, compared to younger adults, are generally not well supported by research data. An example is the setting of calcium allowances for postmenopausal women. Calcium intakes tend to be quite low among older adult and elderly women who suffer the most from skeletal fractures stemming from osteoporosis. Recent published findings show that dietary calcium has little or no effect in preventing or slowing bone loss and osteoporosis in older women, even when high intakes from supplements are ingested.

Setting separate RDAs for the elderly has been more difficult than it would seem. One major difficulty is that the elderly population is highly heterogeneous; individuals vary greatly in their energy and nutrient needs based on their activity levels and other factors. In addition, declines in GI function, especially reduced gastric acid secretion (hypochlorhydria), lead to reduced efficiencies both of digestion and absorption of most nutrients. In the elderly, it is difficult to dissociate nutrient deficiencies due to poor dietary intakes from deficiencies resulting from poor digestion and absorption of nutrients. Poor GI function may also result from declines in the mass of absorbing cells in the small intestines, due to loss of LBM, and other declines, such as in pancreatic secretions. Thus, nutrient intakes may need to be increased to compensate for the decline in GI function.

The RDAs for the elderly have historically been based on limited information or extrapolations from data obtained from young adults. Future studies will need to establish more accurately the nutrient requirements of the elderly. A new set of recommendations is currently in the process of being established for this population. Much research is currently being conducted on micronutrient needs, including antioxidants, of the elderly.

TABLE 11.6
Nutrient Recommendations for Older Adults (70 Years and Older)

Nutrient	RDA or AI (Male)	RDA or AI (Female)	Benefit or Risk of High Intake
Higher Intakes Needed			
Calcium	1,200 mg	1,200 mg	Benefits bone mass (mineral)
Vitamin D*	15 µg	15 µg	Enhances intestinal calcium absorption
Vitamin K	120 µg	90 µg	Improves bone matrix proteins
Magnesium	420 mg	320 mg	Improves enzyme activities
Zinc	11 mg	8 mg	Improves enzyme activities
Lower Intakes Needed			
Sodium	1200 mg	1200 mg	Adverse effects on calcium retention
Phosphorus	700 mg	700 mg	Adverse effects on bone turnover (calcium loss)
Iron	8 mg	8 mg	Increased risk of hemochromatosis
Vitamin A**	900 µg	700 µg	Increased risk of hip fracture

*1 µg of cholecalciferol equals 40 IU of vitamin D. ** 1 IU of vitamin A equals 0.3 µg retinol.
Data from Food and Nutrition Board, Institute of Medicine. *Dietary Reference Intakes.* Washington, DC: National Academies Press; 1997, 2000, 2004, 2011.

Supplementation

Many older adults would benefit from **supplementation**. Numerous studies have documented specific benefits from the supplementation of different nutrients. **Table 11.7** lists several nutrients for which supplemented intakes greater than the nutrient-specific RDAs have produced quantifiably or demonstrably improved physiologic functions in "healthy" elderly subjects. Those who benefit the most have very low intakes from foods,

TABLE 11.7
Benefits of Micronutrient Supplementation by the Elderly

Micronutrient	Improved Function(s)
Vitamin B_6	Aminotransferases and immune response
Vitamin D and calcium	Bone integrity and mass; reduced risk of fractures
Vitamin B_{12}	Cell renewal and cognition
Folate	Cell renewal, methyl donor, and reduced risk of cancer
Vitamin K	Osteocalcin and bone mass retention
Zinc	Many functions, including immune
Magnesium	Many functions, including heart and bone tissue
Omega-3 fatty acids	Immune defense; general

supplementation Usually purified micronutrients in pill form; nutrients consumed through the ingestion of pills or tablets for the purpose of improving nutritional status; protein and energy may also be increased by specific macronutrient supplements; supplements are distinguished from nutrient fortificants, i.e., nutrients added to foods.

typically too little intake from fruits and vegetables, i.e., they are undernourished primarily of micronutrients.

Undernutrition

Some elderly individuals living either in institutions or freely in their homes or apartments have been reported to experience malnutrition, mainly undernutrition. Several issues relating to nutrition of many elderly include poor appetite (anorexia), consumption of fewer than three meals a day, limited purchasing power, limited facilities for preparing meals, loss of transportation and mobility, loss of teeth and chewing ability, and a decrease of taste or smell. Many of the elderly are sarcopenic and osteopenic, and they may look wasted (cachectic) because of tissue losses.

The 4% of the elderly who are institutionalized are less likely to be affected by the availability of food, but the variety of foods available and the way the food is prepared may be totally out of their control (loss of "locus of control")—and they typically do not eat well. Some of the institutionalized elderly may just not like the foods that are prepared for them. They may also have poor appetites or other conditions, such as depression and dementia, which interfere with their eating. Also, regular use of prescription and other drugs may adversely affect appetite. Drug–nutrient interactions are quite common among the elderly. Therefore, it is not at all unusual that nursing homes and intermediary care facilities for the elderly will have a substantial percentage of residents who are truly undernourished and a larger percentage who have intakes that are insufficient, but not deficient, in one or more nutrients. Deficient micronutrients of concern for the elderly include calcium, vitamin D, folate, vitamin B_{12}, vitamin K, omega-3 fatty acids, magnesium, a few other water-soluble vitamins, and occasionally energy or protein (anorexia, kwashiorkor, and marasmus). Undernourished elders are generally at high risk of mortality.

Further changes in diet and lifestyle, especially increasing the intake of fruits and vegetables and physical activities, are needed to continue the declines in death rates from cardiovascular diseases and to decrease the trend of death rates from cancer. Finally, numerous social barriers exist that limit the elderly in obtaining adequate intakes of nutrients. As the average life span of the elderly population continues to increase, nutritional problems of this population will become more common and persistent, and societal responses will need to be expanded, enhanced, and applied globally.

Overnutrition

Overnutrition is a major problem for many Americans, including a modest percentage of the elderly. Excessive portion sizes have been targeted as one of the major

---

FOCUS 11.2   Nutrient Deficiencies in the Diets of the Elderly

Recent NHANES reports have documented a number of nutrient deficiencies in the diets of the elderly in the United States. Practically all of these deficiencies are of micronutrients, specifically calcium, vitamin D, folate, vitamin B_{12}, iron, zinc, pyridoxine, vitamin C, vitamin E, beta-carotene, vitamin K, and magnesium. Most of these micronutrients are found in sufficient amounts in plant foods, with the exception of vitamin B_{12}. This intake pattern suggests that the bulk of these deficiencies exists because of limited food choices that largely exclude plant foods. Balanced intakes of both plant and animal foods in reasonable serving sizes should supply all of the needed micronutrients. Elderly who have these deficiencies may benefit from a micronutrient supplement, as stated earlier. ●

contributors to overeating and overweight or obesity. One expert has said, "Too much fork and too little foot," in reference to our unbalanced energy equation.

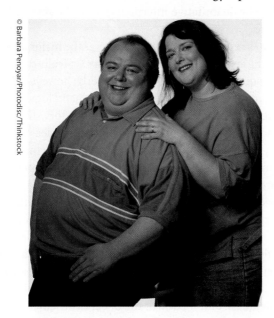

© Barbara Penoyar/Photodisc/Thinkstock

Excessive intakes of nutrients for which adult and elderly consumers need to be concerned include fats, especially saturated fats, sodium (salt), phosphate, omega-6 fatty acids, and possibly vitamin A during the later years. Excessive alcohol consumption has an impact on nutrition in several ways besides contributing to **alcoholism**, a major killer disease.

Diet-Related Chronic Diseases

This section focuses on the dietary risk factors involved in the etiology (or causation) of the more prevalent chronic diseases in the United States and other developed countries. An overview of the epidemiologic, clinical, and quantitative research approaches used by investigators to uncover dietary and other risk factors is beyond this text, but some attention to correlations of risk factors of specific diseases is given. Lastly, potential explanations of the disease processes, (i.e., mechanisms of disease) are offered in brief detail.

Epidemiology

The approach to the study of disease in populations is referred to as epidemiology. **Epidemiology** is the science of the distribution and the determinants or risk factors of diseases and injuries of human populations. The distribution of disease and death in a population is measured by rates, such as the number of deaths per 100,000 population basis per year. Such an index is referred to as a **mortality (death) rate** of a disease in a population for a given time period. **Incidence** (current year) and **prevalence** (existing over time) rates of diseases (**morbidity**) are also frequently used terms. Incidence refers to the number of new cases per year, whereas prevalence is the number of existing cases (new or incident + old or existing) in a population at any point in time.

Epidemiologic studies of diet-related chronic diseases are basically **observational studies** in which dietary variables (energy, nutrients) are measured in a free-living population and associated with disease end points or even death. The approach is to uncover risk factors or determinants of disease and to determine the quantitative importance of

alcoholism Compulsive and uncontrolled consumption of alcoholic beverages, usually to the detriment of the drinker's health, personal relationships, and social standing. It is medically considered a disease, specifically an addictive illness.

epidemiology The quantitative science that examines the risk factors or determinants that contribute to the prevalence of a disease or the incidence of new cases in populations.

mortality (death) rate The annual number of deaths in a population (i.e., deaths per year). Often adjusted for specific factors.

incidence The number of new cases of a disease in a given time frame, such as a year, for a given population.

prevalence The total number of cases of a specific disease existing at any one time; for example, the prevalence rate of CHD would include all individuals with this disease in the United States at a specific time, including both old cases from previous years and any new (incident) cases from the current year.

morbidity Existence of a specific disease in a defined population in a given time frame, such as a year; it can refer to incidence (only new cases) or to prevalence (all cases).

observational study A type of study in which individuals are observed or certain outcomes are measured. No attempt is made to affect the outcome.

❝ Chronic diseases typically have a long period of development, a decade or more, because of the slow progression of cellular pathologic changes that occur in response to the long-term dietary habits and other lifestyle practices. **❞**

❝ Good nutrition helps especially to maintain the immune system as a defense against infections among the elderly. **❞**

all risk factors that contribute to the specific disease. The observational epidemiologic approach does not permit an understanding of specific causation of a disease, but rather provides a relative or quantitative interpretation of the several factors that are associated with a disease.

Chronic diseases replaced infectious diseases as the major killers in the United States by the middle of the last century. Chronic diseases typically occur during the later adult years and become quite common among the elderly; however, they are not the result of aging *per se*. Rather, these diseases occur because of pathologic changes in various tissues as a result of long-term eating patterns, hereditary factors, and other specific **lifestyle risk factors**, such as cigarette smoking and limited physical activity. The etiologies (or, broadly speaking, the causes) of these diseases, therefore, involve several contributing factors or determinants. Chronic diseases typically have a long period of development, a decade or more, because of the slow progression of cellular pathologic changes that occur in response to the long-term dietary habits and other lifestyle practices.

Obesity contributes to several diseases or conditions, especially elevated blood pressure (hypertension), type 2 diabetes, heart and other cardiovascular diseases, gallbladder disease, osteoarthritis, and others, that typically appear during adulthood in the United States, Canada, and many other Western nations. Because obese individuals typically are not physically active, several of these diseases of the metabolic syndrome may coexist in the same individuals, and most will die of cardiovascular complications that occur later in life. The increased incidence of obesity among children and adolescents is an early warning of potential long-term consequences of the chronic diseases later in adult life, if not sooner.

Life Expectancy

The **life expectancy** of Americans has increased considerably, particularly for females, since the end of World War II. This improved health status derives from better preventive health care, especially early in life, better nutrition, better environmental control of sanitation, cleaner water supplies, and better medical care, among other factors. Good nutrition helps to maintain the immune system as a defense against infections among the elderly. **FIGURE 11.7** shows the trends in mean life expectancy from 1930 to 2010.

In the United States, women have an average life expectancy of approximately 80 years of age, and men have an average life expectancy of approximately 75 years. The nations with the greatest mean life expectancy in the world are Japan and Sweden for

lifestyle risk factors A collection of behaviors that can adversely or favorably impact health; for example, cigarette smoking and excessive alcohol consumption (more than two drinks a day on a regular basis) are deleterious risk factors, whereas regular physical activity, a nutritious, balanced diet, and adequate sleep are beneficial risk factors for health.

life expectancy The average lifetime age expected at birth. In the United States, life expectancy is approximately 81 years for females and 76 years for males.

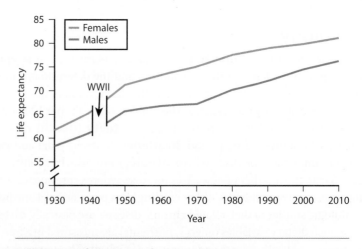

FIGURE 11.7 Life Expectancy by Sex: 1930–2010.

Data from the U.S. Census Bureau.

women and Japan for men. The mean life expectancy of the population of a particular country results to a great extent from the type of diet, eating habits, and activity levels generally followed by that society. Human longevity, in the ideal sense, is estimated to be approximately 110 to 120 years, and some investigators suggest that it can be even longer. If better nutrition and improved preventive services and health care continue, then the trend toward longer lives in the more economically advantaged nations should also continue. Longevity may even reach the **life span** of ~120 years projected for humankind!

A few nutritional risk factors that contribute to morbidity and mortality of the elderly can be easily prevented through the use of nutrient supplements that ensure adequate intakes. This area of prevention among the elderly needs further investigation. Perhaps the factor most limiting to increasing longevity is our knowledge of the aging process. For example, new research findings suggest that several genes exist that contribute to early aging. If we can learn to control those genes, the devastating changes accompanying aging—and even death itself—might be significantly delayed.

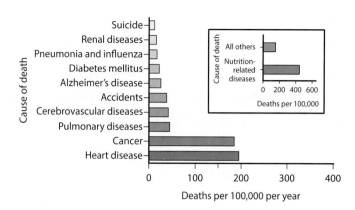

FIGURE 11.8 Top 10 Causes of Death in the United States. Note in the inset that almost 70% of deaths have a nutritional relationship. Age-adjusted rates are per 100,000 population.

Data from *National Vital Statistics Reports*, 60(3); 2011. Available at: www.cdc.gov/nchs/fastats/lcod.htm

Causes of Death in the United States

Everyone must die. Although the causes of death are quite variable, a preponderance of some causes over others does exist. In the United States, Canada, and most Western industrialized nations, the two leading causes of death are cardiovascular diseases and cancer. The U.S. death rates for the 10 leading causes of death are shown in **FIGURE 11.8**. Note that the age-adjusted rates are given per 100,000 population basis.

Since the late 1960s, a marked downward trend in coronary heart (artery) disease death rates has occurred. Although cancer death rates, as a percent of the total, have increased slightly overall, both the cancer incidence and death rate have been falling at about 1% per year since about 1990. **FIGURE 11.9** illustrates the general changes in heart and cancer death rates with time. Death rates from heart disease and cancer each year

> **❝** Death rates from heart disease and cancer each year may become even closer in the twenty-first century if the death rates of cardiovascular diseases continue to decline. **❞**

> **❝** Social drinking, defined as no more than two drinks per day for men and one for women, may contribute as much as 5% of total calories in the diets of U.S. adults. **❞**

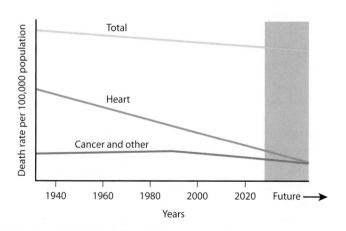

FIGURE 11.9 Trends in Death Rates from Major Chronic Diseases. The decline in total death rate and in other diseases over the last 50 years or so reflects better nutrition and overall health care. For cancer death rates, a slight decrease has occurred over the past two decades.

Modified from Anderson JJB. *Nutrition and Health: An Introduction.* Durham, NC: Carolina Academic Press; 2005.

life span The oldest possible age achievable for the human species. Estimates range from 110 to 130 years; however, few people live to be over 100 years. The number of centenarians in the United States is steadily increasing.

> From a nutritional perspective, a major effect of chronic alcoholism is a reduction of the intestinal absorption of micronutrients and, possibly, an increased elimination of them via the kidneys and hepatic (biliary) routes.

> Undernutrition contributes to the high death rates of alcoholic individuals.

alcohol (ethanol) A simple organic molecule that can cause intoxication. It is metabolized by a two-step process in many cells of the body, but especially in the liver. The metabolism of alcohol yields energy and toxic byproducts.

alcohol metabolism The degradation of alcohol by two enzymatic steps, the first being the slow, or rate-limiting, step requiring alcohol dehydrogenase and the second requiring acetaldehyde dehydrogenase. The final product is acetic acid (acetate), which enters the citric acid (Krebs) cycle after combining with coenzyme A for oxidation to carbon dioxide and water, and some ATP and heat generation.

hypoglycemia The state when plasma glucose concentration is depressed below normal fasting concentration (70 to 110 mg/dL).

alcohol effects Adverse effects on nutritional status and organ systems resulting from excessive intake of alcohol. Alcoholism is typically associated with poor nutritional status.

liver cirrhosis A disease of the liver typically caused by alcoholism in which most of the normal hepatic cells are replaced by scar tissue so that liver function is severely suppressed.

may become even closer in the twenty-first century if death rates from cardiovascular diseases continue to decline.

Alcohol–Diet Interactions

Although not a nutrient *per se*, **alcohol (ethanol)**, which is consumed as a component of alcoholic beverages and some foods, is metabolized by the liver and thereby yields energy in the form of ATP. Thus, molecules of alcohol count as a source of energy in addition to the macronutrients. Alcohol calories contribute 1% to 5% of total energy intake of U.S. adults, but this percentage is a mean for the entire adult population, about 50% of whom consume little or no alcohol. Social drinking, defined as no more than two drinks per day for men and one for women, may contribute as much as 5% of total calories in the diets of U.S. adults. Some individuals may consume up to 30% or so of their calories from alcohol, and the most severe alcoholics get practically all of their calories from alcohol!

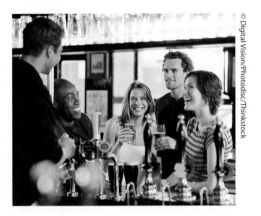

© Digital Vision/Photodisc/Thinkstock

Another important aspect of **alcohol metabolism** is whether reasonably normal food intake accompanies alcohol consumption. If little or no food is eaten by a heavy drinker, then the gluconeogenic pathway of the liver operates to a limited degree, and the alcoholic person can easily become **hypoglycemic** (i.e., low blood glucose). In contrast, if heavy drinking is accompanied by high food intake, an individual may become hyperglycemic because of increased glycogenolysis and, possibly, gluconeogenesis. In fact, several chronic diseases are affected by excessive alcohol intake. Excessive alcohol intake results in elevated blood lipids and hypertension, both of which are risk factors for heart disease/stroke and contributing factors to cancers and other diseases. **Alcohol effects** on the liver may be a major contributor to death.

When alcohol calories exceed 10% of total calories, the liver is unable to quickly degrade all of the alcohol, and the excess alcohol begins to have adverse effects on tissues throughout the body besides the liver. An alcoholic liver typically contains more stored fat in hepatic cells and an increased amount of fibrotic tissue (or **liver cirrhosis**) that replaces liver cells.

When excessive drinking occurs, alcohol calories begin to replace calories from carbohydrates and other macronutrients, and food intake may begin to decline. At that point, the protective actions of micronutrients, now taken in smaller amounts each day, also diminish. From a nutritional perspective, a major effect of chronic alcoholism is a reduction of the intestinal absorption of micronutrients and, possibly, an increased elimination of them via the kidneys and hepatic (biliary) routes. At this point, the disease—alcoholism—most likely exists in an individual. Undernutrition contributes to the high death rates of alcoholic individuals because of low nutrient intakes and poor nutrient metabolism.

SUMMARY

The major compartments of the body—lean body mass (LBM), fat mass, and bone mass—undergo tremendous changes from early life to the elder years. Changes in body composition from 1 year to 20 years of age primarily involve growth and development of the skeleton and musculature. The accumulation of fat tissue by females during the prepubertal period is necessary for the development of reproductive function and the onset of menarche. The accumulation of muscle mass by adolescents, particularly males, in association with pubertal development, especially with the production of testosterone, is closely associated with the increase of skeletal mass. Suboptimal skeletal growth during childhood and adolescence may result from chronically low intakes of calcium.

The major changes in body composition occurring during adulthood are an upward shift in the percentage of body fat and a corresponding downward shift in LBM. All three major components of body composition change in the elderly. Declines in bone mass and continuing declines in LBM, which is reflected by sarcopenia (too little muscle mass), and relatively greater fat mass are usually apparent among the elderly. In the old-old elderly (> 80 years), body weight may decline even more, reflecting significant losses of the fat mass as well as continuing, but smaller, losses of LBM.

Developing healthy food habits early in life is a major step toward prevention of the chronic diseases of later life. Parents or caretakers play a big role in ensuring adequate nutrition in their children and in preventing overweight and obesity during childhood and adolescence years. The nutrient requirements, allowances, and actual intakes by children and adolescents change according to the stage of growth. Food preferences become established early in childhood, and food habits, which are complex in their origin, undergo modification as adolescents begin to emerge as more independent individuals. Undernutrition of children and adolescents is not common in the United States or Canada. Overnutrition, however, as reflected by overweight and obesity in children and adolescents, has become far too prevalent. Excess energy intake contributes to fat accumulation in tissue throughout the body. Health problems affecting children and adolescents in developed countries include obesity, anorexia nervosa, and dental caries. Severe nutrient deficiencies are extremely rare among children and adolescents in developed countries,

but are a problem in poor, developed countries. The major issue of adolescent nutrition remains the imbalance between caloric intake and expenditure because of generally inadequate physical activity.

The nutritional status of adults depends on income, education, social and psychological status, and general health status. Because of declines in most organ systems with increasing age and an overall decline in tissue mass, energy and most nutrient needs decrease with age. Adults need to work at maintaining good health with calorie intake balanced with physical activities. Far too many adults lapse into excessive eating and then into the realm of obesity.

The elderly are a diverse and heterogeneous group of individuals, who gradually undergo decrements in physiological functions and body composition with the course of aging, but at different rates of decline. They typically have decreasing functions of the GI tract that affect adversely the utilization of micronutrients. Therefore, poor GI status may impair nutritional status. Some elderly show consistent deficiencies in the intakes of energy and selected micronutrients, according to national surveys. Supplements of specific micronutrients administered to elderly subjects have generally not been found to result in improved functions specific to the nutrient, which implies that the usual intakes of many elderly are sufficient; truly deficient individuals do need them. Many elderly may improve their health by broad supplementation of micronutrients; however, nutritionists recommend that nutrients be obtained from foods first rather than via supplementation.

Obesity contributes to the etiology of many chronic diseases. If sound dietary habits and regular physical activity are not practiced, obesity and the other chronic diseases will follow in time. In the United States, chronic diseases typically begin in early adulthood (or possibly even earlier) and typically overweight or obesity exists first. Obesity is a risk factor for heart disease and some forms of cancer. Heart disease and cancer remain the two leading causes of death of adults prior to entering the elderly period at age 65. The control of these diseases resides to a great extent within the capability of each individual. However, because of the generally better health of U.S. and Canadian adults, despite the high obesity prevalence, the mean expected life expectancy of men and women has been slowly increasing.

STUDENT ACTIVITIES

1. What is the number one health problem facing children and adolescents in the United States today? Explain why this condition is so prevalent.

2. Which nutrients are poorly consumed by girls beyond age 11 years? What about boys beyond age 11? Explain why adolescents have low intakes of these nutrients

when food availability in the United States is relatively plentiful.

3. Describe the cycle of undernutrition and infectious diseases in young children. How does infection factor into childhood morbidity and mortality rates in developed versus underdeveloped countries?

4. Explain the importance of healthful eating practices and proper dental hygiene to prevent dental caries.

5. How does estrogen status in women affect bone mass and bone density as they proceed through the various stages of adulthood? Explain.

6. Excessive alcohol intake may have adverse health effects. Do you agree or disagree with this statement? Explain in terms of the organs affected.

7. Consider the following statement: "Nutrient supplements are widely recommended for adults." Do you agree or disagree with this statement? Why or why not?

8. For the elderly, calcium and vitamin D recommendations (RDAs) were increased in 2011 by substantial amounts. What is the rationale for this recommendation for adults beyond age 50? Do you agree with these recommendations? Explain.

9. Which nutrients may be affected by low gastric acid production in late life?

10. Today, life expectancy for women in the United States is approximately 80 years, a few years longer than the average life expectancy for men. What health behaviors might contribute to this gender difference in life expectancy? [Hint: Think of lifestyle factors beyond diet that may influence tissue changes, reductions in organ functions, and such.]

WEBSITES FOR FURTHER STUDY

National Institute of Aging
www.nia.nih.gov
Office of Adolescent Health, HHS
www.hhs.gov/ash/oah
National Institute of Child Health and Human Development
www.nichd.nih.gov
USDA/ARS Children's Nutrition Research Center
www.bcm.edu/cnrc

School Meals Programs, Food and Nutrition Service, USDA
www.fns.usda.gov/cnd
Alcoholism Facts from Medicine.net
www.medicinenet.com/script/main/art.asp?articlekey=52888
Elderly Nutrition Program at Nutrition.gov
www.aoa.gov/AoARoot/Press_Room/Products_Materials/pdf/fs_nutrition.doc
Nutrition and the Elderly, SparkPeople.com
www.sparkpeople.com/resource/nutrition_articles.asp?id=869

REFERENCES

Alves C, Lima RV. Dietary supplement use by adolescents. *J Pediatr (Rio J).* 2009;85:287–294.

Calder PC, Yaqoob P. Nutrient regulation of the immune response. In: Erdman JW Jr, MacDonald IA, Zeisel SH (eds.). *Present Knowledge in Nutrition.* 10th ed. Ames, IA: John Wiley & Sons; 2012: 1097–1126.

Gao B, Bataller R. Alcoholic liver disease: pathogenesis and new therapeutic targets. *Gastroenterology.* 2011;141:1572–1585.

Genaro P, de S, Martini LA. Effect of protein intake on bone and muscle mass in the elderly. *Nutr Rev.* 2010;68:616–623.

Hausman DB, Fischer JG, Johnson MA. Nutrition in centenarians. *Maturitas.* 2011;68:203–209.

Maqbool A, Dougherty KA, Parks EP, Stallings VA. Adolescence. In: Erdman JW Jr, MacDonald IA, Zeisel SH (eds.). *Present Knowledge in Nutrition.* 10th ed. Ames, IA: John Wiley & Sons; 2012: 1021–1048.

Meyer F, O'Connor H, Shirreffs SM. International Association of Athletics Federations. Nutrition for the young athlete. *J Sports Sci.* 2007;25(suppl 1):73S–82S.

Narici MV, Maffulli N. Sarcopenia: characteristics, mechanisms and functional significance. *Br Med Bull.* 2010;95:139–159.

Palacios C, Joshipura K, Willett W. Nutrition and health: guidelines for dental practitioners. *Oral Dis.* 2009;15:369–381.

Pelletier DL, Olson CM, Frongillo EA. Food insecurity, hunger, and undernutrition. In: Erdman JW Jr, MacDonald IA, Zeisel SH (eds.). *Present Knowledge in Nutrition.* 10th ed. Ames, IA: John Wiley & Sons; 2012: 1794–1817.

Secher M, Ritz P, Vellas B. Nutrition and aging. In: Erdman JW Jr, MacDonald IA, Zeisel SH (eds.). *Present Knowledge in Nutrition.* 10th ed. Ames, IA: John Wiley & Sons; 2012: 1049–1072.

Suter PM. Alcohol, its role in nutrition and health. In: Erdman JW Jr, MacDonald IA, Zeisel SH (eds.). *Present Knowledge in Nutrition.* 10th ed. Ames, IA: John Wiley & Sons; 2012: 1444–1488.

ADDITIONAL READING

Hadler NM. *Rethinking Aging.* Chapel Hill, NC: University of North Carolina Press; 2011.

Nitzke S, Riley D, Ramminger A, Jacabs G. *Rethinking Nutrition: Connecting Science and Practice in Early Childhood Settings.* St. Paul, MN: Redleaf Press; 2010.

Weil A. *Healthy Aging: A Lifelong Guide to Your Well-Being.* New York: Anchor Books; 2007.

12

Obesity and Weight Control

Obesity, which is now classified as a chronic disease, results primarily from a combination of excessive energy intake from foods and beverages, especially those that are high in calories, and from inadequate physical activity to burn off the excess calories ingested. Weight gain is not influenced by the consumption of any one of the macronutrients alone but by all of them combined! Weight gain is entirely dependent on the total amount of excess calories. A calorie is a calorie, regardless of the source.

Overweight and obesity are characterized by excessive accumulation of fat (triglycerides) in the fat cells (i.e., **adipocytes**) of practically all tissues of the body. Both environmental factors, such as obesity-promoting lifestyle behaviors, and hereditary determinants increase the likelihood of an individual developing obesity. The path to obesity starts with overweight. Part of the widespread increase in body weight in nations throughout the world, especially affluent nations, resides in the change in the food supply—more sugar, fats, and fast foods—that have been promoted by modern marketing strategies targeting children and young people.

One of the great concerns with the obesity epidemic, especially for children and adolescents, is the contribution of obesity to type 2 diabetes mellitus and other chronic diseases of adulthood. In fact, in the United States there is now a double epidemic, sometimes referred to as **diabesity**, reflecting the increased incidence of obesity and diabetes in the same individuals. In 2010, more than 69% of adults in the United States were overweight or obese, and 25.6 million (about 11.3% of adults) had type 2 diabetes! The focus of this chapter is on the prevention of overweight and obesity, but treatment of these conditions is only briefly noted.

Definitions of Overweight and Obesity

Obesity represents an excess accumulation of body fat, or adipose tissue that contains triglycerides. Overweight and obesity can be defined according to body mass index (BMI) as part of a continuum starting with **underweight** and continuing into the range of normal weight up to overweight, and then obesity. BMI has become the most

> **"** Obesity results primarily from a combination of excessive energy intake from foods and beverages, especially those that are high in calories, and from inadequate physical activity to burn off the excess calories ingested. **"**

adipocyte A fat cell. Adipocytes take up fatty acids and glucose in order to synthesize triglycerides and undergo lipolysis to generate glycerol and free fatty acids that diffuse to blood for distribution to other body tissues.

diabesity Term coined to describe the presence of both diabetes and obesity. A metabolic dysfunction that ranges from mild blood sugar imbalance to full-fledged type 2 diabetes that occurs concomitantly with obesity.

underweight Body weight that is 10% or more below the lower range of normal weight (Metropolitan Life or NHANES); also, a BMI of less than 18.5.

> **BMI has become the most common measure used to assess overweight and obesity in adults.**

common measure used to assess overweight and obesity in adults. A calculator for adult BMI is available at http://www.nhlbi.nih.gov/guidelines/obesity/BMI/bmicalc.htm. A BMI calculator for children and adolescents is available at http://apps.nccd.cdc.gov/dnpabmi. **FIGURE 12.1** illustrates the four classes of BMI used in categorizing individuals using arbitrary cutoffs. Recall that individuals who are overweight have a BMI at or greater than 25, and those who are obese have a BMI at or greater than 30—these two classes are of greatest concern to public health.

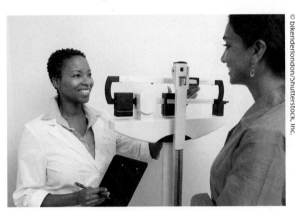

© bikeriderlondon/Shutterstock, Inc.

Adult obesity is associated with adverse health effects. Obesity *per se* can be defined as a disease, and it is also a risk factor for other chronic diseases that may increase mortality. Modest increases in body fat that are within the normal range of BMI (18.5 to 24.9 have little effect on disease risk compared with more significant gains in body weight that move into the overweight range of BMI (25 to 29.9) during adulthood. Research

BMI	19	20	21	22	23	24	25	26	27	28	29	30	31	32	33	34	35
Height									**Weight in Pounds**								
4'10"	91	96	100	105	110	115	119	124	129	134	138	143	148	153	158	162	167
4'11"	94	99	104	109	114	119	124	128	133	138	143	148	153	158	163	168	173
5'	97	102	107	112	118	123	128	133	138	143	148	153	158	163	158	174	179
5'1"	100	106	111	116	122	127	132	137	143	148	153	158	164	169	174	180	185
5'2"	104	109	115	120	126	131	136	142	147	153	158	164	169	175	180	186	191
5'3"	107	113	118	124	130	135	141	146	152	158	163	169	175	180	186	191	197
5'4"	110	116	122	128	134	140	145	151	157	163	169	174	180	186	192	197	204
5'5"	114	120	126	132	138	144	150	156	162	168	174	180	186	192	198	204	210
5'6"	118	124	130	136	142	148	155	161	167	173	179	186	192	198	204	210	216
5'7"	121	127	134	140	146	153	159	166	172	178	185	191	198	204	211	217	223
5'8"	125	131	138	144	151	158	164	171	177	184	190	197	203	210	216	223	230
5'9"	128	135	142	149	155	162	169	176	182	189	196	203	209	216	223	230	236
5'10"	132	139	146	153	160	167	174	181	188	195	202	209	216	222	229	236	243
5'11"	136	143	150	157	165	172	179	186	193	200	208	215	222	229	236	243	250
6'	140	147	154	162	169	177	184	191	199	206	213	221	228	235	242	250	258
6'1"	144	151	159	166	174	182	189	197	204	212	219	227	235	242	250	257	265
6'2"	148	155	163	171	179	186	194	202	210	218	225	233	241	249	256	264	272
6'3"	152	160	168	176	184	192	200	208	216	224	232	240	248	256	264	272	279

FIGURE 12.1 Adult BMI Chart. Locate the height of interest in the leftmost column, and read across the row for that height to the weight of interest. Follow the column of the weight up to the top row that lists the BMI. A BMI of 18.5 to 24.9 is in the healthy range, a BMI of 25 to 29.9 is in the overweight range, and a BMI of 30 and above is in the obese range. Due to rounding, these ranges vary slightly from the NHLBI values. Underweight is less than 18.5.

Reproduced from U.S. Departments of Agriculture and Health and Human Services. *Dietary Guidelines for Americans.* 6th ed. Washington, DC: US Government Printing Office; 2005.

suggests that the healthiest weights exist within the BMI range of 18.5 to 24.9, but recent results have shown that modest adult overweight (BMI of 25 to 27) also may result in low mortality rates. A modest increase in body weight by adults who are fairly active in physical endeavors or exercise may not be disadvantageous. However, individuals with body weights in the obese range (a BMI of 30 or higher) have a greatly increased risk of death and disability from several chronic diseases.

An exception to the general rule about classifying individuals as overweight according to BMI should be made for highly trained athletes who may have extremely well-developed muscles and high LBM (i.e., large muscle mass but less body fat). According to the weight-based BMI calculation, these individuals are considerably above the healthy normal weight BMI range. Yet, they typically are lean and in top physical condition. Muscle mass is denser than fat mass. When a person "trades" fat mass for muscle mass through exercise, he or she may fall in the overweight range of BMI even as his or her visceral (abdominal) fat may decrease in size.

Alternative Weight Assessment Methods

Other methods used to assess weight include **waist circumference** measurements and dual-energy x-ray absorptiometry (DXA). DXA, a highly reproducible method available at major medical and research centers throughout the world, is currently used to assess fat mass. With DXA, data are generated on the two body compartments: fat mass and bone mass. Based on measurements of the fat mass and bone mass, lean body mass (LBM) can be calculated by difference from total body mass (weight). Bone mass is the same as bone mineral content (BMC) in mass units (kilograms), which is used to assess bone health.

> Individuals with body weights in the obese range (a BMI of 30 or higher) have a greatly increased risk of death and disability from several chronic diseases.

PRACTICAL APPLICATIONS **12.1**

Measure Your Waist Circumference

Waist circumference is a fairly good surrogate measurement for BMI calculation, even if it only estimates abdominal girth. Obtain a cloth tape measure (nonexpandable) typically used by tailors and seamstresses. Measure your waist circumference at the belly button (preferably without clothing over the belly). Individuals with a waist circumference greater than 35 inches for women and 40 inches for men are considered overweight, even if their BMI is less than 25. This value serves as your base—and probably lowest—for the remainder of your life! For example, if you are 20 years old, this base value can be used to compare similar waist measurements every 5 or 10 years. Of course, measurements during pregnancy will not be comparable and measurement during severe illness accompanied by weight loss also will not be representative. At all other stages of adult life, however, comparative waist measurements will signify changes in diet and in BMI in both genders, and in most cases reduced physical activity. ■

waist circumference A measure of abdominal girth that is a fairly good surrogate measurement for BMI.

android fat distribution Fat distribution pattern where fat has a greater propensity to distribute around the abdomen as measured by the waist-to-hip ratio (WHR). It is the typical fat distribution pattern in adult males.

Fat Distribution and Body Fat Percentages

The distribution of fat and obesity throughout the body follows two major patterns: an "apple" shape and a "pear" shape (see **FIGURE 12.2**). The apple shape also is called an android fat distribution. **Android fat distribution**, which is more common in males,

> The distribution of fat and obesity throughout the body follows two major patterns: an "apple" or android shape and a "pear" or gynoid shape.

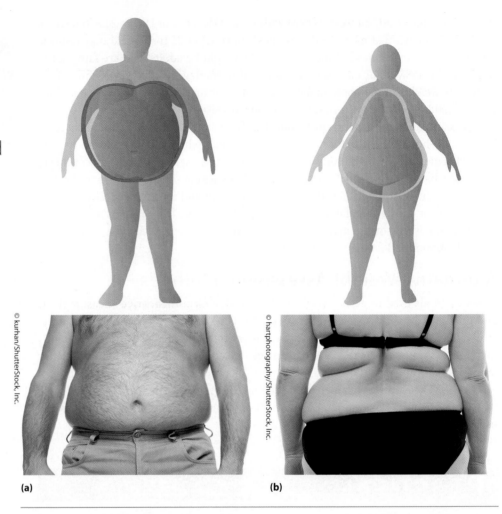

FIGURE 12.2 Apples Versus Pears. Fat distribution typically varies in males and females. Males tend to be apple shaped, with more fat around the midsection. In contrast, females tend to be pear shaped, accumulating fat around the thighs and buttocks.

is characterized by excess fat accumulation in the midsection (waist) of the body. The pear shape also is referred to as gynoid fat distribution. **Gynoid fat distribution**, which is more common in females, is characterized by greater fat deposition around the thighs and buttocks. The waist-to-hip ratio is much greater in android than in gynoid obesity. This fat pattern of android (visceral) obesity has a significant negative impact on several chronic diseases, including type 2 diabetes, coronary heart disease, stroke, and renal failure, as well as metabolic syndrome. Hypertension typically occurs with increased body fat, particularly around the waist.

The visceral (abdominal) fat accumulation found in the android pattern leads to increases in serum free fatty acids and eventually to insulin resistance, a major feature of the metabolic syndrome. The incidence of type 2 diabetes, hypertension, and abnormal blood lipids (LDL-cholesterol) is higher in apple-shaped individuals. Research on clarifying the disease mechanisms linked with these two distinct types of body fat distribution is ongoing.

Body Fat and Aging

Estimated body fat percentages of U.S. adults ages 25 to 75 years are shown in **FIGURE 12.3**. Both males and females gain body fat as they get older. Men tend to add a greater percentage of their weight from ages 20 to 50. Women generally have a period

gynoid fat distribution Fat distribution pattern where fat has a greater propensity to distribute around the hips and thighs as measured by the waist-to-hip ratio (WHR). It is the typical fat distribution pattern in adult females.

of weight gain following menopause (around age 50). As body weight increases because of gains of fat mass, LBM must increase slightly in order to support the fat mass. Therefore, a relative (percentage) decline in LBM occurs as the percentage of fat mass increases.

For example, consider a 60-year-old woman who has gained 3 kilograms since the beginning of menopause. At the start of menopause she weighed 60 kilograms and had 20 kilograms of fat. She has gained approximately 1 kilogram in LBM. Thus, her percent body fat may have increased by almost 5%, but her percent LBM may have decreased by over 2%—even though it increased by a kilogram! These relative changes in the mass of the three body compartments are greatly influenced by any increase in the absolute increase of fat mass because the percent of fat mass typically increases with a gain in total body mass (or body weight).

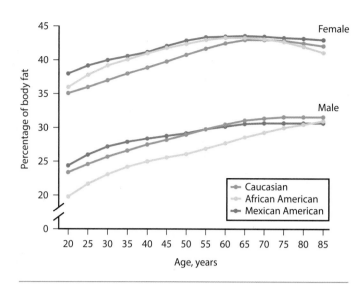

FIGURE 12.3 Estimated Percentages of Body Fat in Adult Males and Females by Age.

Data from Kelly TL, Wilson KE, Heymsfield SB. Dual energy x-ray absorptiometry body composition reference values from NHANES. *PLoS One.* 2009;4:e7038.

Body Fat and Athletes

Athletes typically have less body fat than nonathletes. For example, a typical male college student has 15% to 20% body fat. Many athletes, especially long-distance runners, may have only 5% body fat. Females generally have 5% to 10% more body fat than males during early adulthood. The fat mass of a typical female college student is approximately 25% to 30% of her total weight. Female runners, gymnasts, and basketball players generally have levels of body fat comparable to male athletes (10% to 15%). However, if body fat levels dip too low they may experience fewer menstrual cycles per year (**oligomenorrhea**) or totally stop menstruating (amenorrhea).

> *As body weight increases because of gains of fat mass, LBM must increase slightly in order to support the fat mass.*

PRACTICAL APPLICATIONS 12.2

Body Fat in an Intercollegiate Male Athlete

The percentage of an individual's body weight due to fat accumulation or body fat mass varies with age and sex, as well as with absolute body weight. Athletes generally have low body fat mass because of their increased fitness compared to nonathletes. A DXA scan of an 80-kilogram male distance runner revealed that he had 4 kilograms of body fat (5% body fat) and 1.5 kilograms (~2% bone) of bone mass. His height is 2 meters (well over 6 feet). Calculate this athlete's BMI (BMI = weight ÷ height^2). Based on his BMI, would you classify him as normal weight, overweight, or obese? Explain which compartment of the body (fat, lean, bone) contributes the most to his body composition. ∎

Physiological Changes and Obesity

Obesity results in a number of physiological changes in the body, including increases in the number and size of fat cells. In addition, obesity can result in elevated insulin concentrations, which can then reinforce the obesity or cause additional weight gain.

oligomenorrhea Having fewer menstrual cycles than normal; for example, fewer than nine menses per year.

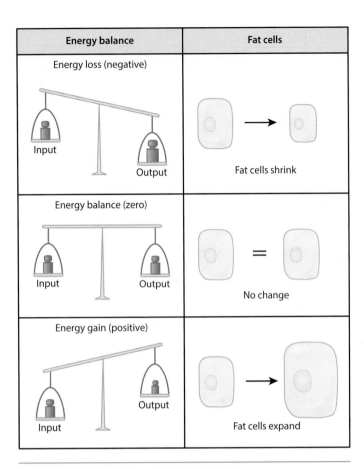

Energy balance	Fat cells
Energy loss (negative)	Fat cells shrink
Energy balance (zero)	No change
Energy gain (positive)	Fat cells expand

FIGURE 12.4 Changes in Fat Cells Based on Energy Intake. With excess energy intake, fat cells increase in size. With decreased energy intake, they shrink.

Increased Fat Cell Recruitment and Size

Excess body fat results in enlarged fat cells (hypertrophy) and possibly an increase in the number of fat cells (hyperplasia). The major distribution of fat cells in the body is largely in place early in life, but excessive consumption of calories can signal first the proliferation (new cell divisions) of precursor **stem cells** in bone marrow and then the recruitment of newly generated preadipocytes in other tissue locations. This system of increasing the pool of adipocytes is quite elastic, and depends on the consumption of food energy in excess of the body's needs.

Once these cells are distributed and relocated to peripheral tissues, they may expand or enlarge with further storage of triglycerides if high calorie intake continues. Excessive cell recruitment and enlargement can potentially result in an extreme state of obesity (BMI greater than 40) known as very severely or morbidly obese. When fat cells expand, the cell membranes enlarge to accommodate the excess triglycerides in storage, and the cell nucleus tends to become more flattened at one side.

The fat cells also may shrink in size when energy intake is substantially reduced over time and triglycerides are degraded and removed. However, once fat cells are produced, even though they may shrink in size, it is assumed that they remain for life and may continue to expand with greater energy consumption.

Three scenarios of energy balance are illustrated in **FIGURE 12.4**. When energy balance becomes positive over a period of a few weeks or longer, fat cells expand; conversely, fat cells shrink if caloric intake is reduced to a state of negative energy balance. In short, hypercaloric diets stimulate the expansion of the fat cells, whereas hypocaloric diets cause them to contract.

Self-Perpetuating Obesity and Elevated Insulin Concentrations

Regardless of its initial cause, obesity may be self-perpetuating because of insulin resistance by the cells of fat tissue and muscle. Our metabolic systems operate in such a way that the fatter we are, the easier it is to become still fatter. Following the addition of new or expansion of existing adipocytes, the body has an increased capacity to store more fat, so long as insulin is available.

Obesity leads to an elevated basal (fasting) insulin concentration (**hyperinsulinemia**) and an enhanced insulin response following a meal or glucose load (challenge). Insulin regulates the storage of lipids in adipose tissue by enhancing glucose entry into adipocytes, and it also enhances fatty acid synthesis in fat cells. Hyperinsulinemia associated with obesity increases the quantity of glucose that is converted to triglycerides and stored in the fat cells. Serum insulin and **leptin** concentrations, both signals of adiposity, increase in obesity, and their increased concentrations *should* inhibit further food (energy) consumption after they enter the parts of the brain that control appetite and food intake. This presumed inhibition, however, functions poorly in obese individuals. In insulin resistance resulting from excessive energy intake, fat cells (and muscle

stem cell An undifferentiated cell that has the potential to develop into one of many different kinds of cells, such as a skin cell, red blood cell, etc.

hyperinsulinemia An abnormally and excessively elevated serum insulin concentration either after a meal or during fasting (overnight); characteristic of type 2 diabetes mellitus and obesity.

leptin A hormone produced by fat cells and released into the blood that inhibits the feeding center of the hypothalamus in the brain and thereby helps regulate body weight.

FOCUS 12.1   Diabesity

Type 2 diabetes typically follows the establishment of overweight or obesity, resulting in *diabesity*. This sequence of overweight leading to diabetes is all too common. Peripheral resistance to insulin, often referred to as glucose intolerance, results when too many triglycerides

become stored, especially in peripheral fat and muscle cells but also in most other cell types. A high percentage of obese individuals develop type 2 diabetes during their lifetimes. ●

cells) no longer can take up the glucose efficiently and the blood glucose concentration rises after a meal and does not return to baseline for considerably more than 3 hours, as occurs in healthy individuals. Serum insulin continues to rise until beta (β) cells start to wear out and do not produce adequate amounts of insulin.

The basal metabolic rate (BMR) in obese people is directly related to their LBM, because fat cells have a relatively low level of metabolic activity. (In spite of the pathways involved in fatty acid synthesis and metabolism, fat cells expend very little energy over a 24-hour period.) Therefore, BMR does not decrease as long as LBM is maintained. In fact, BMR may represent as much as 80% to 90% of total energy expenditure in obese individuals who are very inactive, because so little energy is expended in daily physical activities. This concept is illustrated for three different individuals in **FIGURE 12.5**.

> **"** Obesity leads to an elevated basal (fasting) serum insulin concentration (hyperinsulinemia). **"**

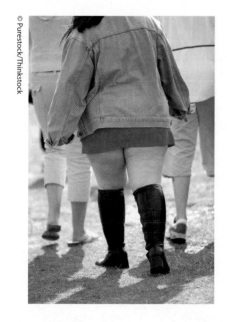

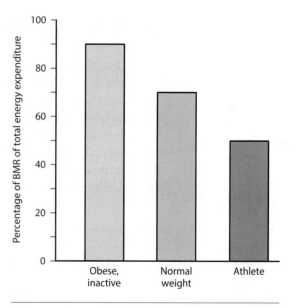

FIGURE 12.5 Percent BMR of Total Energy Expenditure.
Note the much greater percentage of energy used for BMR by obese individuals than by normal weight individuals or athletes.

Etiology of Obesity: Dietary and Other Risk Factors

Obesity has multiple causes. Thus, several types of obesity typically exist in any population. However, it has been estimated that the general cause (adverse risk factors) in about 95% of obese individuals is the same—an imbalance between energy consumption and energy expenditure. In roughly 5% of cases, a clinical hormonal imbalance is implicated as the cause of obesity.

Most obese individuals consume more energy (kilocalories) in the form of food and beverages than they expend in the maintenance of basic biological functions and the

> **"** In roughly 5% of cases, a clinical hormonal imbalance is implicated as the cause of obesity. **"**

> Obesity results from several potential factors, including chronic overconsumption of food, poor dietary choices, overeating in response to stress, sedentary lifestyle, genetic predisposition toward inefficient energy usage, or some combination of these factors.

performance of daily activities. The excess energy that is consumed is transformed into "storage" triglycerides in the adipose tissue. Small amounts of stored fat are regularly degraded as sources of energy to meet metabolic needs during periods of fasting. Some of this burning (oxidizing) of triglycerides is also used for temperature regulation. When energy consumption exceeds energy expenditure over an extended period of time, obesity develops. Television watching and computer use for several hours a day contributes to the development of obesity, including during childhood and adolescence.

This simple explanation of obesity, however, tells us little about the etiologic risk factors that contribute to an individual becoming obese. Obesity results from several potential factors, including chronic overconsumption of food, poor dietary choices, overeating in response to stress, sedentary lifestyle, genetic predisposition toward inefficient energy usage, or some combination of these factors. The factors giving rise to obesity encountered in the environment are shown in **FIGURE 12.6**.

Two major factors have shifted recent U.S. dietary patterns toward excess energy intake: an increase in the number of meals eaten outside of the home, especially at low-cost fast-food restaurants, and an increase in portion sizes. For example, some fast-food sandwiches are loaded with energy-dense components, and their total energy content can be as high as 600 to 800 kilocalories! Energy density is the number of kilocalories per serving of a specific food. In people who do not get enough physical activity, the consumption of several servings of energy-dense foods per day may exceed the amount of energy these individuals are able to expend. In addition, such an eating pattern may not provide sufficient amounts of micronutrients.

Heredity and Obesity

Besides environmental contributions, obesity also may have genetic determinants. Obesity has long been known to run in families, and it has been clearly established that both hereditary and environmental factors are at play with some individuals. An individual with lean parents has only an approximately 9% chance of becoming obese. The frequency of obesity increases to 41% among those with one obese parent and to 71% among individuals with two obese parents. However, the relationship between heredity and obesity is difficult to evaluate, because family kinship implies numerous common practices, in addition to genetic traits, including dietary habits, patterns of physical activity, cultural background, and socioeconomic status.

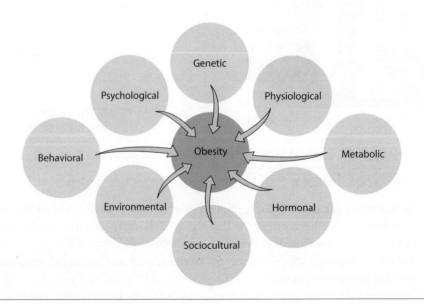

FIGURE 12.6 Obesogenic Factors. A variety of factors contributes to the development of obesity.

However, twin studies indicate that hereditary determinants of obesity are powerful. Twin studies that have compared monozygotic twins (identical twins, who have identical genetic makeup) with dizygotic twins (fraternal twins, who have 50% common genes) have found a strong genetic predisposition toward obesity. However, the environment and individual habits may override this predisposition over time, considering that other studies have found that weight is not as strongly correlated in non-twin siblings over time as their lifestyles tend to diverge.

Given the many genetic factors involved in determining body weight (height, build, and fat distribution), it is thought that as many as 30 different genes may affect the development of obesity. (A genetic trait for leanness also may exist.) Clearly, hereditary factors contribute to overweight and obesity, but research so far has not provided much understanding of the specific genes operating to increase fat accumulation. A newer approach to developing our understanding of the genetic basis for obesity is based on epigenetics, which is the study of how the environment and behavior influence genetic expression.

> Twin studies that have compared monozygotic twins (identical twins, who have identical genetic makeup) with dizygotic twins (fraternal twins, who have 50% common genes) have found a strong genetic predisposition toward obesity.

Increased Prevalence of Overweight and Obesity

Although the prevalence of obesity has been increasing in the United States over the last several decades, obesity is not uniformly distributed in the population. Rather, certain sexes, races, ethnic groups, and socioeconomic groups are more likely to be obese than others, as was demonstrated by the first U.S. National Health and Nutrition Examination Survey (NHANES I) in the early 1970s and in subsequent surveys into the twenty-first century. For example, obesity is more common among African Americans and Hispanics than whites or Asian Americans. It is also higher in those of lower socioeconomic status. Average weight among adults also varies by height and by age group (see Appendix C).

Keep in mind, however, that in recent decades in the United States obesity has been increasing for every gender and ethnic category. It also has been increasing for children and adolescents. Recent estimates suggest that one-third of the adult U.S. population is obese, and that 15% of all children and adolescents are obese. The percentages of those who are overweight or obese are even higher. In the United States, 69% of adults and 30% of children are overweight or obese, but these trends seem to be leveling off. The following are some of the trends in prevalence of obesity in the United States:

> Recent estimates suggest that one-third of the adult U.S. population is obese, and that 15% of all children and adolescents are obese.

- The prevalence of obesity is greater in adult women than in adult men at all ages.
- The prevalence of obesity is greater in adult African American and Hispanic women than in adult white women at all ages.
- The prevalence of obesity increases from age 20 to 70, and after age 70 it declines.

Obesity of Childhood and Adolescence

More and more children in the United States and other developed countries, and even in some developing countries, are becoming overweight and obese. The major reason for the childhood obesity epidemic seems to be the increased amount of time children spend doing sedentary activities, such as watching television, working on the computer, and playing video games, and increased consumption of energy-dense foods.

In the United States, children's diets now include more fast foods, more high-fat snacks, more sugary beverages, and more salty foods. These shifts in dietary intake patterns have been well documented along with the trend of increasing serving sizes of many of these foods, especially at fast-food restaurants. Several factors influencing the eating habits of schoolchildren have been documented in recent years. For example, school lunches have been found to be fairly high in fat and not so high in micronutrients,

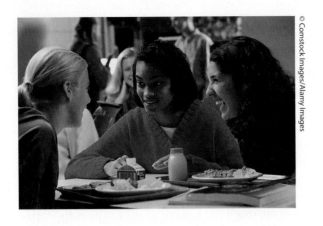

© Comstock Images/Alamy Images

with some lunches featuring energy-dense but nutrient-poor foods such as French fries and soft drinks. Also, soft drinks and other highly sweetened beverages have generally been available in many schools. Finally, many schools do not provide time for recess or physical education, limiting the amount of physical activity for children to engage in.

Recognition of the link between decreased physical activity and the increase in childhood obesity has resulted in the development of a number of programs intended to get children and adolescents to move more. One volunteer program, Girls on the Run, has been popular in many parts of the United States, and the President's Committee on Physical Fitness is another helpful program aimed at reducing widespread overweight and obesity rates in children. Whether these programs will be successful will require about two decades to be established. Improvements in the USDA's School Lunch Program also are anticipated.

The recent obesity epidemic among children and adolescents also is unfortunately associated with increased rates of type 2 diabetes and other morbidities in these populations. In essence, chronic diseases typically found only among adults are now appearing among our youth.

Obesity of Adulthood

As has been discussed, the prevalence of overweight and obesity in American adults has increased tremendously. Overweight and obesity progress over a period of years or decades and can contribute to a number of chronic diseases later in life.

The Development of Overweight and Obesity

The natural progression to adult-onset obesity for a hypothetical male is as follows. During childhood, energy expended during physical activity and intake from food are usually balanced, resulting in a normal body weight. However, in early adulthood the energy balance becomes positive because of excessive caloric intake relative to decreasing levels of energy expenditure. Thus, body weight increases slowly through adulthood, reaching unhealthy levels associated with overweight and obesity. Then, in mid-adulthood, at 50 to 60 years of age or so, energy intake slowly declines but remains nearly in balance as body weight tends to level off. Subsequently, with continuation of reduced physical activity, energy balance may even become negative because of a further reduction of energy intake. As cells (LBM) die and BMR declines, weight usually also declines modestly. However, with a decline in both LBM and physical activity, the percent fat mass usually increases.

For the hypothetical female, the major difference in the progression to obesity, aside from pregnancy and lactation, is the postmenopausal weight gain resulting from the decline in ovarian estrogen production and increased food consumption. As with men, the percent fat mass in women at approximately 10 years postmenopause holds steady or increases.

Morbidity and Mortality and Obesity

> **The obese are at increased risk for a number of metabolic disorders, including type 2 diabetes, coronary artery disease, hypertension, and endocrine disorders.**

The obese are at increased risk for a number of metabolic disorders, including type 2 diabetes, coronary artery disease, hypertension, and endocrine disorders. Individuals with visceral obesity (apple shape) are much more likely to develop the chronic metabolic diseases. These diseases that develop from the state of obesity result largely from the metabolic alterations that the excess fat causes when insulin cannot lower the serum glucose concentration sufficiently and also from other pathologic tissue changes.

Excessive fat tissue is accompanied by an increase in capillary beds supporting adipocytes, and this increase in capillaries makes the heart, especially the left ventricle, pump or work harder to deliver blood to these tissues. Research suggests that death rates from cardiovascular disease are associated in a major way with overweight and obesity.

Obese individuals suffer more from arthritis, joint diseases, and sleep apnea. Obesity also increases the risk of gallbladder disease, typically manifested by **gallstones** (cholesterol), which is almost nine times more common in women than men. Research also suggests that death rates from breast cancer are associated with overweight and obesity. Obesity in pregnancy is associated with increased maternal *and* fetal morbidity and mortality.

The medical risks increase with the degree of obesity. A significant increase in mortality exists in obese individuals (BMI ≥ 30), and severe obesity (BMI ≥ 40) may increase the risk of early death by two- or even threefold (see **FIGURE 12.7**).

However, there is one beneficial health aspect of obesity—bone mass and density may increase modestly because of weight gain. When weight loss occurs in obese subjects, they also will have declines in bone mass and density, and the amount of bone loss depends on the degree of weight loss.

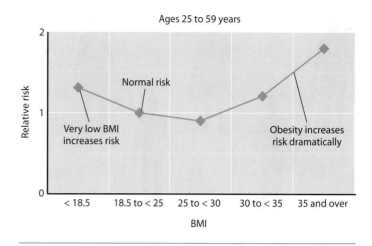

FIGURE 12.7 Mortality Rate Compared to BMI. People with a very high BMI have a higher relative risk of mortality.

Adapted from Flegel KM, Graubard BI, Williamson DF, Gail MH. Excess deaths associated with underweight, overweight, and obesity. *JAMA.* 2005;293:1861–1867.

Weight Loss

Healthy weight loss is slow weight loss. Most experts recommend losses of no more than 1 to 2 pounds per week. **Very low calorie diets (VLCDs)** may produce excessive loss over short time periods, but such losses typically are not sustainable. The three main components that must exist, if weight loss and maintenance of a lower body weight are to be successful, are reduced caloric intake, decreased fat consumption, and regular exercise of 30 minutes or so most days of the week (see **Table 12.1**).

The self-perpetuating nature of obesity may be exacerbated with extreme weight-reduction diets, fasts, and decreased exercise. As a protective function against starvation, the body responds to caloric deprivation with a reduction in BMR. In other words, the body expends less energy in thermogenesis (the production of heat) and the maintenance of basic body functions with decreased energy intake. This metabolic compensation explains why some obese individuals may fail to lose weight on as little as 800 kilocalories per day over periods of weeks or longer. Recent evidence suggests that exercise may prevent this adaptation-to-starvation response, but unfortunately dieting often is accompanied by a decrease in physical activity.

Changes in Body Compartments

Weight loss occurs primarily because of a decline in adipose tissue mass, but both LBM and bone tissues are lost during weight reduction. Losses in LBM result from the degradation of protein-rich tissues, such as skeletal and heart muscle. Free fatty acids from adipose tissue can be used as energy sources by the liver and nearly all other tissues. Amino acids that are part of the structures of LBM tissues are converted to alanine

TABLE 12.1 Recommendations for Weight Loss and Maintenance
• Reduce total caloric intake.
• Decrease fat consumption.
• Engage in regular exercise.

gallstone A crystalline deposit that forms in the gallbladder. Can be as large as a golf ball or as small as a grain of sand.

very low calorie diet (VLCD) A diet that provides approximately 400 to 600 kilocalories per day for the purpose of weight loss (e.g., protein-sparing modified fast).

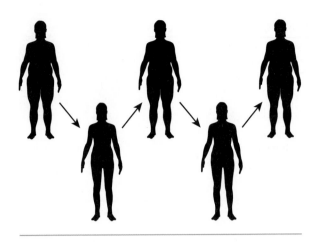

FIGURE 12.8 Yo-Yo Dieting. Yo-yo dieting results in the alternating increase and decrease in size of fat cells.

within the muscle and other cells. Alanine is then degraded for meeting glucose needs via the alanine–glucose cycle, compromising the ability of the tissues to function.

Weight Cycling

Many people who are following a weight-loss diet will stop dieting at one time or another. If they return to their old eating patterns, they usually regain the previous weight lost, often quite rapidly. This down-and-up pattern is called weight cycling, or yo-yo dieting. When they are dieting their shrunken fat cells are often referred to as "being hungry" and will likely gain new triglycerides and fill up again once energy intake increases. **FIGURE 12.8** illustrates the typical pattern of yo-yo dieting along with the relative filling of fat cells under the two extremes of weight gain and loss. However, how much fat mass yo-yo dieters regain during rebound is not clear. One recent report did not find an increase in fat mass after body weight returned to the pre-weight-loss value in a study of obese subjects.

As individuals go through cycles of weight loss and weight regain, they may also lower their LBM (and BMR), which is not a healthy change. The loss of LBM during weight loss leads to sarcopenia, which may be followed by insufficient replacement of muscle of all three types (skeletal, heart, and smooth) during each cycle of regaining weight. Loss of LBM should be avoided during any weight-loss regimen. Although the erratic swings in eating behavior characterized by weight cycling may have adverse effects on dieters' bodies, the precise effects cannot be determined at present.

Approaches to Weight Management

Weight can be managed in a number of ways, depending on the amount of weight that needs to be lost. Current weight management techniques include dietary modification, behavioral approaches, physical activity, medication, and gastric surgery.

Dietary Recommendations

Distinctions exist among the types of weight-loss diets used for weight reduction. Keep in mind, however, that any diet that provides fewer calories than needed for daily activities will result in weight loss, regardless of the nature of the macronutrient mix of the diet. Fasting, a dangerous approach when applied for longer than 24 hours, means that no food is consumed for a period of time (although water is permissible). **Fasting** is generally *not* a safe method for weight loss. Over a period of several days, total fasting results not only in negative energy balance but also in negative balances of nitrogen (from protein), vitamins, and minerals.

Hypocaloric diets (roughly 1,200 kilocalories per day or less) that provide too little energy to meet cellular needs are routinely used for weight reduction. The idea is that the body will use energy from its fat reserves to meet the body's energy needs. Under medical supervision, very restrictive diets (~400 to 600 kilocalories per day) can be used. Most physicians and nutritionists recommend the less severe hypocaloric diets as the recommended approach to sensible weight loss. Weight loss on these types of diets takes time and patience to achieve, but it is the healthiest approach to weight loss.

In moderate restriction, caloric intake may be reduced to 1,200 to 1,600 kcal per day depending on the individual's sex, height, and weight. Fat should be reduced on any low-calorie diet. A well-planned diet at this caloric level can provide the needed nutrients and will usually result in gradual weight loss (1 to 2 pounds per week). More rapid

fasting The absence of food (but not necessarily water or other fluids) for a period of time. For example, an overnight fast typically lasts 12 hours. Fasting becomes total starvation when no food is consumed for 2 days or longer; physiologic mechanisms respond rapidly to fasting to protect vital bodily resources.

weight loss associated with crash diets or fasts is typically associated with excessive loss of lean tissue (LBM) and body fluids. Keeping the weight off also requires some type of maintenance diet that continues the intake of both lower amounts of fat and total energy for a lifetime. Calorie control is usually aided by eating breakfast and smaller meals during the rest of the day in addition to exercise. Behavioral modification employs steps that lead to the extinction of old behaviors and the institution of new healthy behaviors, especially those relating to food selection and serving size in balanced meals.

Hypocaloric diets should include representative foods from the basic food groups each day. **High-protein, low-carbohydrate diets**, such as Atkins, South Beach, and others, and low-fat regimens are hypocaloric and if carefully followed they restrict caloric consumption and reduce body weight. These diets, however, tend to minimize intakes of certain micronutrients, which can be detrimental to health if followed for long periods of time. In contrast, hypocaloric diets such as Weight Watchers and similar diets that encourage consumption of a variety of foods from all the food groups provide all the micronutrients in sufficient amounts.

One aspect of weight reduction is the early phenomenon of water loss as food intake declines. Water loss represents a major component of weight loss during the first few days after beginning a hypocaloric diet, before muscle and adipose tissues adapt their metabolic machinery to the decreased energy consumption. Glycogen, the starch that is stored in the liver and muscles, binds substantial amounts of water. When this glycogen is depleted during the first few days of a hypocaloric diet, this water also is released and excreted. Thus, water loss of several pounds over 7 to 10 days may be encouraging to the dieter, but this loss does not represent fat loss to any important extent.

The simultaneous degradation of fat and protein-rich tissues, such as muscle, becomes significant only 7 to 10 days after starting a hypocaloric diet. Finally, weight loss should not exceed 1 to 2 pounds per week after the initial adjustment period of 7 to 10 days so protein tissue degradation does not become overly excessive.

Weight-loss diets tend to rise and fall in popularity. In recent years, high-protein, low-carbohydrate diets have been quite popular, but interest in these diets seems to be declining because of clinical complications and poor success in keeping the pounds off long term. All of these diets need to be consumed along with fruits and vegetables and dietary fiber in order to maintain a healthy intake of all nutrients.

The best way to prevent obesity, as well as the development of type 2 diabetes, is to maintain body weight within a healthy range by reducing energy consumption and increasing physical activity; that is, modifying both food intake and activity patterns. The caloric distribution of an **obesity-prevention diet** should approximate the values given in **Table 12.2**. Thus, the optimal diet should be low in fats, animal proteins, sugars (except naturally occurring ones present in dairy products and fruits), and alcohol, which contains largely "empty" calories (i.e., calories without micronutrients). Foods with added sugars, sweetened alcoholic beverages, and soft drinks also add extra unneeded or "empty" calories and should be avoided. Consumption of fruit juices in large quantities should also be limited because of their high caloric value. Furthermore, the optimal diet should be high in complex carbohydrates and dietary fibers, focusing on fruits and vegetables. Processed foods that contain excessive amounts of fat, salt, or sugar should be limited. This wholesome diet, in addition to preventing obesity, is also protective against the development of diabetes, dental caries, high blood pressure, coronary disease, and possibly cancer.

The obesity-preventive diet is probably the best all-around diet for all people. This type of diet is used in treating patients who have both obesity and type 2 diabetes as well as other chronic diseases associated with excessive energy consumption. The key to controlling obesity, type 2 diabetes, and the other chronic diseases remains the reduction of body weight to within the normal range of BMI (18.5 to 24.9) through dietary

> ❝ In moderate restriction, caloric intake may be reduced to 1,200 to 1,600 kilocalories per day depending on the individual's sex, height, and weight. ❞

> ❝ The obesity-preventive diet is probably the best all-around diet for all people. ❞

high-protein, low-carbohydrate diet A hypocaloric diet that is proportionally high in proteins and low in carbohydrates in an effort to promote weight loss. Examples include the Atkins Diet and the South Beach Diet. These diets minimize intakes of certain nutrients and therefore can be detrimental if followed for long periods of time.

obesity prevention diet A diet that is low in fats, animal proteins, sugars, and alcohol and high in complex carbohydrates and dietary fibers, with a focus on fruits and vegetables. This diet is also protective against the development of diabetes, dental caries, hypertension, coronary artery disease, and possibly cancer.

TABLE 12.2
Major Components of the Obesity-Preventive Diet

Nutrient Variable	Recommendations
Energy	Achieve/maintain BMI < 25.
Carbohydrates	55–60% of total calories. Consume complex carbohydrates and dietary fiber. Avoid processed carbohydrates.
Fat	≤ 30% of total calories. Consume low-fat dairy foods and reduce other fats.
Protein	≤ 15% of total calories. Reduce number of servings of meat/fish/poultry per day and increase legumes by one to two servings per day.
Beverages	The focus should be on consuming water. Limit alcoholic beverages to only one to two drinks per day. Sugary beverages should be limited so as to consume no more than 30 grams of sugar from such beverages.
Dietary fiber	Consume a variety of plant sources (legumes, whole grains, nuts, seeds, and fruits).
Cholesterol	≤ 300 mg per day.
Micronutrients	Consume five servings of fruits and vegetables per day, especially fresh citrus fruits and dark green, leafy vegetables.

modification and a regular exercise program starting early in life and continuing into adulthood. Professional help may be needed for the chronically obese.

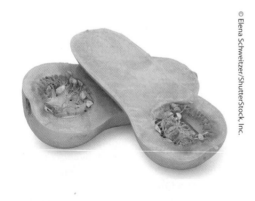

© Elena Schweitzer/ShutterStock, Inc.

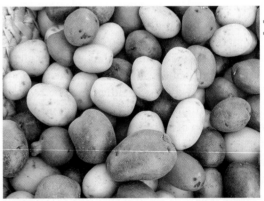
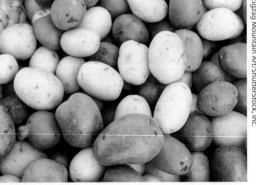

© Zigzag Mountain Art/ShutterStock, Inc.

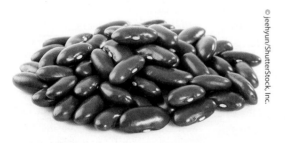

© jeehyun/ShutterStock, Inc.

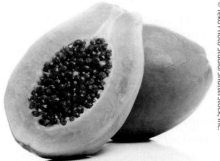

© Yeko Photo Studio/ShutterStock, Inc.

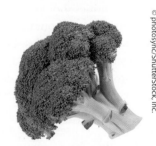

© photosync/ShutterStock, Inc.

FOCUS 12.2   Weight Management and Type 2 Diabetes

The vast majority of subjects with type 2 diabetes are overweight or obese at the time of onset. Usually, they also are over 35 years of age. One of the first steps in the clinical management of a newly recognized diabetic subject is weight loss to achieve a healthy body weight as well as by improvements in other health indicators. In the past, such patients have initially been placed on a calorie-restricted diet (1,200 kilocalories per day for women; 1,600 kilocalories per day for men), with most calories coming from complex carbohydrates. Patients used to be instructed to use diabetic exchange lists in order to adhere to the prescribed energy intake, but the exchange system was so difficult to learn that it has largely been abandoned. Today, many patients are allowed to consume according to their own preferences within the parameters of a healthy diet (i.e., a "no diet" approach). Dietary counseling of diabetic subjects, and their family members, is important in motivating and teaching the subjects to control their weight and hence their diabetes.

When a healthier body weight (normal BMI range or possibly overweight) is achieved, the symptoms of diabetes mellitus disappear in many patients. Glucose tolerance curves, previously abnormal, become improved and even almost normalized, and urinary glucose (sugar) may no longer be detected. Long-term success of dietary modifications, however, depends on the motivation and adherence to healthy eating practices.

In addition to dietary approaches, most patients with type 2 diabetes are treated with drugs to keep their blood glucose concentrations down (but still typically higher than normal). Oral glycosides that help glucose entry into cells are the first-line drugs in treatment. If they are not sufficiently effective in regulating blood glucose, then insulin injections may be employed.

Dietary approaches are recommended to be tried first, but drugs may be preferable because of more immediate results in lowering blood glucose and obesity. Unfortunately, diet therapy requires long periods of modifications of eating patterns and gaining nutrition knowledge before improvement of health status is achieved. Physicians are less likely to emphasize dietary changes and they are more likely to go directly to the use of drugs to treat obesity and altered glucose metabolism and elevated serum insulin concentrations, whereas dietitians favor dietary modifications. Yet, to obtain successful dietary modification, especially the acceptance of a more plant-based diet, patients need to be very willing to modify their diets. Health professionals, especially dietitians and diabetes educators, are needed to serve as change agents in addition to physicians. ●

Physical Activity

As has been discussed, physical activity is a critical component of weight management. Participation in a regular exercise program most days of the week for a minimum of 30 minutes helps insulin move glucose into skeletal muscle tissue and probably other tissues as well. Because of the beneficial impact on insulin utilization and regulation of blood glucose, people with type 2 diabetes are often prescribed exercise. In fact, regular physical activity often can eliminate the need for drug treatment of diabetic patients. The combination of diet and exercise can be successful in reducing body weight and serum glucose concentrations. In addition, frequent physical activity is also associated with decreased appetite and may help to maintain the BMR in the face of decreased caloric intake. Of course, physical activity must be tailored to the abilities of the individual and may require medical supervision.

Behavior Modification Techniques

Behavior modification techniques are used to help individuals achieve successful dietary changes and increase physical activity. Behavioral approaches teach the person to analyze his or her own behavior, to identify those situations and behaviors that contribute to excess weight, and to modify those situations or behaviors so as to produce long-term changes that will promote weight loss and maintenance of a desirable

behavior modification (dietary) The use of psychological techniques for changing individual behaviors related to food consumption, including wise selection of foods, meal planning, and food preparation. Involves unlearning old, unhealthy habits and learning new, healthy behaviors.

weight. Self-monitoring of eating behavior is often a cornerstone of behavioral weight-loss programs.

Self-monitoring approaches differ from just keeping a food diary in that the subject is often asked to record the time and location of eating, associated emotions and activities, and eating companions in addition to food and caloric intake. Such information allows the individual to analyze patterns, such as overeating when stressed or tired, that may contribute to his or her weight problem. Once the subject has identified problem situations, behavioral strategies for solving those problems are devised. These strategies depend on the expertise of the behavioral specialists involved in dietary management.

The presence of a weight plateau in many obese individuals suggests that a hypothalamic set point has been established at some time during early adulthood. The mechanism regulating this set point appears to be genetically controlled and frustrates the most motivated of dieters. Because of this biological set point, it is likely that approaches such as behavioral therapy alone will not help the vast majority of severely obese subjects. In these cases drug therapy may be warranted.

Pharmacologic Therapy

Pharmacologic (drug) therapy is currently used in the treatment of obesity. Anorectic drugs (i.e., appetite suppressants) alter the levels of one or more neurotransmitters in the brain that are thought to be involved in the regulation of eating behavior. Although it is generally held that such drugs suppress appetite, in fact they operate in a variety of ways, and so far they have not been very successful, in part because of major adverse side effects. Drug therapies for obese subjects need to be demonstrated to be both safe and efficacious over fairly long periods of treatment.

Other useful drugs for reducing fat digestion and absorption, and hence body fat, are enzyme inhibitors that act within the lumen of the small intestine. Drugs such as orlistat act within the GI tract by partially blocking the action of lipase enzymes and thereby reducing the amount of fatty acids made available for absorption across the intestinal epithelium. More fat enters the stools in individuals who tolerate the drug well, although some subjects do not tolerate it well. Long-term effects on weight reduction in patients taking these drugs have been modest, yet beneficial.

These new approaches of pharmacologic therapy, combined with other approaches, will continue to be used with overweight and modestly obese individuals. Because anorectic drugs have no impact on the individual's eating habits, environment, and preferences, obese individuals will still need nutrition education or re-education to improve their food selection, portion control, and eating practices. Drug therapy will most likely always be used in conjunction with some form of diet therapy and exercise to control weight. Recent drug discoveries of agents for the treatment of obese subjects suggest that a revolution in the pharmacologic treatment of obesity has just begun.

Gastric Surgery

Surgical treatment has been used as an approach to severe obesity for the past few decades. Because surgical treatments involve considerable medical risk, they are generally restricted to individuals with a BMI of 35 or greater with comorbidities (other diseases) or a BMI of 40 or greater with no comorbidities who have tried and failed at other weight-loss efforts and who are physically able to withstand the medical procedure. Surgical procedures for obesity generally involve bypassing a section of the stomach (see **FIGURE 12.9**). Bypass surgery is designed to limit food intake without seriously interfering with digestion and absorption. In stomach bypass surgery, a small section of stomach is separated from the rest of the stomach with staples and connected to the intestines, which greatly reduces the size of the stomach. The result is greatly reduced consumption of food, because excessive food consumption results in extreme discomfort and vomiting. The gastric procedure may result in rapid loss of up to 55% of a person's excess weight. However, the procedure has a mortality rate of 1% to 2%, and death rates for patients older than age 50 are much higher.

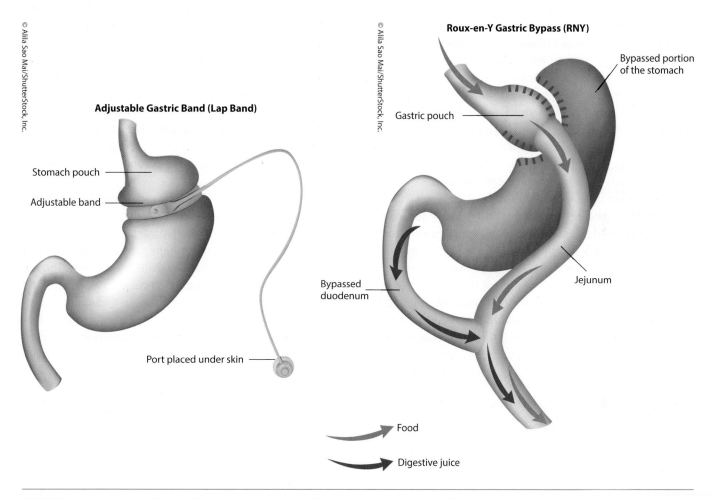

FIGURE 12.9 Gastric Bypass Surgery. With gastric bypass surgery, the stomach's capacity is reduced by approximately 50%.

SUMMARY

With excessive energy intake, fat cells enlarge and the body fat compartment also increases in mass. The changes in body fat distribution are linked, in part, to gender: females have more gynoid distribution and males more android. If expansion of the fat compartment becomes maxed out, new fat cells are generated to accommodate the need for greater storage of energy derived from foods, and this capacity is enormous! High storage capacity of triglycerides in fat cells is uniform throughout adipose tissue and muscle tissue and this condition contributes to insulin insensitivity and a high serum concentration of glucose, which in turn lead to other chronic diseases beyond obesity. Typically, in adulthood the body fat compartment increases in both mass and percentage of total body mass (weight) and BMI increases. BMI serves as a useful estimate of total body fat.

In the United States and many other developed countries, obesity has become a highly prevalent multifactorial disease with serious health consequences. Excess body fat leads to metabolic alterations that contribute to the major chronic diseases so common in affluent societies. In general, the percent fat composition of the body increases with adult age. Overconsumption of food and too little activity represent the major, though not the only, factors involved in the causation of obesity. Other causes of obesity include social and cultural factors such as eating at fast-food restaurants and the increasing amount of time spent performing sedentary activities.

For obesity, type 2 diabetes, and other chronic diseases resulting from excessive energy consumption, dietary modifications that lead to weight loss and stabilization at a healthy body weight can also be effective in reducing the often severely elevated blood glucose concentration. Subject compliance to and acceptance of healthy diets are the most difficult obstacles to successful therapy. The metabolic syndrome is taking on much more significance in the United States in the twenty-first century. An optimal diet for obesity prevention serves also for the prevention of not only type 2 diabetes but for practically all of the other chronic diseases of adults as well.

Responsible dieting involves a steady loss of 1 to 2 pounds a week on a healthy, well-rounded diet coupled with an exercise program. Many dieting strategies have developed, including those that advocate high protein intake and low carbohydrates and those that advocate the opposite. The key is a sustained hypocaloric approach coupled with increased physical activity. For those for whom dieting has been unsuccessful, new drug therapies have been shown to hold promise, but their long-term effectiveness and safety remain to be established. The treatment of severely obese subjects with surgery has been very helpful but has risks.

STUDENT ACTIVITIES

1. Using the current definitions of BMI, define *overweight* and *obesity*.

2. Define *underweight* in terms of BMI. Do underweight and obesity have the same risks?

3. Calculate the BMI of a 60 year-old woman who is 5 feet tall and weighs 180 pounds. Use metric units. Conversions are 1 lb = 0.45 kg; 1 ft = 12 in × 2.54 cm/in.

4. Briefly explain how DXA data of two different compartments of the body (i.e., bone mass of 2 kg and fat mass of 37 kg) can be used to estimate the lean body mass or muscle mass. Use a young adult male 100-kilogram (total body mass) body weight for this calculation.

5. Describe the biological process by which fat cells may be increased in the body.

6. Explain what happens to fat cells when weight loss occurs.

7. Explain why overweight/obesity can so easily lead to type 2 diabetes.

8. Describe the typical distribution of body fat in females and males. Explain why the fat distribution patterns differ.

9. Name three additional chronic diseases that obesity promotes in adults.

10. Speculate on the effect of obesity on death rates of males and females and how the rates increase with age later in life.

11. In one column, list the adverse risk factors for obesity and then in a second column briefly explain how each contributes to obesity.

12. Explain why excessive body fat affects blood flow to organs of the body.

13. Speculate on the meaning of the term *sarcobesity*, which occurs in many older adults.

WEBSITES FOR FURTHER STUDY

American Diabetes Association
www.diabetes.org
American Heart Association: Population-Based Prevention of Obesity
http://circ.ahajournals.org/content/118/4/428.full.pdf
The Obesity Society
www.obesity.org

CDC: Overweight and Obesity
www.cdc.gov/nccdphp/dnpa/obesity
Medline Plus: Obesity
www.nlm.nih.gov/medlineplus/obesity.html
WHO Health Topics: Obesity
www.who.int/topics/obesity/en

REFERENCES

Anderson JJB, Prytherch S, Sparling M, Barrett CH, Guyton JR. Metabolic syndrome. *Nutr Today.* 2006;41:115-122.

Brand-Miller J, Colagiuri S. Insulin resistance and the metabolic syndrome. In: Erdman JW Jr, MacDonald IA, Zeisel SH (eds.). *Present Knowledge in Nutrition.* 10th ed. Ames, IA: John Wiley & Sons; 2012: 1166–1185.

Casazza K, Nagy T. Body composition evaluation. In: Erdman JW Jr, MacDonald IA, Zeisel SH (eds.). *Present Knowledge in Nutrition.* 10th ed. Ames, IA: John Wiley & Sons; 2012: 1557–1573.

Drewnowski A. The real contribution of added sugars and fats to obesity. *Epidemiol Rev.* 2007;29:160–171.

Food and Nutrition Board, Institute of Medicine. *Dietary Reference Intakes for Energy.* Washington, DC: National Academies Press; 2002.

Johnstone AM. Energy intake, obesity, and eating behavior. In: Erdman JW Jr, MacDonald IA, Zeisel SH (eds.). *Present Knowledge in Nutrition.* 10th ed. Ames, IA: John Wiley & Sons; 2012: 1627–1650.

Jenkins DJA, Wolever TM, Taylor RH, et al. Glycemic index of foods: a physiological basis for carbohydrate exchange. *Am J Clin Nutr.* 1981;34(3):362–366.

Katz DL. Competing dietary claims for weight loss: Finding the forest throughout truculent trees. *Ann Rev Public Health.* 2005;21:61–88.

Kelly TL, Wilson KE, Heymsfield SB. Dual energy x-ray absorptiometry body composition reference values from NHANES. *PLoS One.* 2009;4:e7038.

Maqbool A, Dougherty KA, Parks EP, Stallings VA. Adolescence. In: Erdman JW Jr, MacDonald IA, Zeisel SH (eds.). *Present Knowledge in Nutrition.* 10th ed. Ames, IA: John Wiley & Sons; 2012: 1021–1048.

Nicklas TA, Baranowski T, Cullen KW, Berenson G. Eating patterns, dietary quality and obesity. *J Am Coll Nutr.* 2001;20(6):599–608.

Nicklas TA, Yang SJ, Baranowski T, Zakeri I, Berenson G. Eating patterns and obesity in children: The Bogalusa Heart Study. *Am J Prev Med.* 2003;25(1):9–16.

Pedersen SD, Sjödin A, Astrup A. Obesity as a health risk. In: Erdman JW Jr, MacDonald IA, Zeisel SH (eds.). *Present Knowledge in Nutrition.* 10th ed. Ames, IA: John Wiley & Sons; 2012: 1127–1146.

Rolls BJ, Roe LS, Meengs JS. Reductions in portion size and energy density of foods are additive and lead to sustained decreases in energy intake. *Am J Clin Nutr.* 2006;83(1):11–17.

Sahyoun NR, Jacques PF, Zhang XL, Juan W, McKeown NM. Whole-grain intake is inversely associated with the metabolic syndrome and mortality in older adults. *Am J Clin Nutr.* 2006;83(1):124–131.

Zizza C, Siega-Riz AM, Popkin BM. Significant increase in young adults' snacking between 1977–1978 and 1994–1996 represents a cause for concern! *Prev Med.* 2001;32(4):303–310.

ADDITIONAL READING

Brand Miller J, Wolever T. *The New Glucose Revolution.* New York: Marlowe & Company; 2003.

Calle EE, Kaaks R. Overweight, obesity and cancer: Epidemiologic evidence and proposed mechanisms. *Nat Rev Cancer.* 2004;4(8):579–591.

Flegal KM, Graubard BI, Williamson DF, Gail MH. Excess deaths associated with underweight, overweight, and obesity. *JAMA.* 2005;293(15):1861–1867.

Ford ES, Giles WH, Dietz WH. Prevalence of the metabolic syndrome among US adults: Findings from the third National Health and Nutrition Examination Survey. *JAMA.* 2002;287(3):356–359.

Gosnell M. Killer fat. *Discover.* February 2007;48–53.

Motluk A. Supersize surprise. *New Scientist.* 2007;192:34–38.

Reaven, GM. Role of insulin resistance in human disease: Banting Lecture 1988. *Diabetes.* 1988;37(12):1595–1607.

Reaven GM. The metabolic syndrome: Is this diagnosis necessary? *Am J Clin Nutr.* 2006;83:1237–1247.

Shell ER. *The hungry gene: The inside story of the obesity industry.* New York: Grove Press; 2002.

CHAPTER 13

Nutritional Needs for Physically Active Adults and Athletes

For athletes, dancers, or those engaging in moderate exercise or physical activity, optimal performance depends on good nutrition. Intake of adequate amounts of macronutrients, micronutrients, and water are critical in meeting the body's increased demands during physical activity. The energy-yielding macronutrients are primarily carbohydrates and fats, though proteins provide approximately 15% to 17% of total caloric intake each day. Proteins also provide essential amino acids needed for repair of tissues involved in activities such as muscle and tendons. Energy must be consumed in amounts commensurate with energy expenditure in exercise or physical activity, such as sports and dance, in order to maintain body weight. Micronutrients need to be consumed to support a variety of functions, such as increased muscle contractions, which require enzyme cofactors to generate the ATP needed for optimal physical performance. Water intake should be increased to compensate for fluids lost through sweat and urine production. In active individuals, all tissues benefit from optimal intakes of nutrients, phytochemicals, and fluids.

Nutrition and exercise go hand-in-hand in achieving physical fitness and reaping the associated health benefits. Like all people, athletes should maintain their weight at a level that is consistent with good health by balancing energy (calorie) intake from foods with energy expenditure in regular daily activities. Skeletal muscle mass, which constitutes a large fraction of LBM, is maintained predominantly through its use in physical activity. If energy expenditure is high due to increased physical activity, food intake also should generally be increased to meet the body's caloric needs and to ensure adequate intake of all the essential nutrients.

The benefits of regular physical activity and good nutrition are many, including a healthy appearance and increased endurance in performing everyday activities. Advantages to the organ systems of the body also accrue from the combination of good

❝ Nutrition and exercise go hand-in-hand in achieving physical fitness and reaping the associated health benefits. ❞

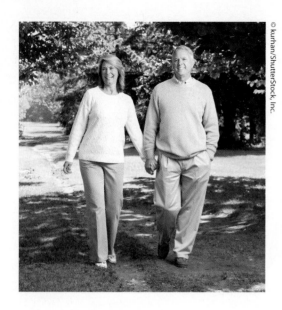

© kurhan/ShutterStock, Inc.

nutrition and regular physical activity. Some of these benefits include increases in cardiovascular function, lung capacity, strength and endurance, and bone mass and integrity. Physical activity can also reduce tension and stress, and, of course, is instrumental in achieving and maintaining one's ideal weight. One of the major benefits of physical activity is improvements in bone density in young males and females, which have been shown to be maintained three to four decades after the high-level physical activity ceases. Physical activity and exercise throughout the life cycle can help to prevent the development of chronic diseases later in life.

This chapter provides an overview of nutrition in relation to exercise. It is divided into two parts. The first part considers the nutrient needs of healthy, moderately active individuals who perhaps engage in recreational sports or other fitness pursuits. The second part examines the nutrient needs of competitive athletes and others who engage in strenuous physical activity, such as dancers. Nutrient intake recommendations are only modestly increased for competitive athletes and very active individuals.

If the amount of physical activity or exercise increases, so will the need for additional nutrients, at least to a modest extent, in order to maintain functional tissues and to maintain weight at the new level of energy expenditure.

Nutrition and Healthy, Active Living

People who exercise regularly are better able to balance their energy intake and energy output. Maintenance of body weight (or BMI) at a healthy level is an important consequence of regular physical activity. Appropriate intake of energy (calories) by moderately active individuals, accompanied by adequate intakes of protein, water, and micronutrients, supports the body's many functions and contributes generally to good health. If the amount of physical activity or exercise increases, so will the need for additional nutrients, at least to a modest extent, in order to maintain tissue function and to maintain weight at the new level of energy expenditure. It is not possible to know precisely how much energy an individual needs until training routines occur and the individual has adapted to the new activity level.

Specific Nutritional Needs for Healthy, Active Adults

The specific nutritional needs of most physically fit individuals can be met by meeting or slightly exceeding the RDAs for the various macronutrients and micronutrients. Most moderately active individuals should be able to meet approximately 100% of their nutritional requirements by consuming the number of food servings recommended by MyPlate. **Table 13.1** lists the RDAs for some of the major essential nutrients and provides additional information on nutrient needs for athletes and moderately active adults. By following these general guidelines, most people should be able to achieve a high level of physical fitness.

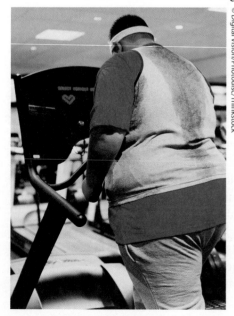

© Digital Vision/Photodisc/Thinkstock

Body weight should remain relatively constant near the desirable weight for height at which each individual is able to maintain a feeling of well-being. Because weight may be affected by greater muscle mass, body weight and BMI may exceed the normal range for those who engage in moderate physical activity, particularly those who engage in sustained weight training. (Excessive overweight does not typically infer fitness, even in competitive athletes who have great strength or power in lifting or moving massive weight but who have excessive abdominal fat accumulation.)

Those individuals engaging in moderate levels of exercise probably do not require additional servings of protein because most North Americans are already ingesting more protein than is needed to meet daily tissue needs. The RDA levels of dietary protein typically remain sufficient to support good health. Protein

TABLE 13.1

Recommended Intakes and Reasons for Increased Intake by Athletes and Moderately Active Adults

Nutrient	Male	Female	Reason for Increased Intake with Physical Activity
Energy	3,000 kcal	2,200 kcal	To support tissue function, especially increased energy needs of skeletal muscle
Protein	60 g	50 g	To replace degraded muscle proteins
Water	—	—	To maintain fluid balance
Iron	10 mg	18 mg	To replace increased losses, especially via the GI tract
Calcium	1,000 mg	1,000 mg	To support increased bone formation
Antioxidants	—	—	To defend against exercise-generated free radicals
Other vitamins and minerals	—	—	To support many tissue and organ functions

Data from Food and Nutrition Board, Institute of Medicine. *Dietary Reference Intakes.* Washington, DC: National Academies Press;1997–2004, 2011.

> Those individuals engaging in moderate levels of exercise probably do not require additional servings of protein because most North Americans are already ingesting more protein than is needed to meet daily tissue needs.

intakes in the United States are typically so high that with adequate energy consumption more than enough protein is regularly ingested.

Needs for many micronutrients, particularly the water-soluble vitamins such as thiamin, niacin, and riboflavin, are increased in some athletes and moderately active individuals, but adequate amounts are consumed with increased food intake. Intakes of certain minerals, such as calcium and iron, may need to be increased to meet the body's needs, especially for female athletes or women engaging in a lot of physical activity. Most vitamins and other minerals also are needed in modestly increased amounts by athletes and moderately active individuals. Fat-soluble vitamins need to be consumed at only 100% of the RDA levels; increases are not needed.

Dietary calcium is absorbed to replace calcium lost in urine and sweat each day. It also is used to replace bone mineral lost in normal bone turnover. In individuals who put more strain on their bones during physical activity, however, more calcium ions are incorporated into the bone as a result of new bone formation. Little or no gain in bone mass and density occurs with moderate activity, but the bone that is renewed or repaired by exercise is healthier. Thus, maintaining an adequate intake of calcium at RDA levels should accompany any activity pattern because of the protection against microscopic fractures and the maintenance of bone strength that result from the combination of adequate intakes of calcium, other nutrients, and exercise. Phosphate is typically sufficient in all diets if enough food is consumed. Magnesium intake may need to be increased slightly, especially if dietary plant sources are low. Recall that dark green, leafy plants are the major sources of this mineral. Potassium also is an important nutrient for people who exercise regularly since sweat contains measurable amounts of potassium and most

> Intakes of fluids and electrolytes typically need to be increased. Adequate intakes of water and other fluids are important for active individuals.

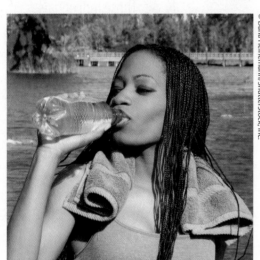

© Dana Heinemann/ShutterStock, Inc.

Americans do not consume RDA levels of this critical mineral. Orange juice, bananas, and potatoes contain substantial amounts of potassium. Sodium in modest amounts may need to be increased because it also is lost in sweat.

Iron is needed to replace the iron lost as a result of the normal degradation of hemoglobin in red blood cells, myoglobin in skeletal muscle, and many enzymes throughout the body. Iron needs are usually higher among competitive athletes but are increased only minimally among moderately active individuals. However, if iron consumption from iron-rich or iron-fortified foods is too low, iron intake from supplements may need to be increased. Iron status monitoring with hematocrit or hemoglobin measures and possibly with serum ferritin measurements may be recommended by a physician prior to iron supplementation.

Antioxidant vitamins, namely vitamin C (ascorbic acid), vitamin E, and the carotenoids, are generally needed in increased amounts by athletes and those engaging in moderate physical activity through the consumption of plant foods and other foods rich in these vitamins. If moderately active individuals take a daily supplement at RDA levels, that extra security over and above their food intake should provide ample amounts of antioxidants that protect against the oxygen-based free radicals generated as a normal consequence of cellular metabolism as a result of oxygen utilization.

Selenium and zinc, two antioxidant minerals, also need to be consumed in RDA amounts on a daily basis by moderately active adults. Selenium is needed by the enzyme glutathione peroxidase, which helps protect cells from free radicals. Zinc is part of a few enzymes that also help to neutralize free radicals. Intakes of selenium and zinc at 100% of their RDAs should be sufficient.

Intakes of fluids and electrolytes typically need to be increased. Adequate intakes of water and other fluids are important for active individuals. Phytochemicals are needed especially for their antioxidants.

Energy Intake for Active Living

Energy is the critical component for optimal physical performance and fitness. Protein, of course, is an important energy source, but calories from carbohydrates and fats drive the muscle activities necessary for physical performance. Energy needs should be met so that individuals retain approximately the same body weight over the time frame of their activity. The more energy that is expended in activities, the more dietary calories that are needed to support the energy-requiring steps of metabolism—up to some reasonable limit.

The three major components of energy expenditure are resting energy expenditure (REE or BMR), diet-induced thermogenesis (DIT), and exercise-induced thermogenesis (EIT), which is also called the thermic effect of exercise. For athletes and others who engage in fairly rigorous physical activity, the percentage of total energy expenditure in these physical activities (EIT) over 24 hours exceeds the estimated 15% expended by individuals involved in light or moderate activities. This 15% EIT is built into the energy DRIs for adults of 3,000 kilocalories per day for males and 2,400 kilocalories for females. For more active individuals, EIT might represent 20% to 30% of total daily expenditures, but no hard-and-fast rule governs this variable level of expenditure.

FIGURE 13.1 compares the daily energy expenditure of an average young adult male, a male collegiate athlete in an endurance sport (e.g., cross-country running), and a moderately active adult male. Figure 13.1 illustrates three points about energy expenditure. First, the REE in absolute kilocalories of the collegiate athlete is almost twice that of the less active male, which reflects a significant increase in metabolism, especially in muscle tissue, even though the REE (%) of total energy expenditure per day is only 60%. Second, the actual amount of energy expended in athletic activities is only about 1,000 kilocalories per day greater than for less active men. Third, although DIT (% of energy) remains approximately 10% for each of the men, the actual energy expended in digestive processes is about 450 kilocalories per day, almost 75% higher in the athlete than in the less active men, because the athlete must consume and digest greater amounts of food to support his daily expenditures.

Energy Systems of the Body

The major calorie-consuming metabolic pathways during exercise are anaerobic and aerobic metabolism (respiration) in all cells of the body but especially in skeletal and heart muscle. The burning of glucose with the addition of oxygen (aerobic metabolism) generates much of the cellular energy (in the form of ATP) needed for muscle contraction and other functions. **FIGURE 13.2** illustrates the relative amounts of ATP generated by aerobic versus anaerobic metabolism.

In contracting skeletal muscle, the demand for oxygen typically increases greatly during the performance of most athletic activities other than sprinting or short-burst lifting. Skeletal muscle contains myoglobin that stores additional oxygen for use during short-burst activities. This protein is especially important during anaerobic activities, but endurance aerobic athletes also may benefit from more efficient oxygen storage on myoglobin gained during training. If an activity lasts for long periods, such as running a marathon, the muscle stores of glycogen are largely depleted in the first hour and the use of fatty acids by muscles for energy increases while the use of glucose declines (see **FIGURE 13.3**). Typically, most athletes and other moderately active individuals use both anaerobic and aerobic metabolic pathways.

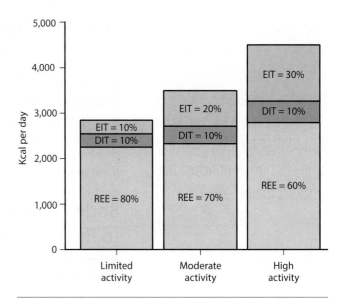

FIGURE 13.1 Daily Energy Expenditure and Physical Activity. Comparison of the daily energy expenditure of an average young adult male, a moderately active adult in his mid-30s, and a male collegiate athlete in an endurance sport.

Modified from Anderson JJB. *Nutrition and Health: An Introduction.* Durham, NC: Carolina Academic Press; 2005.

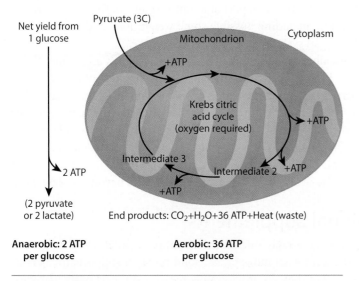

FIGURE 13.2 Relative Amounts of ATP Generated by Aerobic Versus Anaerobic Metabolism.

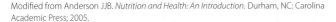

Modified from Anderson JJB. *Nutrition and Health: An Introduction.* Durham, NC: Carolina Academic Press; 2005.

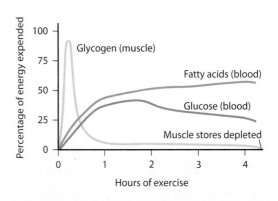

FIGURE 13.3 Glucose and Fatty Acids as Energy Sources. The use of glucose and fatty acids as energy sources changes over time in physical activity.

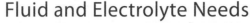

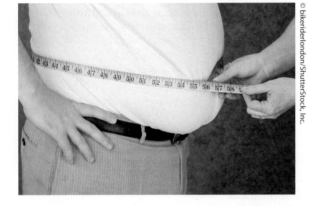
© bikeriderlondon/ShutterStock, Inc.

> Because of electrolyte losses during an event or physical activity, electrolyte balance can only be maintained by additional intake, especially from electrolyte-enriched fluids or sports drinks.

> Major changes in the three compartments of body composition typically follow: fat mass will decline, LBM will increase, and waist circumference will decrease, resulting in a body that appears to be fitter.

sports drink Electrolyte-enriched fluid that is formulated to replace electrolytes lost during a sporting event or physical activity.

Fluid and Electrolyte Needs

Active individuals typically need fluid (water) and electrolyte replacement prior to, during, and after exercise. Exercise increases sweat production in order to dissipate heat from the body. Increased sweat production results in the loss of both water and electrolytes. Both sensible and insensible water losses must be replaced. Because of electrolyte losses during an event or physical activity, electrolyte balance can only be maintained by additional intake, especially from electrolyte-enriched fluids or **sports drinks**. Many individuals do not recognize these electrolyte losses and do not replace them sufficiently through normal food intake or mineral supplements.

Body Composition and Metabolic Adaptations to Regular Exercise

Adaptations of body composition, especially the LBM compartment representing skeletal muscle, follow the level of performance of athletes or activity of more moderately active individuals. Weight adjustments may also occur, but typically an increase in LBM is observed along with a decline in the fat mass in moderately active people who typically maintain their body weight after a sufficient period of training. Any gain in LBM, even a small gain, is a definite plus that hopefully can be maintained for many years by the continuation of regular physical activity. Age and inactivity will eventually contribute to the erosion of LBM, but hopefully any early life gains in functions of the heart, lungs, and other organs can be reasonably conserved.

Individuals of different body weights expend energy in direct relation to their body weight while exercising. To perform the same task—for example, jogging or running a mile—a 200-pound person will expend almost twice as many calories as a 100-pound individual. If this specific exercise is practiced over and over again for weeks to months, modest changes in body weight will typically occur in these adults. Major changes in the three compartments of body composition typically follow: fat mass will decline, LBM will increase, and waist circumference will decrease, resulting in a body that appears more fit. Moderate physical activity, when part of a routine pattern, thus has a positive impact on body composition, including possibly some weight loss, and improves the functioning of the body's organ systems (see **FIGURE 13.4**).

The bone mass of physically active adults may be increased slightly after 6 months or more of moderate activity. Premenopausal women have been shown to obtain this skeletal benefit so long as participation is consistent. Also, older women can maintain—but not necessarily increase—bone mass with regular physical activity. The same holds for middle-aged and older men. Even more impressive gains occur in girls and boys who participate in regular weight-bearing exercises during both pre- and postadolescent stages of growth and development. The skeletal benefits gained early in life have been shown by Swedish investigators to be maintained for as many as 40 years beyond adolescence!

Role of Nutritional Supplements

Active adults may benefit from a daily micronutrient supplement at levels no greater than 100% of current RDAs for each nutrient. No solid research supports the beneficial effects of supplements, but they do provide a degree of insurance, particularly for moderately active individuals. Other types of supplements, such as herbal products, are not recommended.

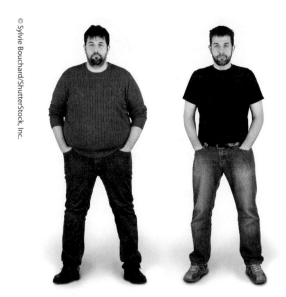

FIGURE 13.4 Body Composition and Exercise. As a person with a higher BMI exercises and converts fat mass to lean mass, the BMI may not change, but health will definitely improve.

> No solid research supports the beneficial effects of supplements.

Nutrition for Competitive Athletes

Competitive athletes and others who engage in vigorous physical activity, such as top-level dancers, have modest increases in nutrient needs during the highly active periods of practice or performance. They also have increased requirements for energy. Although the RDAs for energy, protein, and micronutrients are set for moderately active individuals, not for highly active athletes, the increments above the RDAs needed by very active adults are only modestly greater.

Refer back to Table 13.1 for the RDAs of nutrients and energy for healthy adult males and females. Consider these RDAs to be the lower limits of amounts needed by competitive athletes and dancers. Greater amounts of food than normally consumed provide greater than 100% of the RDAs of most nutrients. Supplements of micronutrients would increase intakes well beyond recommendations and could possibly lead to toxic intake levels.

> Although the RDAs for energy, protein, and micronutrients are set for moderately active individuals, not for highly active athletes, the increments above the RDAs needed by very active adults are only modestly greater.

Energy Intake

Competitive athletes obviously need more calories each day than moderately active individuals. Thus, top-level athletes will typically exceed the age- and sex-specific energy RDAs for both average moderately active individual (i.e., the basis for the energy RDAs), and for relatively inactive individuals. Athletes should meet their increased caloric needs by increasing their carbohydrate intake to 55% or more of total energy consumption. As recommended for all adults, most of these calories should be from complex carbohydrates, not sugars.

In a sustained athletic event such as a long endurance race (running, skating, cycling), the body first burns stored carbohydrates (i.e., glycogen). As glycogen stores run low, the body burns a declining percentage of carbohydrates and starts burning an increasing percentage of fats (see Figure 13.3). However, fat does not generate energy as efficiently as glycogen, and thus athletic performance may suffer in later stages of an endurance event. Although glycogen stores in muscle tissue are greatly reduced

> Athletes should meet their increased caloric needs by increasing their carbohydrate intake to 55% or more of total energy consumption.

PRACTICAL APPLICATIONS 13.1

Calculate the Approximate Daily Energy Needs of a Distance Runner

Assume that a healthy 21-year-old female distance runner covers 70 miles a week at a pace of about 7 to 8 minutes per mile. She is 68 inches tall and weighs 120 pounds. From the RDA table, obtain her age-specific daily energy allowance in kilocalories. Then, estimate her energy expenditure (in kilocalories) from running and add this amount to her RDA for energy (in kilocalories). The total is her estimated daily requirement of energy intake to meet her increased expenditure in exercise. Explain whether you think that this young woman is actually consuming this estimated total amount of calories each day if she is maintaining her weight. ■

over the time of the endurance event, they typically do not become 100% depleted. **Carbohydrate loading** to boost glycogen stores through the consumption of high-starch meals (70% carbohydrate) for a few days prior to a major event helps to prolong the burning of carbohydrates for a longer period during endurance activities and may improve performance. Both muscle and liver glycogen stores are improved.

Protein

> *Generally speaking, this slight need for increased protein is more than met by the increase in food quantities eaten by an active athlete who is already consuming a diet high in protein.*

The protein needs of competitive athletes are modestly higher than those of nonathletes because of increased muscle tissue damage and repair that must occur in order to keep the body in top working condition. In addition, some new protein synthesis of muscle fibers occurs each day. Therefore, athletes should consume one to two additional servings of protein a day. Modest increases in protein intake greater than the RDAs are safe. However, supplemental protein (i.e., protein powder) is not recommended unless protein from foods is insufficient, which may be an issue for vegetarian athletes. Generally speaking, this slight need for increased protein is more than met by the increase in food quantities eaten by an active athlete who is already consuming a diet high in protein.

Fluid and Electrolytes

Fluid needs are greater for competitive athletes and high-level dancers. These active individuals expend so much more energy than moderately active adults that they lose more water from sweat during their activities and for a half-hour or so afterward. Fluid loss that leads to dehydration has serious adverse effects on performance. During competition, athletes with water imbalance may develop muscle cramps, and their muscles may become less efficient.

It is extremely important to protect against the possibility of dehydration and poor performance or inability to perform at all by consuming water as often as possible before, during, and after physical activity. Water is needed to help with heat dissipation, especially in trained athletes, via sweat and other routes (urine and stools), which is critical in protecting against hyperthermia and its damaging effects. Sports medicine personnel working with athletic teams and other athletes are always encouraging athletes to replace fluids so as to prevent heat stroke, heat prostration (collapse), or other complications of water imbalance.

Large male athletes with a low ratio of body surface area to body mass (generally those weighing more than 250 pounds) are particularly vulnerable to heat-related problems because they have poor cooling via sweat evaporation under conditions of high humidity and high temperature. Recent deaths of football players remind us of this vulnerability of excessive body weight in high temperatures. These athletes need cold-water

carbohydrate (glycogen) loading A technique used by endurance athletes to increase muscle glycogen before an event. It involves consuming high-carbohydrate (starch-based) meals several days (typically 6) prior to an event while at the same time decreasing training time.

tubs to jump in for more effective cooling or very cold fans blowing on them. Their major problem is too high a body core temperature resulting from their activities and inefficient cooling by sweat evaporation. Hyperthermia alone may cause severe damage to several tissues, including muscle and brain. Hyperthermia can also result in death.

Electrolytes, namely sodium and potassium, are lost in sweat by competitive athletes and they need to be replaced with meals, generally not by salt pills. Hot, humid environments contribute to even greater electrolyte losses along with fluids. Along with fluids, electrolyte replacement may be recommended if an athlete loses a substantial amount of body weight, roughly 10 pounds or 3% to 7% of body weight, during a practice or a game. For example, large football players practicing in the hot, humid summer months may easily lose this amount of weight (water loss) in a single session. Thus, they will need to replace electrolytes as well as fluids lost in sweat. Athletes especially need to ensure that they consume adequate amounts of potassium from beverages and foods because this electrolyte is critical for the function of skeletal muscle. Severe electrolyte imbalance requires medical care, and this life-threatening condition may be difficult to reverse!

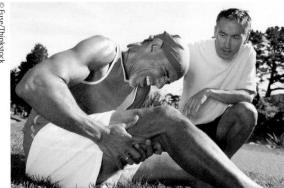

Alcoholic beverages are not recommended for the replacement of lost fluids, even though small amounts (one to two drinks) of alcohol may have an ergogenic effect (see the section on nutritional ergogenic aids).

The maintenance of both water and electrolyte balance permits optimal performance in an activity. Thirst still remains the best guide for water replacement, but athletes often need to be reminded to ingest enough fluids. Sports drinks designed to replace losses remain important aids.

Vitamins and Minerals

As with moderately active adults, vitamins and minerals are generally needed in amounts that reach or modestly exceed 100% of their RDAs. Calcium and iron are highlighted here because of the increased need for these two minerals by competitive athletes. The requirements for athletes for these two minerals have been investigated extensively.

Calcium intake must be at or slightly above RDA levels in order to maintain (or improve) bone mass during periods of physical training. Female athletes in particular are at risk of calcium deficiency because their intake of calcium-rich foods is often low. Calcium deficiency is prevalent among female athletes. Calcium-deficient nonmenstruating (amenorrheic) female athletes who are not producing estrogens are at an increased risk of developing low bone mass, which can result in stress fractures. Cross-country runners, gymnasts, ballet dancers, and other athletes competing at high levels are at particular risk for problems resulting from low calcium intake.

Iron intake may need to be increased to prevent deficiency, or even worse, iron deficiency anemia. Endurance athletes who consume little or no meat, fish, or poultry are at particular risk for developing iron deficiency. In addition, endurance athletes, especially runners, may lose blood (and iron) through the GI tract as a result of stress on the gut tissue from the jarring nature of the activity. Female runners in particular may need an iron supplement.

After heavy training for a period of several months, the body gets tired and somewhat stressed because tissues, especially muscle, require repair. A furlough may be needed. If weight loss and feelings of tiredness occur, the athlete should consider improving his or her dietary habits, perhaps incorporating a supplement; increasing the amount of sleep; and perhaps seeing a physician for an iron status assessment (i.e., hematocrit, hemoglobin) and a physical examination.

Eating for Endurance Training

Refer to a food composition table and find at least five high-carbohydrate foods, especially complex carbohydrates (or combination meals or mixed dishes), that can help distance runners maintain weight during training regimens. List the amount of carbohydrates in one serving of each of the five foods. Then estimate how many servings of each food are required to provide 2,000 kilocalories per day, a large fraction of a female's total daily energy needs. Also, state which micronutrients are provided by each of the five foods in amounts that meet 20% of the RDAs. What can you conclude about the nutritional value of these carbohydrate sources, aside from their supply of energy? ■

Phytomolecules and Dietary Fiber

An RDA exists for dietary fiber but not for any other phytomolecules, many of which act as antioxidants. Fiber aids in the passage of nutrients and waste products through the digestive system as well as in promoting the secretion of bile from the liver and gallbladder. Fiber slows gastric emptying, and thereby nutrient absorption following a meal, but it speeds up colonic transit of materials that are destined for fecal elimination. The many non-nutrient antioxidants in plant foods add to the nutrient antioxidants provided by the diet, all of which help to reduce the presence of potentially damaging free radicals in the cells. With normal or modestly elevated antioxidant intakes, lower blood and urine concentrations of oxidation reaction products are observed in athletes compared to those with low intakes of antioxidants. This benefit of antioxidants requires further research to provide data in support of additional intakes.

Supplements

As a general rule, athletes and other active individuals may benefit from a daily vitamin-mineral supplement that provides micronutrients at 100% of the PDVs (labels for supplements do not use RDAs). Such supplements typically only provide about 10% to 20% of the daily calcium recommendation, but they usually contain 100% RDA amounts for iron and most B vitamins and vitamins C and A (or beta-carotene). These supplements are cheap and provide reasonable assurance of adequate intakes. Calcium intakes may need to be increased by a separate supplement if intake from dairy and other calcium-rich foods does not reach 500 milligrams per day.

Megadoses (doses greater than RDAs or food label PDVs) of micronutrient supplements are not recommended. Megadoses may be harmful and may even interfere with physical performance. Adverse alterations of metabolism may result from chronic high doses of a few micronutrients. Athletes, as well as others, should avoid taking high doses of any vitamin or mineral without a physician's prescription. RDA or PDV amounts of essential micronutrients in a vitamin-mineral supplement, however, are considered safe.

Protein supplements or caloric supplements (see **FIGURE 13.5**) are not generally recommended for athletes; food in sufficient amounts should provide all the needed macronutrients and energy. However, some athletes who wish to increase their body weight may not be able to do so from typical intake of food alone. These individuals are often advised to supplement their regular diet

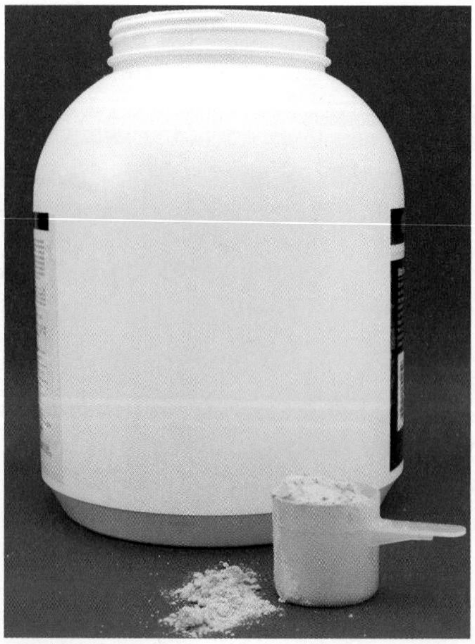

FIGURE 13.5 **Protein Supplements Require Caution.** Consumption of excessive amounts of protein from supplements can result in kidney damage.

© Clifford Farrugia/ShutterStock, Inc.

with energy-rich foods, such as milkshakes, in order to try to increase calorie intake. Continuing caloric supplements after achieving the desired increase in body weight, however, is not recommended. Protein supplements or excessive egg consumption are not recommended, even for power and weight lifters, because of potential adverse effects to the kidneys from excessive nitrogen-containing waste products and of damage to the arterial walls from high circulating levels of cholesterol. It is a myth that athletes require much larger amounts of protein than do nonathletes.

Nutrition-Related Issues Affecting Athletes

Several problems of nutrition are associated with competitive athletic performance. These issues include dehydration, anorexia of running, amenorrhea and the female athlete triad, the use of anabolic steroids and other drugs, and iron deficiency anemia.

Dehydration

Dehydration, a common problem of athletes and others engaging in strenuous activity, often goes unrecognized. Dehydration can lead to a decrease in blood volume and loss of mental concentration, which can adversely affect athletic performance. Fluid intakes should, of course, equal water losses through excretions and losses from body surfaces, especially the high losses from the head and neck. The thirst response, which is activated by a decrease in blood volume or an increase in serum sodium concentration, redresses both the water balance and sodium balance. Sweat losses through evaporation rid the body of the excess heat that accumulates as a result of activity.

On hot, humid days, it is difficult to exchange the heat from the body to the hot, muggy air. The sweat mechanism, however, continues to try to dissipate heat from the body. On such days, water losses can amount to 5% or more of body weight. On cool, windy days, activity continues to generate heat, which is also lost via perspiration. Although water losses on these types of days are usually not appreciated at a conscious level, dehydration still results. Being in air-conditioned rooms or airplanes for long hours also will contribute to dehydration if water and nonalcoholic or noncaffeinated drinks are not consumed.

Anorexia of Running

A new syndrome, known as **anorexia of running**, has recently been described, but it has not been adequately investigated. The loss of appetite and tissue wastage with this condition are not nearly as severe as in advanced anorexia nervosa. This anorexia occurs in men and women who are distance (endurance) runners, typically logging 80 to 100 miles of running a week. The prevalence of anorexia of running and its severity are not well understood at this time because these "anorexic" runners have no apparent adverse effects other than suppressed appetites. These runners typically have low percentages of body fat, and their energy intakes are high in carbohydrates and usually greater than the RDAs that are based on moderate activity rather than the high expenditure levels of distance runners. The appetites of these runners, however, are not as high as expected because some inhibition of the food intake center of the brain is speculated, though not yet supported by research findings.

Amenorrhea and Oligomenorrhea

Amenorrhea is the cessation of the menstrual cycle due to weight loss and a concomitant decline in percentage body fat (i.e., below 10% to 15%). It is defined as the absence of menstrual cycles for 6 consecutive months or longer due to athletic training and losses in body fat. Oligomenorrhea, or fewer than eight menstrual cycles a year, is more common than amenorrhea among female athletes. This suspension of reproductive

> **"** The prevalence of anorexia of running and its severity are not well understood at this time because these "anorexic" runners have no apparent adverse effects other than suppressed appetites. **"**

dehydration Excessive loss of fluids from the body that contributes to water imbalance.

anorexia of running Loss of appetite and tissue wastage in endurance runners who are running 80 to 100 miles per week. Prevalence and severity are not currently well understood.

cycling is common among female athletes who are training intensively, including distance runners, swimmers, gymnasts, basketball players, ballet dancers, and others. Preadolescent girls who because of their sport activities do not achieve menarche by age 13 may go until their late teens before doing so.

Though the precise mechanism is unknown, the inhibition of the menstrual cycle by exercise appears to occur due to decreased estrogen production by the ovaries and significant falls in serum estrogen concentrations. This inhibition likely is initiated in brain centers that lead to reduced hormone secretion that normally supports ovarian function. Exercise-related amenorrhea is associated with low circulating levels of both estrogens and progesterone as well as a low percentage of body fat. In one study of recreational female distance runners, nearly all developed menstrual changes consisting mainly of oligomenorrhea, but none developed amenorrhea. Total body weight did not change in these athletes, but they became leaner when they increased their running distance from the start of serious training (baseline) by 50 miles per week. A second study assessed reproductive hormones of amenorrheic, oligomenorrheic, and eumenorrheic (i.e., those with normal menstrual cycles) women runners and nonrunning controls with daily blood sampling over a 21-day period. Significantly decreased estradiol and progesterone concentrations were found in the oligomenorrheic and amenorrheic runners compared with nonrunning controls and eumenorrheic runners.

Bone loss is commonly found in amenorrheic and oligomenorrheic athletes, especially runners. Bone loss results in osteopenia (i.e., too little bone mass). The loss of bone mass in amenorrheic and possibly oligomenorrheic athletes probably relates to the reduction of serum estrogens. When estrogen levels fall in female athletes, they begin to lose bone mass, as measured by DXA. This loss may be slightly accelerated in females who do not consume adequate amounts of calcium and vitamin D. In some cases the bone loss is so great that exercise-associated stress fractures occur. When stress fractures affect the proximal femur (shaft but not the hip), athletes must take months to recuperate before they can typically compete again.

Following sufficient weight gain and cessation of heavy training, menstrual cycles normally start within a few months. However, some women may not resume their menstrual cycle; these women may require induction of their cycles by drugs or hormones under care of a physician. The reproductive consequences of athletic amenorrhea, in terms of reduced fertility and inability of becoming pregnant, are not clear at this time.

Women who are amenorrheic are at increased risk of injury. Amenorrheic women who run great distances each week have low bone mass of the vertebrae and of the entire skeleton, especially at sites of trabecular bone tissue, which may result from low circulating estrogen concentrations. They also frequently suffer from stress fractures of the femur shaft but not of the hip. These young female runners would have the bone mass roughly equivalent to values of postmenopausal women. Less is known about the adverse effects of oligomenorrhea on the skeleton or in the development of musculoskeletal injuries related to athletic performance rather than to amenorrhea.

Female Athlete Triad

The **female athlete triad** consists of the concurrent medical problems of disordered eating, amenorrhea (or oligomenorrhea), and osteopenia, often accompanied by **stress fractures** (see **FIGURE 13.6**). Disordered eating refers to poor eating practices, such as insufficient calories plus limited amounts of fat and animal protein, rather than to anorexia nervosa. The triad affects female competitive athletes, especially those in endurance or running sports. The poor eating patterns are self-determined and treatment by dietitians and other professionals typically involves restructuring food selection and consuming balanced intakes of acceptable foods that support competitive performance in physical activities.

❝ Amenorrheic women who run great distances each week have low bone mass of the vertebrae and of the entire skeleton. They also frequently suffer from stress fractures of the femur shaft but not of the hip. ❞

❝ The female athlete triad consists of the concurrent medical problems of disordered eating, amenorrhea (or oligomenorrhea), and osteopenia, often accompanied by stress fractures. ❞

female athlete triad A condition occurring among some female athletes that is characterized by amenorrhea or oligomenorrhea, poor eating habits (but not true anorexia), and osteopenia (and possibly stress fractures).

stress fracture A small bone fracture, especially in the femur and feet, that may occur in athletes, especially runners, due to the strain of forces at specific sites; such fractures are often difficult to find on x-rays because they are so small.

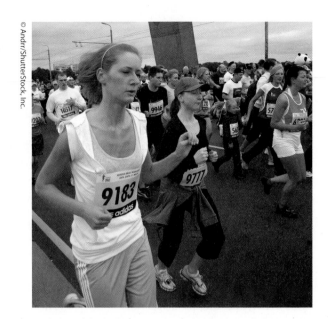

Disordered
eating

Female
athlete
triad

Amenorrhea
(or oligomenorrhea)

Osteopenia
(fractures)

FIGURE 13.6 Female Athlete Triad. The
female athlete triad consists of disordered
eating, amenorrhea (or oligomenorrhea),
and osteopenia.

Reproduced from Anderson JJB. *Nutrition and
Health: An Introduction.* Durham, NC: Carolina
Academic Press; 2005.

Anabolic Steroids and Other Performance-Enhancing Drugs

Anabolic steroids and other drugs used by athletes to improve performance may
have severe adverse effects. Anabolic steroids are similar in many respects to testosterone, the male sex hormone, but these drugs have a more powerful stimulatory action
on muscle development. Muscle mass will increase with exercise or use under the
appropriate training conditions without steroid drugs, but greater muscle mass clearly
results from a combination of the training and steroids.

The problem is that these drugs have adverse effects that are very detrimental to
health. One of these negative effects is that use of steroids can increase blood cholesterol levels well into the unhealthy range (i.e., greater than 240 mg/dL). Other adverse
alterations occur in the metabolism of the liver, gonads, and brain. Behavioral effects
such as rage are also common.

The use of steroid drugs is usually illegal, and athletes in most national and international sports are banned from using them because of the dangers associated with them.
Similarly, other drugs, such as diet pills and "epo" (erythropoietin), that are used by
athletes in attempts to improve their performance are banned and are not considered
safe by medical authorities.

Strict Vegetarian (Vegan) Diets

Strict vegetarians may not obtain sufficient amounts of all nutrients for optimal athletic
performance without additional intake of micronutrient supplements. Vegans, in particular, may find it difficult to get enough energy and all essential nutrients in the amounts
needed for optimal athletic performance because they consume large amounts of fiber
each day with complex carbohydrates in largely unprocessed plant foods. Excessive
fiber intake limits the quantity (volume) of food that can be consumed and, hence, the
amounts of essential micronutrients and phytochemicals. This problem may be overcome if essential micronutrients at 100% RDA levels are consumed from supplements.

Balanced lacto-ovo-vegetarian diets that carefully follow recommendations should
provide all the nutrients in the amounts needed for high-level athletic performance.
Lacto-ovo-vegetarians are usually able to meet their protein needs by consuming dairy
products and eggs. However, athletes in strength sports, such as wrestling, weight lifting,
and others, may need additional protein to maintain their muscle mass and strength in
addition to their body weight.

> *Vegans, in particular,
> may find it difficult to get
> enough energy and all essential
> nutrients in the amounts
> needed for optimal athletic
> performance because they
> consume large amounts of
> fiber each day with complex
> carbohydrates in largely
> unprocessed plant foods.*

anabolic steroid Commonly used
term for synthetic steroid molecules
used by bodybuilders and power
athletes to improve their muscle
mass, muscle definition, or strength.
These drugs are illegal for these
purposes, but they can be used
clinically to improve strength and
bone mass of elderly subjects.

PRACTICAL APPLICATIONS 13.3

Female Vegan Athletes

A healthy 21-year-old female intercollegiate cross-country runner consumes approximately 3,000 kilocalories each day. Because she is a vegan, she typically consumes the following foods each day: eight servings of cereals (breads and grains), four servings of vegetables, three servings of fruit, three 8-ounce cups of soy milk, two servings of nuts, and usually one energy bar (150 kilocalories). One of her vegetable servings is soy (prepared as a burger in a bun) and one of her fruits is a serving of fresh orange juice (6 ounces). Use a food composition table or other sources to determine how her intake of energy and protein compares to the RDAs. Is she getting enough energy and protein to meet her body's needs? ■

Iron Deficiency of Distance Runners

Iron deficiency and iron deficiency anemia disproportionately affect female athletes, especially if they continue to have regular menstrual periods. This deficit of iron results because of the heavy demand for iron by muscle tissue and the poor absorption efficiency of nonheme iron present in vegetables and grains. The major reason for the loss of iron stores by most women is almost invariably a poor diet coupled with menstrual losses. Female athletes may benefit from iron supplements as well as supplements for other micronutrients. Young vegetarian athletes are especially vulnerable to iron deficiency and to the more serious iron-deficiency anemia.

For both genders, excessive running, especially the pounding on hard surfaces, may contribute to gastrointestinal losses of blood and, hence, iron. How widespread these losses are remains uncertain, but they are sufficient that all distance runners should consume additional iron through dietary means or iron supplements. Distance athletes should have their hemoglobin and serum ferritin levels checked.

> **❝** Young vegetarian athletes are especially vulnerable to iron deficiency and to the more serious iron-deficiency anemia. **❞**

Nutritional Ergogenic Aids

Nutritional **ergogenic aids** are substances or mixtures of substances that enhance physical performance. They contain energy (calories) and nutrients that speed up metabolic pathways, thus yielding more metabolic energy for muscular work. Ergogenic aids are intended to help athletes in their specific sports because of their energy-enhancing properties. Honey, glucose, and various sugar or carbohydrate solutions legitimately fit

ergogenic aid Substances that improve physical performance or exercise; nutritional ergogenic aids typically are substances found in common foods, but that are provided in larger quantities to provide a druglike dose; other types of ergogenic aids also exist.

FOCUS 13.1　The Critical Role of Iron in the Diets of Distance Athletes

Iron is a structural component of heme in red blood cells. It also is needed for myoglobin in the muscle and is a structural component of many of the body's enzymes. Enzymes in the mitochondria require iron to generate ATP from glucose. ATP is the energy currency of cells, especially the mitochondria-rich muscle cells that use so much ATP in the contraction of muscle fibers. If iron deficiency occurs, individuals will have too little energy or "pep" to participate in activities. Thus, iron in the diet is critical for maintaining energy for cellular metabolism. Adequate iron intake also may help prevent stress fractures in distance runners. ●

TABLE 13.2
Nutritional Substances Marketed as Ergogenic Aids

Energy-Providing Sources	Other Potential Aids
Sugars (e.g., glucose, fructose, sucrose)	Caffeine
Synthetic carbohydrates	Alcohol
Dextrins	Creatine phosphate
Polycose	B vitamins

Reproduced from Anderson JJB. *Nutrition and Health: An Introduction.* Durham, NC: Carolina Academic Press; 2005.

into this category. Many other bizarre substances do not. A wide variety of substances has been marketed as ergogenic aids (see **Table 13.2**). Most foods provide energy, and therefore are naturally ergogenic.

Carbohydrate-containing sports beverages are the most commonly marketed ergogenic aids, but some precautions are warranted. Because of their high sugar concentrations (and osmotic forces), they attract water to them from body fluids after they enter the GI tract. Thus, some sugar-rich drinks may induce diarrhea, adversely affecting performance. However, when supplied as dilute solutions (i.e., 5% to 7%) these sports beverages may be the most effective of all ergogenic aids. The calories in energy-containing drinks are designed primarily for endurance athletes, but other athletes in sports requiring short bursts of energy, such as sprinting or wrestling, may also benefit from them. Moderately active adults also may benefit from these diluted sugar-based beverages, especially if they contain some electrolytes. Several of these sports drinks are available in the marketplace.

Recall that the energy for most activities is derived primarily from glycogen stores in muscle, rather than from fat stores in adipose tissue, although the utilization of fatty acids increases with time in competitive endurance events. In extended activities, the muscle glycogen supply becomes depleted—as do the liver stores of glycogen—so another source of glucose must be provided. The usual source of energy for muscle functions during extended exercise is blood glucose that is derived from liver gluconeogenesis. When hepatic gluconeogenesis becomes a significant source of energy in an endurance event, dilute glucose solutions will help the athlete keep blood glucose up so that a high level of athletic performance can be maintained. Marathon runners who have utilized all of their glycogen stores by the 18th or 20th mile need glucose replacement as well as fluids after this point, if not sooner, to keep up their pace and finish the race. Well-trained athletes are well adapted to the demands for glucose because their metabolic systems operate at optimal levels.

Other ergogenic aids, such as caffeine and alcohol, may also improve athletic performance in small amounts, but little is known about how they act in the body's exercise-related metabolism. Caffeine may enhance the performance of distance runners when taken just prior to an event, but its benefit compared with a carbohydrate drink may be nil. In general, practically all studies show that if caffeine does have a positive effect on exercise or sport performance, it is not very large.

When supplied as dilute solutions (i.e., 5% to 7%) these sports beverages may be the most effective of all ergogenic aids.

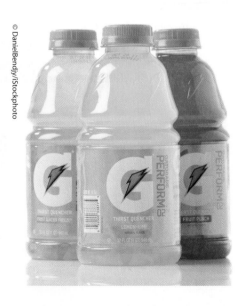

© DanielBendjy/iStockphoto

Protein is not usually considered an ergogenic aid, but nearly all amino acids derived from proteins can be converted to glucose by gluconeogenesis. Therefore, protein may help competitive athletes by sparing the energy needs of higher amounts of carbohydrates for muscle contraction and other processes.

Caution about the hype surrounding ergogenic aids is needed because of the potentially adverse effects that may result from the use of these aids—and the monetary cost may also be high! A major concern about the marketing of these products is the potential quackery relating to them; hucksterism runs rife in this area because of our limited knowledge—"gray areas"—that make it difficult for consumers to recognize the limited science behind these products. For example, a decade or so ago chromium picolinate was being pushed as being essential for optimal performance by athletes and others. Now, it is creatine phosphate (phosphocreatine) that is being touted as the "in" ergogenic aid needed to enhance skeletal muscle performance because of its role in energy storage in muscle cells. There is no evidence of any beneficial effects of phosphocreatine in athletic performance. In fact, too much phosphate with creatine may be detrimental because a high serum phosphate concentration alters calcium homeostasis, which leads to PTH-directed bone resorption and net bone loss. Therefore, the use of creatine phosphate is not recommended.

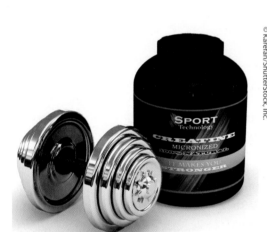

© Karefan/ShutterStock, Inc.

Ergogenic aids will continue to be used by high-level and recreational athletes who believe in them. However, little scientific evidence supports any beneficial effects of ergogenic aids except as an energy source, almost exclusively derived from carbohydrates.

Body Composition of Competitive Athletes

The body composition of successful competitive athletes varies greatly in the proportion of the lean and fat compartments. For example, female athletes who lose fat mass may have declines in estrogen and begin to lose bone mineral. Large athletes, such as football linemen, heavyweight wrestlers, and lifters, generally have a relatively high percentage of body fat compared with endurance athletes. Some of these athletes with large amounts of body fat are obese, even though they also have a high LBM. **Table 13.3** gives representative examples of the variety and ranges of body compositions of intercollegiate athletes of both sexes. Female athletes whose artistic or sport-specific performance requires low body fat, such as gymnasts and ballerinas, may also be amenorrheic, and need to be exceedingly lean in order to perform at a high level.

> Ergogenic aids will continue to be used by high-level and recreational athletes who believe in them. However, little scientific evidence supports any beneficial effects of ergogenic aids except as an energy source, almost exclusively derived from carbohydrates.

TABLE 13.3
Typical Body Composition of Intercollegiate Athletes

Sport	Percentage of Fat Mass	
	Males	Females
Cross-country and running sports	5–10	10–15
Basketball	10–15	10–20
Gymnastics	5–10	10–15
Strength sports and weight lifting	15–40	20–45

SUMMARY

Active adults maintain better health as a result of a regular exercise program because all of the organ systems operate with greater efficiency. Nutrients typically are better utilized. Body composition changes, although typically modest, represent slight decreases in fat mass and slight increases in LBM. Bone mass typically changes very little, if any. Typically, cardiorespiratory performance, muscle strength, and bone integrity all improve. Exercise also reduces the risk of several chronic diseases. Engaging in physical activity throughout the life cycle has a great health benefit in supporting a healthy and active body.

As with all people, active individuals should follow a balanced diet with foods from all of the food groups to achieve and maintain optimal health. Large food servings and meals are not recommended, and high-dose supplements are not needed (more than 100% of RDAs). If supplements are taken by active individuals, the individual nutrients, with the exception of calcium, should be consumed at 100% of the RDAs (or PDVs, which are used in labeling of supplements).

Sound nutrient intakes by athletes, dancers, and other highly active individuals are critical for the support of optimal physical performance. Energy, protein, water, electrolytes, and other micronutrients have been reviewed in relation to their use in the support of physical performance. The RDAs remain the best estimates of intakes that meet nutritional requirements. Athletes and other active individuals should be starting at 100% of the recommendations and increase their intake of energy, protein, and micronutrients as needed. Several ergogenic aids that are nutritional have been highlighted in terms of improving performance, and nutritional supplements have also been recommended for the same reasons. Good food choices for athletes are important, and they should be based on MyPlate and the *Dietary Guidelines for Americans*. Energy remains the critical dietary component that must be increased by highly active individuals, aside from the obvious need for protein, micronutrients, and fluids.

Endurance athletes need, above all other active individuals, fluids, calories, and other nutrients. They expend so much energy in training and competition that they can gradually lose weight over a season of their sport. Therefore, endurance athletes should increase their energy intake from carbohydrate-rich foods, especially complex carbohydrates, to maintain body weight for maximal performance. Athletes also must replace the fluids lost in sweat by drinking water or other liquids, other than alcoholic beverages, in order to prevent dehydration. The sense of thirst may not be sufficiently sensitive to inform the body that it needs more water, but it helps to ensure adequate water balance in the resting period after practice or performance. Juices from citrus fruits or vegetables are especially good for fluid replacement because they also contain electrolytes. If total caloric consumption remains low for any athlete, especially for females, then it is possible that too little of the micronutrients will also be consumed.

STUDENT ACTIVITIES

1. What major differences in body composition typically distinguish athletes from nonathletes?

2. Identify three problem nutrients for athletes, especially female athletes. Explain why deficits in these nutrients can be detrimental to athletic performance.

3. Explain what a nutritional ergogenic aid is.

4. Describe the relationship among disordered eating, osteopenia, and iron deficiency. How does this relationship impact the athletic performance and bone tissue of female athletes?

5. Why might distance runners become iron deficient or develop iron deficiency anemia?

6. Explain why athletes, but not moderately active adults, may benefit from micronutrient supplements.

7. How can vegan athletes obtain sufficient nutrients and energy to support their physical activity? Explain. [Hint: Think of high fiber intake.]

8. Explain how the turnover of body protein, especially muscle fibers (proteins), influences an athlete's need for dietary protein.

9. Use a food composition table to calculate the approximate amount of iron provided by a 2,000-kilocalorie diet of a female vegan athlete.

10. Do you think that male athletes such as distance runners should be taking a daily nutrient supplement of micronutrients? Explain.

11. Athletes typically generate more free radicals because of their higher rates of energy metabolism than inactive people. What effect does a typical diet have in defending against these free radicals? Explain.

12. Why may high intakes of creatine phosphate, an ergogenic aid, be a health concern? Explain.

WEBSITES FOR FURTHER STUDY

Healthy Eating for an Active Lifestyle, USDA
www.choosemyplate.gov/food-groups/downloads/TenTips
/DGTipsheet25HealthyEatingActiveLifestyle.pdf
Dietary Guidelines for Americans
www.cnpp.usda.gov/dgas2010-policydocument.htm
American College of Sports Medicine
www.acsm.org

Vegan Diets for Athletes
www.livestrong.com/article/190288-vegan-diets-for-athletes
Podiatry Today: **Recognizing and Preventing Dehydration in Athletes**
www.podiatrytoday.com/article/3331

REFERENCES

Anderson JJB, Stender M, Rondano P, Bishop L, Ducket AB. Nutrition and bone in physical activity and sport. In: Wolinsky I (ed.), *Nutrition in Exercise and Sport,* 3rd ed. Boca Raton, FL: CRC Press; 1997:219–244.

Barrack MT, Van Loan MD, Rauh MJ, Nichols JF. Physiologic and behavioral indicators of energy deficiency in female adolescent runners with elevated bone turnover. *Am J Clin Nutr.* 2010;92:652–659.

Burke LM. Sports nutrition. In: Erdman JW Jr, MacDonald IA, Zeisel SH (eds.), *Present Knowledge in Nutrition.* 10th ed. Ames, IA: John Wiley & Sons; 2012:1073–1096.

Das SK, Roberts SB. Energy metabolism in fasting, fed, exercise, and re-feeding states. In: Erdman JW Jr, MacDonald IA, Zeisel SH (eds.), *Present Knowledge in Nutrition.* 10th ed. Ames, IA: John Wiley & Sons; 2012:117–133.

Dornemann TM, McMurray RG, Renner JB, Anderson JJB. Effects of high-intensity resistance exercise on bone mineral density and muscle strength of 40–50 year old women. *J Sports Med Phys Fitness.* 1997;37:246–251.

Food and Nutrition Board, Institute of Medicine. *Dietary Reference Intakes.* Washington, DC: National Academies Press; 1997–2004, 2011.

Harp JB, Hecht L. Obesity in the National Football League. *JAMA.* 2005;29:1061–1062.

Maughan RJ, Shirreffs SM, Ozgünen KT, et al. Living, training, and playing in the heat: challenges to the football player and strategies for coping with environmental extremes. *Scand J Med Sci Sports.* 2010;20(suppl 3):117–124.

Nattiv A, Loucks AB, Manore MM, et al. The female athlete triad: a position stand by the American College of Sports Medicine. *Med Sci Sports Exer.* 2007;39:1867–1882.

Nieman DC. Immunonutrition support for athletes. *Nutr Rev.* 2008;66:310–320.

Rodriguez NR, DiMarco NM, Langley S. Nutrition and athletic performance: a joint position statement of the American College of Sports Medicine, the American Dietetic Association, and the Dietitians of Canada. *Med Sci Sports Exer.* 2009;41:709–731.

Tam N, Nolte HW, Noakes TD. Changes in total body water content during running races of 21.1 km and 56 km in athletes drinking *ad libitum. Clin J Sport Med.* 2011;21:218–225.

Tarnopolsky MA. Caffeine and creatine use in sport. *Ann Nutr Metab.* 2010;57(suppl 2):1–8.

Thrash L, Anderson JJB. The female athlete triad. *Nutr Today.* 2000;35:168–174.

Tveit M, Rosengren BE, Nilsson J-A, et al. Bone mass following physical activity in young years: a mean 39-year prospective controlled study in men. *Osteopor Int.* 2013;24:1389–1397.

ADDITIONAL READING

McArdle WD, Katch FI, Katch VL. *Exercise Physiology: Energy, Nutrition, and Human Performance.* 6th ed. Philadelphia: Lippincott, Williams & Wilkins; 2007.

Williams MH. *Nutrition for Health, Fitness, and Sport.* 9th ed. Boston: McGraw-Hill; 2010.

Wolinsky I (ed.). *Nutrition in Exercise and Sport.* Boca Raton, FL: CRC Press; 1998.

CHAPTER 14

Diet-Related Cancers and Other Chronic Diseases

Diet is strongly correlated with the development of certain diseases. This chapter presents overviews of a few of the more common diet-related diseases, including specific cancers, such as those of the breast, prostate, and colon; metabolic syndrome; diseases affecting the eye and the brain; and arterial calcification. These conditions affect millions of North Americans and others throughout the world, especially the elderly. This chapter also explores the role of nutrition in maintaining a healthy immune system.

Diet-Related Cancers

The diet-related cancers are more prevalent in developed countries. Dietary and other etiologic risk factors are considered to contribute to the development of these cancers. The major diet-related cancers are those affecting the breast tissue, the prostate, and the colon. Diet may be influential in promoting or preventing these cancers and, possibly, others.

What Is Cancer?

A **cancer** is a cluster of cells that have run amok—too many cells without any function! Cell **proliferation** is an increase in the number of cells as a result of cell growth and cell division. Cell **differentiation** is the normal process by which a cell matures to possess a more distinct form and function. Cell proliferation is normally regulated by intracellular mechanisms and by hormones or other factors that act on the cell to govern the balance between proliferation and differentiation. In cancer, excessive cell divisions occur when a cell loses its ability to control cell proliferation. The aberrant or abnormal cells that are produced do not undergo the steps to become mature functional

cancer A disease of uncontrolled cell growth (proliferation). Cancer cells do not conduct the normal functions characteristic of their cell type, but they do keep the general characteristics of their tissue of origin. Cancer cells exist in varying degrees of undifferentiation; they may be contained or some may break away from their point of origin and spread (metastasize) to other tissues of the body. Cancer is the second most common cause of death in the United States.

proliferation An increase in the number of cells as a result of cell growth and cell division. Cancer is a disease characterized by uncontrolled cell proliferation.

differentiation The characteristic (normal) changes of cells as they mature from newly formed daughter cells (via cell division) to functional cells in a tissue (or organ). Cancer cells do not undergo normal differentiation.

> In cancer, excessive cell divisions occur when a cell loses its ability to control cell proliferation. The aberrant cells that are produced do not undergo the steps to become mature functional cells that are characteristic of their tissue or organ (i.e., differentiation).

> The utilization of bloodborne glucose and other nutrients feed the cancer and allow abnormal cells to grow without the limits of normal cells.

metastasis The spread of malignant cancer cells from the original site of production via lymphatics and blood vessels to distant tissues (e.g., lung, liver, or bone), where secondary growth occurs; characterized by invasiveness.

genome The genetic material of an organism that consists of tens of thousands of different genes coding for specific proteins.

mutation A change in the DNA within a gene that changes the gene's genetic role; the change could be beneficial, but it usually is not. A mutation can contribute to the development of cancer.

carcinogenesis The process of cancer cell formation and growth.

carcinogen A cancer-causing molecule that may or may not result in a gene mutation. Carcinogens can act by either initiating cancer through mutations or through the promotion of cancer cells that have already been initiated. In general, refers to any molecule that causes cancer.

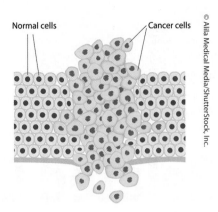

Normal cells   *Cancer cells*

© Ailia Medical Media/ShutterStock, Inc.

FIGURE 14.1 Cancer Cells vs. Normal Cells. Compared to normal cells, cancer cells are much more variable in size, have an abnormal shape, and often look ugly.

cells that are characteristic of their tissue or organ (i.e., differentiation). As shown in **FIGURE 14.1**, cancer cells differ greatly in appearance from normal cells. Excess cells pile up in an organ and interfere with its normal function. In addition, cancer cells may leave their tissue of origin and spread through the blood to other locations in the body without the restraints of normal cells, a process known as **metastasis**.

Normal cells perform roles that are unique to the tissue they are part of. At some stage of their development, these cells or their precursors must multiply. Normal cells increase in number or proliferate only to the extent necessary to perform their function in the body. Following proliferation, cells differentiate into cells unique to the tissue in which they exist. Typically, at this late stage precursor cells divide only as needed, perhaps only rarely. Epithelial cells that line body tubes and the lungs, however, divide throughout life. Cancer cells are undifferentiated cells that do not perform any normal function in the body, but they proliferate without regulation and, in most types, may break away and via the blood circulation spread to other locations in the body without the restraints of normal cells. The uncontrolled cell proliferation and growth of cancers are limited only by the formation of new arteries and capillaries for vascular supply of nutrients and oxygen. The utilization of bloodborne glucose and other nutrients feed the cancer and allow the abnormal cells to grow without the limits of normal cells.

The processes of cell growth and differentiation and other cellular functions are controlled by the genetic material, deoxyribonucleic acid (DNA), which resides within the cell nucleus. The totality of all the genes is known as the **genome**, which consists of tens of thousands of different genes coding for specific proteins. Proteins carry out cell functions of maintenance and growth within the cell. Among their many roles, proteins may be secreted by the cell to communicate with other cells, to provide structural support, or to serve as enzymes. A single alteration in the DNA code—that is, a **mutation**—may cause a change in the RNA that is read from the DNA, which may eventually change the specific protein array of linear amino acids. Such changes may reduce or eliminate the ability of the protein to function. These abnormal proteins are just excess baggage in a cell. Abnormal changes in the synthesis of a protein in cells may be the beginning of **carcinogenesis** (i.e., excessive proliferation without differentiation).

Although any cell type in the body may develop into a cancerous cell, the vast majority of cancers arise in epithelial tissues, which normally undergo frequent cell divisions and are most exposed to **carcinogens** (i.e., cancer-causing agents). Epithelial cell types are found in the gastrointestinal tract, the respiratory tree, the urinary tract, and the reproductive organs. In addition, stem cells in bone marrow may divide too rapidly, such as in leukemias affecting the white blood cells and other blood-related cancers.

The cellular differences necessary to transform a normal cell into a cancer cell begin with the accumulation of one or more mutations in DNA. These changes require time to result in fully transformed and invasive cancer cells. In most cases, the abnormal DNA in a cell is detected within the cell itself and then repaired or the cell is deleted via programmed cell death (also known as apoptosis). The risk of developing cancer increases with age, but for unknown reasons cancer may also develop in children, and typically cancerous cells proliferate much more rapidly in children than in adults. The alterations in cell physiology that occur during the formation of a cancer cell are illustrated in **FIGURE 14.2**.

Cancer Causation: Etiologic Risk Factors

The "causes" of cancer—that is, the initiating factors in the etiology of cancer—are not known with certainty, but environmental variables such as cigarette smoke, asbestos, numerous chemicals, and ionizing radiation are well-established initiating agents. The oxygen that we breathe also generates free radicals in our cells that contribute to DNA mutations. Once genetic changes have occurred, nutrients and non-nutrients obtained from foods and beverages can have a significant influence on whether a cancer (or neoplasm) will grow large enough to be a threat to life. The roles of nutrients as both **promoters** of cancer development and as preventers of cancer are considered to be

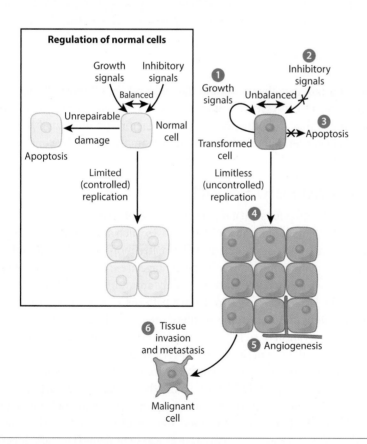

FIGURE 14.2 Changes That Occur During the Formation of a Cancer Cell. The loss of control of cell division results in excessive proliferation of abnormal cells that have the capability of leaving the original site of cancer and metastasizing to distant tissues via the blood circulation. A feature of cancer cells is that they do not anchor to a connective tissue base like normal cells, which makes it possible for them to travel to other parts of the body. Angiogenesis, the formation of new blood vessels, is necessary to provide blood flow to the tumor.

Reproduced from Anderson JJB. *Nutrition and Health: An Introduction.* Durham, NC: Carolina Academic Press; 2005.

promoter (of cancer) A dietary or environmental molecule or endogenous hormone/factor that promotes cancer development, including its progression and promotion.

> *The roles of nutrients as both promoters of cancer development and as preventers of cancer are considered to be extremely important.*

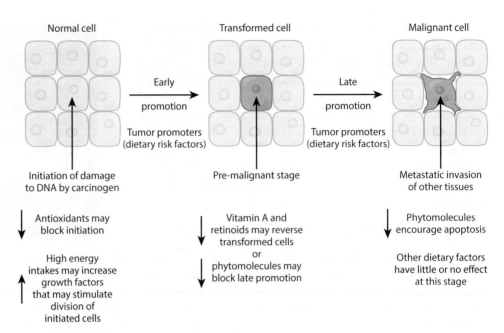

FIGURE 14.3 The Stages of Cancer Development Influenced by Dietary Factors. Nutrients may alter cell metabolism by aiding the actions of promoters or antipromoters. An example of one cell becoming highly undifferentiated ("ugly") is shown here. When many of these cells are present as part of a clone of abnormal cells, a cancer or malignancy is said to exist.

Reproduced from Anderson JJB. *Nutrition and Health: An Introduction.* Durham, NC: Carolina Academic Press; 2005.

extremely important (see the section on the Doll and Peto Report). The stages of cancer development, i.e., **initiation** (carcinogenic insult) and **promotion** (continuing growth of tumor), that are influenced by dietary factors are illustrated in **FIGURE 14.3**. **Progression** of cancer is another term used that simply means the continuous growth in size of a cancer.

The Doll and Peto Report

In 1981, Doll and Peto published a report on 12 possible risk factors for cancer in which they specified percentages for the avoidable causes, such as cigarette smoking and poor diets. These estimates remain the best-guesstimates more than three decades later! By far the largest contributors to cancer by percentage are from tobacco and the diet (see **Table 14.1**). Cancer incidence rates vary widely around the world, which may result, in part, from the large differences in dietary patterns as well as other lifestyle factors or behaviors among cultures. Some of these dietary differences include methods of food storage, preservation (e.g., salt and other additives), cooking (e.g., open flame and excessive heat), and the use of raw foods and seasonings.

Other risk factors for cancer that reflect environmental contributions are pollutants, industrial products, x-rays and radiation from other devices, and bacteria and viruses. Physical activity is generally considered to be a protective factor, but it was not considered in the review by Doll and Peto. Good sources of information about substances, especially chemicals, that are known to cause cancer in humans (i.e., carcinogens) can be found on the websites of the International Agency for Research on Cancer (IARC) and the National Toxicology Program's (NTP) Report on Carcinogens. Another source of general information on cancer and its prevention and treatment is the National Cancer Institute (NCI) website. Recommendations on diet and cancer prevention can be found on the American Institute for Cancer Research (AICR) website.

initiation (of cancer) The first stage of a cancer that is characterized by damage to DNA; generally irreversible.

promotion (of cancer) The second stage of a cancer that is characterized by development of a population of abnormal cells through the support of a cocarcinogen or promotor (e.g., dietary factors).

progression (of cancer) The final stage in the development of a cancer. Changes in a tumor, such as increased rates of cell division, abnormal microscopic appearance of cells, and malignant or invasive characteristics.

TABLE 14.1
Causes of Cancer Deaths by Percentage

Factor	Percentage of All Cancer Deaths	
	Best Estimate	Range of Estimates
Diet	35	20–60
Tobacco	30	25–40
Infection	10	> 1
Reproductive/sexual behavior	7	1–13
Occupation	4	2–8
Alcohol	3	2–4
Geophysical factors (e.g., radon, elevation)	3	2–4
Pollution	2	< 1–5
Medicines/medical procedures	1	0.5–3
Industrial products	< 1	< 1–2
Food additives	< 1	–5*–2

* Possible protective role for natural and synthetic antioxidants (e.g., BHT, BHA) used as additives.
Data from Doll R, Peto R. The causes of cancer: quantitative estimates of avoidable risks of cancer in the United States today. *J Natl Cancer Inst.* 1981;66:1191–1308.

> **Cancer incidence rates vary widely around the world, which may result, in part, from the large differences in dietary patterns as well as other lifestyle factors or behaviors among cultures.**

The most thoroughly studied cause of cancer is cigarette smoking, which gives rise to lung cancer in smokers around the world. The risk of lung cancer in nonsmokers, even in heavily industrialized and atmospherically polluted nations, is low, but secondary smoke does carry some risk for nonsmokers. The etiologic factors contributing to cancers of the large bowel (colon), breast, and prostate are less well understood. These three cancers, common in industrialized nations, are associated with affluence and a "rich" dietary intake in terms of energy and protein, but they are not entirely linked to industrialization. For example, in industrialized Japan breast cancer rates are low, whereas they are high in New Zealand, a largely agricultural nation. Industrial and agricultural chemicals and pollutants have had a limited, though measurable, impact on cancer rates in industrialized nations. For example, agricultural carcinogens are thought to increase the cancer rates of exposed farm workers and their families.

The general nature of the environment, including the ways people live and eat, appear to have more bearing on cancer rates than place of origin or ethnic (genetic) heritage. Critical environmental factors affecting all of us include the following: (1) air, (2) drinking water, (3) types of foods and their storage, (4) methods of food preparation, (5) food portions (serving sizes), (6) infectious diseases, and (7) radiation from sunlight and other sources. Poor sanitation and suboptimal personal hygiene are also factors, but they generally decrease in significance as nations become more industrialized and mean individual income rises. Nevertheless, estimation of the contribution of any of these environmental factors to the overall cancer rates of a nation remains difficult because biological markers resulting from cancer cell production, especially early in cancer development (hidden or unknown), are not detectable.

> **The general nature of the environment, including the ways people live and eat, appears to have more bearing on cancer rates than place of origin or ethnic (genetic) heritage.**

TABLE 14.2
Comparison of Diet-Cancer Patterns of Typical Western and Asian Nations

Dietary Pattern	Common Cancers	Nondietary Contributors to Cancer
Western Nations		
High meat, fish, poultry	Lung	Inactivity
High dairy	Colon and rectum	Cigarette smoking
Low vegetable and fruit	Breast	Air pollution
Low grain	Endometrium (uterus)	Obesity
High protein (animal)	Prostate	Radiation
High fat (total and saturated)	Ovary	Hormonal replacement therapy
Low carbohydrate	Pancreas	
Low dietary fiber		
Moderate sodium (salt)		
Typical Asian Nations		
High grain	Stomach	Infections (esp. viral)
High vegetable	Liver	Cigarette smoking
Low meat, fish, poultry	Mouth	Poor food preservation
Low dairy	Larynx	Air pollution
High carbohydrate	Lung	Poor hygiene
High dietary fiber	Esophagus	Cooking on open flame
Low fat (total and saturated)		Nitrosamine products
Low protein (animal)		
High sodium (salt)		

Reproduced from Anderson JJB. *Nutrition and Health: An Introduction.* Durham, NC: Carolina Academic Press; 2005.

> Doll and Peto have estimated that the avoidable risk of cancer in the United States could be reduced by one-third through the adoption of a healthier diet and another third by total abolition of smoking of all types of tobacco.

Differences in dietary patterns between Western and Asian nations may provide clues about adverse dietary variables and cancer (see **Table 14.2**).

Doll and Peto also have estimated that the avoidable risk of cancer in the United States could be reduced by one-third through the adoption of a healthier diet and another third by total abolition of all types of tobacco. Those estimated reductions are largely based on the sharp decline in U.S. stomach cancer rates observed over the 20th century, a drop related to a higher quality of food and reductions in the consumption of salt-preserved foods. In Japan, gastric cancer rates have declined greatly over the last several decades, a change attributed to a decrease in the use of salt-preserved foods, especially fish, and an increase in the use of refrigerators for cold preservation of fish and other seafood.

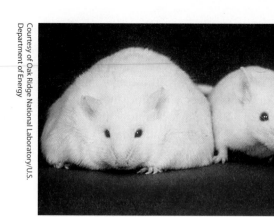

Courtesy of Oak Ridge National Laboratory/U.S. Department of Energy

Excessive Energy and Diet-Related Cancers

Findings from experimental animal studies, from human migration studies, and from other epidemiologic studies have established a strong association between dietary factors and a few cancers. High caloric intake (from all macronutrients) is a risk factor for cancers of the colon, breast, prostate, and possibly others. Calorie-restricted diets in experimental studies with animals have clearly resulted in decreased tumor rates and increased longevity, but human studies have not been clear on potential tumor inhibition or regression from calorie restriction. Excessive body weight resulting from high caloric intake has been shown in epidemiologic studies to contribute to increased cancer rates, but linkages with specific dietary variables have not been consistently found.

The data from animal studies on dietary fats may be clearer: High-fat intakes contribute to increased tumor rates, especially if the fat is high in polyunsaturated fatty acids. Human studies, however, have not provided data that clearly link dietary fat, either saturated or polyunsaturated fatty acids, and cancer. Some reports suggest a link between high-fat intakes, especially from animal foods, and cancer. However, several large cohort studies in the United States, including the Women's Health Initiative and the Nurses' Health Study, have failed to find a significant link between dietary fat and breast cancer. Obesity from excessive energy intake relative to energy expenditure in activities has been hypothesized as a major factor in the development of cancers of the breast (postmenopausal), prostate, and colon, but additional evidence is needed to establish the validity of this hypothesis.

Protein intakes at high levels (i.e., 20% or more of total energy consumption) have not been found to be consistently and independently associated with cancer rates in epidemiologic studies. Red meat intake alone, which contains both fat and protein, has been found to be associated only with increased rates of colon cancer. The red meat–cancer link remains a viable hypothesis, however, because vegetarian populations typically have lower rates of diet-related cancers. In terms of postulated mechanisms, insulin and insulin-like growth factors (IGFs) are known to promote growth when energy intakes or protein intakes (or both) are high because the hormones may overstimulate some rapidly dividing cells into hyperproliferation and subsequent cancer. Human evidence on this association, however, is largely limited to speculation. Potential mechanisms of action of the dietary macronutrients are not offered here because of their complex involvement in cancer causation.

Micronutrients, Phytochemicals, and Fiber and Diet-Related Cancers

The micronutrients are considered to be protective against most cancers. Those dietary components that protect against the development of cancer are known as

> Calorie-restricted diets in experimental studies with animals have clearly resulted in decreased tumor rates and increased longevity, but human studies have not been clear on potential tumor inhibition or regression from calorie restriction.

> Obesity from excessive energy intake relative to energy expenditure in activities has been hypothesized as a major factor in the development of cancers of the breast (postmenopausal), prostate, and colon, but additional evidence is needed to establish the validity of this hypothesis.

> Red meat intake alone, which contains both fat and protein, has been found to be associated only with increased rates of colon cancer.

anticarcinogens because they either counteract the action of carcinogens or they prevent the activation or expression of carcinogens. Consistent linkages between micronutrients and cancer have not been documented, but antioxidant micronutrients and phytochemicals most likely are important anticarcinogens. Those micronutrients with known antioxidant activity (vitamins C and E, beta-carotene, zinc, and selenium) have received more research attention than others. Many phytochemicals also have roles as antioxidants that act to prevent cancer. (See the section on antioxidants.) Dietary fiber, both soluble and insoluble, may also be protective against cancer by decreasing the absorption of carcinogens across the GI tract. See **Table 14.3** for good food sources of micronutrients and phytochemicals.

Micronutrients

Among the B vitamins, deficiency of at least one has been shown in epidemiologic investigations to be associated with disorders of the colon, including the type of cancer known as an adenoma. Folic acid or folate appears to have a protective role against cancer initiation. Other B vitamins that act as antioxidants also have roles in the prevention of cancer. These vitamins need to be consumed at RDA levels, and phytochemicals in plant foods also need to be ingested in reasonable amounts on a regular basis in order to protect against the development of diverse cancers.

Selenium and zinc have roles as antioxidants in animal models and, possibly, in humans. Zinc acts as part of enzymes involved in controlling free radicals and may help support immune function and thereby assist in the prevention of cancer. Selenium plays an active role in the antioxidant enzyme glutathione peroxidase.

Iron deficiency may be related to increased rates of gastric cancers in humans, but insufficient data exist to make a definitive statement about the role of iron deficiency in cancer development.

Deficient intakes of calcium or vitamin D may also be related to colon cancer and possibly to prostate cancer. Results of a few trials suggest that the potential protective roles of additional dietary calcium or vitamin D against colon cancer, and possibly others, may be related to an effective antiproliferative action of calcium or vitamin D.

Choline, a methyl-group donor in liver and other cell types, may also help in preventing the development of cancer in the liver and other tissues. Methyl donors such

> *The micronutrients are considered to be protective against most cancers. Those dietary components that protect against the development of cancer are known as anticarcinogens because they either counteract the action of carcinogens or they prevent the activation or expression of carcinogens.*

TABLE 14.3
Good Sources of Micronutrients and Phytochemicals

Food Group	Micronutrients	Phytochemicals
Meat, fish, poultry, eggs	Iron, zinc, PFA, vitamins	None
Dairy (milk, yogurt, cheese)	Calcium, B vitamins, vitamin D	None
Cereals, whole grains	Vitamins and minerals	Some antioxidants
Fruits	Vitamin C and others	Rich in antioxidants
Vegetables	Vitamins and minerals	Rich in antioxidants
Nuts and seeds	Vitamins and minerals	Rich in antioxidants
Vegetable oils	Vitamin E	Very low in any phytochemicals

Plant foods also contain dietary fiber.

FOCUS 14.1   Free Radicals and the Development of Cancer

Free radicals result from the normal metabolic activities of cells that involve oxygen. Several types of highly reactive chemical species are generated in these metabolic pathways, especially those operating in mitochondria. Free radicals such as superoxides (O_2^-) and hydroxyl radicals (OH^-) are potent species with highly reactive electrons that can react with and damage DNA, proteins, and other macromolecules and thereby initiate changes that may eventually lead to cancer. Free radicals are normally rapidly neutralized in cells by protective enzyme systems that use antioxidants. Cells contain several mechanisms to inactivate and eliminate free radicals (i.e., quenching them), but these systems require several micronutrients as well as non-nutrient phytochemical antioxidants to provide the best protection against free radicals. ●

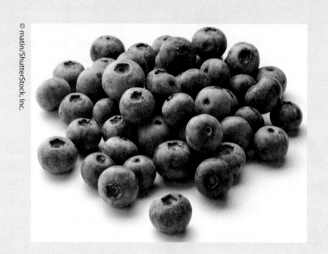

© matin/ShutterStock, Inc.

as choline and folate may help prevent cancer by protecting DNA through addition of methyl groups.

Besides acting as an antioxidant, ascorbic acid (vitamin C) also prevents the conversion of carcinogen precursors to carcinogens, for example, by blocking the modification of nitrites or nitrates to nitrosamines in the stomach. It also serves as an antioxidant in cells, and it plays a role in immune defense. Some data suggest that lower cancer incidence rates, especially gastric and esophageal, are associated with reasonable consumption of foods containing vitamin C, but a potential protective role of vitamin C against breast cancer and other hormone-dependent cancers has not been supported by epidemiologic findings. In addition to inhibiting carcinogens in the oral cavity, stomach, and esophagus, vitamin C may help prevent cancer development in the lungs and bladder. Clearly, much more work is needed on the vitamin C–cancer linkage.

Alpha-tocopherol, a form of vitamin E, acts as an antioxidant by protecting membranes against damaging attacks by free radicals. (BHT and BHA, antioxidant food additives, are thought to act in a similar manner.) Adults have difficulty obtaining RDA amounts of vitamin E in their diets, but reported deficiency of this vitamin in the United States is rare.

Beta-carotene and other carotenoids may have anticarcinogenic effects, but less evidence has been established for these antioxidants. The consumption of foods with these vitamin A precursors reduces the risk of cancer by conversion to forms of vitamin A that promote a normal pattern of differentiation. In animal and human experiments, treatment with retinoids (synthetic) or modified vitamin A molecules has been demonstrated to reduce a variety of cancers, but vitamin A intake *per se* has not been shown to reduce the rates of these cancers. Research among smokers has shown that beta-carotene in pill form actually increases the risk of lung cancer by about 20%. Plant sources of carotenoids are probably most beneficial because they supply good amounts of not only beta-carotene but also other phytochemicals, such as lycopene, and other antioxidants.

Anticarcinogens include antioxidants such as beta-carotene (a precursor of vitamin A), vitamin C (ascorbic acid), vitamin E, antioxidant food additives, selenium, many phytochemicals, and possibly other micronutrients. Examples of vegetables that

" Cells contain several mechanisms to inactivate and eliminate free radicals, but these systems require several micronutrients (vitamins and minerals) as well as non-nutrient phytochemical antioxidants to provide the best protection against free radicals. "

anticarcinogen A molecule that blocks the action of a carcinogen or reverses the promotion of an initiated cell.

FOCUS 14.2   Supplements: Helpful or Harmful?

Large prospective studies in the United States and Finland using beta-carotene supplements did not show any improvements in lung cancer rates after several years. Antioxidant supplements were not helpful in reducing cancers in older men, and in one report beta-carotene may have actually increased lung cancer development! In general, results of supplement studies have been disappointing. Good diets rich in fruits, vegetables, and whole grains remain as the most effective approach to lowering the risk of cancer, along with other healthy lifestyle behaviors. ●

> *Antioxidants prevent or delay the oxidative steps that are necessary before normal cells convert to cancer cells.*

are good sources of beta-carotene, vitamin C, or vitamin E are provided in Table 14.3. Antioxidants prevent or delay the oxidative steps that are necessary before normal cells convert to cancer cells. Risks of cancer are higher, according to this reasoning, when such naturally occurring antioxidants as beta-carotene, vitamins C and E, and trace minerals, including selenium, zinc, or others, are low. Thus, an individual's nutritional status becomes critical for protection against the development of cancers. The latency period or delay from initiation of one cancer cell to the time of its detection as a sizeable cancer or neoplasm may be extended by good nutrition (i.e., during the early cancer promotion stage), but good nutrition alone cannot eliminate the cancer.

Vitamin E is found in cells in the fat-soluble portions of membranes, both the enveloping and internal membranes. Vitamin E molecules that are modified after taking on highly reactive oxygen species (i.e., free radicals) must be regenerated at the membrane surface or interface by vitamin C molecules, which, in turn, become modified. Vitamin C molecules are in solution in the cell water of the cytoplasm, and other enzyme systems in the cell may regenerate vitamin C by combining with the free radicals. This partnering of vitamins E and C allows free radicals from lipid membranes to be removed and deactivated in the cytoplasm of the cell.

Dietary Fiber

Dietary fiber, which consists of both soluble and insoluble molecules derived from plant cell walls and other structural elements, appears to have a role to play in reducing colon, breast, and prostate cancers. Good sources of dietary fiber in the U.S. diet are listed in **Table 14.4**. Although processed wheat products (i.e., white bread, rolls, and crackers) contain relatively little dietary fiber, they are a major source of fiber in the U.S. diet because so many of these items are consumed on a daily basis. Epidemiologic findings, however, have been inconsistent and contradictory in finding associations between dietary fiber and cancer. One human investigation reported that consumption of pentosans (five-carbon, or pentose, sugars linked in a polysaccharide) found in the water-soluble fraction of fiber derived from whole wheat and other products was associated with a lower incidence of colon cancer. A few other epidemiologic reports have found significant associations between low fiber intakes and higher rates of colon adenoma (precancerous lesion). Prospective human clinical trials have failed, however, to find a significant association between supplemental fiber and colon cancer. Further studies are needed to investigate specific fiber components.

Phytochemicals

Thousands of different molecules derived from plants, known as polyphenols because they possess several hydroxyl groups on aromatic rings, have antioxidant properties that benefit human health and likely reduce cancer development (see **Table 14.5**). Although much remains to be learned about the protective roles of the non-nutrient phytochemicals found in plants, many chemopreventive mechanisms have been described. The

TABLE 14.4
Dietary Fiber Content of Common Foods

Food Item	Quantity	Fiber Content (g)
Split peas (cooked)	1 cup	16.3
Red kidney beans (boiled)	1 cup	13.1
Raspberries (raw)	1 cup	8.0
Whole-wheat spaghetti	1 cup	6.3
Oat bran muffin	1 medium	5.2
Broccoli (boiled)	1 cup	5.1
Oatmeal (cooked)	1 cup	4.0
Green beans (cooked)	1 cup	4.0
Brown rice (cooked)	1 cup	3.5
Apple (with skin)	1 medium	3.3
Popcorn (air popped)	2 cups	2.4
Whole-wheat bread	1 slice	1.9
White bread	1 slice	0.6

Data from U.S. Department of Agriculture, Agricultural Research Service. 2011. USDA National Nutrient Database for Standard Reference, Release 24. Nutrient Data Laboratory Home Page. www.ars.usda.gov/ba/bhnrc/ndl.

Dietary fiber, which consists of both soluble and insoluble molecules derived from plant cell walls and other structural elements, appears to have a role in reducing colon, breast, and prostate cancers.

TABLE 14.5
Common Phytochemicals and Their Modes of Action and Common Food Sources

Mode of Action	Phytochemical Examples	Common Food Sources
Antioxidants	Carotenoids, curcumin, flavonoids, isothiocyanates	Broccoli, carrots, sweet potatoes, tomatoes, tumeric, blueberries, grapes, tea, Brussels sprouts, cabbage, kale
Anti-inflammatory	Curcumin, resveratrol	Tumeric, red wine, grapes
Estrogenic	Isoflavones, lignans	Soybeans, tofu, soy milk, flaxseed
Blood thinning	Capsaicin, resveratrol	Hot peppers, red wine, grapes
Carcinogen metabolism	Flavonoids, indoles, isothiocyanates, monoterpenes, allyl sulfides	Blueberries, grapes, tea, Brussels sprouts, cabbage, kale, citrus fruit, garlic, onions
Apoptosis inducers	Resveratrol, allyl sulfides	Red wine, grapes, garlic, onions
Slow cell proliferation	Flavonoids, resveratrol, saponins	Blueberries, grapes, tea, red wine, lentils, red beans
Lipid lowering	Allicin, stanol esters	Garlic, onions, stanol ester–fortified margarine

Data from Anderson JJB. *Nutrition and Health: An Introduction.* Durham, NC: Carolina Academic Press; 2005.

> *Thousands of different molecules derived from plants, known as polyphenols because they possess several hydroxyl groups on aromatic rings, have antioxidant properties that benefit human health and likely reduce cancer development.*

functions performed by phytochemicals in protecting against development of cancer include enhancement of enzymes to detoxify or excrete potential carcinogens, stimulation of antioxidant mechanisms, direct interference with the actions of carcinogens on cells, and inhibition of tumor growth.

PRACTICAL ACTIVITY **14.1**

Dietary Phytochemicals as Antioxidants

Many phytochemicals exist in the lipid compartments of cells (i.e., cell membranes) that can take on oxygen free radicals and help prevent the generation of carcinogens within cells. In which of the major food groups in your usual diet are any of these phytochemicals found? ■

In summary, the micronutrients, particularly the antioxidant nutrients (vitamins C and E, beta-carotene, zinc, and selenium), antioxidant phytochemicals, and dietary fiber may play a protective role against most cancers, but further study, especially in humans, is needed. Other micronutrients have minimal beneficial effects in lowering cancer risk.

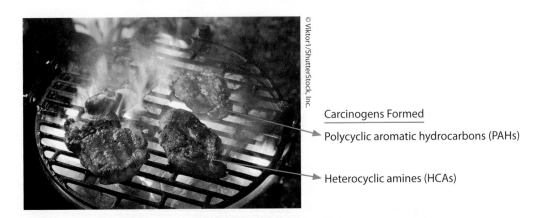

© Viktor1/ShutterStock, Inc.

Carcinogens Formed

→ Polyclic aromatic hydrocarbons (PAHs)

→ Heterocyclic amines (HCAs)

Carcinogenic Agents: Food Components and Non-Nutrient Food Additives

Some foods have compounds that either indirectly or directly damage the genetic material (DNA) of cells; that is, they act as **mutagens**. These food components may be naturally occurring or contaminants. For example, **aflatoxins** are toxic molecules produced by fungi (*Aspergillus flavus*) that grow on stored grains (corn) and legumes (peanuts, soybeans) that contain high levels of moisture. Aflatoxins are potent liver carcinogens. Several organic molecules in smoked and charred meats and fish also are mutagenic, and two separate classes of these mutagenic molecules—polycyclic aromatic hydrocarbons (PAHs) and heterocyclic amines (HCAs)—are recognized as carcinogens in animal models. Many naturally occurring chemicals in foods, including mushrooms, also can cause cancer in animal models. **Table 14.6** lists both naturally occurring food-related carcinogens and the additives that have been reported to cause cancer.

Food additives are being increasingly consumed in our highly processed food supply. These additives are of two kinds: intentional substances (3,000) and unintentional additives (12,000). Only a few additives, including Red Dye #2 and cyclamates, have been

mutagen An agent, chemical or physical, that initiates a mutation to DNA within a gene by direct damage to nuclear DNA; the result often is a gene that is dysfunctional. May lead to cancer in some instances.

aflatoxin Toxic molecule produced by fungi that grow on moist grains, peanuts, and other legumes in storage. These mycotoxins are potentially cancer promoting because they act as mutagens.

TABLE 14.6
Carcinogenic Components of Foods: Both Natural and Induced

Carcinogen	Source
Aflatoxins	Fungus growing on food
Heterocyclic amines (HCAs)*	Grilled meats
Polycyclic aromatic hydrocarbons (PAHs)*	Broiled meats
Nitrosamines	Processed meats with added nitrates or nitrites
Hydrazines	Mushrooms
Tannins	Tea, coffee, and cocoa
Pyrrolizidine alkaloids (PAs)	Herbs and herbal teas
Estrogenic substances	Soybeans, some cereals
Acrylamide*	Cooked starch-based foods

* Carcinogens with asterisks are from the cooking method or packaging process.
Data from International Agency for Research on Cancer, World Health Organization. *National Toxicology Program Report on Carcinogens.* Lyon, France: WHO.

> Several organic molecules in smoked and charred meats and fish also are mutagenic, and two separate classes of these mutagenic molecules—polycyclic aromatic hydrocarbons (PAHs) and heterocyclic amines (HCAs)—are recognized as carcinogens in animal models.

removed because of their carcinogenicity. Saccharin, a non-nutritive sweetener, which tests have shown to be carcinogenic to the urinary bladder of rats by a mechanism that is not relevant to humans, remains available for use although it has largely been replaced by aspartame. In general, use of food additives has not been shown to increase the risk of human cancers at this time. If adverse effects of additives do exist, they are too small to detect at the level of sensitivity of current epidemiologic methods.

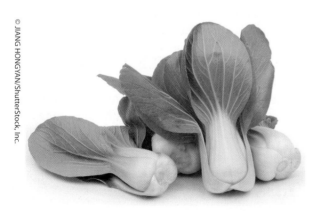

© JIANG HONGYAN/ShutterStock, Inc.

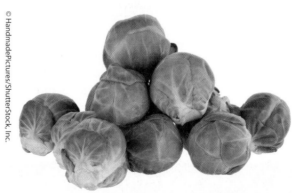

© HandmadePictures/ShutterStock, Inc.

Nitrosamines are considered to be carcinogenic in human subjects as well as in animal models. Nitrites and nitrates, used in the curing and preservation of meats, have been found to form nitrosamines, especially in the upper gastrointestinal tract, by reacting with primary or secondary amines present in foods. A pH of about 3 is required for this reaction. Ascorbic acid in the stomach or upper small bowel may inhibit nitrosamine formation, but the exact mechanism for this protective effect is not known. The mechanism of carcinogenesis of nitrosamines is related to alterations in the control

nitrosamines Molecules resulting from the combination of a nitrate or nitrite with a protein in foods or tissues. In meats, the combination of nitrite with the secondary amine groups of myoglobin or other muscle proteins results in potentially carcinogenic nitrosamines.

of the renewal of epithelial cells. For example, the Japanese have a high rate of stomach cancer. The cause of this gastric cancer is not fully understood, but it seems to be related to high salt consumption or to other dietary factors. For example, the Japanese consume fish stored in vinegar at a low pH, which may contribute to the development of gastric cancer.

Other environmental contaminants are inadvertently present in the food supply at very low levels. The contribution of these contaminants to increased risk of cancer is, as with food additives, difficult to detect. Too little information currently exists to draw conclusions about the quantities of well-known contaminants ingested or inhaled by humans or about potential interactions.

It is easy to be skeptical of the safety of our food supply and worry about all the additives and chemicals and pesticides in our foods and the effects that they may be having on us and our children. Nevertheless, the risk attributed to any chemical or class of chemical in our food or environment is quite small. Choosing foods that claim to have less pesticides and chemicals on them may be beneficial, but the proof of lower risk is difficult to establish. The American and Canadian food supplies are generally very safe, and, when a new chemical of concern becomes a public issue of concern, the responsible agencies do usually move into action, though usually more slowly than some would like. By far the highest risks from the foods we eat are from the effects the foods themselves have on us through the development of obesity and the acute infections of microorganisms that cause food poisoning.

Cancer Death Rates in the United States

In general, cancer death rates have been slowly declining in the United States. However, of the diet-related chronic disease, deaths from cancer now rank number one, just ahead of coronary heart diseases. Cancer currently accounts for approximately 23% of all deaths each year! Except for colon, lung, and breast cancers, death rates from cancer have held remarkably steady throughout the last half of the 20th century. However, within the last few years, breast cancer death rates have declined even though breast cancer incidence (morbidity) rates remain steady. This is due, in part, to earlier diagnosis and improved medical treatment. With the obesity epidemic, breast cancer incidence, not death rates, may begin to rise.

Because colon, breast, and prostate cancers have strong dietary determinants, dietary modifications may prove helpful in preventing or delaying development of these specific cancers, as well as others. Prudent dietary practices by adults with respect to the consumption of animal foods and to the maintenance of desirable body weight remain reasonable goals for lowering the risk of the diet-related cancers (see **Table 14.7**). The lower prevalence rates of most cancers among lacto-ovo-vegetarian Seventh-Day Adventists and among meat-eating Latter-Day Saints (Mormons) compared with other omnivores

> *In general, cancer death rates have been slowly declining in the United States. However, of the diet-related chronic diseases, deaths from cancer now rank number one, just ahead of coronary heart disease.*

FOCUS 14.3 Vegetarianism and Cancer Prevention

Studies that support the benefits of a vegetarian diet in the prevention of cancer have often been conducted among the Seventh-Day Adventists, a religious group in the United States and worldwide that emphasizes a healthy lifestyle that avoids alcohol, tobacco, pork and other meats, caffeine-containing beverages, and highly refined foods.

More than half of U.S. Adventists are lacto- or ovo-vegetarians or eat meat less than once a week. Epidemiologic studies among Adventists have pointed to a relationship between a plant-based diet and lower rates of cancer of the colon, pancreas, and lung. ●

TABLE 14.7
Postulated Mechanisms of Actions of Macronutrients and Dietary Fiber in the Development of Colon and Breast Cancers

Macronutrients	Postulated Mechanisms in Promotion of Cancers
Total calories	Excess energy supports cell growth and promotion of carcinogenesis.
Fat	Provides excess energy for cell growth, solubilizes fat-soluble carcinogens, promotes growth and differentiation of cells, and serves as a source of free radicals.
Carbohydrate	Serves as an energy source. Glucose increases postprandial insulin, a cell growth factor.
Protein	Increases production of growth factors that may stimulate cell growth, including abnormal cell division.
Dietary fiber	Low fiber intakes increase transit time and carcinogen exposure time in large bowel and modify metabolic activity of fecal flora, possibly leading to increase in colon cancer.

Reproduced from Anderson JJB. *Nutrition and Health: An Introduction.* Durham, NC: Carolina Academic Press; 2005.

> The lower prevalence rates of most cancers among lacto-ovo-vegetarian Seventh-Day Adventists and among meat-eating Latter-Day Saints (Mormons) compared with other omnivores in the United States suggest that lifestyle variables, primarily the plentiful intake of plant foods, may be important in cancer prevention.

in the United States strongly suggest that lifestyle behaviors, primarily the plentiful intake of plant foods, may be important in cancer prevention.

Major Diet-Related Cancers and Potential Mechanisms

Cancer is a complex disease, and the etiology behind the development of cancer differs based on the affected tissue or organ system.

Breast Cancer

Abnormal growth of breast tissue is, in part, hormone dependent. Breast cancer has the highest incidence of any cancer among women in Western nations. Risk factors for breast cancer include early menarche, a late first pregnancy (over age 30), few pregnancies or none, high energy intake, and obesity.

Vegetarians in Western nations have lower rates of breast cancer than nonvegetarians. Vegetarians are afforded some protection against the development of breast tumors because they have lower circulating estrogen concentrations, especially when they also consume a low-energy diet. Low consumption of fruits, vegetables, and dietary fiber has been implicated in the development of breast cancer because of low intake of antioxidants, other anticarcinogens, and dietary fiber.

> Vegetarians in Western nations have lower rates of breast cancer than nonvegetarians. Vegetarians are afforded some protection against the development of breast tumors because they have lower circulating estrogen concentrations, especially when they also consume a low-energy diet.

Prostate Cancer

Prostate cancer is similar to breast cancer in that it is hormone dependent. Prostate cancer is more common among older men than younger men. Data reported by Finnish researchers suggest that vitamin E may be protective against prostate cancer. Plant antioxidants from diverse sources may help slow the conversion from benign hyperplasia of the prostate, which is common in older men, to cancer. Protective roles for calcium or vitamin D remain unclear.

Colon Cancer

Epidemiologic studies have found that colon cancer is associated with the typical Western diet. This diet is high in fat and protein but low in phytochemicals and fiber. Colon cancer rates are high in economically developed nations, with the exception of Japan. Colon cancer rates are lower in developing countries, in part because of much higher daily fiber consumption among those populations. Red meat consumption has been found to be clearly associated with increased colon cancer risk. Researchers are also examining whether low calcium intake may also be a risk factor for colon cancer.

Stomach (Gastric) Cancer

The etiology of gastric cancer is complex. The diverse cell types found in this organ are directly exposed to nutrients, non-nutrients, and contaminants in the food supply, and they are also continually exposed to stomach acid. Nitrosamines that form in meats and fish following the binding of nitrogen groups with proteins in these foods are potent carcinogens that require the low pH of the stomach for their formation. However, a serving of vitamin C in the same meal protects against excessive nitrosamine formation. High gastric cancer rates have historically occurred in the Japanese population because of their preference for salt-preserved or pickled vegetables and seafood. The high salt content of these foods enhances nitrosamine production, and thus cancer onset.

Worldwide Variability in Cancer Morbidity and Mortality Rates

Both hereditary and environmental factors contribute to cancer. The focus of this chapter has been on environmental factors, mainly dietary factors. The varying incidences of the different types of cancers throughout the world point to the importance of environmental factors in the development of cancer. The customs, habits, and dietary practices of a region may be more significant than genetics. For example, migration studies of Japanese individuals who have moved from Japan to Hawaii or California have shown changes in the incidence rates of different cancers after relocation, in large part because of dietary changes. Such migration studies also provide data that specific types of cancer are potentially preventable.

> Epidemiologic studies have found that colon cancer is associated with the typical Western diet. This diet is high in fat and protein but low in phytochemicals and fiber.

> For example, migration studies of Japanese individuals who have moved from Japan to Hawaii or California have shown changes in the incidence rates of different cancers after relocation, in large part because of dietary changes.

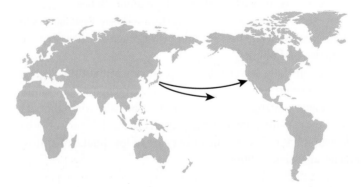

U.S. cancer incidence rates are listed in **Table 14.8** for the most prevalent cancers by estimated numbers of new cases. Potential nutrient factors involved in the etiology of these specific cancers are also given. Recall that incidence rates represent new cases of disease (morbidity) in a year, but not death or mortality rates.

TABLE 14.8
Most Common Cancers in the United States and Possible Dietary Risk Factors

Type of Cancer	Estimated New U.S. Cases (2011)	Possible Dietary Risk Factors
All cancers	1,596,670	Overweight and obesity, low fruit and vegetable consumption, limited consumption of whole grains and legumes
Prostate cancer	240,890	Low lycopene and selenium intake; high calcium intake
Breast cancer	230,480	High alcohol consumption; overweight and obesity
Lung cancer	221,130	Low fruit intake, high arsenic intake, beta-carotene supplements
Colorectal cancer	141,210	Diet high in processed foods and red meat, low fiber intake, high alcohol consumption, low calcium intake
Other cancers	762,960	Unknown

Data from SEER Stat Fact Sheets. Surveillance Epidemiology and End Results (SEER). Available at: http://seer.cancer.gov/statfacts/index.html.

Dietary Recommendations for Cancer Prevention

Current recommendations for the prevention of cancer, from a global perspective, provided by the international cancer research groups AICR and WCRF are noted below:

- Be as lean as possible to reduce body fatness (BMI between 18.5 and 25).
- Be physically active as part of everyday life.
- Limit consumption of energy-dense foods and avoid sugary drinks to avoid weight gain.
- Eat mostly foods of plant origin.
- Limit intake of red meat and avoid processed meats (typically with additives).
- Limit alcoholic drinks to two a day for men and one a day for women.
- Limit consumption of salt and avoid moldy cereals (grains) or pulses (legumes).
- Aim to meet nutritional needs through diet alone; try to avoid supplement use.
- Special: Mothers should breast-feed; infants should be breast-fed.
- Special: Cancer survivors need to follow the recommendations for prevention of additional cancer.

Although no specific diet has been recommended, these guidelines focus on an increase in the consumption of plant foods and weight management throughout adult life.

Other Nutrition-Related Chronic Diseases

In addition to diet-related cancers, several other chronic diseases have a nutrition component. Here we review four of those conditions: metabolic syndrome, diseases affecting the eye and brain, arterial calcification, and immune suppression. These conditions have not typically been described in introductory texts as having nutritional determinants in their causation, but recent research findings support the diet–disease connections of these seemingly diverse conditions. Metabolic syndrome is probably the best understood of these conditions.

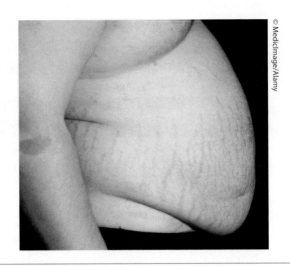

FIGURE 14.4 Fat Accumulation and Metabolic Syndrome. People with metabolic syndrome often have increased fat accumulation in the abdomen, liver, muscle, and subcutaneous (skin) tissue.

> A person is designated as having metabolic syndrome if he or she has three of the following five abnormalities: (1) abdominal obesity, (2) prediabetes, (3) high blood pressure, (4) low serum HDL-cholesterol, and (5) elevated serum triglycerides.

Metabolic Syndrome

Metabolic syndrome (MetS) is a cluster of several medical conditions, or comorbidities, namely central (visceral) obesity, hypertension, insulin resistance, and abnormal lipid metabolism, which together increase the risk of type 2 diabetes mellitus and cardiovascular disease. A person is designated as having the metabolic syndrome if he or she has three of the following five abnormalities: (1) abdominal obesity (see **FIGURE 14.4**), (2) prediabetes, (3) high blood pressure, (4) low serum HDL-cholesterol, and (5) elevated serum triglycerides (see **Table 14.9**). An important feature of the syndrome is that multiple biological alterations are occurring in an individual at the same time. These changes typically begin during middle age and increase in prevalence with age.

According to the CDC, approximately 68 million U.S. adults have metabolic syndrome, or roughly 35% of all U.S. adults. Because of the obesity epidemic, this number

metabolic syndrome A complex of conditions that results from overweight or obesity and insulin resistance; contributes to several chronic diseases (the "deadly quartet"). Characterized by a large waist, low HDL-cholesterol, high fasting triglycerides, high fasting glucose, and high blood pressure.

TABLE 14.9
Diagnosis of Metabolic Syndrome Requires Three of the Following Five Criteria

Abnormality	Criteria
Elevated waist circumference	Men: > 40 inches Women: > 35 inches
Elevated triglycerides	≥ 150 mg/dL
Reduced HDL ("good") cholesterol	Men: < 40 mg/dL Women: < 50 mg/dL
Elevated blood pressure	≥ 130/85 mm Hg or use of medication for hypertension
Elevated fasting glucose	≥ 100 mg/dL or use of medication for hyperglycemia

Modified from Grundy SM, Cleeman JI, Daniels SR, et al. Diagnosis and management of the metabolic syndrome: an American Heart Association/National Heart, Lung, and Blood Institute scientific statement: executive summary. *Circulation*. 2005;112:e285–e290.

will likely increase. Maintaining a healthy body weight is most critical for preventing the metabolic syndrome. The presence of multiple chronic diseases in the same individual decreases one's chances of survival over time. The U.S. healthcare system must increasingly cope with this common syndrome and the high economic costs associated with it.

Dietary recommendations to help counter the development of metabolic syndrome are based on healthy eating patterns, including matching calorie consumption with calorie expenditure, eating fewer processed foods, consuming less sugar and salt, avoiding soft drinks and sugary beverages, and including more fish and plant foods (i.e., vegetables, fruits, whole grains, nuts and seeds) in the diet. Decreased energy intakes should be accompanied by a reduction in saturated fat intake (i.e., animal products) and smaller portions of food. The DASH diet, the Mediterranean eating pattern, and the Okinawa diet represent healthy dietary approaches to prevent obesity and the metabolic syndrome. These diets include ample amounts of plant foods plus fish and other seafood.

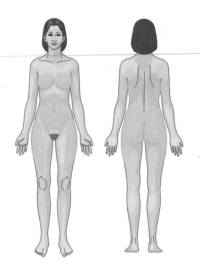

Eye Diseases: Age-Related Macular Degeneration and Cataracts

Visual function is affected by two major chronic diseases of the eyes: **age-related macular degeneration (AMD)** and **cataracts (opacities)**. AMD involves cell damage to a small area (~¼ inch in diameter) in the middle portion of the retina, called the *macula*, which captures images like a camera and relays them via the optic nerve to the visual cortex for processing of the information (see **FIGURE 14.5**). Oxidative damage via free radicals to the macula reduces its capability to transmit sharp images to the brain. Insufficient intake of antioxidants and phytochemicals from plant foods is hypothesized to strongly contribute to the suboptimal repair of damage from free radicals.

In addition to oxidative damage, additional deterioration of the optical nerve because of protein glycation, resulting from high serum glucose concentration, reduces the performance of nerve conduction from the eye to the brain. Nerve damage results from glucose molecules that complex nonenzymatically with proteins in the nerve membranes, thereby reducing nerve function. This latter effect results from the chronic high serum glucose concentrations that occur during prediabetic conditions or in type 2 diabetes mellitus.

A cataract is the clouding of the lens of the eye, leading to decreased vision. Cataracts are also affected by free radicals, but other factors may have major adverse effects on the lens, such as direct exposure to sunlight or other harsh light, pollutants, radiation, and cigarette smoke.

> " Dietary recommendations to help counter the development of metabolic syndrome are based on healthy eating patterns, including matching calorie consumption with calorie expenditure, eating fewer processed foods, consuming less sugar and salt, avoiding soft drinks and sugary beverages, and including more fish and plant foods in the diet. "

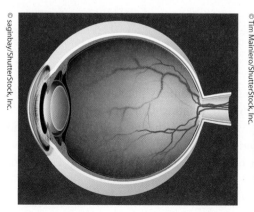

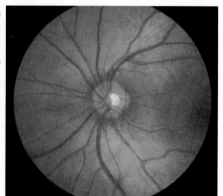

age-related macular degeneration Condition characterized by cell damage to a small portion of the retina (i.e., the macula), which captures images and relays them via the optic nerve to the brain. Oxidative damage via free radicals to the macula reduces its ability to transmit sharp images to the brain.

cataract Clouding of the eye, leading to decreased vision.

Prevention of both of these chronic eye conditions may result from good nutritional intakes. Carotenoids, omega-3 fatty acids, zinc, and other micronutrients have

■■ Oxidative damage via free radicals to the macula reduces its capability to transmit sharp images to the brain. Insufficient intake of antioxidants and phytochemicals from plant foods is hypothesized to strongly contribute to the suboptimal repair of damage from free radicals. ■■

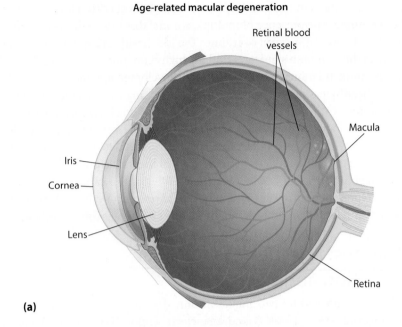

FIGURE 14.5 Anatomic Location of Macula Portion of Retina. (a) With AMD, the macula becomes damaged, affecting the ability of the eyes to capture and process visual images. (b) Cataracts result from clouding of the lens of the eye, leading to decreased vision.

memory loss Unusual forgetfulness. Occurs in some people as part of the normal aging process, or it may signal the onset of dementia caused by a disease process such as Alzheimer's disease.

dementia Loss of cognitive ability that results in problems with memory, language, and thinking. May be temporary or permanent, depending on the condition or disease causing it. Alzheimer's disease is a type of dementia resulting from plaques that form on the brain.

been experimentally shown to improve these eye conditions, but not to correct them to their optimal state. Recent studies have shown that antioxidant supplements can play a small but significant role in preventing AMD. However, these same researchers found that zeaxanthin and lutein, two carotenoids widely thought to have special protective effects, did not improve prevention over beta-carotene, and that omega-3 fatty acids play no protective role.

Brain Diseases

Memory loss, **dementia**, and Alzheimer's (dementia) disease are commonly found in older adults. The origin of these conditions remains largely a mystery, but arterial changes, such as fatty plaque formations that later calcify, may be involved in their etiology. Unhealthy dietary intakes may influence the development of these disorders, and healthy diets may delay them or even prevent them from ever occurring. A recent large investigation of U.S. adults found a beneficial effect of the Mediterranean diet in the reduction of incident (new) cases of dementia.

Vascular depression, one form of depression that involves damage to major arteries of the brain, may have a strong linkage to diets that promote arterial plaque formation, which begins much earlier in life than when the depression is clinically identified. Diets high in energy, fat, sugar, and animal products, plus insufficient amounts of plant foods and fish, may contribute to plaque formation. New evidence also suggests calcium supplements (i.e., large loads in a single dose) may contribute to arterial damage in the brain. Whether mineralization of plaque occurs in the brain arteries has not yet been established, but the carotid arteries in the neck on both sides have been shown to undergo calcification. So, similar pathological events that occur in the carotid arteries are presumed also to occur in the brain itself. **FIGURE 14.6** shows scans of a brain with vascular lesions.

Additional studies have reported that memory loss and dementia in elderly individuals may be decreased through increased intake of omega-3 fatty acids, especially DHA. The balance between the intake of omega-3 and omega-6 fatty acids seems to take on a greater importance for the maintenance of brain function than previously recognized. Healthy intakes of antioxidant micronutrients and phytochemicals most likely also benefit cells in various parts of the brain. Eye nerves are an extension of the brain, and healthy nutrient intakes may benefit the nervous tissue of both the brain and the eye in a similar way.

Arterial Calcification

Calcification or mineralization of several major arteries and the heart valves typically occurs in late life, even in those with good kidney function. Calcifications occur in the medial layer of an artery as a result of fatty deposits or atherosclerotic plaque in the intimal layer that affect the smooth muscle cells of the media. Calcification results when smooth muscle cells in the medial layer convert to bone cells that make new bone that hardens, a process known as arteriosclerosis. The net results are a narrowing of

> **❝** Memory loss, dementia, and Alzheimer's disease are commonly found in older adults. The origin of these conditions remains largely a mystery, but arterial changes, such as fatty plaque formations that later calcify, may be involved in their etiology. **❞**

> **❝** Vascular depression, but not necessarily other forms of depression, may have a strong linkage to diets that promote arterial plaque formation, which begins much earlier in life than when the depression is clinically identified. **❞**

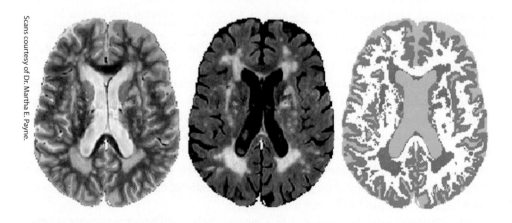

Scans courtesy of Dr. Martha E. Payne.

FIGURE 14.6 Brain Lesions in Vascular Depression. Proton density image (left), fluid-attenuated inversion recovery image (center), and tissue classification image (right; lesions in red). These lesions have been cross sectionally associated with higher calcium intakes.

Reproduced from Payne ME, Anderson JJB, Steffens DC. Calcium and vitamin D intakes may be positively associated with vascular brain lesions in both depressed and nondepressed elders. *Nutr Res.* 2008;28(5):285–292.

vascular depression A form of depression resulting from damage to the major arteries of the brain. May have a strong linkage with diets that promote arterial plaque formation, which generally occurs much earlier in life than when the depression is clinically identified.

> Calcification results when smooth muscle cells in the medial layer convert to bone cells that make new bone that hardens, a process known as arteriosclerosis. The net results are a narrowing of the arterial lumen, stiffening of the artery, and a disturbance in blood flow dynamics.

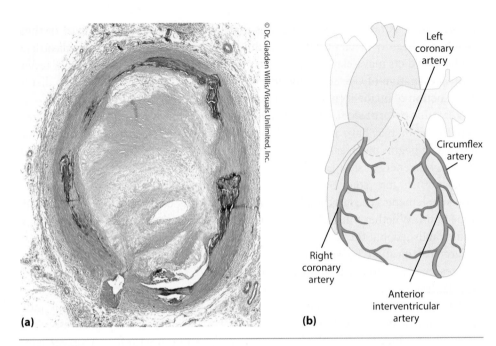

FIGURE 14.7 Arterial Calcification in Coronary Artery. With arteriosclerosis, calcium deposits form in the arterial wall, appearing as darker-stained streaks in the medial part of the arterial wall (a). The normal anatomy of the coronary arteries is shown in (b).

> A number of factors have been identified as possibly promoting arterial calcification, including calcium loading, elevated serum phosphate concentrations, use of the anticoagulant warfarin or Coumadin, elevated parathyroid hormone, and most heart disease risk factors.

calcium loading High intakes of supplemental calcium. Research suggests that it may promote arterial calcification, and thus increase the risk of cardiovascular disease.

the arterial lumen, stiffening of the artery, and a disturbance in blood flow dynamics. For example, the rigidity of the arteriosclerotic aorta does not permit normal back-flow of blood after each heart contraction so that the coronary arteries do not receive enough nutrients and oxygen-enriched blood to support healthy heart function. Clots are much more likely to form at narrowed, calcified sites. These physical changes, in turn, increase the risk of myocardial infarction (heart attack) and also stroke (brain attack) in affected individuals. Calcification represents a serious threat to life. **FIGURE 14.7** demonstrates sites of calcification in a scan of a coronary artery.

A number of factors have been identified as possibly promoting arterial calcification, including **calcium loading** (supplemental intake), elevated serum phosphate concentrations, use of the anticoagulant warfarin or Coumadin, elevated parathyroid hormone, and most heart disease risk factors. Of the heart disease risk factors, hyperlipidemia associated with LDL-cholesterol may be the most prominent. In addition, a few inhibitory factors of calcification have been identified, but it is presumed that they become less potent or blocked or they may be secreted in lesser amounts late in life.

Besides calcium loading, an elevation of serum phosphate may also be a significant risk factor in late life. Small declines—often undetected—in renal function that help reabsorb and hence retain more phosphate than desirable usually accompany aging. Processed foods, including luncheon meats, bakery products, and phosphorylated cola beverages, typically contain phosphate additives. These phosphorus-rich foods can be reduced or eliminated. Keeping the serum concentrations of both calcium and phosphate ions within the normal ranges means that the ratio of calcium to phosphorus of foods (and the total diet) will remain optimal.

An enigma observed in people with osteoporosis is the presence of increasing arterial calcification as aging progresses. These two pathological states seem to operate in parallel with the arterial calcification feeding off the loss of calcium and phosphate ions from the skeleton via bone resorption in addition to the dietary provision of these mineral ions, especially the use of calcium supplements or loads in fairly high doses (~500 milligrams or more). So, the overall calcium balance probably remains slightly negative with respect to bone losses in older adults but positive once arterial calcification is factored in. This predicament of coexisting diseases is difficult to overcome, but it can be minimized by wise eating practices and healthy behaviors.

Calcium supplements may accelerate the calcification process in late life, but as yet the evidence to confirm this has been lacking.

Immune System Health

The immune system, especially the cell-mediated aspect (cellular immunity), is sensitive to deficiencies of nutrients, particularly protein, several vitamins, trace elements, and phytochemicals. Chronic depression of the immune system because of such nutrient deficits may diminish the efficacy of the immune system in two important ways; that is, the neutralization and removal of precancerous and cancerous cells. Similarly, viruses such as the hepatitis and human papilloma viruses and other infectious agents are less well defended against by the humoral aspect (immunoglobulins or antibodies and other related molecules in blood) of the immune defense mechanism when nutrition is not optimal. **FIGURE 14.8** illustrates the components of immune defense in the body. The involvement of the immune system in cancer development is complex, but good nutrition supports the immune system in its protective roles against both cancer and infectious organisms.

Protein of reasonably high quality, vitamins, and minerals help support the synthesis of the components of the immune system and supply immune cells, such as white blood cells, with the needed nutrients for their diverse functions.

> An enigma observed in people with osteoporosis is the presence of increasing arterial calcification as aging progresses. These two pathological states seem to operate in parallel with the arterial calcification feeding off the loss of calcium and phosphate ions from the skeleton via bone resorption in addition to the dietary provision of these mineral ions.

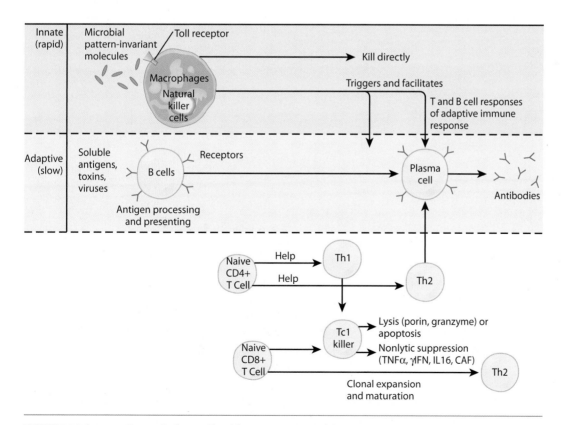

FIGURE 14.8 Immune System Defenses. The different components of the immune system are responsible for protecting the body from pathogens. B cells produce antibodies and T-cells secrete various factors, both of which help neutralize and often kill foreign agents in a complex array of actions in body fluids.

❝ The immune system, especially the cell-mediated aspect (cellular immunity), is sensitive to deficiencies of nutrients, including protein and antioxidants, especially several vitamins, trace elements, and phytochemicals. ❞

Several dietary factors may improve the function of the cells of the immune system:

- Maintain adequate protein intake, but avoid excessive intake, from both plant and animal sources.
- Increase intake of a wide range of fruits and vegetables for their antioxidants and other beneficial components.
- Use herbs, such as garlic.
- Consider consuming probiotics in yogurt.
- Limit alcohol use to established recommendations.

Foods rich in antioxidants and other micronutrients help the immune system defend against cancer and bacteria, viruses, and other microorganisms. Plant foods rich in antioxidants include berries and other fruits; cabbage, broccoli, spinach, garlic, and other vegetables; almonds; mushrooms; and teas, both green and black. One animal product, live-culture yogurt, also supports defense of a healthy immune system. Lifestyle factors that may help support the immune system include engaging in regular physical activity, getting adequate sleep, laughing, not smoking, and regularly washing hands with soap and hot water.

SUMMARY

Induction of carcinogenesis has been determined from animal studies to be a multiple-step sequence that begins with an initiating event in which mutagens or carcinogens may interact in some manner with DNA. The consumption of carcinogen-laden, salt-cured, and smoked foods is not recommended, but micronutrients and phytochemicals in plant foods may have preventive roles against cancer. Modifications of food consumption patterns could potentially contribute to significant reductions of cancer rates in the United States and Canada.

Cancer cells no longer maintain a balance between growth and inhibitory factors that control the proliferation of normal cells. Diet–cancer associations have been clearly demonstrated in animal studies, but the human linkages have not been as well documented, except for gastric cancer. According to the estimates of Doll and Peto, the risk of cancer can be decreased about a third through dietary modifications, especially for colon, breast, and prostate cancers, and by increasing daily intakes of micronutrients and phytochemicals. Dietary fiber from wheat and bran may protect against colon and other cancers. Improved dietary habits, including better food selection and a reduction in the rate of obesity,

would contribute greatly to a reduction in the risk for these specific cancers and perhaps for nearly all other cancers.

A group of seemingly unrelated chronic diseases that especially affect older adults was highlighted. In the United States, metabolic syndrome affects approximately 35% of all adults, and as the obesity trend continues, metabolic syndrome will likely increase in prevalence as well. These conditions are currently areas of considerable research interest because of their prevalence among the elderly and because so little is known about their etiologies and treatment strategies. Inadequate dietary intakes may be significant, but clearly other lifestyle factors and genetic factors may make important contributions to these disorders. Changing dietary habits to incorporate healthier foods in normal serving sizes, less processed food, and the use of healthier preparation methods into the usual pattern of eating remain an important approach to delaying or preventing these conditions. Several micronutrients, such as calcium, vitamin D, potassium, zinc, antioxidant vitamins, selenium, vitamin A and carotenoids, as well as omega-3 fatty acids, and phytochemicals need to be reemphasized because of their health benefits.

STUDENT ACTIVITIES

1. Describe cancer in terms of (a) one cell gone "bad" and then (b) a clone of this one "bad" cell.

2. Briefly explain initiation, promotion, progression, and metastasis with regards to cancer.

3. List the four most common cancers in the United States and state which of these have a strong linkage with diet.

4. Why might cancer morbidity and mortality be somewhat lower in both Seventh-Day Adventists and LDS (Mormons) compared to the rest of the U.S. population?

5. Briefly describe how each of the following nutrients influence cancer: energy, fat, antioxidants, fiber.

6. Describe the interaction between vitamin C and vitamin E in cells.

7. Define the term *free radical*, and explain how nutrients may reduce free radicals.

8. How are polyphenols protective against the development of cancer?

9. List three dietary factors that can influence the onset of breast cancer. Then briefly note how each factor operates in breast epithelial cells.

10. List at least five nutrients or related dietary variables that act to prevent the development of cancer. Briefly explain how each of these helps to prevent cancer.

11. Metabolic syndrome is characterized by abnormal alterations of a minimum of three major measurable variables. List three of these five variables.

12. Which one risk factor seems to have had the greatest impact on the metabolic syndrome? [Hint: the contribution of several risk factors leading to the development of the metabolic syndrome were uncovered by the Framingham (Heart Study) investigators.]

13. State three dietary recommendations to reduce the risk of metabolic syndrome in individuals.

14. Age-related macular degeneration (AMD) is considered to result from the consumption of insufficient amounts of antioxidants. Name a few micronutrients and two non-nutrient phytochemicals that act as antioxidants.

15. Briefly explain how antioxidants act within cells of the macula.

16. Vascular depression appears to result from arterial damage in the brain. How can diet contribute to the development of arterial damage in the brain? Explain.

17. Atherosclerotic damage of brain arteries may be further affected by mineralization or arteriosclerotic changes. Briefly state what is different between these two types of vascular pathology. [Hint: Think of adverse changes of heart arteries in older adults.]

18. Explain how arterial calcification can adversely affect blood flow within arteries.

19. Do you think that calcium from supplements versus dietary calcium from foods behaves differently in the body? How might supplements increase the risk of arterial calcification?

20. Immune defense involves two major components: antibodies and cellular immunity relating especially to lymphocytes. Briefly note how each arm of immunity operates. Then state how low intakes of specific nutrients might reduce the effectiveness of the immune response to infectious agents.

WEBSITES FOR FURTHER STUDY

American Cancer Society
www.cancer.org
CA: Cancer Journal for Clinicians
http://onlinelibrary.wiley.com/journal/10.3322/(ISSN)1542-4863
American Institute for Cancer Research (AICR)
www.aicr.org/ser
International Agency for Research on Cancer (IARC)
www.iarc.fr
National Toxicology Program's (NTP) Report on Carcinogens
http://ntp-server.niehs.nih.gov

National Cancer Institute
www.cancer.gov
PubMed Health: Metabolic Syndrome
www.ncbi.nlm.nih.gov/pubmedhealth/PMH0004546
Macular Degeneration Research
www.ahaf.org/macular/?gclid=CKeR59TbrrECFQeR7QodlxgAgg
Linus Pauling Institute: Nutrition and Immunity
http://lpi.oregonstate.edu/ss10/nutrition.html

REFERENCES

The Age-Related Eye Disease Study 2 (AREDS2) Research Group. Lutein + zeaxanthin and omega-3 fatty acids for age-related macular degeneration: the Age-Related Eye Disease Study 2 (AREDS2) randomized clinical trial. *JAMA*. 2013;309:2005–2015. doi:10.1001/jama.2013.4997.

Akbaraly TN, Brunner EJ, Ferrie JE, et al. Dietary pattern and depressive symptoms in middle age. *Br J Psychiatry*. 2009;195:408–413.

Alberti KG, Eckel RH, Grundy SM, et al. Harmonizing the metabolic syndrome: a joint interim statement of the International Diabetes Federation Task Force on Epidemiology and Prevention; National Heart, Lung, and Blood Institute; American Heart Association; World Heart Federation; International Atherosclerosis Society; and International Association for the Study of Obesity. *Circulation* 2009;120:1640–1645.

Allison MA, His S, Wassel CL, et al. Calcified atherosclerosis in different vascular beds and the risk of mortality. *Arterioscler Thromb Vasc Biol*. 2012;32:140–146.

Anderson JJB. Calcium, vitamin D, and bone health: how much do adults need? *Nutr Food Sci*. 2009;39:337–341.

Anderson JJB. Osteoporosis. In: Erdman JW Jr, MacDonald IA, Zeisel SH (eds.). *Present Knowledge in Nutrition*. 10th ed. Ames, IA: John Wiley & Sons; 2012: 833–842.

Anderson JJB, Prytherch SA, Sparling M, et al. The metabolic syndrome: a common hyperinsulinemic disorder with severe health effects. *Nutr Today*. 2006;41:115–122.

ATBC Study Group. Incidence of cancer and mortality following alpha-tocopherol and beta-carotene supplementation: a post-intervention follow-up. *JAMA*. 2003;290:476–485.

ATBC Study Group. The effect of vitamin E and beta-carotene on the incidence of lung cancer and other cancers in male smokers. *New Engl J Med*. 1994;330:1029–1035.

Axelsson TG, Chmielewski M, Lindholm B. Kidney disease. In: Erdman JW Jr, MacDonald IA, Zeisel SH (eds.). *Present Knowledge in Nutrition*. 10th ed. Ames, IA: John Wiley & Sons; 2012: 1384–1406.

Bazzano LA, Li TY, Kamudi J, et al. Intake of fruit, vegetables, and fruit juices and risk of diabetes in women. *Diabetes Care.* 2008;31:1311–1317.

Bolland MJ, Barber PA, Doughty RN, et al. Vascular events in healthy older women receiving calcium supplementation: randomized controlled trial. *BMJ.* 2008;336:262–266.

Bolland MJ, Grey A, Avenell A, et al. Calcium supplements with or without vitamin D and risk of cardiovascular events: reanalysis of the Women's Health Initiative limited access dataset and meta-analysis. *BMJ.* 2011;342:d2040.

Brand-Miller J, Colagiuri S. Insulin resistance and the metabolic syndrome. In: Erdman JW Jr, MacDonald IA, Zeisel SH (eds.). *Present Knowledge in Nutrition.* 10th ed. Ames, IA: John Wiley & Sons; 2012: 1166–1185.

Buchman AL, McClave SA. Nutrition and gastrointestinal illness. In: Erdman JW Jr, MacDonald IA, Zeisel SH (eds.). *Present Knowledge in Nutrition.* 10th ed. Ames, IA: John Wiley & Sons; 2012: 1360–1383.

Calder PC, Albers R, Antoine J-M, et al. Inflammatory disease processes and interactions with nutrition. *Br J Nutr.* 2009;101(suppl 1):1S–45S.

Cheynier V. Polyphenols in foods are more complex than often thought. *Am J Clin Nutr.* 2005;81(suppl):223S–229S.

Chiu C-J, Milton RC, Klein R, et al. Dietary compound score and risk of age-related macular degeneration in the Age-Related Eye Disease Study. *Ophthalmology.* 2009;116:939–946.

Chong EW-T, Robman LD, Simpson JA, et al. Fat consumption and its association with age-related macular degeneration. *Arch Ophthalmol.* 2009;127:674–680.

Clinton SK, Giovannucci EL, Miller EC. Nutrition in the etiology and prevention of cancer. In: Kufe KW, Pollock RE, Weichselbaum RR, et al. (eds.). *Cancer Medicine.* 6th ed. Hamilton (ON): BC Decker; 2003.

Demer L. Skeleton in the atherosclerosis closet. *Circulation.* 1995;92:2029–2032.

Detrano R, Guerci AD, Carr JJ, et al. Coronary calcium as a predictor of coronary events in four racial or ethnic groups. *N Engl J Med.* 2008;358:1336–1345.

Doll R. The lessons of life: keynote address to the Nutrition and Cancer Conference. *Cancer Res.* 1992;52:2024S–2029S.

Doll R, Peto R. The causes of cancer: quantitative estimates of avoidable risks of cancer in the United States today. *J Natl Cancer Inst.* 1981;66:1191–1308.

Duncan AM. The role of nutrition in the prevention of breast cancer. *AACN Clin. Issues.* 2004;15:119–135.

Eng SM, Gammon MD, Terry MB, et al. Body size changes in relation to postmenopausal breast cancer among women on Long Island, New York. *Am J Epidemiol.* 2005;162:229–237.

Esposito K, Marfella R, Ciotola M, et al. Effect of a Mediterranean-style diet on endothelial dysfunction and markers of vascular inflammation in the metabolic syndrome. *JAMA.* 2004;292:1440–1446.

Feart C, Samieri C, Rondeau V, et al. Adherence to a Mediterranean diet, cognitive decline, and risk of dementia. *JAMA.* 2009;302:638–648.

Ford ES, Giles WH, Dietz WH. Prevalence of the metabolic syndrome among US adults: Findings from the third National Health and Nutrition Examination Survey. *JAMA.* 2002;287:356–359.

Fraser GE. *Diet, Life Expectancy, and Chronic Disease: Studies of Seventh-Day Adventists and Other Vegetarians.* New York: Oxford University Press; 2003: 85–108.

Grundy SM, Cleeman JI, Daniels SR, et al. Diagnosis and management of the metabolic syndrome: an American Heart Association/National Heart, Lung, and Blood Institute scientific statement: executive summary. *Circulation.* 2005;112:e285–e290.

He FJ, Nowson CA, Lucas M, et al. Increased consumption of fruit and vegetables is related to a reduced risk of coronary heart disease: meta-analysis of cohort studies. *J Hum Hypertens.* 2007;21:717–728.

Hedelin M, Klint A, Chang ET, et al. Dietary phytoestrogen, serum enterolactone and risk of prostate cancer: the cancer prostate Sweden study (Sweden). *Cancer Causes Control.* 2006;17:169–180.

Hermsdorf HHM, Zulet MA, Abete I, Martinez JA. Discriminated benefits of a Mediterranean dietary pattern within a hypocaloric diet program on plasma RBP4 concentrations and other inflammatory markers in obese subjects. *Endocrinology.* 2009;36:445–451.

Holligan SH, Berryman CE, Wang L, et al. Atherosclerotic cardiovascular disease. In: Erdman JW Jr, MacDonald IA, Zeisel SH (eds.). *Present Knowledge in Nutrition.* 10th ed. Ames, IA: John Wiley & Sons; 2012: 1186–1277.

Hu FB. Plant-based foods and prevention of cardiovascular disease: an overview. *Am J Clin Nutr.* 2003;78(suppl 3):544S–551S.

Karuppagounder SS, Pinto JT, Xu H., et al. Dietary supplementation with resveratrol reduces plaque pathology in a transgenic model of Alzheimer's disease. *Neurochem Int.* 2009;54:111–118.

Knoops KTB, de Groot LC, Kromhout D, et al. Mediterranean diet, lifestyle factors, and 10-year mortality in elderly European men and women: the HALE project. *JAMA.* 2004;292:1433–1439.

Knopman DS. Mediterranean diet and late-life cognitive impairment. *JAMA.* 2009;302:686–687.

Lee MM, Gomez SL, Chang JS, et al. Soy and isoflavone consumption in relation to prostate cancer risk in China. *Cancer Epidemiol Biomarkers Prev.* 2003;12:665–668.

Lichtenstein AH, Appel LJ, Brands M, et al. Diet and lifestyle recommendations revision 2006: a scientific statement from the American Heart Association Nutrition Committee. *Circulation.* 2006;114:82–96.

Manach C, Scalbert A, Morand, C, et al. Polyphenols: food sources and bioavailability. *Am J Clin Nutr.* 2004;79:727–747.

Martinez-Gonzalez MA, de la Fuente-Arrillaga C, Nunez-Cordoba JM, et al. Adherence to Mediterranean diet and risk of developing diabetes: prospective cohort study. *BMJ.* 2008;336:1348–1351.

Matalas A-L, Zampelas AZ, Stavrinos V (eds.). *The Mediterranean Diet: Constituents and Health Promotion.* Boca Raton, FL: CRC Press; 2001.

McClain CJ, Hill DB, Marsano L. Liver disease. In: Erdman JW Jr, MacDonald IA, Zeisel SH (eds.). *Present Knowledge in Nutrition*. 10th ed. Ames, IA: John Wiley & Sons; 2012: 1407–1443.

Mozumdar A, Liguori G. Persistent increase of prevalence of metabolic syndrome among U.S. adults: NHANES III to NHANES 1999–2006. *Diabetes Care*. 2011;34:216–219.

Munoz M-A, Fito M, Marrugat J, et al. Adherence to the Mediterranean diet is associated with better mental and physical health. *Br J Nutr*. 2009;101:1821–1827.

Nicastro H, Milner JA. Cancer. In: Erdman JW Jr, MacDonald IA, Zeisel SH (eds.). *Present Knowledge in Nutrition*. 10th ed. Ames, IA: John Wiley & Sons; 2012: 1336–1359.

Payne ME, Anderson JJB, Steffens DC. Calcium and vitamin D intakes may be positively associated with brain lesions in depressed and nondepressed elders. *Nutr Res*. 2008;28:285–292.

Payne ME, Haines PS, Chambless LE, et al. Food group intake and brain lesions in late-life vascular depression. *Int Psychogeriatrics*. 2006;19:295–305.

Payne ME, Hybels CF, Bales CW, Steffens DC. Vascular nutritional correlates of late-life depression. *Am J Geriatr Psychiatry*. 2006;14:787–795.

Pineo CE, Anderson JJB. Cardiovascular benefits of the Mediterranean Diet. *Nutr Today*. 2008;43:114–120.

Potter JD, Steinmetz K. Vegetables, fruits and phytoestrogens as preventive agents. *IARC Sci Publ*. 1996;139:61–90.

Raggi P, Kleerekoper M. Contribution of bone and mineral abnormalities to cardiovascular disease in patients with chronic kidney disease. *Clin J Am Soc Nephrol*. 2008;3:836–843.

Razquin C, Martinez JA, Martinez-Gonzales MA, et al. A 3 years follow-up of a Mediterranean diet rich in virgin olive oil is associated with high plasma antioxidant capacity and reduced body weight gain. *Eur J Clin Nutr*. 2009;63:1387–1393.

Sabate J, Ang Y. Nuts and health outcomes: new epidemiologic evidence. *Am J Clin Nutr*. 2009;89(suppl):1643S–1648S.

Sahyoun NR, Jacques PF, Zhang XL, et al. Whole-grain intake is inversely associated with the metabolic syndrome and mortality in older adults. *Am J Clin Nutr*. 2006;83:124–131.

Sanchez-Villegas A, Delgado-Rodriguez M, Alonso A., et al. Association of the Mediterranean dietary pattern with the incidence of depression. *Arch Gen Psychiatry*. 2009;66:1090–1098.

Scarmeas N, Stern Y, Mayeux R, et al. Mediterranean diet and mild cognitive impairment. *Arch Neurol*. 2009;66:216–225.

Scarmeas N, Stern Y, Mayeux Y, Luchsinger JA. Mediterranean diet, Alzheimer disease, and vascular mediation. *Arch Neurol*. 2006;63:1709–1717.

Schroeder H. Protective mechanisms of the Mediterranean diet in obesity and type 2 diabetes. *J Nutr Biochem*. 2007;18:149–160.

Serra-Majem L, Roman B, Estruch R. Scientific evidence of interventions using the Mediterranean Diet: a systematic review. *Nutr Rev*. 2006;64:27S–47S.

Sparling MC, Anderson JJB. The Mediterranean diet and cardiovascular diseases: translating research findings to clinical recommendations. *Nutr Today*. 2009;44:124–133.

Sram RJ, Farmer P, Singh R, et al. Effect of vitamin levels on biomarkers of exposure and oxidative damage—The EXPAH study. *Mutation Res*. 2009;672:129–134.

Stein K. After the media feeding frenzy: whither the Women's Health Initiative Dietary Modification Trial? *J Am Diet Assoc*. 2006;106:794–800.

Tan JSL, Wang JJ, Flood V, Mitchell P. Dietary fatty acids and the 10-year incidence of age-related macular degeneration. *Arch Opththalmol*. 2009;127:656–665.

Trichopoulou A, Bamia C, Trichopoulos D. Anatomy of health effects of Mediterranean diet: Greek EPIC prospective cohort study. *BMJ*. 2009;338:2337–2345.

Tsivgoulis G, Judd S, Letter AJ, et al. Adherence to a Mediterranean diet and risk of incident cognitive impairment. *Neurology*. 2013;80:1684–1692.

Vishwanathan R, Johnson EJ. Eye disease. In: Erdman JW Jr, MacDonald IA, Zeisel SH (eds.). *Present Knowledge in Nutrition*. 10th ed. Ames, IA: John Wiley & Sons; 2012: 1489–1531.

World Cancer Research Fund and American Institute of Cancer Research. *Food, Nutrition, Physical Activity and the Prevention of Cancer: A Global Perspective*. Washington, DC: AIRC; 2007.

Wright ME, Lawson KA, Weinstein SJ, et al. Higher baseline serum concentrations of vitamin E are associated with lower total and cause-specific mortality in the Alpha-Tocopherol, Beta-Carotene Cancer Prevention Study. *Am J Clin Nutr*. 2006;84:1200–1207.

Wu X, Beecher GR, Holden JM, et al. Lipophilic and hydrophilic antioxidant capacities of common foods in the United States. *J Agric Food Chem*. 2004;52:4026–4037.

CHAPTER 15

Nutrition and Hunger: A Global Problem

Aside from the more affluent nations, typified by the United States, Canada, Australia, New Zealand, Japan, and those of Western Europe, many countries have occasional **food shortages** that affect the nutritional status and disease rates of their populations. Such shortages are typically local in nature, but in times of crop failures, pestilence (i.e., widespread infectious diseases), and war they are much more critical for a nation and life-threatening for many of its people, especially the very young and very old who have depressed immune system defenses. The poorest of the poor countries of the world have a high and persistent prevalence of hunger that contributes to malnutrition and disease. Food availability and sufficient purchasing power are essential for obtaining food in sufficient amounts and of reasonable nutritional quality for the support of a healthy population.

When food is in short supply, hunger and undernutrition soon follow. To overcome food shortages, nations need to maintain food stores, receive **food assistance** from countries with surpluses, and appeal for help from international agencies, including the United Nations. Oddly, food shortages sometimes occur in nations, such as India and Bangladesh, that also are experiencing increases in overweight and obesity among their more affluent citizens. "**Globesity**," a term coined by the World Health Organization to refer to global obesity trends, is increasing in most nations of the world because the emerging middle classes have the purchasing power to consume more than adequate amounts of food plus the means to limit much of the physical activity previously required for everyday living. This change from suboptimal nutrition to overnutrition is referred to as the **nutrition transition**. Nevertheless, even in the face of major pockets of overweight and obesity, undernutrition remains an enormous burden in many nations of the world.

food shortages Shortages in food supplies that are typically local in nature due to crop failures and armed conflicts. These shortages can affect the nutritional status and disease rates of a population. They can be life-threatening for many people, especially the very young and very old who have depressed immune systems.

food assistance Food provided by countries with food surpluses to countries that are experiencing food shortages. International organizations such as the United Nations are often responsible for identifying areas in need of assistance and in coordinating the delivery of supplies.

globesity A term coined by the World Health Organization to refer to global obesity trends.

nutrition transition Global phenomenon whereby the emerging middle classes in many developing countries are attaining the purchasing power to consume more than adequate amounts of food and achieving the means to limit much of the physical activity previously required for everyday living, resulting in an increasing prevalence of overweight and obesity.

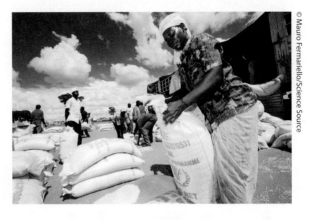

> "Globesity," a term coined by the World Health Organization to refer to global obesity trends, is increasing in most nations of the world because the emerging middle classes have the purchasing power to consume more than adequate amounts of food plus the means to limit much of the physical activity previously required for everyday living.

This chapter focuses on the issues of world **hunger** and undernutrition in those nations that are typically referred to as being economically underdeveloped. Topics covered include malnutrition, food production, overpopulation, the continuing **Green Revolution** involving new genetic strains of rice and other crops, the vicious **undernutrition–infection cycle**, and food security. Emphasis is placed on cooperation among nations and international agencies to help reduce hunger and its severe health consequences.

Types of Malnutrition

Many people around the world—as many as 1 billion—are broadly defined as malnourished. This number fluctuates depending on world grain prices and climatic events. Most cases of malnutrition result from a simple lack of most any kind of food.

Protein–Energy Malnutrition

In many underdeveloped countries, protein–energy malnutrition (PEM) is a serious problem. In children, these forms of protein–energy malnutrition are called marasmus (starvation) and kwashiorkor (see **FIGURE 15.1**). Often, the diets of those who are impoverished are relatively high in inexpensive starches and water, but low in protein and typically several micronutrients. When a young child exists on such a diet and without breast milk or other quality protein sources for months or longer, kwashiorkor will likely develop because of the extremely low protein intake. A classic sign of this form

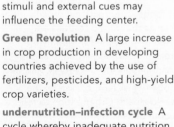

hunger Basic physiologic drive for finding and consuming food that is under the control of the feeding center of the brain; various internal stimuli and external cues may influence the feeding center.

Green Revolution A large increase in crop production in developing countries achieved by the use of fertilizers, pesticides, and high-yield crop varieties.

undernutrition–infection cycle A cycle whereby inadequate nutrition depresses the immune system, thus reducing the body's ability to respond to invading organisms. During sickness, the body responds by decreasing appetite, digestion of ingested nutrients, and utilization of absorbed nutrients and increasing mobilization and wasting of the body's stored nutrients, which further decreases the body's immune response, further driving the cycle.

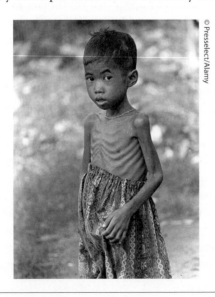
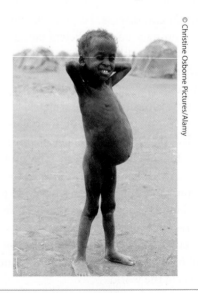

FIGURE 15.1 Marasmus and Kwashiorkor. Lack of calories and nutrients leads to marasmus (a), while extremely low protein intake can led to kwashiorkor (b).

TABLE 15.1
Comparison of Symptoms of Marasmus and Kwashiorkor in Children*

Clinical Symptom	Marasmus	Kwashiorkor
Growth failure	Present	Present
Edema	Absent	Present (bloated belly)[†]
Mental changes	Uncommon	Present
Liver enlargement	Uncommon	Common
Hair dyspigmentation	Uncommon	Common
Skin changes	Absent	Common
Appetite	Present	Poor
Anemia	Common	Common

* Gradations between these extremes also exist. Marasmus usually affects infants in the first 6 months of life, whereas kwashiorkor develops later in the first year or the second year of life, after the child has been fully weaned (and typically replaced by another nursing infant). [†] A bloated belly is a hallmark characteristic of kwashiorkor in children.

of protein–energy deficiency is reddish, curly, brittle hair. In marasmus, children are deficient in all macronutrients and, hence, energy. The different symptoms in children seen with these two types of protein-energy malnutrition are described in **Table 15.1**.

Micronutrient Deficiencies

Micronutrient deficiencies vary globally based on a region's soil mineral content and the types of crops grown. Even when calories and protein intakes are improved, certain micronutrients may still be deficient. For example, in parts of India and central Africa vitamin A deficiency overlaps with other nutritional problems. Chronic vitamin A deficiency can lead to blindness, especially in children. Approximately 200,000 children each year go blind due to vitamin A deficiency. Fortunately, vitamin A deficiency is preventable.

Another serious deficiency is of iron, which leads to anemia. Far too many females of reproductive age, primarily menstruating women, as well as young children, are iron deficient. Anemia during pregnancy is a risk factor for death during childbirth for both

FOCUS 15.1 Prevention of Blindness

Prevention of permanent eye damage of infants and children who consume vitamin A–deficient diets, such as in India, Indonesia, and Bangladesh, can be effectively achieved with massive doses of vitamin A (50,000 to 100,000 IU) given orally once or twice a year. These high doses are not toxic when taken by those who are deficient because cells of the liver and, to a lesser extent, fat tissue, can take up nearly 100% of this dose and put it in temporary storage. Such doses are very effective in preventing blindness, infections, and even death. An estimated half million children, especially in the South Asian subcontinent, die each year because of vitamin A deficiency. Typically, these deaths result from the undernutrition–infection cycle (i.e., poor defense against bacteria and viruses because of a sluggish immune response). The resulting diseases, such as respiratory infections, diarrhea, and measles, greatly deplete nutrient stores and further decrease disease resistance. ●

the mother and the infant. The more severe iron deficiency anemia leads to poor learning in school and poor performance at work.

Iodine deficiency, which may result in goiter and mental retardation, is common in many regions of the world. It may easily be overcome through fortification of salt with iodine. The United Nations is working to iodinate salt supplies in all countries of the world.

Zinc deficiency, which slows growth and sexual development during adolescence, is another nutritional problem in a few less developed nations, but it is more difficult to detect and diagnose. Zinc deficiency has been slow to be recognized as a serious problem. Estimates are that many millions of people are zinc insufficient.

Food Production and Distribution

The agricultural production of plant foods—grains, fruits, and vegetables—requires adequate amounts of arable land, sufficient water, and weather conditions that support reasonable crop yields and stable markets year after year. However, grains contain protein of only moderate quality, and more than one protein source is necessary to provide the protein quality needed to support human growth and development and the maintenance of body tissues. This mixing of protein sources, or complementation, ensures that all essential amino acids are consumed in amounts sufficient to support the body's needs. The most commonly consumed grain in the world is rice, which is low in protein, vitamins, and minerals but high in carbohydrates. Thus, complementing two or more protein sources each day improves the intake of all essential amino acids and most micronutrients.

Energy Requirements for Protein Production

Producing protein from plant crops typically requires a tenth of the energy from fossil fuels compared with that required to raise livestock for meat. In the United States, the costs of producing poultry and cattle are significantly higher than those for producing an equivalent amount of legumes, especially soybeans, or grains (raw with little or no processing). Because of the efficiencies of our mass agricultural system, however, the costs of chicken and beef in the American marketplace are generally quite low. The irony is that affluent nations have reasonably low-cost animal products readily available, but developing nations do not—and these populations are the ones that typically need greater intakes of high- to moderate-quality protein sources. So, in developing nations, especially very poor countries or those involved in civil wars or other conflicts, diets consist of low-quality protein plant sources that are low in essential micronutrients needed to support healthy active lives.

Deforestation, Soil Exhaustion, and Desertification

A major problem relating to food production in developing and poor nations is the erosion of topsoil over large land areas. Deforestation in some areas and overproduction of crops in others have led to a reduction in the number of acres of land available for productive agriculture. Deforestation and **soil exhaustion** result in the gradual loss of nutrients from soils, especially nitrogen and minerals, which has had a negative impact on crop yields. Farmers in many of these poor or developing countries do not practice crop rotation (i.e., the practice of alternating crops, such as soy and corn, in order to rejuvenate the soil with nitrogen-fixing plants or legumes). Lower crop yields due to soil exhaustion have contributed to the migration of many poor farmers from rural areas to urban areas.

Declining average annual rainfall has also been an adverse factor in semiarid regions. An example is the **desertification** that has occurred over the last century in the Sahel of Africa, a huge tract just south of the Sahara that encompasses several nations. The reduction in **crop yields** has put additional pressure on many of these nations because

soil exhaustion Condition that occurs when the same crops are grown multiple times in the same location, leading to depletion of soil nutrients and eventual loss of the ability of the soil to support crops or other plant life. Can be prevented by crop rotation and application of fertilizer.

desertification The process through which fertile land becomes a desert due to poor agricultural methods, drought, deforestation, or climate change.

crop yields Average production of a specific crop, such as bushels of corn, per acre or hectare.

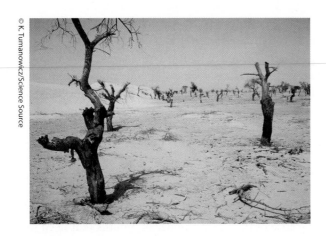

© K. Tumanowicz/Science Source

FIGURE 15.2 Desertification in Sub-Saharan Africa. The replacement of cropland by desert in the Sahel region has meant displacement for many people.

of continuing population increases. Decreased crop yields combined with wars and other conflicts often result in famine in these areas. **FIGURE 15.2** illustrates the desertification of former cropland in Sub-Saharan Africa.

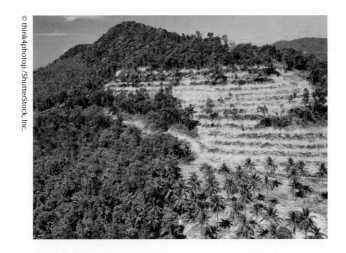

© think4photop /ShutterStock, Inc.

> Deforestation in some areas and overproduction of crops in others has led to a reduction in the number of acres of land available for productive agriculture.

Improving Food Production and Distribution

When food production is low and distribution of foods within a nation is haphazard or diverted (even stolen), then poverty, disease, and undernutrition are likely to follow. This scenario has been repeated many times over the last century in several nations in Africa, South Asia, the Middle East, and Latin America. A convergence of circumstances may hold a country or region in poverty. These deterrents may include a culture of lawlessness and corruption, continuing civil war, climatic crises (hurricanes or droughts), lack of natural resources, environmentally impoverished land (e.g., deforestation), lack of international investments, endemic diseases (malaria or dengue fever), and more recent diseases (e.g., HIV, the Ebola virus). National crises are compounded by impoverished governments that provide limited medical services, little or no basic sanitation, insufficient roads and infrastructure, an inadequate educational system, and an unstable rule of law. Such a combination of factors would make it difficult for any country to escape the cycle of poverty, malnutrition, and disease.

> Such a combination of factors would make it difficult for any country to escape the cycle of poverty, malnutrition, and disease.

The World Bank, the International Monetary Fund, and other agencies provide loans to developing and poor nations to improve agricultural practices and to improve food distribution as well as for other economic purposes. Occasionally, loans to the poorest of nations have been written off; yet many poor countries remain in crisis regarding producing enough food for their populations.

Efficient crop production and food distribution are critical for maintaining a healthy population. When these functions no longer operate efficiently, hunger will contribute to disease and death among large segments of a population, especially in children younger than 5 years.

Population Growth

Although world **population growth** has been slowing over the past two decades, a common problem in the poorest developing nations is high population growth. High rates of population growth in many developing countries have exacerbated problems of food shortages because of the sheer number of mouths that need to be fed, especially infants and children. In affluent countries, population growth rates have steadied at about 1.0% to 1.5% per year or less; however, growth rates in some developing nations still range between 3% and 5% per year.

Table 15.2 shows the distribution of nations by income. The poorer, rapidly growing developing nations are typically much younger (mean age ~20 to 25 years) compared with developed nations (mean age ~35 to 45 years) (see **FIGURE 15.3**). These low-income nations also have the most rapidly growing populations because of the high birth rates. With greater per-person income, nations typically transition to declining death rates and then later to reductions in birth rates and a lower rate of population growth. Increasing birth rates and slowing death rates among the older segments of a population can continue to generate health problems for a country if food shortages and undernutrition are not corrected by governmental intervention. The great numbers of people coupled with poor crop production contributes to a population–food dilemma for some of the poorest nations, and this dilemma is compounded because infectious diseases are also high in nutritionally compromised infants and children.

TABLE 15.2
Examples of Countries in Different Income Classifications

Lowest Income	Next-Lowest Income	Moderate Income	Highest Income
Afghanistan	Bolivia	Algeria	Australia
Bangladesh	Cameroon	Argentina	Canada
Ethiopia	Egypt	Azerbaijan	France
Haiti	India	Brazil	Germany
Malawi	Morocco	China	Japan
Nepal	Nicaragua	Dominican Republic	Russian Federation
North Korea	Nigeria	Iraq	South Korea
Somalia	Paraguay	Jordan	Sweden
Tanzania	Sri Lanka	Mexico	United Kingdom
Uganda	Ukraine	Turkey	United States

Data from the World Bank.

population growth Increases in population over time. Population growth can be problematic for poor developing nations, which often lack the resources to feed more people.

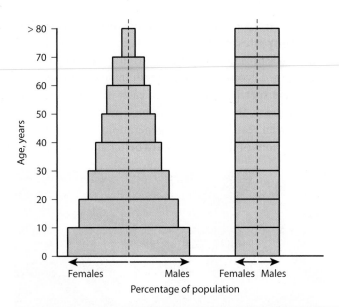

FIGURE 15.3 Ten-Year Age Breakdowns of Populations/Nations. Countries with high birth rates and rapid growth have a pyramid shape (left). Countries with slow or no growth have a chimney shape (right). The contrast of growth rates is based mainly on greater birth rates in the pyramid nations followed by greater death rates in later decades, a characteristic of poor nations with limited food security.

PRACTICAL APPLICATIONS 15.1

Analyze the Cost of the Imbalance of Food Production with Population Growth

Azuriana is a small landlocked mountainous country with a population of 20 million. It has relatively little arable land for crop production, but it has grazing lands that support limited livestock production. If you assume that Azuriana, one of the poor nations of the world, needs twice as much grain for breads and baked goods as it produces (but no more meat), then it must import this amount at a fairly high cost from a producer-nation. The question is how can Azuriana import the needed food when its gross national product is insufficient to pay for 100% of the cost? What steps can the government of Azuriana take to feed its population? ■

> High rates of population growth in many developing countries have exacerbated problems of food shortages because of the sheer number of mouths that need to be fed, especially infants and children.

Birth control by whatever effective methods are culturally acceptable is needed in many nations where food production is not meeting demand and where infant and child death rates remain excessively high. Typically, the birth rates of nations with improving nutrition will decline after a period of one to two decades when the need for more children, mainly boys for the workforce on farms or elsewhere, declines. During the transition period from higher to lower rates of reproduction, however, the population may have a burst of an increase because of the survival of more children into adulthood. Thus, the life expectancy of the population lengthens because adults and the elderly live longer when nutritional and environmental conditions improve.

Better nutrition, of course, results from better economic conditions within a nation. Improved economic status, a higher standard of nutrition, and higher level of education, especially of women, all help promote birth control so that high rates of births per year (5%) decline to more moderate rates (2% to 3% per year) and, possibly, to low rates (1% to 2% per year). (A few European nations are experiencing negative rates of growth with low fertility rates and limited population growth only through immigration.) Birth control measures follow these trends in developing countries that transition into more developed economies. The length in years of these changes, however, varies according to the specific conditions of each nation. For some of the poorest nations of the world today, the process of change may be just a dream, whereas for others changes have been real. Only future generations will know the outcome of the transitions of many nations of the world toward better and fully sustaining economies.

> **"** Better nutrition, of course, results from better economic conditions within a nation. **"**

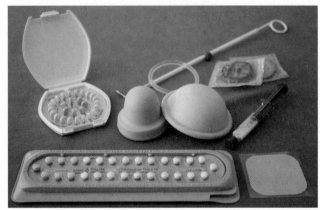

© Jones & Bartlett Learning. Photographed by Kimberly Potvin

Urbanization

Urbanization is a major trend in the world, especially in economically undeveloped nations. In rural areas in poor and developing countries, it is extremely difficult to sustain a living. Many farming families migrate to urban areas, usually the country's capital city, in search of employment opportunities. Because of shortages of housing, poor water supplies, inadequate sanitation, and limited finances, many of these migrant families have been forced to live in so-called shanty towns, which are called *barrios* in Latin America. Substandard nutrition and sanitation in these new shanty towns increase the spread of infectious disease, especially among children. Thus, infant and child mortality rates are typically high in these crowded areas.

> **"** Because of shortages of housing, poor water supplies, inadequate sanitation, and limited finances, many families have been forced to live in so-called shanty towns, which are called *barrios* in Latin America. **"**

These new developments around big cities typically improve as more money becomes available—and as the governments begin to provide improved basic services, such as water and sanitation. Many large cities have grown considerably larger, with outlying rings of shanty towns, as a result of this urbanization and have become megacities. Some of the largest cities in the world, with 10 to 20 million people, also have the largest populations of people living in shanty towns, including Mexico City, Mexico; Karachi, Pakistan; and Lagos, Nigeria.

urbanization An increase in the number of people living in urban areas. In many poor and developing countries, the rural poor migrate to urban areas in search of employment opportunities. Urbanization often results in the development of so-called shanty towns that are characterized by substandard nutrition and sanitation.

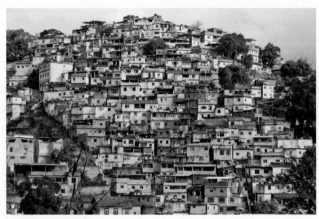

© Publio Furbino/ShutterStock, Inc.

Even with the new numbers of people living in poverty in the cities of developing countries, three-quarters of the billion malnourished people in the world still live in rural areas. Living in rural areas means that markets are farther away, health care is often inaccessible, and fortified foods such as iodized salt or iron additives in cereals may be unattainable.

Poverty–Disease Cycle

The societal causes and the results of malnutrition can be described as part of a *poverty–disease cycle* (see **FIGURE 15.4**). This cycle helps explain why it is difficult for families, villages, and even nations to escape from the grip of poverty and its grinding consequences. People remain in poverty because of several social factors, such as illiteracy, limited skills, lack of property or other assets, and political and economic instability. These conditions may lead to malnutrition because of limited food availability and insufficient purchasing power. Environmental degradation and limited water supplies also contribute to the poverty–disease cycle. **Water quality** is desperately unsatisfactory in many highly populated areas of the world.

About 6 to 7 million children younger than 5 years of age die each year from infectious diseases, including diarrhea, respiratory infections, measles, and neonatal (newborn) causes. Of these deaths, it has been estimated that between 35% and 55% are related to malnutrition. Undernourished children typically grow poorly and often enter adulthood handicapped both physically and mentally. Iron, iodine, zinc, and vitamin A deficiencies contribute to disease and disability that affect many children and adults living in poverty. If children survive to become adults, repetition of the poverty–disease cycle typically follows, often for several generations.

This cycle operates at a national level as well as at the local level. Chronic undernutrition and severe deficiencies of specific micronutrients reflect poor infrastructure, including inadequate public health measures of disease prevention and treatment, limited

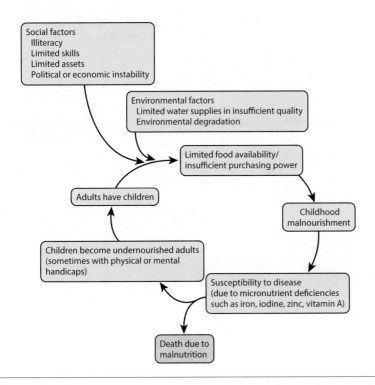

FIGURE 15.4 Poverty–Disease Cycle. The poverty–disease cycle includes medical, economic, and social factors that keep poor people entrenched in poverty.

poverty–disease cycle People living in poverty are often unable to purchase adequate amounts of food, which may eventually lead to malnutrition and disease. Poor people who suffer from disease and malnutrition are often unable to work, thus making it even more difficult for them to escape poverty.

water quality A measure of the condition of water in an area and its ability to be used by people. In many parts of the world, water may be contaminated by chemicals or sewage, making it unsuitable for human use.

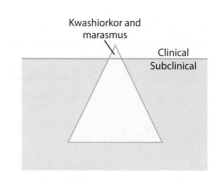

FIGURE 15.5 Many Cases of Undernutrition Remain Unidentified. Subclinical cases of moderate or mild growth disturbances related to protein–energy undernutrition are typically not recognized and treated. The vast majority of these cases of severe undernutrition occur in developing nations.

Reproduced from Anderson JJB. *Nutrition and Health: An Introduction.* Durham, NC: Carolina Academic Press; 2005.

> One of the major reasons for undernutrition in many poor and developing nations is the limited variety of foods available for consumption, most of which are high in carbohydrates, mainly starches.

water quantity and quality (i.e., potability), and high infant mortality rates. Critical cases of undernutrition only represent the tip of an iceberg (see **FIGURE 15.5**). International aid agencies face all of the complexities of dysfunctional governmental bureaucracy in many poorer nations as their workers try to overcome the stumbling blocks to provide better nutrition, safe water, and public health programs, such as immunizations.

Food Shortages and Undernutrition

Low food availability and undernutrition are worldwide problems (see **FIGURE 15.6**). One of the major reasons for undernutrition in many poor and developing nations is the limited variety of foods available for consumption, most of which are high in

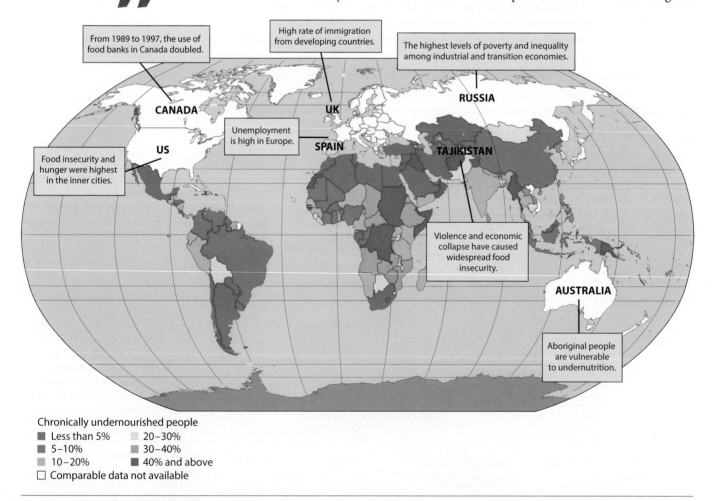

From 1989 to 1997, the use of food banks in Canada doubled.

High rate of immigration from developing countries.

The highest levels of poverty and inequality among industrial and transition economies.

Food insecurity and hunger were highest in the inner cities.

Unemployment is high in Europe.

Violence and economic collapse have caused widespread food insecurity.

Aboriginal people are vulnerable to undernutrition.

CANADA · US · UK · SPAIN · RUSSIA · TAJIKISTAN · AUSTRALIA

Chronically undernourished people
- ■ Less than 5%
- ■ 5–10%
- ■ 10–20%
- □ Comparable data not available
- ■ 20–30%
- ■ 30–40%
- ■ 40% and above

FIGURE 15.6 Low Food Availability and Undernutrition. Food insecurity is a worldwide problem.

Reproduced from Food and Agriculture Organization of the United Nations, 2012. Hunger: Interactive world hunger map. www.fao.org/hunger/en.

FOCUS 15.2   Declines in Seafood

Seafoods contain high-quality protein plus minerals and many vitamins, which make them highly nutritious. A recent scarcity of freshwater fish, not to mention the declines in marine fish, has lead to severe shortages of high-quality protein in several nations, including Nigeria and Bangladesh. This shortfall has resulted from overfishing and the failure to restock lakes with fingerling fish. Because of this widespread decline in freshwater fish, international conferences have been called to try to alleviate this problem in providing high-quality protein in areas with otherwise low protein intakes. ●

carbohydrates, mainly starches. **Staple foods** in much of the world, mainly rice, cassava, wheat, or corn, are high in carbohydrates and energy, but low in protein and micronutrients. Legumes or pulses, when available, provide high-quality protein and many micronutrients. In countries where freshwater fish provide protein, water shortages also negatively impact protein availability.

Protein–energy deficiency diseases remain quite rare among young children in the United States and Canada, but cases nevertheless do appear from time to time because of poverty; poor prenatal care, especially by teenage mothers; or for other reasons. The discovery of such cases should result in prompt medical intervention with the administration of intravenous nutrition (parenteral nutrition) in a hospital or clinic. Recovery of the child typically takes from several weeks to months, and the provision of nutrition education to the mother or caregiver is essential. However, malnutrition is far more common, even occasionally routine, in developing countries, and the number of malnourished children increases greatly during war, drought, and other periods of disaster.

FOCUS 15.3   Severe Undernutrition and Low Serum Protein Concentration

If dietary protein intake in growing children is not sufficient to support normal growth, and typically protein quality is not adequate under these conditions, then essential amino acids are not available for protein synthesis throughout the body. As a result, skeletal growth (collagen and other bone proteins) is compromised, muscle growth is limited, and the synthesis of all body proteins, including serum proteins, is reduced. Serum concentrations of proteins, especially albumin, are typically low when protein undernutrition exists. ●

Although protein is not the only nutrient deficient in the diets of many living in the developing world, it is the key macronutrient needed for reasonable growth and development from the time of conception through adolescence. (Recall that high-quality protein foods also contain many other essential micronutrients.) Nearly all of the developing nations are in the southern hemisphere, especially in the tropics. Because of their location, these nations have relatively limited amounts of land for crop production and often they have poor quality soil conditions. The crops that can be easily produced by farmers in tropical countries are, unfortunately, high in energy but low in protein. Furthermore, major animal livestock production does not generally occur in most of these areas, and fish or seafood cultivation is limited or nonexistent.

Most children of the developing world get too little dietary protein relative to energy, which often means that they do not achieve their maximal adult height. Children with inadequate protein often have short legs and arms relative to their trunk. This disproportionate

staple foods A food that is eaten routinely and in large quantities such that it constitutes the large portion of the diet of a population. In much of the world, rice, cassava, wheat, or corn are staples. Many staple foods, such as rice, are high in carbohydrates and energy but low in many other nutrients.

seafood A staple food in many coastal areas that is a source of high-quality protein plus minerals and many vitamins.

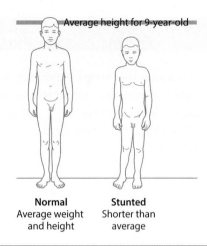

FIGURE 15.7 The Long-Term Effects of Undernutrition.
Children who experience malnutrition during critical periods of
growth will often have stunted growth reflected in long torsos and
relatively short legs.

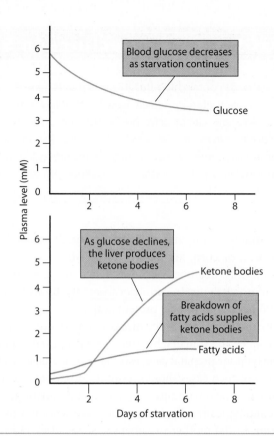

FIGURE 15.8 Energy Sources During Starvation. During starvation, the
sources of energy change as blood glucose declines and production of ketone
bodies from breakdown of fatty acids provide energy to the nervous system.

> Brain development
> may also be compromised by
> undernutrition *in utero* and
> during the first year of life.
> However, unlike other organs
> and tissues, brain mass does
> not shrink with undernutrition;
> rather, the brain simply does
> not grow in size.

immune cells Class of white
blood cells or leukocytes named
lymphocytes that are responsible
for specific immune effects. Consist
primarily of two types: B cells and
T cells. Other cells involved in
immune defense secrete cytokines
that enhance the activities of
lymphocytes.

length of the body torso compared with the short legs results from undernourishment
during critical periods of growth, and this shape remains for life (see **FIGURE 15.7**). Energy
sources change during starvation (**FIGURE 15.8**). As blood glucose is depleted, tissues,
such as the brain and central nervous system that require glucose, can utilize ketone bodies produced by breakdown of fatty acids. This shift in energy sources helps to preserve
body protein.

Brain development may also be compromised by undernutrition *in utero* and during
the first year of life. However, unlike other organs and tissues, brain mass does not shrink
with undernutrition; rather, the brain simply does not grow in size. Another effect of
undernutrition in children is that the immune system may not develop sufficiently; especially, the **immune cell** numbers remain low. Common infectious diseases are much more
virulent among undernourished children because the cells of their immune systems are
not able to effectively combat the infections. (Depressed immune defense is also common
among the elderly who are undernourished.) Death rates among infants and children are
typically much greater in developing nations than for children living in affluent nations.

Undernutrition and Infectious Diseases: A Vicious Cycle

The presence of undernutrition in infants and children makes them far more vulnerable
to the infectious diseases of childhood caused by bacteria and viruses. Undernourished
children do not defend well against infections, such as measles, that contribute greatly
to the much higher childhood morbidity and mortality rates in the developing world.

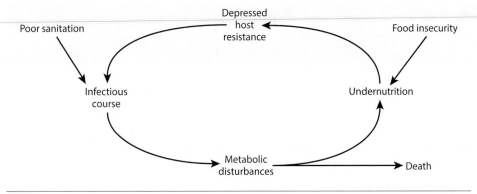

FIGURE 15.9 The Undernutrition–Infection Cycle. This cycle is common among poor infants and children of the developing world.

Reproduced from Anderson JJB. *Nutrition and Health: An Introduction*. Carolina Academic Press; Durham, NC: 2005.

Measles, a viral disease of no great consequence among American children because of vaccination efforts, has deadly consequences among undernourished children of developing nations in Africa. In South Asia and Central Africa, infectious diseases are more prevalent because of poor intakes of nutrients, such as vitamin A. Low or practically zero intakes of vitamin A (or carotenoids), for example, have very adverse effects on the immune system's ability to defend against viruses and bacteria.

The relationship between undernutrition and depressed resistance to infection is often called the *undernutrition–infection cycle*. In this cycle, inadequate nutrition depresses the immune system response, especially the number of immune cells produced, thus reducing the body's ability to respond adequately to the invading organisms. Immunoglobulins (antibodies) may not, however, be affected in defending against these microorganisms. During sickness, the body, in turn, responds by decreasing appetite, the absorptive efficiency of ingested nutrients, and the utilization of nutrients that are absorbed and by increasing the mobilization and wasting of the body's stored nutrients in tissues through an increase in excretion. The unavailability of nutrients decreases immune function, further driving the cycle. The undernutrition–infection cycle can be represented as a reinforcing circle, with death as a potential end result (see **FIGURE 15.9**).

In undernourished children, the severity of a common infectious disease illustrates the terrible vicious cycle between undernutrition and infectious disease. In the United States and other technologically advanced nations, measles may affect children, but they typically recover within a week or so if they have not been vaccinated. (Because most children are vaccinated, this disease is quite rare in the United States.) In these more affluent nations, measles occurs almost exclusively in children, and it results in low or

> The relationship between undernutrition and depressed resistance to infection is often called the *undernutrition–infection cycle*. In this cycle, inadequate nutrition depresses the immune system response, especially the number of immune cells produced, thus reducing the body's ability to respond adequately to the invading organisms.

FOCUS 15.4 Effects of Undernutrition on the Immune System

The immune system has two major components that help it to defend against foreign organisms: antibodies (immunoglobulins such as IgG, IgA, and others) and immune cells (cell-mediated immunity). Undernutrition affects the production and function of the immune cells, especially lymphocytes. Lymphocytes consist of T cells, B cells, and natural killer cells. The subtypes of lymphocytes, such as helper T cells, need a good supply of nutrients to meet their needs for renewal (cell divisions) and to synthesize and secrete molecules that help conduct the interlinked concert of the many diverse cells involved in immune defense. If nutrition is not adequate, the effectiveness of these immune cells declines, even to the point of being overwhelmed by foreign organisms, especially viruses. Low protein intake greatly limits

(continues)

FOCUS 15.4   Effects of Undernutrition on the Immune System (*continued*)

immunoglobulin synthesis as well as the formation of additional immune cells. Death may occur if the body loses its race with the growth of the infectious agents. Undernutrition in the very young and children as well as the elderly is most devastating because these populations already have weaker immune system defenses. The key nutrients needed for support of immune cells are protein, vitamin A, zinc, and, possibly, vitamin D; others may also be critical. ●

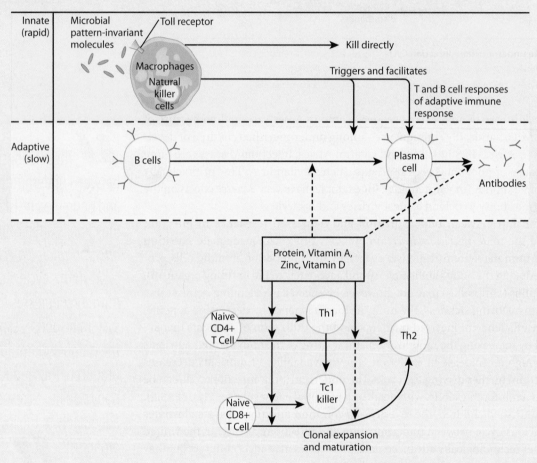

zero mortality rates. After their short-term illness, then, children can return to school and participate in normal activities. In developing countries, however, the children may be ill for several weeks, and in many cases may die (high mortality rate) because of the great virulence of the measles virus in poorly nourished children. The major difference between well-nourished versus undernourished children, then, is that the immune system cannot adequately fight common infectious agents, and the infections linger and may further limit growth, even if a child survives.

One of the major reasons for continuing or intercurrent infections in infants and children in poor and developing countries is contaminated water supplies. Because of poor sanitation, many sources of water contain parasites, viruses, and bacteria from human waste and, when consumed by those with weak immune defenses compromised by poor nutrition, infections easily develop. This factor alone—poor quality water—contributes greatly to the death rates of infants and children in poor nations. Communities that protect their water supplies and separate their sewage systems from their water sources typically have much lower death rates. A good water supply is important for health and elimination of the deadly cycle of infection, undernutrition, and death. Good hygiene, adequate nutrition, clean water, and other survival tools can help those families with young children who are most likely to suffer, but education and usually money, often from international agencies, are needed to break this cycle.

The Green Revolution and Genetically Modified (GM) Foods

Increased food supplies are needed to meet the needs of the world's growing population and to reduce poverty and hunger. The development of new genetic varieties, first by traditional plant breeding methods and relatively recently through the development of **genetically modified** organisms, has been and will continue to be the basis of meeting the need for food energy and nutrients in the developing world. The new genetically modified (GM) or biotech plant varieties have increased resistance to specific crop diseases as well as improved nutritional value. Some of these food items even have longer shelf-lives than non-GM products.

The use of genetic engineering to create new GM crops enables scientists to create new, healthier strains much more quickly than traditional methods of breeding crops and then selecting for desirable traits. The use of genetic engineering has great potential to extend the benefits of the Green Revolution to increase the production of critical crops, such as rice, wheat, and other grains, many-fold, which should permit the accumulation of much needed stores in all undernourished regions of the world in the future (see **FIGURE 15.10**). In addition, some GM foods can have genes built into their DNA that govern the synthesis of new or increased amounts of vitamins, such as beta-carotene in rice.

The Extension of the Green Revolution

GM foods represent the greatest advance—at least theoretically, if not practically—in agriculture since the Green Revolution of the 1960s and 1970s. In 2011, almost 10% of the world's arable land was used for GM crops, such as soybeans, corn, and canola (rapeseed). Although the technical aspects of producing new genetic varieties is beyond the scope of this text, suffice it to say that modifying the genome of a specific plant used in food production, especially grains, enhances the plant's resistance to potentially damaging pests, increases the production of usable food per hectare (a metric unit equal to approximately 2.5 acres), and even reduces the size of the stalk (stem) and nonfood components that will be wasted or used as fertilizer.

" The use of genetic engineering to create new GM crops enables scientists to create new, healthier strains much more quickly than traditional methods of breeding crops and then selecting for desirable traits. "

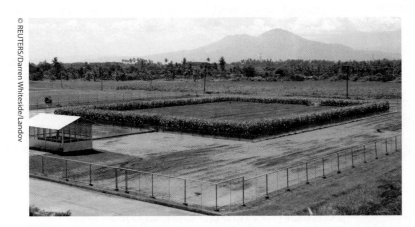

FIGURE 15.10 GM Crops. GM crops have the potential to greatly increase crop yields and food supplies in developing countries.

genetically modified Development of new varieties of plants or animals that have had changes made to their DNA through genetic engineering methods. Allows for the rapid development of new varieties that have increased resistance to specific crop diseases as well as enhanced nutritional value (e.g., golden rice that has enhanced vitamin A content).

FOCUS 15.5 Development of Golden Rice

In the Philippines, "golden rice" containing beta-carotene added via changes in the rice genome has been developed to improve the vitamin A status of populations in Asia (see **FIGURE A**). Beta-carotene acts as a provitamin to vitamin A, splitting into two retinol molecules in the gastrointestinal tract. The beta-carotene in the rice gives it a golden or orange-like hue. This genetic modification is being hailed as a great humanitarian contribution from the genetic revolution of plant engineering. Hopefully, this golden rice will be available in sufficient amounts so blindness can be greatly reduced on the Indian subcontinent and in other parts of Asia where vitamin A is deficient in the diet. ●

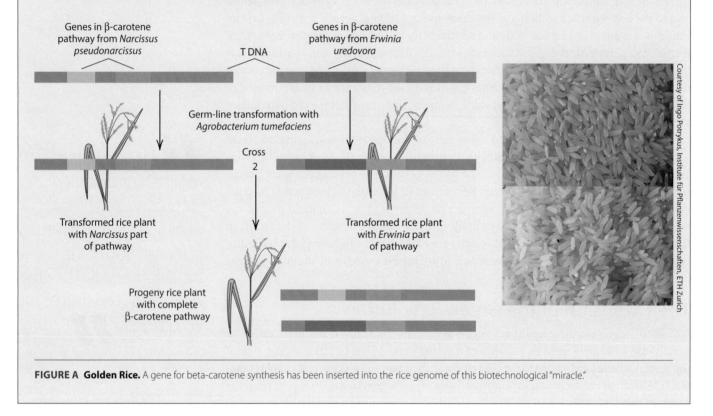

Genes in β-carotene pathway from *Narcissus pseudonarcissus*

T DNA

Genes in β-carotene pathway from *Erwinia uredovora*

Germ-line transformation with *Agrobacterium tumefaciens*

Cross 2

Transformed rice plant with *Narcissus* part of pathway

Transformed rice plant with *Erwinia* part of pathway

Progeny rice plant with complete β-carotene pathway

Courtesy of Ingo Potrykus, Institute für Pflanzenwissenschaften, ETH Zurich

FIGURE A **Golden Rice.** A gene for beta-carotene synthesis has been inserted into the rice genome of this biotechnological "miracle."

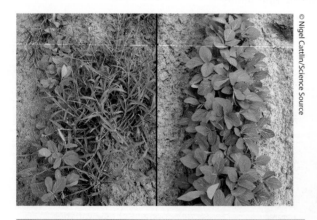

© Nigel Cattlin/Science Source

FIGURE 15.11 Test Plot of GM vs. Non-GM Soybeans. The non-GM soybean plants on the left have not been sprayed with glyphosate to suppress weeds, because that herbicide would also kill the soybeans. The GM plants on the right are free of weeds because they have had a new gene inserted into their genome that protects the plants against the herbicide, which has killed only the weeds.

The production of GM foods has increased tremendously over the last decade. In the United States, the largest GM crops include soybeans and corn. GM soybeans are also being grown in Brazil, Argentina, Canada, and China. The biggest boosts in production have occurred in developing nations, many of which are reducing or eliminating food shortfalls.

GM foods have widespread penetration in the U.S. food markets for human use as well as for animal feeds. Planting of GM soybeans in the United States, for example, has greatly surpassed the acreage of non-GM soybeans (see **FIGURE 15.11**). Many GM foods, such as GM tomatoes and lettuce, are being produced that have higher nutrient quality and a longer shelf-life. New breeds of pigs with lower fat content are being developed. Cows that produce low-fat milks are also being introduced.

Concerns About GM Crops

The major concern of many consumers and health professionals about GM foods is their safety. Basically, these novel products are made through the use of recombinant DNA technologies such as gene splicing. The quality of foods made with these techniques must be proven before the FDA will approve them for commercial markets. The USDA also has a big role in the safety of foods that go on the table. Such safeguards must also be in place before full consumer acceptance of these items is achieved. The nutrient composition of these foods should be similar to non-GM foods of the same type, but some components, such as fat content, may be improved.

The genetic enhancement of plant and animal varieties is generally widely accepted, although many consumers and watchdog groups have reservations about GM products. So far, no adverse effects—either environmental or for human health—from the production of GM crops have been verified. GM foods are now generally considered to be safe and wholesome for human consumption. However, because of concerns about their safety, little production of GM crops has occurred in Europe. The absolute proof of safety still awaits the long-term experience of GM production as well as the introduction of other GM crops.

A few years ago, claims were made that the life cycle of the Monarch butterfly was significantly interfered with by the Monsanto GM soy product, but these claims have recently been disproven. In addition, some had claimed that honeybees were negatively impacted by GM crops. However, recent evidence suggests that honeybees are not affected by biotechnologically produced proteins, and no toxicities have been found. Therefore, despite the introduction of new genes into many plant genomes, a healthy ecological interaction exists among GM crops and the butterflies and honeybees that fertilize many of them.

The USDA's Animal and Plant Health Inspection Service (APHIS) has stringent regulations for field-testing of new GM plants that will be used in foods for human consumption. One concern is that pollen and seed from GM crops may potentially contaminate non-GM crops that may be growing in nearby fields. The FDA cooperates closely with USDA to prevent this from happening.

In summary, the major benefits of GM foods are increased crop yields or efficiency of production and introduction of micronutrients that are deficient in a population, such as beta-carotene for vitamin A deficiency. In the United States, the production of GM crops has increased substantially. For example, approximately 85% of U.S. corn and 91% of U.S. soybean production today involves GM crops. The remarkable success so far, after only about one and a half decades, has spread to the development of many other GM crops and to their use by many poor nations of the world in addition to more affluent countries. Consumer acceptance has been good, but the lack of labeling as "GM food" on packaging remains an issue for concerned citizens that will most likely arise from time to time. Remain alert on this issue, as the media and popular press report new updates on GM foods. More information will emerge on the benefits—and perhaps the disadvantages—of GM crops in the future.

The United Nations and International Relief Agencies

International efforts to relieve hunger and extended famines are typically slow unless an area with undernutrition gets great media coverage in the United States and other developed countries. Humanitarian organizations, including church-related agencies, typically arrive first in an affected area because the media of many affluent nations often ignore or only superficially cover the food distribution problems of nutritionally deprived areas. Then, often much later, the United Nations (UN), wealthy nations, and additional relief organizations respond with food and assistance from health

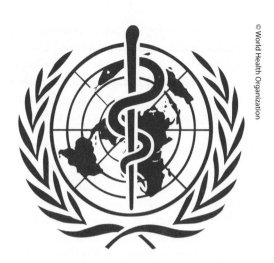

professionals. However, the governments of several affluent nations, such as Sweden and others, provide support in personnel, food, and money to the beleaguered nations through an early response system. The U.S. government, however, is typically slow in responding to the crisis needs of undernourished pockets of the world.

The World Health Organization (WHO) is the unit of the United Nations that is responsible for monitoring global health. It has identified several health issues that have strong nutritional linkages and has called for programs to reduce the burden of these conditions. In addition to undernutrition and underweight, increased risks of several diseases or conditions are especially of concern because of deficiencies of vitamin A, iron, zinc, and a few other nutrients. Further aspects of nutrition-related problems that have recently emerged are overweight, elevated serum cholesterol, and other chronic diseases resulting from changes in traditional eating patterns, in particular increased intakes of fast foods and excessive energy intakes. Experts at WHO estimate that life expectancy worldwide may be increased by 5 to 10 years with the consumption of healthier diets.

In general, the relief agencies, Doctors Without Borders, World Food Program, and other groups do heroic work in helping undernourished people in the nations affected by famines, especially where wars, droughts and other natural disasters, and intentional isolation of people for political reasons have occurred. Medical teams have typically worked hand-in-hand with the food dispensers and other health personnel. Nevertheless, all too frequently far too many deaths occur before these teams can be mobilized in full force to overcome food shortages. In the future, improved response times will be increasingly important for saving lives. Adequate funding also remains a key obstacle.

Combating Food Insecurity

The means to grow adequate supplies of food to support the health of a nation or region is often challenging, in part because of politics and in part because of limited consumable water and arable land. Too many children remain hungry and undergo the undernutrition–infection cycle, leading to death. International agencies represent only one means of aid in the developing world. These multifactorial problems require multifaceted solutions that link and coordinate efforts of local, national, and international agencies. World crop production keeps improving and increasing in tons available, yet populations continue to increase in developing nations while the availability of potable water and arable lands continues to decrease.

In the United States, **food insecurity** affects too many people, especially since the global recession of 2008–2009. In addition to the "old" homeless or "street people" who have largely dropped out of society, the "new" homeless include those whose homes

> ❝ Experts at WHO estimate that life expectancy worldwide may be increased by 5 to 10 years with the consumption of healthier diets. ❞

food insecurity Condition when people do not have adequate access to safe, nutritious foods to meet their dietary needs and to sustain an active, healthy life.

have been foreclosed. These people are trying to provide for their families the best they can, typically without jobs and often living in vans or campers. Food kitchens and local commodity warehouses are having increasing difficulty keeping enough food on hand to meet the needs of the newly homeless and poor. The aftereffects of the recession will likely linger, causing more hunger and starvation than a rich nation such as the United States should have. Many people will require government assistance and help from private agencies well into the future.

Future of the Nutrition–Population Dilemma

Because the coupling of hunger and limited purchasing power leads to population growth, the opposite pattern—improving nutritional status and increased purchasing power—leads to a reduction in population growth and even eventually to population control. Thus, the burden on the world's nations and the United Nations is to ensure sufficient food production, to distribute the food to storage sites for use in local marketing networks, to reduce undernutrition, and to improve the health and nutritional status of the populations within the affected nations. The solution to the **nutrition–population dilemma** sounds simple, but the governments of the world are not meeting the objectives needed to achieve this idealistic goal. Much needs to be done before this small planet we call earth can serve truly as a "mother" for all people so that they can be healthy and live in a more harmonious idealistic way.

Another more recent problem facing some of the developing nations is an increase in the percentage of the population that is older (over 50 years of age) because of somewhat improved diets and better health care. As a result of the "graying" of these populations, a greater demand for healthcare services and drugs has emerged. The aging segments of these populations have increased rates of the many chronic diseases that also afflict developed nations. Therefore, obesity, type 2 diabetes mellitus, and cardiovascular disease rates are on the rise in these nations. A general correlate is that as infant and child survival rates improve in developing nations, the number of older adults as a percentage of the population increases, along with rates of chronic diseases.

If the spiral of increasing population and poor nutrition continues in many economically developing nations, then these problem nations could theoretically destabilize the surrounding regions, possibly leading to hostilities or worse. Several adverse scenarios could be postulated. So, it is crucial that the world's nations come closer together in sharing resources and wealth.

nutrition–population dilemma The global problem of producing and distributing food to the world's poor in order to improve their nutritional status and reduce undernutrition.

SUMMARY

Linkages between undernutrition and population growth in poor nations of the world are noted in terms of poor food production and availability coupled with high population growth rates. Birth rates are the highest in the poorest countries. The poverty-disease cycle and the undernutrition–infection cycle are related to the limited availability of quality diets—energy, protein, and micronutrients—mainly in Africa, Asia, and Latin America. Food shortages, for whatever reason, must be prevented by various agencies in order to provide critical and often emergency relief to nations or regions of the world in crisis. With better overall nutrition and healthier living environments, populations in many of these nations may be able to move from the poorest to less poor categories with declines in growth rates. Some of these same issues (e.g., food insecurity) apply to pockets of the poor in advanced nations like the United States.

Advances in food production, notably the extension of the Green Revolution that is based on genetically modified organisms and their GM food products, is still needed in many nations of the world today, and undernutrition and hunger coupled with high population growth rates will likely continue for several decades unless poor countries are able to develop economically. Only then will the nutritional status of these populations be enhanced and population growth rates reduced. Better nutrition will clearly herald advances in health.

STUDENT ACTIVITIES

1. Explain what happens in a nation in terms of health, death rates, birth rates, and so on when food production remains constant in the face of population increases. When food production declines, what happens to the population growth rate? [Assume no outside support or food.]

2. Why are international agencies so important in situations where food production declines below needed levels? Explain.

3. Define undernutrition in broad terms. Then, define marasmus and kwashiorkor and identify a few specific changes that occur in appearance with each condition.

4. When protein intake is insufficient and then deficient, how does the body respond?

5. If you were able to measure one serum component to assess nutritional status, what would you measure? [Hint: Think of the major protein circulating in blood.]

6. Briefly note how the immune system is compromised by deficient protein intake. How important is this for infants and children? For the elderly?

7. Draw a diagram and explain the cycle of undernutrition and infectious disease.

8. Distinguish between crop production resulting from the Green Revolution versus that from GM crops.

9. What is the name of the biochemical process in plants that is essential for the support of human and animal life in addition to the plants themselves? Which specific environmental variable(s) does this process depend on? [Hint: Think of what plants do.]

10. In poor countries of the world, how does food availability influence growth and development of children and the overall health of the nation? Explain.

11. In addition to protein, what other nutrients are typically low or deficient in poor nations?

12. Which nutrients are critical for the growth acceleration that occurs during adolescence?

WEBSITES FOR FURTHER STUDY

Colorado State University Department of Soil and Crop Sciences (Transgenic Crops)
http://cls.casa.colostate.edu/TransgenicCrops/what.html
Doctors Without Borders
www.doctorswithoutborders.org

UN Food and Agriculture Organization (Globally Important Agricultural Heritage Systems)
www.fao.org/nr/giahs/en
Gapminder
www.gapminder.org

The Millennium Development Goals Report
www.un.org/en/development/desa/publications
/mdg-report-2012.html
UN Food and Agricultural Organization
www.fao.org
University of Michigan (GM Crops: Costs and Benefits)
http://sitemaker.umich.edu/sec006group5/home

Genetically Engineered Crops in the US, USDA
www.ers.usda.gov/data-products/adoption-of-genetically-
engineered-crops-in-the-us/documentation.aspx
World Bank
www.worldbank.org
World Health Organization
www.who.int/en

REFERENCES

Aggrey N, Wambugu S, Karugia J, Wanga E. An investigation of the poverty–environmental degradation nexus: a case study of Katonga Basin in Uganda. *Res J Envir Earth Sci.* 2010;2:82–88.

Pearce EN. Monitoring and effects of iodine deficiency in pregnancy: still an unsolved problem. *Eur J Clin Nutr.* 2013;67:481–484.

Pelletier DL, Frongillo EA. Changes in child survival are strongly associated with changes in malnutrition in developing countries. *J Nutr.* 2003;133:107–119.

Pelletier DL, Olson CM, Frongillo EA. Food insecurity, hunger, and undernutrition. In: Erdman JW Jr, MacDonald IA, Zeisel SH (eds.). *Present Knowledge in Nutrition.* 10th ed. Ames, IA: John Wiley & Sons; 2012: 1794–1817.

Popkin BM, Adair LS, Ng SW. Global nutrition transition and the pandemic of obesity in developing countries. *Nutr Rev.* 2012;70:3–21.

Sachdev HPS, Gera T. Preventing childhood anemia in India: iron supplementation and beyond. *Eur J Clin Nutr.* 2013;67:475–480.

Struble MB, Aomari LL. Position of the American Dietetic Association: addressing world hunger, malnutrition, and food insecurity. *J Am Diet Assoc.* 2003;103:1046–1057.

Swaminathan S, Edward BS, Kurpad AV. Micronutrient deficiency and cognitive and physical performance in Indian children. *Eur J Clin Nutr.* 2013;67:467–474.

Whitman DB. Genetically modified foods: harmful or helpful? Available at: www.csa.com/discoveryguides/gmfood/overview.php.

World Bank. *The World Development Report: Agriculture for Development.* Washington, DC: Author; 2008.

Young H, Sadler K, Borrel A. Public nutrition in humanitarian crises. In: Erdman JW Jr, MacDonald IA, Zeisel SH (eds.). *Present Knowledge in Nutrition.* 10th ed. Ames, IA: John Wiley & Sons; 2012: 1818–1855.

ADDITIONAL READING

Collier P. *The Bottom Billion: Why the Poorest Countries Are Failing and What Can Be Done About It.* New York: Oxford University Press; 2008.

Dando WA. *The Geography of Famine.* London: Edward Arnold; 1980.

Keys A. (ed.). *Biology of Starvation.* (2 vols.) Minneapolis: University of Minnesota Press; 1950.

Kidder T. *Mountains Beyond Mountains.* New York: Random House; 2004.

Lappé FM, Collins J, Rosset P. *World Hunger: Twelve Myths.* New York: Grove Press; 1998.

Stein Z, Susser M, Saenger G, Marolla F. *Famine and Human Development: The Dutch Hunger Winter of 1944–1945.* New York: Oxford University Press; 1975.

16

Human Nutrition: Healthy Options for Life

Healthy eating patterns provide the "oomph" for our bodies to function at peak performance, and good eating habits need to be practiced on a regular basis. Good health results from optimal nutrition as well as other lifestyle factors, a worthy goal that is seldom achieved. Consider a competitive distance runner who is running near the best times in his or her event. You know that this athlete will need sufficient energy, protein, micronutrients, and phytochemicals to keep the body running at its highest level of operation. Optimal body function requires reasonable amounts—within fairly broad windows—of all the nutrients obtained from a variety of foods from the various food groups. Water also is needed to keep the body operating efficiently. Healthy eating patterns, then, permit the human machine—our bodies—to function at an optimal level for life.

This chapter provides an overview of the benefits of healthy eating patterns throughout life. These patterns are largely plant based, but animal products should be consumed in modest amounts. Both plant and animal foods provide protein, energy, and essential micronutrients. Healthy eating patterns promote optimal growth and development early in life, and, when coupled with regular physical activity, they reduce the risks of developing common chronic diseases later in life. No single "healthy" eating pattern exists, but rather several patterns of sound eating practices may contribute to healthy growth and development in early life, maintenance in mid-life, and then the prevention or delay of the chronic diseases with strong dietary linkages in later life. Healthy eating patterns may exist in any nation, but typically affluent populations have sufficient purchasing power to be able to consume optimal diets.

> *Healthy eating patterns provide the "oomph" for our bodies to function at peak performance, and good eating habits need to be practiced on a regular basis.*

> *Healthy eating patterns promote optimal growth and development early in life, and, when coupled with regular physical activity, they reduce the risks of developing common chronic diseases later in life.*

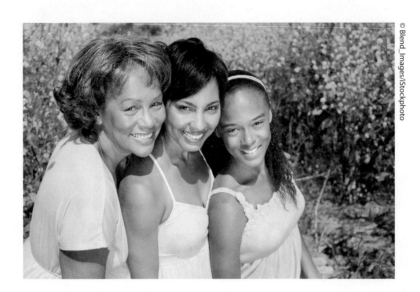

Healthy Eating Patterns for Health Promotion and Disease Prevention

The selection of nutrient-dense foods should be coupled with regular physical activity in order to balance energy intake with expenditure and thus maintain an ideal body weight. Both undernutrition (BMI < 18.5) and overnutrition (i.e., BMI > 25) have adverse health effects. Balanced nutrition and a body weight within the healthy range typically contribute to optimal nutritional status and health and freedom from disease. Institutionalization of sound nutritional knowledge and concepts about healthy eating patterns should last a lifetime.

Good nutrition and other healthy lifestyle behaviors, besides supporting a healthy BMI, can help to reduce the risk of developing chronic diseases such as obesity, type 2 diabetes mellitus, hypertension, heart disease and stroke, diet-related cancers, and osteoporosis. Overnutrition promotes overweight, obesity, metabolic syndrome, and the other chronic diseases just mentioned. Obesity has become highly prevalent in the United States, affecting approximately 35% of the adults and more than 18% of children and adolescents. The prevalence of type 2 diabetes also remains high despite the wealth of information about the dietary and lifestyle risks of this disease. In the United States, type 2 diabetes affects about 11.3% of adults. This rate is somewhat lower in Canada, which has less of an obesity problem than the United States. The combination of these two diseases has aptly been called "diabesity."

Although identifying people who are obese may seem easy, locating the linkages between obesity and the chronic diseases has taken decades of research. In fact, a full understanding of the relationship between obesity and the development of chronic disease still remains to be uncovered. However, it is now understood that accumulated body fat, especially around the abdomen (visceral fat), tends to be associated with high blood pressure, insulin resistance, elevated liver production of triglycerides, and decreased serum HDL-cholesterol levels. These major components of the metabolic syndrome contribute to the development of not only type 2 diabetes mellitus but also cardiovascular disease (CVD) and other chronic diseases.

In the United States, Canada, and other affluent nations, overnutrition—with its concomitant overweight and obesity—has become the focus of much nutrition research

> **"** Both undernutrition (BMI < 18.5) and overnutrition (i.e., BMI > 25) have adverse health effects. Balanced nutrition and a body weight within the healthy range typically contribute to optimal nutritional status and health and freedom from disease. **"**

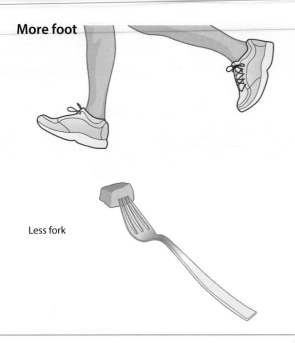

More foot

Less fork

FIGURE 16.1 **Balance of Energy Intake and Energy Expenditure.** The key to weight maintenance is the balancing of energy intake and energy expenditure.

> Researchers are now saying that, aside from assuring good moderate-calorie diets, physical activity has been a largely neglected element in controlling energy balance.

as well as of public health programs intended to reduce overweight and obesity. So far, little progress has been achieved, but changes in USDA food programs are attempting to improve the health of children and adults and preventing even greater rates of childhood obesity.

Researchers are now saying that physical activity has been a largely neglected element in controlling energy balance. New approaches are attempting to link exercise with nutrition in order to reduce weight gain in adults and to prevent weight gain among children and adolescents (see **FIGURE 16.1**). Whether these programs will be successful remains unclear, but in the United States lack of physical activity is a clear contributor to the obesity epidemic. Without major lifestyle changes, this epidemic of obesity coupled with type 2 diabetes will continue.

Food Guides and Dietary Recommendations

Emphasis on good nutrition through the use of food guides is intended to ensure that a variety of foods and sufficient numbers of servings are consumed from different food groups each day. Education, whether formal or informal, is needed to promote consumer awareness of the importance of the various food guidance systems and recommendations. In the United States, nutrition education reaches most schoolchildren and some college students, but it misses large segments of the population, especially the poor or low-income families who qualify for USDA food programs, such as the food stamp program (SNAP) and the School Lunch Program.

General recommendations for promoting health and preventing disease include MyPlate and guidelines from several independent associations (see **Table 16.1**). Harvard University's Healthy Eating Plate is another food guidance system. Compare the Healthy Eating Plate with USDA's MyPlate in **FIGURE 16.2**. The Harvard recommendations go a bit farther than those of the USDA, suggesting that grains be mostly whole grains, that protein sources not be red meat or processed meat, that the number of servings

TABLE 16.1
Recommendations for Adult Macronutrient and Energy Intakes from the USDA and Several Nonprofit Organizations

Macronutrient	USDA MyPlate	Percentage of Total Energy Intake		
		NIH Clinical Guidelines for Overweight and Obesity	National Cholesterol Education Program (ATP III)	American Diabetes Association (ADA)
Carbohydrate	53%	~55%	50–60%	60–70%
Fat	29%	~30%	25–35%	15–20%
Protein	18%	~15%	~15%	15–20%
Fatty Acids				
Saturated	7.8%	8–10%	< 7%	< 10%*
Monounsaturated	10.7%	< 15%	< 20%	< 10%
Polyunsaturated	8.9%	< 10%	< 10%	~10%
Cholesterol	230 mg	< 300 mg	< 200 mg	< 300 mg†

* Trans fats are not recommended; no alcohol recommendations are given. † These values are reduced to 7% and 200 mg per day when LDL-cholesterol is > 100 mg/dL
Data from the American Diabetes Association.

of vegetables be much more (about double) than the number of servings of fruit, that vegetables not include French fries, that the preferred drink be water and not milk, and that healthy oils such as olive and canola be used in cooking. The Healthy Eating Plate also supports consumption of seafood, red wine, and nuts.

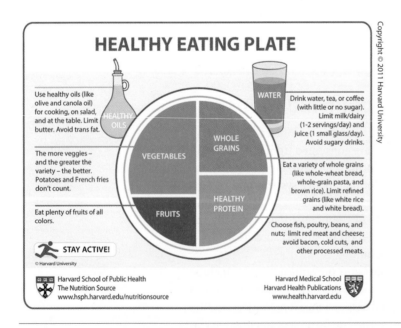
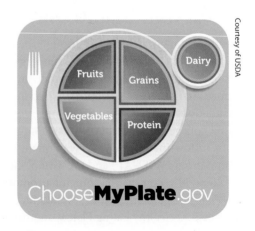

FIGURE 16.2 Harvard University's Healthy Eating Plate vs. the USDA's MyPlate. A variety of food guidance systems and recommendations have been offered to promote health and longevity.

Nutrition for a Lifetime: Nutrients and Phytochemicals

Obtaining the essential nutrients and energy from foods is the primary purpose of eating, plain and simple. Specific macronutrients, micronutrients, and phytochemicals have been linked to the support of various body functions. Requirements and allowances (RDAs) for macronutrients and micronutrients vary with growth or maintenance and different stages of life and gender. Phytochemicals, though not nutrients *per se*, from a variety of plants have also been recommended for the support of optimal body function.

In addition to obtaining nutrients from foods, many people in the United States take a daily supplement to ensure adequate micronutrient intake. Such nutrient supplements, however, do not provide the diverse types of phytochemicals found in plant foods that act as significant health promoters! In addition, nutrient supplements are almost always taken in a large load or dose, which may have adverse effects when consumed in such high amounts. Calcium loading exemplifies the potential problems of supplements because of its postulated enhancement of arterial calcification (see below).

Because nutrient requirements vary across the life cycle, energy intakes by older adults may need to be lower than those for more active, younger adults. However, older adults still need to consume about the same amounts of micronutrients and phytochemicals each day as younger adults. It is therefore especially important that older adults consume *nutrient-dense* and *energy-reduced* foods. Junk or low-quality foods and highly processed foods do not generally satisfy the requirements of nutrients of adults, especially older adults. The best rule is to take on good healthy eating habits early in life—get a good start—and maintain these habits throughout life!

> In addition to obtaining nutrients from foods, many people in the United States take a daily supplement to ensure adequate micronutrient intake. Such nutrient supplements, however, do not provide the diverse types of phytochemicals found in plant foods that act as significant health promoters!

Caution Regarding the Use of Supplements

In the last few years, cautions have been raised about relying on supplements to provide essential nutrients. Nutrients that are concentrated and not in the normal matrix of their food origins behave differently in the body after they are ingested as a load and then absorbed. The use of nutrients in fortified foods is not the same, however, because the additional or enriched nutrients are absorbed more slowly and then distributed throughout the body by the blood circulation. For example, the value of multivitamin supplements, long considered part of a "health insurance" packet, has recently been questioned, with some believing that they may actually have adverse health effects. Supplementation with too much folate or too much calcium may have deleterious actions, folate by reducing immune defenses and calcium by promoting arterial calcification. Vitamin D supplements in excess have also been cited for their potential harm. Yet meeting adult requirements for these micronutrients with appropriate intakes from foods fortified with folate may help to prevent fetal abnormalities, and appropriate intakes of vitamin D and calcium-fortified foods may benefit the body, particularly in the maintenance of bone health.

> The value of multivitamin supplements, long considered part of a "health insurance" packet, has recently been questioned, with some believing that they may actually have adverse health effects.

Established Healthy Dietary Patterns

The traditional Mediterranean dietary pattern has been widely recommended as a healthy way of eating for life (see **FIGURE 16.3**). The general concept behind the Mediterranean diet is to follow the general diet that has contributed to the good health and longevity of many Mediterranean peoples. No one specific Mediterranean diet exists because the different Mediterranean countries all have their own dietary preferences.

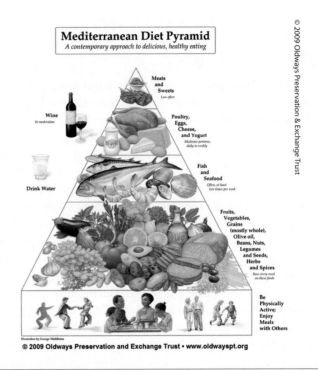

FIGURE 16.3 The Mediterranean Diet Pyramid.

However, the diets of the different countries of the region do have some general similarities. Specifically, a typical Mediterranean diet is rich in fruits, vegetables, and whole grains but low in high-fat meats and dairy products. Those meats that are consumed are generally low in fat (e.g., chicken). Dairy products include low-fat cheese and live-culture yogurt. In addition, in many of these countries around the Mediterranean, sea fish and other seafood, red wine, and olive oil have traditionally been important parts of the typical diet. **Table 16.2** highlights the major food components of the Mediterranean diet in four countries.

TABLE 16.2
Major Components of the Mediterranean Diet in Four Different Countries

Nation	Grains or Starches	Fats	Dairy	Meat, Poultry Fish,	Vegetables	Fruits	Beverages
Italy	Pasta, rice, potatoes, bread	Olive oil, lard	Cheese, butter	Fish, beef	Tomatoes, eggplants	Oranges, grapes	Wine, coffee
Croatia	Rice, goulash, pasta	Olive oil	Cheese, yogurt	Beef, seafood, lamb	Tomatoes, onion, cabbage	Lemons	Coffee
Greece	Bread, potatoes, barley	Olive oil	Cheese, yogurt	Fish, beef, nuts	Tomatoes, okra, peppers	Lemons, oranges	Wine, ouzo, coffee, tea
Morocco	Pasta, couscous	Olive oil	Yogurt	Fish, lamb, beef	Eggplant, tomatoes, peppers, chickpeas	Dates	Green mint tea

Data from Noah A, Truswell AS. Commodities consumed in Italy, Greece and other Mediterranean countries compared with Australia in 1960s and 1990s. *Asia Pacific J Clin Nutr.* 2001;10:2–9.

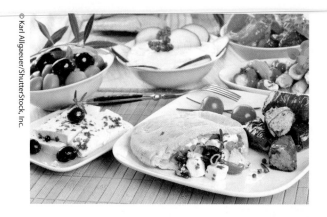

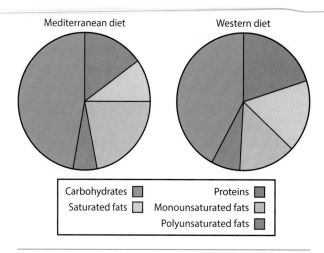

FIGURE 16.4 Macronutrient Compositions of a Typical Mediterranean Diet and a Typical Western Diet. These diets differ in the amounts of fats and carbohydrates consumed.

FIGURE 16.4 compares the macronutrient composition of the typical Western diet with the traditional Mediterranean dietary pattern. Non-Mediterranean populations can adapt their eating to the Mediterranean way and have healthy outcomes. For example, in Australia people who adhered closely to the Mediterranean diet reduced their risk of death by almost 50% compared to those Australians who did not follow this diet (see **FIGURE 16.5**).

The Okinawa diet, which also is characterized by seafood, vegetables (especially seaweed), and fruits, has also been shown to have positive health effects that lead to great longevity. The same may be said for the other Asian diets, mainly when serving sizes are not excessive and dietary intake of energy is balanced with regular physical activity. See **FIGURE 16.6** for foods typical in an Asian diet.

> The traditional Mediterranean dietary pattern has been widely recommended as a healthy way of eating for life. The general concept behind the Mediterranean diet is to follow the general diet that has contributed to the good health and longevity of many Mediterranean peoples.

FIGURE 16.5 Reduction in Risk of Mortality After Switching from an Australian Diet to a Mediterranean Diet for 6.5 years. Those who adhered well to the Mediterranean diet (fourth quartile) had the greatest reduction of risk of death compared with the less adherent groups (first through third quartiles).

Data from Barzi1 F, Woodward M, Marfisil RM, Tavazzi L, Valagussa F, Marchioli R, on behalf of GISSI-Prevenzione Investigators. Mediterranean diet and all-causes mortality after myocardial infarction: results from the GISSI-Prevenzione trial. *Eur J Clin Nutr.* 2003;57:604–611.

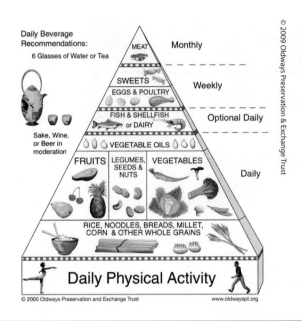

FIGURE 16.6 The Asian Diet Pyramid. An Asian diet is packed with seafood, vegetables, and fruits.

Although not an established diet of any nation, the **Dietary Approaches to Stop Hypertension (DASH) diet** has been formulated by scientists and physicians to reduce high blood pressure in the United States. This diet not only reduces sodium intake, but it also controls the amount of food energy consumed by using low-fat dairy products, lean meats, and limited amounts of carbohydrates from breads and cereals. Processed foods and fried foods are strictly limited, and plant foods other than potatoes are emphasized. The DASH diet has been successful in not only reducing blood pressure but also body weight and serum glucose concentrations.

Superfoods

Steven Pratt and Kathy Matthews, in their book, *SuperFoods*, identify 14 foods as being "superfoods." These foods have been designated as being "super" because they contain so many nutrients in amounts that support good function and health (see **FIGURE 16.7**). The plant foods they have identified are especially rich in potassium and very low in sodium. They also are rich in many vitamins, trace elements, and phytochemicals. These specific foods certainly are good for all of us, but many other foods also could be categorized as superfoods. The 14 designated "superfoods" are listed in **Table 16.3**. These foods alone—at the number of recommended servings per week—should provide all the essential nutrients and support good health.

The point of this listing of superfoods is really to get away from fast foods, heavily processed foods, and foods that are rich in fat, sugar, or salt. Superfoods are nutrient dense; too many of the foods in the Western diet are energy dense or rich in problem nutrients, such as sodium, sugar, phosphate, or saturated or trans fatty acids. Additional foods beyond the 14 items listed in **Table 16.3** also may satisfy the criteria for being a "superfood," but those listed demonstrate that focusing on plant foods is the best way to obtain the essential nutrients and phytochemicals that promote health and prevent chronic diseases.

A problem with limiting a diet to these 14 foods is that some are only available seasonally, except perhaps at very high costs. As an example, blueberries, which can be

Dietary Approaches to Stop Hypertension (DASH) diet Diet formulated by scientists and physicians to reduce hypertension. This diet is low in saturated fat, cholesterol, and total fat and focuses on fruits, vegetables, and fat-free or low-fat dairy products. Contains less sugar and red meat than the typical American diet. This diet also promotes maintenance of a healthy weight and can help to prevent the development of chronic diseases such as type 2 diabetes and cardiovascular disease.

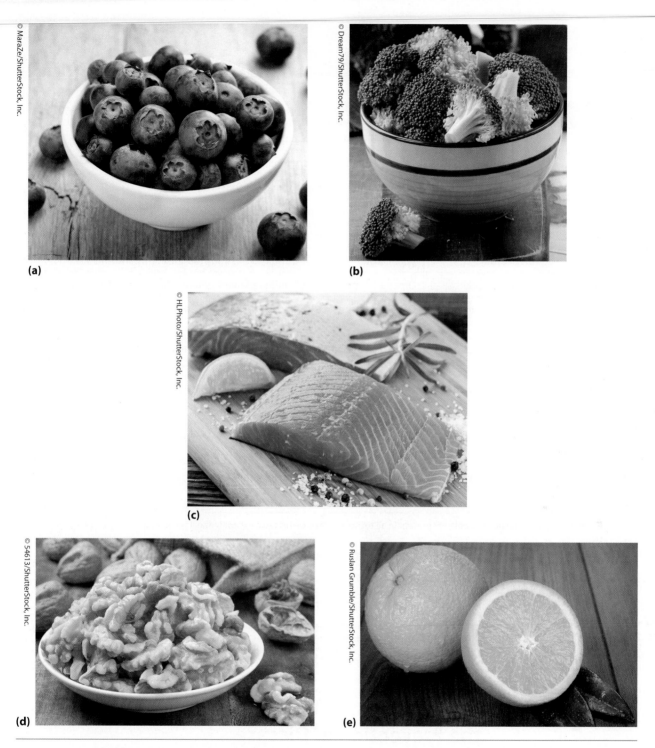

FIGURE 16.7 Superfoods. Superfoods are nutrient dense, and many are good sources of the phytochemicals that are instrumental in preventing the development of chronic diseases. They include (a) blueberries, (b) broccoli, (c) salmon, (d) walnuts, and (e) oranges.

added relatively easily to almost any meal and many mixed dishes, become very pricey by mid to late winter in the northern hemisphere. Other foods, such as wild salmon, can also be very expensive. Thus, this list of 14 foods may fit the purchasing power of the affluent, but not that of most families, who generally have a much more limited food budget. Also, note that three of the foods—wild salmon, turkey, and yogurt—are not derived from plants. Nevertheless, keep in mind the core concept of how plant foods, including the superfoods listed, readily fit most of the food guides for consumers and

TABLE 16.3
Fourteen Superfoods

Food	Servings	Nutrients Contained in Good Amounts*
Beans	0.5 cup/week	Protein, B vitamins, iron, potassium, magnesium
Blueberries	1–2 cups/day	Carotenoids, B vitamins, vitamins C and E, potassium, magnesium
Broccoli	0.5–1 cup/day	Folate, calcium, vitamin C, beta-carotene, vitamin K
Oats	5–7 servings/day	Protein, magnesium, potassium, zinc, copper, selenium, thiamin
Oranges	1 serving/day	Vitamin C, folate, potassium
Pumpkin	~0.5 cup/day	Beta-carotene, vitamins C and E, potassium, magnesium, pantothenic acid
Salmon (wild)	2–4 times/week	Omega-3 fatty acids, B vitamins, selenium, vitamin D, potassium, protein
Soy	15 g soy protein/day	Omega-3 fatty acids, vitamin E, potassium, folate, magnesium, selenium, protein
Spinach	~1 cup steamed/day or 2 cups raw/day	Beta-carotene, vitamins C and E, B vitamins, minerals (calcium, magnesium, zinc, others)
Tea (green or black)	~1 or more cups/day	Fluoride
Tomatoes	1 or more servings/day	Lycopene, vitamin C, beta-carotene, B vitamins, chromium, biotin
Turkey	3–4 servings/week of 3–4 oz	Protein, niacin, vitamins B_6 and B_{12}, iron, selenium, zinc
Walnuts	1 oz/5 times a week	Vitamin E, magnesium, protein, potassium, vitamin B_6
Yogurt	2 cups/day	Protein, calcium, riboflavin, vitamin B_{12}, potassium, magnesium, zinc

* Phytochemicals, including fiber and polyphenols, are present in all the foods listed in this table except in the animal foods, salmon, turkey, and yogurt.
Data from Pratt S, Matthews K. *SuperFoods: Fourteen Foods That Will Change Your Life.* New York: Morrow/HarperCollins; 2004.

> A core of foods, especially plant sources, needs to serve as the basis for any good diet.

offer a host of potential health benefits. A core of foods, especially plant sources, needs to serve as the basis for any good diet.

Specific Dietary Approaches to the Prevention of Disease

The prevention of disease goes beyond diet; it also involves lifestyle and behavior, topics that are largely beyond the scope of this text. Suffice it to say that being physically active, not smoking, consuming alcohol in moderation or not at all, and practicing other good health behaviors are important for health promotion and disease prevention. However, hereditary factors cannot yet be overcome even by the most optimal dietary pattern. Three specific ways of eating may provide optimal nutrient intakes: the Mediterranean diet and the Okinawa diet generally satisfy all dietary recommendations. The DASH diet also serves well. By building these dietary approaches into your daily patterns of living and incorporating physical activity, you will likely optimize health. New information based on solid scientific investigations, such as the impact of increased intakes of omega-3 fatty acids on health, may, however, mean that one or another of the current recommendations will require adjustment or tinkering.

Major concerns about the highly processed Western diet continue to be raised because of increased rates of obesity, diabetes, heart disease, and other chronic diseases. For example, the typical U.S. diet is high in fat, sugar, and calories. It contains too few daily servings of fruits and vegetables. Legumes, including soybeans and soy-based products, and nuts are consumed by small percentages of the population on a daily basis. Limited physical activity puts extra pressure on the appropriate reduction of caloric intake, which is rarely matched, as witnessed by the high rate of adult overweight and obesity of roughly 65%! For many, weight fluctuations are a common occurrence. The promotion of healthy diets for extending optimal function and increasing life expectancy fits in well with other beneficial lifestyle practices.

Fortification of foods with nutrients has had a major impact in reducing disease and in promoting the healthy growth of fetuses and infants and children, but concerns have been raised about the beneficial effects of supplements on adult health. Food fortification programs in many nations have corrected serious health problems and have even prevented deaths. Folate fortification has reduced neural tube defects in babies; selenium fortification has practically eliminated cardiomyopathy, or an enlarged heart, in China; and thiamin, riboflavin, niacin, and iron fortification have been instrumental in promoting healthy growth in children and maintaining health in adults in the United States and other nations. Fortification, and possibly the use of supplements, has had a major impact in reducing micronutrient deficits in the North American diet. Nevertheless, potassium and vitamin K intakes still remain too low because of the consumption of too few servings of fruits and vegetables!

Dietary Guidelines for Americans

The *Dietary Guidelines for Americans* is published approximately every 5 years by the U.S. Departments of Agriculture and Health and Human Services to help consumers make sound food choices in their everyday lives. The current edition is the result of deliberations by a committee of experts known as the Dietary Guidelines Advisory Committee. Their recommendations are generally accepted as a proactive guide for maintaining or improving health outcomes in children and adults, but they are not without controversy because of the limited or inconsistent scientific support for a few of the major guidelines. For example, great uncertainty exists about the healthy percentages or proportions of macronutrients that should be consumed at the recommended caloric intake level for an individual (see **Table 16.4**).

The common recommended macronutrient percentages are 50% of total energy from dietary carbohydrates, 35% from fats, and 15% from proteins, with no recommendation for alcohol calories for North Americans who are maintaining a healthy body weight and good health. These recommendations stand, with some fluctuations up or down around each number, but the science supporting the health benefits of these figures is very meager. Thus, there is controversy surrounding them. In fact, these numbers are actually obtained from the current usual eating practices of the U.S. population! For overweight or obese individuals in the United States and Canada, the recommended percentages of a low-calorie diet should differ from the optimal diet percentages recommended above because of the consumption of a low-carbohydrate diet. These percentages should be closer to 38% carbohydrate, 37% fat, and 25% protein, with protein intakes remaining at about 1.0 g per kilogram body weight per day. Some aspects of the *Dietary Guidelines* are less controversial (see **Table 16.4**), such as the control of body weight by diet and physical activity.

> **"** The typical U.S. diet is high in fat, sugar, and calories. It contains too few daily servings of fruits and vegetables. Legumes, including soybeans and soy-based products, and nuts are consumed by small percentages of the population on a daily basis. **"**

> **"** Fortification, and possibly the use of supplements, has had a major impact in reducing micronutrient deficits in the North American diet. **"**

TABLE 16.4
The Scientific Evidence Behind the *Dietary Guidelines for Americans*: Noncontroversial vs. Controversial

Noncontroversial	Controversial
The amount of total calories needed to maintain a healthy weight	The percentages of macronutrients needed to maintain a healthy weight
The increase in total energy intake results almost entirely from carbohydrates	Whether a diet low in carbohydrates or low in fats is better for weight reduction
A high-carbohydrate diet is linked to type 2 diabetes via disordered carbohydrate metabolism	The linkage between a high-fat diet and type 2 diabetes
Dietary fiber from whole (unprocessed) foods improves health outcomes	
Dietary fiber recommendations are difficult to meet on a low-carbohydrate diet	
Plant-based diets provide sufficient high-quality protein to support health	
Physical activity is needed to counter an increase in caloric intake for weight maintenance	

Data from Hite AH, Feinman RD, Guzman GE, et al. In the face of contradictory evidence: Report of the *Dietary Guidelines for Americans* Committee. *Nutrition.* 2010;26:915–924.

Table 16.5 presents several recommendations for routine food selection that should help eliminate excessive consumption of macronutrients while at the same time increasing intakes of micronutrients. Micronutrient deficiencies are much more common in those whose diets are low in plant foods and high in processed baked goods and animal products. Such diets are not only low in micronutrients (i.e., most vitamins and minerals), but they also tend to be low in phytochemicals and fiber.

TABLE 16.5
Recommendations for Routine Food Selections That Help Overcome Macronutrient Excesses and Micronutrient Deficiencies: Healthy-Weight Individuals

Food	Overcoming Macronutrient Excess	Overcoming Micronutrient Deficiency
Fruits and vegetables	Total fat	Most vitamins and minerals; fiber and phytochemicals
Whole grains	Total fat	Most vitamins and minerals; fiber and phytochemicals
Legumes (beans and peas)	Total fat	B vitamins and some minerals; fiber and phytochemicals
Seafood	Saturated fat	B vitamins and some minerals
Vegetable oils	Saturated fat	Vitamins A and D, some phytochemicals
Low-fat dairy	Saturated fat	Some vitamins; calcium and some other minerals

The *Dietary Guidelines*, despite their limitations, are well intended and seek to improve dietary intakes of the U.S. population. They are updated every 5 years based on new knowledge and understandings gained from research investigations. Other guidelines, such as Mediterranean, Okinawan, and DASH diets or the Healthy Eating Plate, may be more successful in achieving long-term health, but any guide that increases a variety of daily plant servings has to be considered beneficial to health.

Populations with Healthy Lives into Old Age

A few populations of the world are known for their longevity. These populations typically have diets rich in plant foods and are characterized by a lot of physical activity, such as from farming, walking, and climbing hillside paths to and from homes and villages. They also are characterized by the total absence of fast foods. Meats are not avoided, but typically plant foods provide the bulk of meals of these superannuated populations! Individuals in these populations, however, may consume wine on a regular basis and possibly have a few undesirable behaviors for health, but their diets are good and they may also have beneficial genes and strong immune defenses that help in protecting against the common chronic diseases and infectious diseases. A few examples of these healthy elderly populations illustrate why they may be so healthy. Corsicans who live on the relatively small island of Corsica in the Mediterranean Sea are generally Italian in origin, and they eat one type of a Mediterranean diet that is rich in seafood, vegetables, and fruit. They also consume a unique variety of red wine. Other Mediterranean nations benefit similarly from their special patterns of eating. Many Okinawans of Japanese background have long lives—many are centenarians—because they consume a healthy diet based on seafoods and green vegetables. Finally, Seventh-Day Adventists (SDA) in Southern California and elsewhere in the world typically consume plant-rich diets, including nuts, which enable them to be healthier and to live longer than most of the non-SDA populations around them. These diverse populations may have healthy dietary patterns, in addition to other healthy habits, that permit greater longevity and less of the chronic disease burden than for other populations.

Foods for Life

Consuming a healthy group of foods, including fortified foods (but not supplements), is the most optimal way for promoting growth, tissue repair, and body maintenance for life. We eat foods for both enjoyment and the nutrients and phytochemicals they contain; we do not eat foods for their nutrients *per se*. Remember that foods, primarily plant foods, are greater than their nutrient content alone because they contain phytochemicals and dietary fiber molecules that support human functions. Findings from research investigations examining food and disease relationships over the last few decades clearly favor the consumption of whole foods or minimally processed foods that are rich in nutrients and plant chemicals.

> Micronutrient deficiencies are much more common in those whose diets are low in plant foods and high in processed baked goods and animal products. Such diets are not only low in micronutrients (i.e., most vitamins and minerals), but they also tend to be low in amounts of phytochemicals and fiber.

> Any guide that increases a variety of daily plant servings has to be considered beneficial to health.

SUMMARY

A healthy diet results from a balanced intake of foods in appropriate portions so that energy intake equals energy expenditure in daily activities. The *Dietary Guidelines* serve as a useful source for achieving this balance. This balanced intake, preferably of a variety of whole foods or at least minimally processed items, provides the essential protein, fatty acids, micronutrients (vitamins and minerals), and phytochemicals and fiber that support the organ systems of the body and, hence, good health. The list of 14 superfoods is an example of foods that support health because they are rich in many nutrients. Several healthy dietary patterns, including the Mediterranean diet and the Okinawan diet, have evolved over the last millennium, and these eating patterns, based largely on plant foods, have contributed to longer lives and reasonable delays in most chronic diseases, including "diabesity," that are so prevalent in Western nations—and rising in less developed nations at present. Emphasis is placed here on the consumption of more plant foods and less total energy, coupled with physical activity and other healthy lifestyle behaviors—or smaller fork and larger foot!

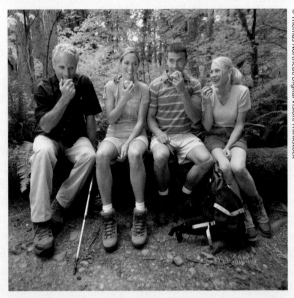

© Thomas Northcut/Digital Vision/Thinkstock

STUDENT ACTIVITIES

1. Identify one plant superfood and one animal superfood (see Table 16.3) that is rich in protein.

2. Identify one superfood that is rich in the following micronutrients: vitamins A, E, D, and K; calcium; and iron (see Table 16.3).

3. From Table 16.3, identify two specific phytochemicals and the superfoods in which they occur.

4. Specify three common features of the diverse Mediterranean diets that are instrumental in health promotion and disease prevention.

5. Explain why obtaining sufficient dietary fiber on a diet rich in animal products is difficult. [Hint: Consider foods that contain dietary fiber, not supplements.]

6. Which type of diet would be more beneficial for obtaining sufficient fiber in the diet: low fat or low carbohydrate? Explain.

7. Extended longevity in some nations can be attributed to specific lifestyle variables that operate independently of hereditary determinants. State two healthy lifestyle variables, other than a healthy diet, that impact favorably or adversely on health and longevity.

8. Of the two calorically excessive diets, high-carbohydrate or high-fat, which is more likely to contribute to type 2 diabetes? Explain.

9. To maintain a healthy adult weight, which two lifestyle variables, including diet, play important roles in weight maintenance? Explain.

10. Of the 14 superfoods listed in the text, identify those that you consume in your own personal diet on a daily or weekly basis. Which ones do you not consume at all? Which foods are of plant or animal origin? What is your ratio of animal to plant foods for these 14 superfoods?

WEBSITES FOR FURTHER STUDY

Stanford Prevention Research Center, Quest for the Optimal Diet
http://camps.stanford.edu/documents/Health-Faire-Optimal-Diet-Talk.pdf
CDC: Fruits and Veggies Matter
www.fruitsandveggiesmatter.gov
Dietary Guidelines for Americans, 2010
http://health.gov/dietaryguidelines/2010.asp
NIH News in Health, What Is Healthy Eating?
http://newsinhealth.nih.gov/2007/March/docs/01features_01.htm
NIH Weight-Control Information Network

http://win.niddk.nih.gov/publications/better_health.htm
National Institute on Aging, What's On Your Plate? Smart Food Choices for Healthy Aging
www.nia.nih.gov/health/publication/whats-your-plate-smart-food-choices-healthy-aging
National Women's Health Information Center: Food and Nutrition Center
http://answers.usa.gov/system/templates/selfservice/USAGov/#!portal/1012/article/3737/Food-and-Nutrition-Information-Center
USDA ChooseMyPlate
www.choosemyplate.gov

REFERENCES

Acheson KJ. Diets for body weight control and health: the potential of changing the macronutrient composition. *Eur J Clin Nutr.* 2013;67:462–466.

de Lorgeril M, Salen P, Martin JL, et al. Mediterranean diet, traditional risk factors, and the rate of cardiovascular complications after myocardial infarction: Final report of the Lyon Diet Heart Study. *Circulation.* 1999;99:779–785.

Esposito K, Marfella R, Ciotola M, et al. Effect of a Mediterranean-style diet on endothelial dysfunction and markers of vascular inflammation in the metabolic syndrome. *JAMA.* 2004;292:1440–1446.

Estruch R, Ros E, Salas-Salvado J, et al. Primary prevention of cardiovascular disease with a Mediterranean diet. *N Engl J Med.* 2013;368:1279–1290.

Fulgoni VL III, Keast DR, Bailey RL, Dwyer J. Foods, fortificants, and supplements: Where do Americans get their nutrients? *J Nutr.* 2011;141:1847–1854.

He FJ, Nowson CA, Lucas M, MacGregor GA. Increased consumption of fruit and vegetables is related to a reduced risk of coronary heart disease: meta-analysis of cohort studies. *J Hum Hypertension.* 2007;10:1–12.

Hite AH, Feinman RD, Guzman GE, et al. In the face of contradictory evidence: Report of the *Dietary Guidelines for Americans* Committee. *Nutrition.* 2010;26:915–924.

Jacobs DR, Tapsell LC. Food, not nutrients, is the fundamental unit of nutrition. *Nutr Reviews.* 2007;65:439–450.

Noah A, Truswell AS. There are many Mediterranean diets. *Asia Pacific J Clin Nutr.* 2001;10:2–9.

Ogden CL, Carroll MD, Curtin LR, et al. Prevalence of overweight and obesity in the United States, 1999–2004. *JAMA.* 2006;295:1549–1555.

Pineo CE, Anderson JJB. Cardiovascular benefits of the Mediterranean diet. *Nutr Today.* 2008;43:114–120.

Pratt S, Matthews K. *SuperFoods: Fourteen Foods That Will Change Your Life.* New York: Morrow/HarperCollins; 2004.

Sparling MC, Anderson JJB. The Mediterranean diet and cardiovascular diseases. *Nutr Today.* 2009;44:124–133.

Vincent-Baudry S, Defoort C, Gerber M, et al. The Medi-RIVAGE study: reduction of cardiovascular disease risk factors after a 3-month intervention with a Mediterranean-type diet or a low-fat diet. *Am J Clin Nutr.* 2005;82:964–971.

ADDITIONAL READING

Anon. *Food, Nutrition, Physical Activity and the Prevention of Cancer: A Global Perspective.* Washington, DC: World Cancer Research Fund and American Institute of Cancer Research; 2007.

Fraser GE. *Diet, Life Expectancy, and Chronic Disease.* New York: Oxford University Press, 2003.

Heller M. *The DASH Diet: Action Plan.* New York: Grand Central Life & Style; 2007.

Willcox BJ, Willcox DC. *The Okinawa Program.* New York: Three Rivers Press; 2001.

Willcox BJ, Willcox DC, Suzuki M. *The Okinawa Diet Plan: Get Leaner, Live Longer, and Never Feel Hungry.* New York: Three Rivers Press; 2005.

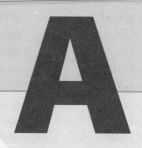

Abbreviations

A list of abbreviations commonly used in this text:

aa (or AA)	amino acid	**CoA**	coenzyme A
ADL	activity of daily living	**CRBP**	cellular retinol-binding protein
AI	Adequate Intake	**CT**	computerized tomography (or computerized axial tomography)
AT	active transport		
ATP	adenosine triphosphate	**CV**	coefficient of variation
BEE	basal energy expenditure	**CVD**	cardiovascular disease
BMC	bone mineral content	**cyto**	cytosol (cytoplasm)
BMD	bone mineral density	**DIT**	diet-induced thermogenesis
BMI	body mass index	**dL**	deciliter
BMR	basal metabolic rate	**DM**	diabetes mellitus
BV	biological value	**DBP**	vitamin D–binding protein
C (or c)	cholesterol or cup; carbon (with capital C only)	**DRI**	Dietary Reference Intake
		DXA	dual-energy x-ray absorptiometry
Ca	calcium	**EFA**	essential fatty acid
Ca:P	ratio of calcium to phosphorus (dietary)	**EHC**	enterohepatic circulation
		EIT	exercise-induced thermogenesis
CA	cancer	**en**	energy
CAD	coronary artery disease	**EPA**	eicosapentaenoic acid
Carbo	carbohydrate	**ER**	endoplasmic reticulum
CE	cholesterol ester (fatty acid)	**ERT**	estrogen replacement therapy
C-H	carbon-hydrogen bond	**FA**	fatty acid
CHD	coronary heart disease	**FAD**	flavin adenine dinucleotide
CHO	carbohydrate molecules (various)	**FAS**	fetal alcohol syndrome
chylo(s)	chylomicron(s)	**Fe**	iron
Cl	chlorine or chloride	**FSH**	follicle-stimulating hormone
C-N	carbon-nitrogen bond	**g**	gram

g/kcal	grams per kilocalorie
GH	growth hormone
GI	gastrointestinal
GnRH	gonadotropin-releasing hormone
GRAS	generally recognized as safe
GTT	glucose tolerance test
H	hydrogen
HBP	high blood pressure
HFCS	high-fructose corn syrup
HDL	high density lipoprotein
HP/DP	health promotion and disease prevention
H-P-A	hypothalamic-pituitary-adrenal (axis)
H-P-O	hypothalamic-pituitary-ovarian (axis)
H-R	hormone-receptor (interaction)
HRT	hormone replacement therapy
IBW	ideal body weight
IDDM	insulin-dependent diabetes mellitus
IF	intrinsic factor
IGF	insulin-like growth factor
IU	International Unit
K	potassium
kcal	kilocalorie
kcal/g	kilocalorie per gram
kg	kilogram
LBM	lean body mass
LCD	low calorie diet
LDL	low density lipoprotein
LH	luteinizing hormone
LOV	lactoovovegetarian
m	meter
MCT	medium-chain triglyceride
MFA	monounsaturated fatty acid
mg	milligram
mL	milliliter
N	nitrogen
Na	sodium
NAD	nicotinamide adenine dinucleotide
NIDDM	non-insulin–dependent diabetes mellitus
NPU	net protein utilization
O	oxygen
OAA	oxaloacetate (oxaloacetic acid)
ox	oxidation
oz	ounce

P	phosphorus or phosphate (ion)
PBM	peak bone mass
PC	phosphatidyl choline (lecithin)
PFA	polyunsaturated fatty acid
PGE	prostaglandin E series
pH	log of the hydrogen ion concentration
PIR	poverty index ratio
PL	phospholipids
pro	protein
P/S	ratio of polyunsaturated to saturated fatty acids
PSMF	protein-sparing modified fast
PTH	parathyroid hormone
QFFQ	quantitative food frequency questionnaire
RA	retinoic acid
RBC	red blood cell
RBP	retinol-binding protein
RD	Registered Dietitian
RDA	Recommended Dietary Allowance
REE	resting energy expenditure (see BMR)
SCAA	sulfur-containing amino acids
SCFA	short-chain fatty acid
SERM	selective estrogen receptor modulator (drug)
SES	socioeconomic status
SFA	saturated fatty acid
T3	triiodothyronine (with 3 iodine atoms)
T4	thyroxin (with 4 iodine atoms)
TC	total cholesterol
TC:HDL-C	ratio of total cholesterol to HDL cholesterol
TG	triglycerides
TIA	transient ischemic attack (ministroke)
TPN	total parenteral nutrition
UFA	unsaturated fatty acid
UL	Upper Tolerable Limit
µg	microgram
US RDI	U.S. Recommended Dietary Intake (for food and supplement labeling)
UV (or UVL)	ultraviolet light
VLCD	very low calorie diet
VLDL	very low density lipoprotein
W-H (or WHR)	ratio of waist to hip
WIC	women, infants, and children

Organizational Acronyms

A list of acronyms commonly used in this text:

AHA	American Heart Association
AMA	American Medical Association
AND	Academy of Nutrition and Dietetics
APHA	American Public Health Association
ARS	Agriculture Research Service (part of the USDA)
ASN	American Society for Nutrition
CDC	Centers for Disease Control and Prevention
CNS/SCN	Canadian Nutrition Society/La Société Canadienne de Nutrition
DHHS	Department of Health and Human Services
FAO	Food and Agricultural Organization (part of the UN)
FDA	Food and Drug Administration
HFCS	Household Food Consumption Survey (part of the USDA)
LRC	Lipid Research Clinics Program (part of the NIH)
MRFIT	Multiple Risk Factor Intervention Trial (part of the NIH)
NAS	National Academy of Sciences
NCEP	National Cholesterol Education Program (part of the NIH)
NCHS	National Center for Health Statistics
NHANES	National Health and Nutrition Examination Survey (part of the PHS)
NIH	National Institutes of Health
NRC	National Research Council (part of the NAS)
UN	United Nations
USDA	U.S. Department of Agriculture
WHO	World Health Organization (part of the UN)

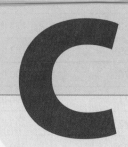

Average Weights for Men and Women by Age Group and Height: United States, 1999–2000

Men

	Age Groups in Years						
Height	**21–30**	**31–40**	**41–50**	**51–60**	**61–70**	**71–80**	**> 80**
60"	134 lbs	141 lbs	146 lbs	146 lbs	144 lbs	138 lbs	128 lbs
61"	139 lbs	146 lbs	150 lbs	151 lbs	149 lbs	143 lbs	133 lbs
62"	144 lbs	151 lbs	156 lbs	156 lbs	154 lbs	148 lbs	138 lbs
63"	149 lbs	157 lbs	161 lbs	162 lbs	159 lbs	153 lbs	143 lbs
64"	154 lbs	162 lbs	166 lbs	167 lbs	164 lbs	158 lbs	149 lbs
65"	160 lbs	167 lbs	172 lbs	173 lbs	170 lbs	164 lbs	154 lbs
66"	165 lbs	173 lbs	177 lbs	178 lbs	176 lbs	169 lbs	160 lbs
67"	171 lbs	179 lbs	183 lbs	184 lbs	181 lbs	175 lbs	166 lbs

Estimated values are from regression equations of weight on height for specified age groups.

68"	177 lbs	185 lbs	189 lbs	190 lbs	187 lbs	181 lbs	172 lbs
69"	183 lbs	191 lbs	195 lbs	196 lbs	194 lbs	187 lbs	178 lbs
70"	190 lbs	197 lbs	202 lbs	202 lbs	200 lbs	194 lbs	184 lbs
71"	196 lbs	204 lbs	208 lbs	209 lbs	206 lbs	200 lbs	191 lbs
72"	203 lbs	210 lbs	215 lbs	215 lbs	213 lbs	207 lbs	197 lbs
73"	210 lbs	217 lbs	221 lbs	222 lbs	220 lbs	214 lbs	204 lbs
74"	216 lbs	224 lbs	228 lbs	229 lbs	227 lbs	220 lbs	211 lbs
75"	223 lbs	231 lbs	235 lbs	236 lbs	234 lbs	227 lbs	218 lbs
76"	231 lbs	238 lbs	243 lbs	243 lbs	241 lbs	235 lbs	225 lbs

Data from NHANES 1999–2000.

Women

	Age Groups in Years						
Height	**21–30**	**31–40**	**41–50**	**51–60**	**61–70**	**71–80**	**> 80**
56"	125 lbs	133 lbs	137 lbs	138 lbs	135 lbs	129 lbs	119 lbs
57"	129 lbs	137 lbs	141 lbs	142 lbs	139 lbs	133 lbs	124 lbs
58"	134 lbs	141 lbs	146 lbs	146 lbs	144 lbs	138 lbs	128 lbs
59"	138 lbs	146 lbs	150 lbs	151 lbs	148 lbs	142 lbs	133 lbs
60"	143 lbs	151 lbs	155 lbs	156 lbs	153 lbs	147 lbs	138 lbs
61"	148 lbs	156 lbs	160 lbs	161 lbs	158 lbs	152 lbs	143 lbs
62"	153 lbs	161 lbs	165 lbs	166 lbs	163 lbs	157 lbs	148 lbs
63"	158 lbs	166 lbs	170 lbs	171 lbs	168 lbs	162 lbs	153 lbs
64"	164 lbs	171 lbs	176 lbs	176 lbs	174 lbs	168 lbs	158 lbs
65"	169 lbs	177 lbs	181 lbs	182 lbs	179 lbs	173 lbs	164 lbs
66"	175 lbs	183 lbs	187 lbs	188 lbs	185 lbs	179 lbs	170 lbs
67"	181 lbs	189 lbs	193 lbs	194 lbs	191 lbs	185 lbs	175 lbs
68"	187 lbs	195 lbs	199 lbs	200 lbs	197 lbs	191 lbs	181 lbs
69"	193 lbs	201 lbs	205 lbs	206 lbs	203 lbs	197 lbs	187 lbs
70"	199 lbs	207 lbs	211 lbs	212 lbs	209 lbs	203 lbs	194 lbs

Data from NHANES 1999–2000.

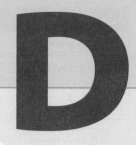

Energy Expenditures in Diverse Physical Activities

Energy Expenditures

Activity	Kcal per Minute per Pound	Kcal per Minute per Kilogram
Archery	0.029	0.065
Basketball	0.063	0.138
Baseball	0.031	0.069
Boxing (sparring)	0.063	0.138
Canoeing (leisure)	0.020	0.044
Climbing hills (no load)	0.055	0.121
Cleaning	0.027	0.060
Cooking	0.020	0.045
Cycling		
5.5 mph	0.029	0.064
9.4 mph	0.045	0.100
Racing	0.077	0.169

Activity	Kcal per Minute per Pound	Kcal per Minute per Kilogram
Dance (modern)	0.038	0.083
Eating (sitting)	0.010	0.023
Farming		
Barn cleaning	0.061	0.135
Driving tractor	0.017	0.037
Feeding animals	0.030	0.065
Forking straw bales	0.063	0.138
Milking by machine	0.010	0.023
Shoveling grain	0.039	0.085
Field hockey	0.061	0.134
Fishing	0.028	0.062
Football	0.060	0.132
Gardening		
Digging	0.057	0.126
Mowing	0.051	0.112
Raking	0.024	0.054
Golf	0.039	0.085
Gymnastics	0.030	0.066
Horseback riding		
Galloping	0.062	0.137
Trotting	0.050	0.110
Walking	0.019	0.041
Judo	0.089	0.195
Knitting (sewing)	0.010	0.022
Marching, rapid	0.064	0.142
Music playing (sitting)	0.018	0.040
Painting (outside)	0.035	0.077
Racquetball	0.065	0.143
Running, cross-country	0.074	0.163
11.5 min. per mile	0.061	0.135
9 min. per mile	0.088	0.193
8 min. per mile	0.094	0.208
7 min. per mile	0.104	0.228
6 min. per mile	0.114	0.252
5.5 min. per mile	0.131	0.289

Activity	Kcal per Minute per Pound	Kcal per Minute per Kilogram
Sailing	0.020	0.044
Scrubbing floors	0.050	0.109
Skiing		
Snow, downhill	0.064	0.142
Water	0.052	0.114
Skating (moderate)	0.038	0.083
Soccer	0.059	0.131
Squash	0.096	0.212
Swimming		
Backstroke	0.077	0.169
Breast stroke	0.074	0.162
Crawl, fast	0.071	0.156
Crawl, slow	0.058	0.128
Butterfly	0.078	0.171
Table tennis	0.031	0.068
Tennis	0.050	0.109
Volleyball	0.022	0.050
Walking (normal pace)	0.036	0.080
Wrestling	0.085	0.188
Writing (sitting)	0.013	0.029

Data from Bannister EW, Brown SR. The relative energy requirements of physical activity. In: HB Falls, ed, *Exercise Physiology.* New York: Academic Press; 1968; Howley ET, Glover ME. The caloric costs of running and walking one mile for men and women. *Medicine and Science in Sports.* 1974;6:235–237; and Passmore R, Durnan GA. Human energy expenditure. *Physiological Reviews.* 1955;35:801–840.

General Classifications for Activities Not Listed Above

Activity	Kcal per Minute per Pound	Kcal per Minute per Kilogram
Very light (i.e., typing, driving)	0.010	0.023
Light (i.e., shopping)	0.021	0.046
Moderate (i.e., dancing, bowling)	0.032	0.070
Heavy (i.e., football, running)	0.062	0.137

Data from Food and Nutrition Board, National Research Council. *Recommended Dietary Allowances* (8th ed.). Washington, DC: National Academy of Sciences; 1974.

Growth Charts

Birth to 36 months: Boys
Length-for-age and Weight-for-age percentiles

NAME _____

RECORD # _____

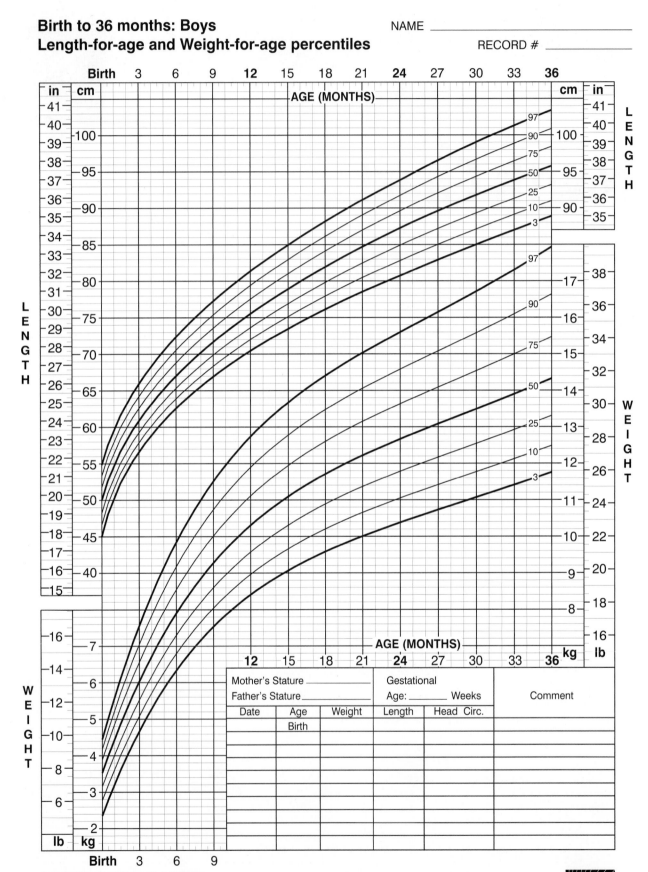

Published May 30, 2000 (modified 4/20/01).
SOURCE: Developed by the National Center for Health Statistics in collaboration with
the National Center for Chronic Disease Prevention and Health Promotion (2000).
http://www.cdc.gov/growthcharts

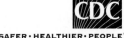

SAFER · HEALTHIER · PEOPLE™

Birth to 36 months: Boys
Head circumference-for-age and
Weight-for-length percentiles

NAME _____

RECORD # _____

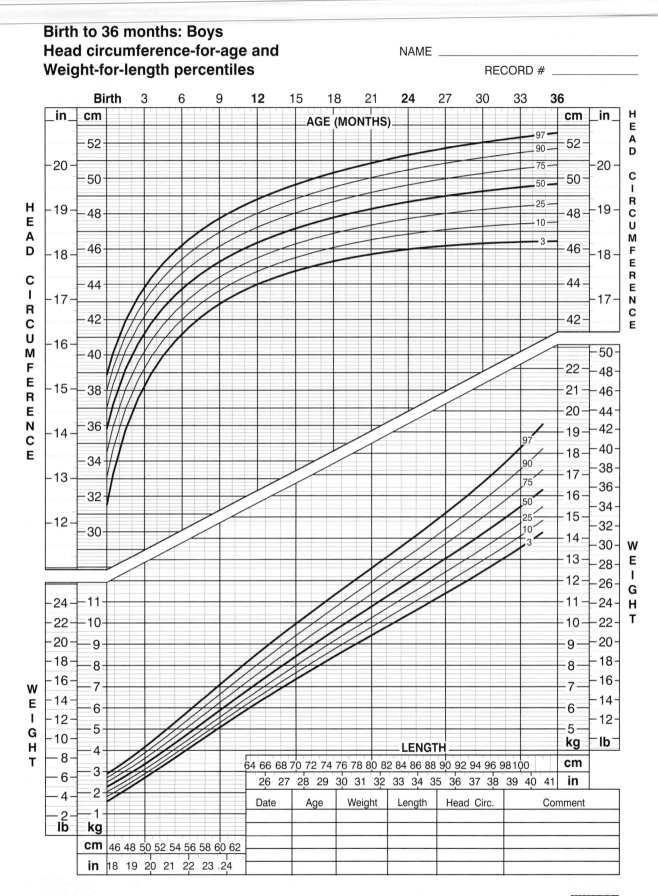

Published May 30, 2000 (modified 10/16/00).
SOURCE: Developed by the National Center for Health Statistics in collaboration with
the National Center for Chronic Disease Prevention and Health Promotion (2000).
http://www.cdc.gov/growthcharts

SAFER · HEALTHIER · PEOPLE™

Birth to 36 months: Girls
Length-for-age and Weight-for-age percentiles

NAME _____

RECORD # _____

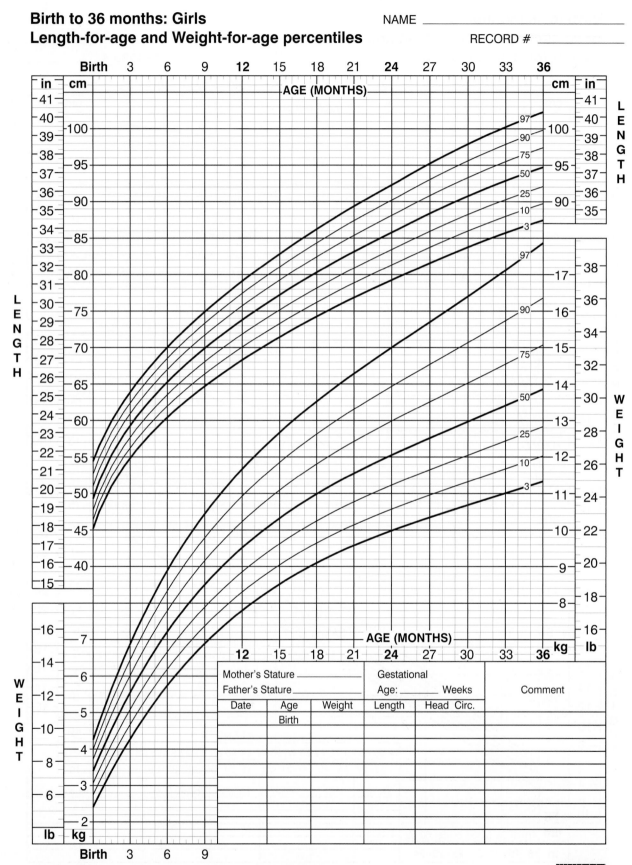

Published May 30, 2000 (modified 4/20/01).
SOURCE: Developed by the National Center for Health Statistics in collaboration with
the National Center for Chronic Disease Prevention and Health Promotion (2000).
http://www.cdc.gov/growthcharts

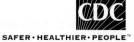

SAFER · HEALTHIER · PEOPLE™

Birth to 36 months: Girls
Head circumference-for-age and
Weight-for-length percentiles

NAME _____

RECORD # _____

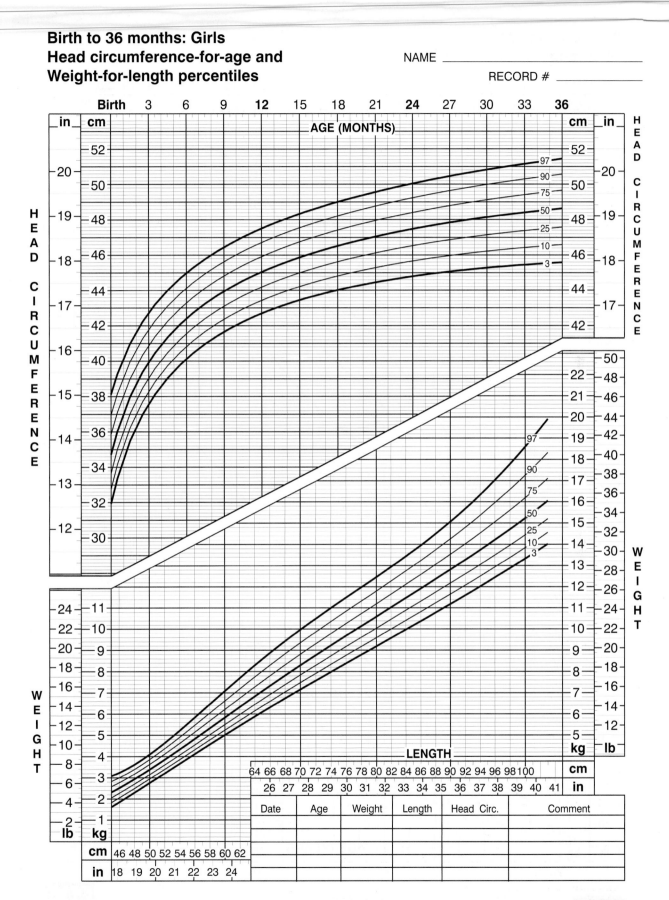

Published May 30, 2000 (modified 10/16/00).
SOURCE: Developed by the National Center for Health Statistics in collaboration with
the National Center for Chronic Disease Prevention and Health Promotion (2000).
http://www.cdc.gov/growthcharts

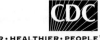

2 to 20 years: Boys
Stature-for-age and Weight-for-age percentiles

NAME _____

RECORD # _____

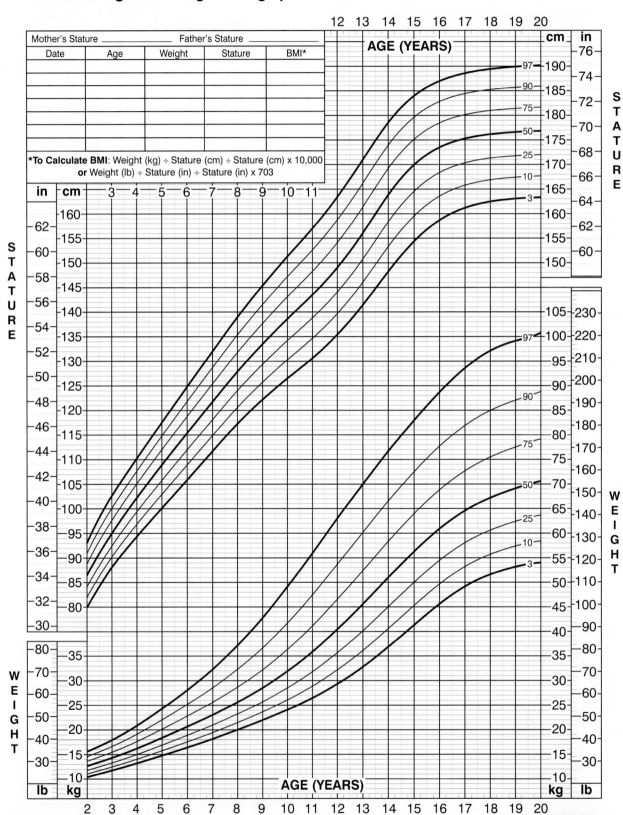

Published May 30, 2000 (modified 11/21/00).
SOURCE: Developed by the National Center for Health Statistics in collaboration with
the National Center for Chronic Disease Prevention and Health Promotion (2000).
http://www.cdc.gov/growthcharts

SAFER · HEALTHIER · PEOPLE™

2 to 20 years: Girls
Stature-for-age and Weight-for-age percentiles

NAME _____

RECORD # _____

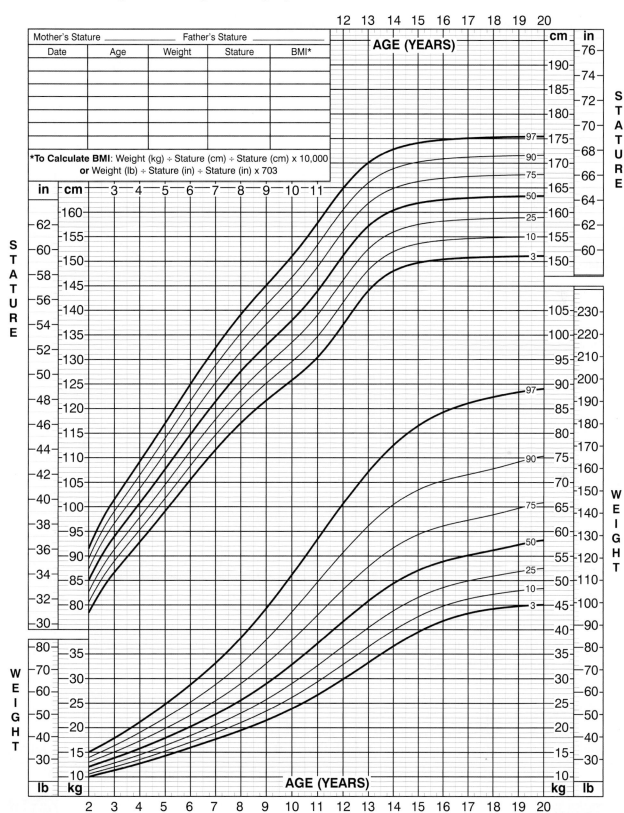

Published May 30, 2000 (modified 11/21/00).
SOURCE: Developed by the National Center for Health Statistics in collaboration with
the National Center for Chronic Disease Prevention and Health Promotion (2000).
http://www.cdc.gov/growthcharts

SAFER • HEALTHIER • PEOPLE™

2 to 20 years: Boys
Body mass index-for-age percentiles

NAME _____

RECORD # _____

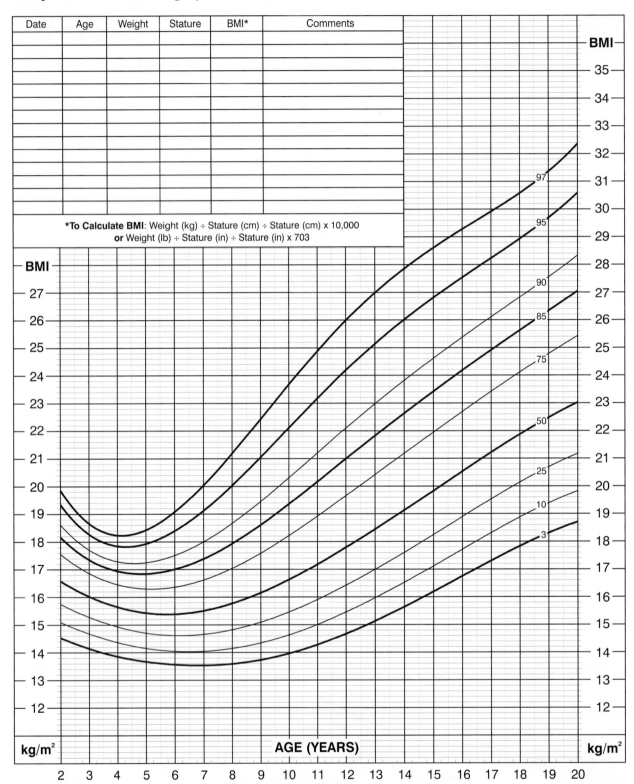

*To Calculate BMI: Weight (kg) ÷ Stature (cm) ÷ Stature (cm) x 10,000
or Weight (lb) ÷ Stature (in) ÷ Stature (in) x 703

AGE (YEARS)

Published May 30, 2000 (modified 10/16/00).
SOURCE: Developed by the National Center for Health Statistics in collaboration with
the National Center for Chronic Disease Prevention and Health Promotion (2000).
http://www.cdc.gov/growthcharts

CDC

SAFER · HEALTHIER · PEOPLE™

2 to 20 years: Girls
Body mass index-for-age percentiles

NAME _____

RECORD # _____

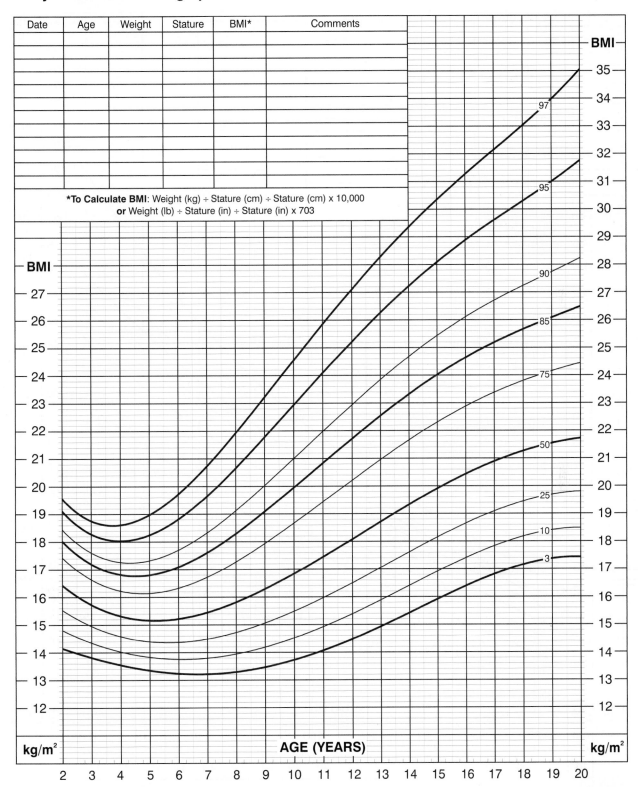

Date	Age	Weight	Stature	BMI*	Comments

*To Calculate BMI: Weight (kg) ÷ Stature (cm) ÷ Stature (cm) x 10,000
or Weight (lb) ÷ Stature (in) ÷ Stature (in) x 703

AGE (YEARS)

kg/m²

Published May 30, 2000 (modified 10/16/00).

SOURCE: Developed by the National Center for Health Statistics in collaboration with
the National Center for Chronic Disease Prevention and Health Promotion (2000).
http://www.cdc.gov/growthcharts

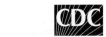

SAFER · HEALTHIER · PEOPLE™

Weight-for-stature percentiles: Boys

NAME _____

RECORD # _____

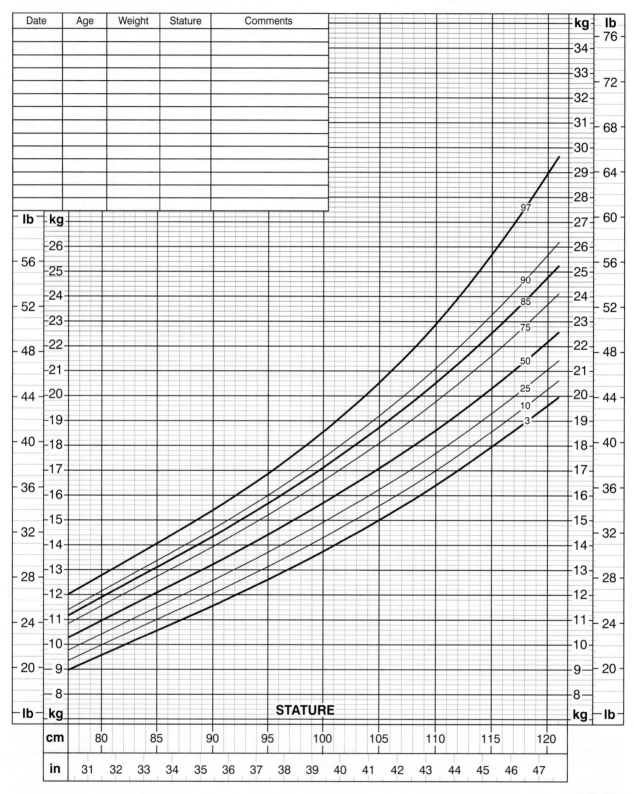

Date	Age	Weight	Stature	Comments

Published May 30, 2000 (modified 10/16/00).
SOURCE: Developed by the National Center for Health Statistics in collaboration with
the National Center for Chronic Disease Prevention and Health Promotion (2000).
http://www.cdc.gov/growthcharts

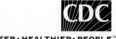

SAFER • HEALTHIER • PEOPLE™

NAME _____

Weight-for-stature percentiles: Girls

RECORD # _____

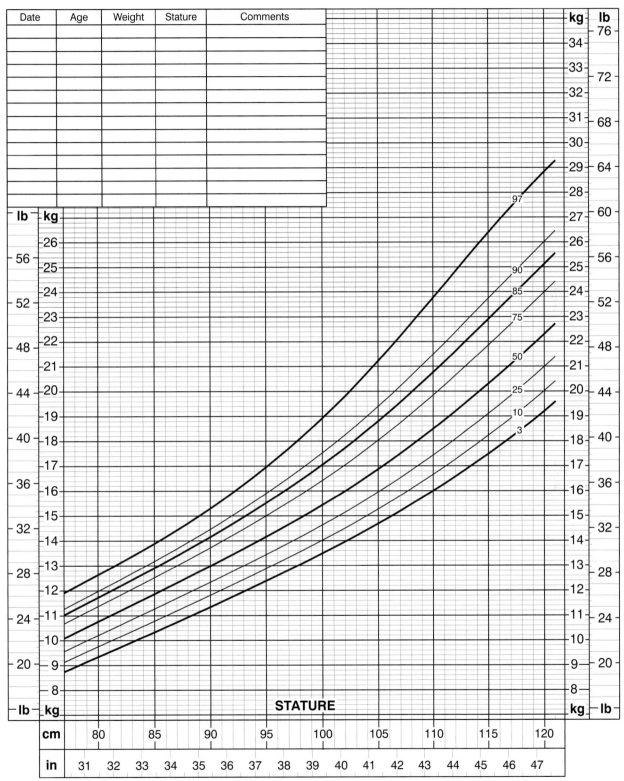

Date	Age	Weight	Stature	Comments

STATURE

Published May 30, 2000 (modified 10/16/00).

SOURCE: Developed by the National Center for Health Statistics in collaboration with
the National Center for Chronic Disease Prevention and Health Promotion (2000).
http://www.cdc.gov/growthcharts

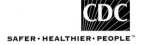

SAFER · HEALTHIER · PEOPLE™

APPENDIX

F

Meal Plans for Weight Gain, Weight Loss, Vegetarianism

High-Carbohydrate Meal Pattern

Breakfast:

6 oz. orange juice (or other)
¾ cup dry cereal
8 oz. low-fat milk
1 egg, fried (or whole)
2 slice whole-wheat bread, toasted
  2 tsp. margarine
  2 tsp. jelly

Lunch:

1 cheese sandwich
  2 slices whole wheat bread
  1 oz. American cheese (2 slices)
  2 pieces of lettuce
  1 slice of tomato, large
  1 tsp. mayonnaise
1 banana

8 oz. low-fat milk

Dinner:

6 oz, baked fish with lemon juice

1 baked potato, large

   2 tsp. margarine

½ cup green beans

½ cup coleslaw

2 pieces cornbread (or other roll)

   2 tsp. honey

1 piece pound cake (or other cake or pie)

8 oz. low-fat milk

Snacks:

1 serving fruit

crackers with 2 Tbsp. peanut butter

Approximate kcal: 3,000

Weight-Loss Meal Pattern

1,800-Calorie Meal Pattern

Breakfast:

¾ cup orange juice

¾ cup cereal

8 oz. low-fat milk

1 slice whole wheat toast

   1 tsp. margarine

Lunch:

1 peanut butter and banana sandwich

   2 slices bread

   1 Tbsp. peanut butter

   ½ banana

5–7 carrot sticks

1 peach

8 oz. low-fat milk

Dinner:

1 hamburger patty (4 oz.)

   1 hamburger bun (or other bread)

1 cup tossed green salad

   1 Tbsp. salad dressing

8 oz. low-fat milk

½ cup ice cream

Snacks:

1 apple or 20 grapes

2 graham crackers (or other low-salt)

2,400-Calorie Meal Pattern

Breakfast:

6 oz. orange juice

1 slice toast

¾ cup cereal

8 oz. low-fat milk

Lunch:

1 slice cheese pizza (plain)

1 cup tossed green salad

   1 Tbsp. dressing

8 oz. low-fat milk

Dinner:

1 cup macaroni and cheese

½ cup lima beans

1 cup tomato and cucumber slices

   I Tbsp. salad dressing

1 dinner roll (or other)

   1 tsp. margarine

8 oz. low-fat milk

Snacks:

1 banana

½ cup raisin and peanut mix

½ cup apple juice

½ cup sherbet

1 granola cookie

Weight-Gain Meal Pattern

6,000-Calorie Meal Pattern

Breakfast:

6 oz. orange juice

1 cup hot cereal

   2 tsp. sugar

1 egg, fried

1 slice whole wheat toast

   1 tsp. margarine

   1 tsp. jelly

1 peanut butter and jelly sandwich
   2 slices bread
   2 Tbsp. peanut butter
   2 tsp. jelly
½ cup raisins
8 oz. apple juice
8 oz. milk (whole)

Lunch:
1 ham and cheese sandwich
   2 slices bread
   1 oz. ham
   1 Tbsp. mayonnaise
1 serving French fries
1 cup tossed green salad
   2 Tbsp. dressing
1 bagel
   2 tsp. margarine
   2 Tbsp. cream cheese
1 cup sweetened applesauce
6 oz. grape juice
10 oz. chocolate milkshake
4 oatmeal cookies

Dinner:
2 pieces baked chicken (7 oz.)
1 cup rice
   1 tsp. margarine
1 cup collard greens
½ cup candied sweet potatoes
2 pieces cornbread
   1 Tbsp. margarine
1 banana
½ cup peanuts
8 oz. chocolate milk (whole)
8 oz. milk (whole)
1 slice apple pie
   ½ cup ice cream

4,000-Calorie Meal Pattern

Breakfast:
6 oz. orange juice
1 cup hot cereal
   2 tsp. sugar
1 egg, fried

1 slice whole wheat toast
  1 tsp. margarine
  1 tsp. jelly
8 oz. milk (whole)

Lunch:

1 ham and cheese sandwich
  2 slices bread
  1 oz. cheese
  1 oz. ham
  1 Tbsp. mayonnaise
1 serving French fries
1 cup tossed green salad
  2 Tbsp. dressing
10 oz. chocolate milkshake
4 oatmeal cookies

Dinner:

2 pieces baked chicken (7 oz.)
1 cup rice
1 cup collard greens
  1 tsp. margarine
½ cup candied sweet potatoes
8 oz. milk (whole)
1 slice apple pie
  ½ cup ice cream
2 pieces cornbread
  1 Tbsp. margarine

Lacto-Ovo-Vegetarian Meal Pattern

Breakfast:

6 oz. orange juice (other)
1 egg, poached (or sunny-side up)
2 slices whole-wheat bread, toasted (or hot cereal)
  2 tsp. margarine
  2 tsp. honey
1 banana
8 oz. low-fat milk

Lunch:

1 cup vegetable soup (homemade)
1 serving crackers (low-salt)

1 peanut butter and jelly sandwich
  2 slices bread
  2 Tbsp. peanut butter
  2 tsp. jelly
7–8 carrot sticks (sliced)
1 apple (or other fruit)
8 oz. low-fat milk

Dinner:

1 cup pinto beans and rice, with mushrooms and spices (cooked)
1 cup collard greens (or other) (cooked)
2 pieces cornbread
  2 tsp. margarine
1 cup tossed salad:
  lettuce pieces
  tomato slices
  onion slices
  green pepper
  bean sprouts
  1 Tbsp. salad dressing
8 oz. low-fat milk

Snacks:

1 piece of fruit
1 oatmeal cookie or ½ cup raisin and nut mix
Approximate kcal: 3,000

Pre-Event and Pre-Game Meal (Single) Pattern

500-Calorie Meal: Breakfast Type

6 oz. orange juice (or other)
Either:
  ½ cup dry cereal (non-sweetened)
    1 tsp. sugar
  1 slice whole-wheat bread, toasted
    1 tsp. margarine
    1 tsp. honey (or jelly or other)
Or:
  2 pancakes
    1 tsp. margarine
    2 Tbsp. syrup
8 oz. low-fat milk
water ad libitum

600–700-Calorie Meal: Lunch or Dinner Type

1 cup vegetable soup (or other)

Either:

    1 chicken or turkey sandwich

        2 slices whole-wheat bread, toasted

        2 oz. breast or leg

        1 oz. American Cheese (one slice)

        1 tsp. margarine

Or:

    1 cup spaghetti noodles (cooked)

        ½ cup tomato sauce (lightly spiced)

        1 Tbsp. mozzarella cheese

    1 slice Italian bread

        1 tsp. margarine without garlic

½ cup sherbet

8 oz. low-fat milk

1 sugar cookie (or other)

water ad libitum

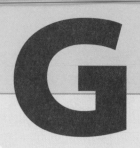

Nutritive Value of Foods

Susan E. Gebhardt and Robin G. Thomas

Introduction

An 8-oz glass of milk, a 3-oz slice of cooked meat, an apple, and a slice of bread. What food values does each contain? How much cooked meat will a pound of raw meat yield? How much protein should a healthy 14-year-old boy get each day?

Consumers want ready answers to questions like these so they can plan nutritious diets for themselves and their families. Also, nutritionists, dietitians, and other health professionals use this type of information in their daily work.

In response, the U.S. Department of Agriculture published the first edition of this bulletin in 1960. USDA nutrition researchers have revised it many times since to reflect our expanded knowledge, to add or subtract specific values, and to update the ever-growing list of available, commonly used foods.

Literature Cited in This Appendix

American Institute for Cancer Research. 2001. The New American Plate. On the American Institute for Cancer Research. Available at: www.aicr.org/nap2.htm

Food and Nutrition Board, Institute of Medicine. *Dietary Reference Intakes for Calcium, Phosphorus, Magnesium, Vitamin D, and Fluoride.* Washington, DC: National Academies Press; 1997.

Food and Nutrition Board, Institute of Medicine. *Dietary Reference Intakes for Thiamin, Riboflavin, Niacin, Vitamin B_6, Folate, Vitamin B_{12}, Pantothenic Acid, Biotin, and Choline.* Washington, DC: National Academies Press; 1998.

Food and Nutrition Board, Institute of Medicine. *Dietary Reference Intakes for Vitamin C, Vitamin E, Selenium, and Carotenoids.* Washington, DC: National Academies Press; 2000.

Schuster, Ellen, compiler. 1997. Making Sense of Portion Sizes. On the Oregon State University Extension Family & Community Development. Available at: http://osu .orst.edu/dept/ehe/nutrition.htm

Subcommittee on the Tenth Edition of the RDAs, Food and Nutrition Board, Commission on Life Sciences, National Research Council. *Recommended Dietary Allowances.* 10th ed. Washington, DC: National Academies Press; 1989.

U.S. Department of Agriculture, Agricultural Research Service. USDA Nutrient Database for Standard Reference, Release 13. Washington, DC: Government Printing Office; 2000.

U.S. Department of Agriculture and U.S. Department of Health and Human Services. *Nutrition and Your Health: Dietary Guidelines for Americans.* Washington, DC: Government Printing Office; 2000.

U.S. Food and Drug Administration. 1999. Food Labeling. Code of Federal Regulations, Title 21, part 101. Available at: www.access.gpo.gov/nara/cfr /waisidx_99/21cfr101_99.html

Equivalents by Volume and Weight

This table contains some helpful volume and weight equivalents. Following is an example that illustrates how you can use the table.

Example: For milk, the nutrient profile covers a 1-cup serving. Let's say you use 2 tablespoons of milk in your coffee. In Table 1, you see that 1 cup equals 16 tablespoons, so the 2 tablespoons you consume are two-sixteenths or one-eighth of 1 cup. To find out the nutritive value of the amount you actually consume—2 tablespoons—you need to divide the nutrient values listed for milk by 8.

TABLE 1
Equivalents by Volume and Weight

Volume	
1 gallon (3.786 liters; 3,786 ml)	4 quarts
1 quart (0.946 liter; 946 ml)	4 cups or 2 pints
1 cup (237 ml)	8 fluid ounces, ½ pint, or 16 tablespoons
2 tablespoons (30 ml)	1 fluid ounce
1 tablespoon (15 ml)	3 teaspoons
1 pint	2 cups
Weight	
1 pound (16 ounces)	453.6 grams
1 ounce	28.35 grams
3.5 ounces	100 grams

Tips for Estimating Amount of Food Consumed

This table lists some handy tips to help you estimate the amount of food you eat when you cannot measure or weigh it.

TABLE 2
Tips for Estimating Amount of Food Consumed

Breads and Grains	
½ cup cooked cereal, pasta, rice	volume of cupcake wrapper or half a baseball
4-oz bagel (large)	diameter of a CD
medium piece of cornbread	medium bar of soap
Fruits and Vegetables	
medium apple, orange, peach	tennis ball
¼ cup dried fruit	golf ball or scant handful for average adult
½ cup fruit or vegetable	half a baseball
1 cup broccoli	light bulb
medium potato	computer mouse
1 cup raw leafy greens	baseball or fist of average adult
½ cup	6 asparagus spears, 7 or 8 baby carrots or carrot sticks, or a medium ear of corn
Meat, Fish, and Poultry, Cooked	
1 oz	about 3 Tbsp. meat or poultry
2 oz	small chicken drumstick or thigh
3 oz	average deck of cards, palm of average adult's hand, half of a whole, small chicken breast, medium pork chop
Cheese	
1 oz hard cheese	average person's thumb, 2 dominoes, 4 dice
Other	
2 Tbsp. peanut butter	Ping-Pong ball
⅓ cup nuts	level handful for average adult
½ cup	half a baseball or base of computer mouse
1 cup	tennis ball or fist of average adult

Note: The serving size indicated in the USDA Food Guide and on food labels is a standardized unit of measure and may not represent the portion of food a person actually eats on one occasion.
Data from Schuster (1997), American Institute of Cancer Research (2001).

Yield of Cooked Meat per Pound of Raw Meat as Purchased

From the time it is purchased to the time it is eaten, meat undergoes certain losses. These include evaporation of moisture and loss of fat in the drippings during cooking and removal of parts such as bone, gristle, and fat before or after cooking. This table shows, for several retail cuts, the yield of cooked meat from 1 pound of raw meat. Yield is given as ounces of:

- Cooked meat with bone and fat
- Cooked lean and fat
- Cooked lean only

Among the factors influencing meat yield is the proportion of fat and lean. Many cuts have an outside layer of fat extending all or part way around. The thickness of this fat layer varies depending on the cutting and trimming practices in the market. The information on yield in Table 3 and on nutritive value in Table 9 applies to retail cuts

TABLE 3
Yield of Cooked Meat per Pound of Raw Meat as Purchased

Retail Cut and Method of Cooking	Parts Weighed	Yield After Cooking, Less Drippings, Weight (oz)
Chops or Steaks for Broiling or Frying		
With bone and relatively large amount fat, such as pork or lamb chops; beef rib; sirloin, or porterhouse steaks	Lean, bone, and fat	10–12
	Lean and fat	7–10
	Lean only	5–7
Without bone and with very little fat, such as round of beef or veal steaks	Lean and fat	12–13
	Lean only	9–12
Ground meat for broiling or frying, such as beef, lamb, or pork patties	Patties	9–13
Roast for Oven Cooking (No Liquid Added)		
With bone and relatively large amount of fat, such as beef rib, loin, chuck; lamb shoulder, leg; pork, fresh or cured	Lean, bone, and fat	10–12
	Lean and fat	8–10
	Lean only	6–9
Without bone	Lean and fat	10–12
	Lean only	7–10
Cuts for Pot Roasting, Simmering, Braising, or Stewing		
With bone and relatively large amount of fat, such as beef chuck, pork shoulder	Lean, bone, and fat	10–11
	Lean and fat	8–9
	Lean only	6–8
Without bone and with relatively small amount of fat, such as trimmed beef, veal	Lean with adhering fat	9–11

trimmed according to typical market practices. Deposits of fat within a cut may be extensive. They are not usually affected by retail trimming but may be discarded after cooking.

Recommended Daily Dietary Intakes

Table 4 shows recommended daily levels of calories and several nutrients essential for maintenance of good nutrition in healthy, normally active persons. The Recommended Dietary Allowances (RDAs) are currently being revised by the National Academy of Sciences. The new recommendations are called Dietary Reference Intakes (DRIs) and include two sets of values that serve as goals for nutrient intake—RDAs and Adequate Intakes (AIs). The right side of Table 4 presents the DRIs published in 1997–2000, with AIs indicated by a dagger (†). The left side of the table includes the 1989 RDAs. More detailed information about DRIs may be obtained from the table's sources. Table 4 includes only the nutrients contained in Table 9.

TABLE 4
Recommended Daily Dietary Intakes

	Dietary Reference Intakes (DRI)							
Life-Stage Group	Protein (g)	Vitamin A (µg RAE)	Iron (mg)	Calcium† (mg)	Thiamin (mg)	Riboflavin (mg)	Niacin‡ (mg)	Vitamin C (mg)
Infants (mo)								
0–6	9.1	400	0.3†	200	0.2†	0.3†	2†	40†
7–12	11.0	500	11	260	0.3†	0.4†	4†	50†
Children (yr)								
1–3	13	300	7	700	0.5	0.5	6	15
4–8	19	400	10	1,000	0.6	0.6	8	25
Males (yr)								
9–13	34	600	8	1,300	0.9	0.9	12	45
14–18	52	900	11	1,300	1.2	1.3	16	75
19–30	56	900	8	1,000	1.2	1.3	16	90
31–50	56	900	8	1,000	1.2	1.3	16	90
51–70	56	900	8	1,000	1.2	1.3	16	90
> 70	56	900	8	1,200	1.2	1.3	16	90
Females (yr)								
9–13	34	600	8	1,300	0.9	0.9	12	45
14–18	46	700	15	1,300	1.0	1.0	14	65
19–30	46	700	18	1,000	1.1	1.1	14	75
31–50	46	700	18	1,000	1.1	1.1	14	75
51–70	46	700	8	1,200	1.1	1.1	14	75
> 70	46	700	8	1,200	1.1	1.1	14	75
Pregnancy (yr)								
14–18	71	750	27	1,300	1.4	1.4	18	80
19–30	71	770	27	1,000	1.4	1.4	18	85
31–50	71	770	27	1,000	1.4	1.4	18	85
Lactation (yr)								
14–16	71	1,300	10	1,300	1.4	1.4	17	115
19–30	71	1,300	9	1,000	1.4	1.6	17	115
31–50	71	1,300	9	1,000	1.4	1.6	17	120

†Values represent Adequate Intake.
‡Expressed as niacin equivalents. 1 mg niacin = 60 mg tryptophan; 0–6 months = preformed niacin, not niacin equivalents.
Note: RDAs and DRIs should not be confused with reference values for food labels established by the U.S. Food and Drug Administration, as follows: vitamin A = 5,000 IU; iron = 18 mg; calcium = 1,000 mg; thiamin = 1.5 mg; riboflavin = 1.7 mg; niacin = 20 mg; vitamin C = 60 mg.
Data from Food and Nutrition Board, Institute of Medicine. *Dietary Reference Intakes*. Washington, DC: National Academies Press; 1998, 2000, 2001, 2002, 2011.

Food Sources of Additional Nutrients

Table 5 lists foods that are of special value in supplying six vitamins and four minerals not shown in Tables 4 and 9. Foods are considered to be of special value as a nutrient source if the food serving is high in the nutrient compared with other foods.

TABLE 5
Food Sources of Additional Nutrients

Vitamins	Vitamins	Minerals
Vitamin B$_6$	**Vitamin E**	**Iodine**
Bananas	Margarine	Iodized salt
Fish (most)	Nuts and seeds	Saltwater fish and shellfish
Liver	Peanuts and peanut butter	**Magnesium**
Meat	Vegetable oils	Cocoa and chocolate
Nuts and seeds	Wheat germ	Dark green vegetables (most)
Potatoes and sweet potatoes	Whole-grain and fortified cereals	Dry beans, peas, and lentils
Poultry	**Folate**	Fish
Whole-grain and fortified cereals	Dark green vegetables	Nuts and seeds
Vitamin B$_{12}$	Dry beans, peas, and lentils	Peanuts and peanut butter
Eggs	Enriched grain products	Whole grains
Fish and shellfish	Fortified cereals	**Phosphorus**
Fortified cereals	Liver	Dry beans, peas, and lentils
Meat	Orange juice	Eggs
Milk and milk products	Wheat germ	Fish
Organ meats	Yeast	Meat
Vitamin D	**Vitamin K**	Milk and milk products
Egg yolk	Broccoli	Nuts and seeds
Fortified cereals	Brussels sprouts	Poultry
Fortified milk	Cabbage	Whole grains
Liver	Leafy green vegetables	**Zinc**
High-fat fish	Mayonnaise	Dry beans, peas, and lentils
	Soybean, canola, and olive oils	Meat
		Poultry
		Seeds
		Shellfish
		Whole-grain and fortified cereals

Daily Values

Daily Values have been established by the Food and Drug Administration as references to help consumers use information on food labels to plan a healthy overall diet. The Daily Values provide a reliable guide for most people. It is helpful to know that a 2,000-calorie level is about right for moderately active women, teenage girls, and sedentary men, and 2,500 calories is the target level for many men, teenage boys, and active women.

Many older adults, children, and sedentary women need fewer than 2,000 calories a day and may want to select target levels based on 1,600 calories a day. Some active men and teenage boys and very active women may want to select target levels based on 2,800 calories per day. The Daily Values for sodium and cholesterol are the same for everyone, regardless of total calories consumed, so you do not have to make adjustments based on your caloric needs.

TABLE 6
Daily Values

Nutrient	Calories	2,000	2,500
Total fat*	Less than	65 g	80 g
Saturated fat[†]	Less than	20 g	25 g
Cholesterol	Less than	300 mg	300 mg
Sodium	Less than	2,400 mg	2,400 mg
Total carbohydrate		300 g	375 g
Dietary fiber		25 g	30 g
Potassium		3,500 mg	3,500 mg

*Total fat values are based on 30% of calories. [†] Saturated fat values are based on 10% of calories.
Your Daily Values may be higher or lower depending on your calorie needs. The Daily Values are based on expert dietary advice about how much, or how little, of some key nutrients you should eat each day, depending on whether you eat 2,000 or 2,500 calories a day.
Data from U.S. Food and Drug Administration (1999).

Amount of Total Fat That Provides 30 Percent of Calories and Saturated Fat That Provides 10 Percent

Several scientific groups suggest that Americans moderate the amount of fat in their diets. Some recommend that fat be limited to amounts that will provide no more than 30 percent of calories. Table 7 lists the amount of fat that provides 30 percent of calories for diets at different total daily calorie levels. For example, a woman wishing to moderate her fat intake to 30 percent of her 2,000-calorie diet is advised to select foods that total no more than 65 grams of fat per day. She can use Table 9 to estimate the grams of fat in the foods she eats.

Table 7 also shows the amount of saturated fat that provides 10 percent of calories for diets at several different daily calorie levels. The amounts of saturated fat are given in upper limits because of that type of fat's ability to raise blood cholesterol levels.

TABLE 7
Amount of Total Fat That Provides 30 Percent of Calories and Saturated Fat That Provides 10 Percent

Total Calories per Day	Total Fat (g) (No More Than 30% of Total Calories)	Saturated Fat (g) (No More Than 10% of Total Calories)
1,600	53	18
2,000*	65	20
2,200	73	24
2,500*	80	25
2,800	93	31

*Percent Daily Values on Nutrition Facts Labels are based on a 2,000-calorie diet. Values for 2,000 and 2,500 calories are rounded to the nearest 5 g to be consistent with the label.
Data from U.S. Department of Agriculture and Department of Health and Human Services (2000).

Caffeine Values

Caffeine is a compound found mostly in coffee, tea, cola, cocoa, chocolate, and in foods containing these. Table 8 lists the amounts of caffeine found in these beverages and foods.

TABLE 8
Caffeine Values

Food	Serving Size	Caffeine (mg)
Beverages		
Chocolate milk, includes malted milk	8 fl oz	5-8
Chocolate shake	16 fl oz	8
Cocoa, prepared from powder		
Regular	6 fl oz	4-6
Sugar-free	6 fl oz	15
Coffee, regular		
Brewed	6 fl oz	103
Prepared from instant	6 fl oz	57

(continues)

TABLE 8
Caffeine Values (*continued*)

Coffee, decaffeinated		
Brewed	6 fl oz	2
Prepared from instant	6 fl oz	2
Coffee liqueur	1.5 fl oz	14
Cola or Dr. Pepper–type, with caffeine	12 fl oz	37
Diet cola, with caffeine	12 fl oz	50
Tea, regular		
Brewed	6 fl oz	36
Instant, prepared	8 fl oz	26–36
Tea, chamomile	6 fl oz	0
Tea, decaffeinated, brewed	6 fl oz	2
Chocolate Foods		
Baking chocolate, unsweetened	1 square (1 oz)	58
Brownies	1	1–3
Candies		
Dark chocolate	1.45-oz bar	30
Milk chocolate bar	1.55-oz bar	11
Semisweet chocolate chips	1/4 cup	26–28
Chocolate with other ingredients (nuts, crisped rice, etc.)	about 1.5 oz	3–11
Cereal (containing cocoa)	1 oz	1
Cocoa powder, unsweetened	1 Tbsp.	12
Cookies (chocolate chip, devil's food, chocolate sandwich)	1	1
Chocolate cupcake with chocolate frosting	1	1–2
Frosting	1/12 pkg (2 Tbsp.)	1–2
Fudge	1 piece (about 3/4 oz)	2–3
Ice cream/frozen yogurt	1/2 cup	2
Pudding		
Prepared from dry mix	1/2 cup	3
Ready-to-eat	4 oz	6
Syrup		
Thin-type	1 Tbsp.	3
Fudge-type	1 Tbsp.	1

Data from U.S. Department of Agriculture, Agricultural Research Service (2000).

Nutritive Value of the Edible Part of Food

Table 9 lists the nutritive values of foods commonly consumed in the United States and makes up the bulk of this publication. The data source is USDA Nutrient Database for Standard Reference, Release 13 (U.S. Department of Agriculture, Agricultural Research Service 2000). Most differences in values between this table and the Standard Reference are due to rounding.

Foods are grouped under the following headings:

- Beverages
- Dairy products
- Eggs
- Fats and oils
- Fish and shellfish
- Fruits and fruit juices
- Grain products
- Legumes, nuts, and seeds
- Meat and meat products
- Mixed dishes and fast foods
- Poultry and poultry products
- Soups, sauces, and gravies
- Sugars and sweets
- Vegetables and vegetable products
- Miscellaneous items

Most of the foods listed are in ready-to-eat form. Some are basic products widely used in food preparation, such as flour, oil, and cornmeal. Most snack foods, a separate food group in the Standard Reference, are found under Grain Products.

Measures and Weights

The approximate measure given for each food is in cups, ounces, pounds, some other well-known unit, or a piece of a specified size. The measures do not necessarily represent a serving, but the unit given may be used to calculate a variety of serving sizes. For example, nutrient values are given for 1 cup of applesauce. If the serving you consume is ½ cup, divide the values by 2 or multiply by 0.5.

For fluids, the cup measure refers to the standard measuring cup of 8 fluid ounces. The ounce is one-sixteenth of a pound, unless "fluid ounce" is indicated. The weight of a fluid ounce varies according to the food. If the household measure of a food is listed as 1 ounce, the nutrients are based on a weight of 28.35 grams, rounded to 28 grams in the table. All measure weights are actual weights or rounded to the nearest whole number.

The table gives the weight in grams for an approximate measure of each food. The weight applies to only the edible portion (part of food normally eaten), such as the banana pulp without the peel. Some poultry descriptions provide weights for the whole part, such as a drumstick, including skin and/or bone. Keep in mind that the nutritive values are only for the edible portions indicated in the description. For example, item 877, roasted chicken drumstick, indicates a weight of 2.9 oz (82 grams) with the bone and skin. But note that the weight of one drumstick, meat only, is listed as 44 grams (about ½ oz). So the skin and bone equal 38 grams (82 minus 44). Nutrient values are always given for the gram weight listed in the column Weight—in this case, 44 grams.

Food Values

Values are listed for water; calories; protein; total fat; saturated, monounsaturated, and polyunsaturated fatty acids; cholesterol; carbohydrate; total dietary fiber; four minerals (calcium, iron, potassium, and sodium); and five vitamins (vitamin A, thiamin, riboflavin, niacin, and ascorbic acid, or vitamin C). Water content is included because the percentage of moisture is helpful for identification and comparison of many food items. For example, to identify whether the cocoa listed is powder or prepared, you could check the water value, which is much less for cocoa powder. Values are in grams or milligrams except for water, calories, and vitamin A.

Food energy is reported as calories. A calorie is the unit of measure for the amount of energy that protein, fat, and carbohydrate furnish the body. Alcohol also contributes to the calorie content of alcoholic beverages. The official unit of measurement for food energy is actually kilocalories (kcal), but the term "calories" is commonly used in its place. In fact, "calories" is used on the food label.

Vitamin A is reported in two different units: International Units (IU) are used on food labels and in the past for expressing vitamin A activity; Retinol Equivalents (RE) are the units released in 1989 by the Food and Nutrition Board for expressing the RDAs for vitamin A.

Values for calories and nutrients shown in Table 9 are the amounts in the part of the item that is customarily eaten—corn without cob, meat without bones, and peaches without pits. Nutrient values are averages for products presented here. Values for some nutrients may vary more widely for specific food items. For example, the vitamin A content of beef liver varies widely, but the values listed in Table 9 represent an average for that food.

In some cases, as with many vegetables, values for fat may be trace (Tr), yet there will be numerical values listed for some of the fatty acids. The values for fat have been rounded to whole numbers, unless they are between 0 and 0.5; then they are listed as trace. This definition of trace also applies to the other nutrients in Table 9 that are rounded to whole numbers.

Other uses of "trace" in Table 9 are:

- For nutrients rounded to one decimal place, values falling between 0 and 0.05 are trace.
- For nutrients rounded to two decimal places, values falling between 0 and 0.005 are trace.

Thiamin, riboflavin, niacin, and iron values in enriched white flours, white bread and rolls, cornmeals, pastas, farina, and rice are based on the current enrichment levels established by the Food and Drug Administration. Enrichment levels for riboflavin in rice were not in effect at press time and are not used in Table 9. Enriched flour is used in most home-prepared and commercially prepared baked goods.

Niacin values given are for preformed niacin that occurs naturally in foods. The values do not include additional niacin that may be formed in the body from tryptophan, an essential amino acid in the protein of most foods.

Nutrient values for many prepared items were calculated from the ingredients in typical recipes. Examples are biscuits, cornbread, mashed potatoes, white sauce, and many dessert foods. Adjustments were made for nutrient losses during cooking. Nutrient values for toast and cooked vegetables do not include any added fat, either during preparation or at the table. Cutting or shredding vegetables may destroy part of some vitamins, especially ascorbic acid. Since such losses are variable, no deduction has been made.

Values for cooked dry beans, vegetables, pasta, noodles, rice, cereal, meat, poultry, and fish are without salt added. If hot cereals are prepared with salt, the sodium content ranges from about 324–374 mg for Malt-O-Meal, Cream of Wheat, and rolled oats. The sodium value for corn grits is about 540 mg; sodium for Wheatena is about 238 mg. Sodium values for canned vegetables labeled as "no salt added" are similar to those listed for the cooked vegetables.

The mineral contribution of water was not considered for coffee, tea, soups, sauces, or concentrated fruit juices prepared with water. Sweetened items contain sugar unless identified as artificially sweetened.

Several manufactured items—including some milk products, ready-to-eat breakfast cereals, imitation cream products, fruit drinks, and various mixes—are included in Table 9. Such foods may be fortified with one or more nutrients; the label will describe any fortification. Values for these foods may be based on products from several manufacturers, so they may differ from the values provided by any one source. Nutrient values listed on food labels may also differ from those in Table 9 because of rounding on labels.

Nutrient values represent meats after they have been cooked and drained of the drippings. For many cuts, two sets of values are shown: meat including lean and fat parts, and lean meat from which the outer fat layer and large fat pads have been removed either before or after cooking.

In the entries for cheeseburger and hamburger in Mixed Dishes and Fast Foods, "condiments" refers to catsup, mustard, salt, and pepper; "vegetables" refers to lettuce, tomato, onion, and pickle; "regular" is a 2-oz patty, and large is a 4-oz patty (precooked weight).

Table 9. Nutritive Value of the Edible Part of Food

Food No.	Food Description	Measure of edible portion	Weight (g)	Water (%)	Calories (kcal)	Pro-tein (g)	Total fat (g)	Fatty acids		
								Satu-rated (g)	Mono-unsatu-rated (g)	Poly-unsatu-rated (g)

Beverages

Alcoholic
  Beer

1	Regular	12 fl oz	355	92	146	1	0	0.0	0.0	0.0
2	Light	12 fl oz	354	95	99	1	0	0.0	0.0	0.0

  Gin, rum, vodka, whiskey

3	80 proof	1.5 fl oz	42	67	97	0	0	0.0	0.0	0.0
4	86 proof	1.5 fl oz	42	64	105	0	0	0.0	0.0	0.0
5	90 proof	1.5 fl oz	42	62	110	0	0	0.0	0.0	0.0
6	Liqueur, coffee, 53 proof	1.5 fl oz	52	31	175	Tr	Tr	0.1	Tr	0.1

  Mixed drinks, prepared from recipe

7	Daiquiri	2 fl oz	60	70	112	Tr	Tr	Tr	Tr	Tr
8	Pina colada	4.5 fl oz	141	65	262	1	3	1.2	0.2	0.5

  Wine
    Dessert

9	Dry	3.5 fl oz	103	80	130	Tr	0	0.0	0.0	0.0
10	Sweet	3.5 fl oz	103	73	158	Tr	0	0.0	0.0	0.0

    Table

11	Red	3.5 fl oz	103	89	74	Tr	0	0.0	0.0	0.0
12	White	3.5 fl oz	103	90	70	Tr	0	0.0	0.0	0.0

Carbonated*

13	Club soda	12 fl oz	355	100	0	0	0	0.0	0.0	0.0
14	Cola type	12 fl oz	370	89	152	0	0	0.0	0.0	0.0

  Diet, sweetened with aspartame

15	Cola	12 fl oz	355	100	4	Tr	0	0.0	0.0	0.0
16	Other than cola or pepper type	12 fl oz	355	100	0	Tr	0	0.0	0.0	0.0
17	Ginger ale	12 fl oz	366	91	124	0	0	0.0	0.0	0.0
18	Grape	12 fl oz	372	89	160	0	0	0.0	0.0	0.0
19	Lemon lime	12 fl oz	368	90	147	0	0	0.0	0.0	0.0
20	Orange	12 fl oz	372	88	179	0	0	0.0	0.0	0.0
21	Pepper type	12 fl oz	368	89	151	0	Tr	0.3	0.0	0.0
22	Root beer	12 fl oz	370	89	152	0	0	0.0	0.0	0.0

Chocolate flavored beverage mix

23	Powder	2-3 heaping tsp	22	1	75	1	1	0.4	0.2	Tr
24	Prepared with milk	1 cup	266	81	226	9	9	5.5	2.6	0.3

Cocoa
  Powder containing nonfat dry milk

25	Powder	3 heaping tsp	28	2	102	3	1	0.7	0.4	Tr
26	Prepared (6 oz water plus 1 oz powder)	1 serving	206	86	103	3	1	0.7	0.4	Tr

  Powder containing nonfat dry milk and aspartame

27	Powder	½-oz envelope	15	3	48	4	Tr	0.3	0.1	Tr
28	Prepared (6 oz water plus 1 envelope mix)	1 serving	192	92	48	4	Tr	0.3	0.1	Tr

Coffee

29	Brewed	6 fl oz	178	99	4	Tr	0	Tr	0.0	Tr
30	Espresso	2 fl oz	60	98	5	Tr	Tr	0.1	0.0	0.1
31	Instant, prepared (1 rounded tsp powder plus 6 fl oz water)	6 fl oz	179	99	4	Tr	0	Tr	0.0	Tr

*Mineral content varies depending on water source.

Choles-terol (mg)	Carbo-hydrate (g)	Total dietary fiber (g)	Calcium (mg)	Iron (mg)	Potas-sium (mg)	Sodium (mg)	Vitamin A (IU)	Vitamin A (RE)	Thiamin (mg)	Ribo-flavin (mg)	Niacin (mg)	Ascor-bic acid (mg)	Food No.
0	13	0.7	18	0.1	89	18	0	0	0.02	0.09	1.6	0	1
0	5	0.0	18	0.1	64	11	0	0	0.03	0.11	1.4	0	2
0	0	0.0	0	Tr	1	Tr	0	0	Tr	Tr	Tr	0	3
0	Tr	0.0	0	Tr	1	Tr	0	0	Tr	Tr	Tr	0	4
0	0	0.0	0	Tr	1	Tr	0	0	Tr	Tr	Tr	0	5
0	24	0.0	1	Tr	16	4	0	0	Tr	0.01	0.1	0	6
0	4	0.0	2	0.1	13	3	2	0	0.01	Tr	Tr	1	7
0	40	0.8	11	0.3	100	8	3	0	0.04	0.02	0.2	7	8
0	4	0.0	8	0.2	95	9	0	0	0.02	0.02	0.2	0	9
0	12	0.0	8	0.2	95	9	0	0	0.02	0.02	0.2	0	10
0	2	0.0	8	0.4	115	5	0	0	0.01	0.03	0.1	0	11
0	1	0.0	9	0.3	82	5	0	0	Tr	0.01	0.1	0	12
0	0	0.0	18	Tr	7	75	0	0	0.00	0.00	0.0	0	13
0	38	0.0	11	0.1	4	15	0	0	0.00	0.00	0.0	0	14
0	Tr	0.0	14	0.1	0	21	0	0	0.02	0.08	0.0	0	15
0	0	0.0	14	0.1	7	21	0	0	0.00	0.00	0.0	0	16
0	32	0.0	11	0.7	4	26	0	0	0.00	0.00	0.0	0	17
0	42	0.0	11	0.3	4	56	0	0	0.00	0.00	0.0	0	18
0	38	0.0	7	0.3	4	40	0	0	0.00	0.00	0.1	0	19
0	46	0.0	19	0.2	7	45	0	0	0.00	0.00	0.0	0	20
0	38	0.0	11	0.1	4	37	0	0	0.00	0.00	0.0	0	21
0	39	0.0	19	0.2	4	48	0	0	0.00	0.00	0.0	0	22
0	20	1.3	8	0.7	128	45	4	Tr	0.01	0.03	0.1	Tr	23
32	31	1.3	301	0.8	497	165	311	77	0.10	0.43	0.3	2	24
1	22	0.3	92	0.3	202	143	4	1	0.03	0.16	0.2	1	25
2	22	2.5	97	0.4	202	148	4	0	0.03	0.16	0.2	Tr	26
1	9	0.4	86	0.7	405	168	5	1	0.04	0.21	0.2	0	27
2	8	0.4	90	0.7	405	173	4	0	0.04	0.21	0.2	0	28
0	1	0.0	4	0.1	96	4	0	0	0.00	0.00	0.4	0	29
0	1	0.0	1	0.1	69	8	0	0	Tr	0.11	3.1	Tr	30
0	1	0.0	5	0.1	64	5	0	0	0.00	Tr	0.5	0	31

Table 9.   Nutritive Value of the Edible Part of Food

Food No.	Food Description	Measure of edible portion	Weight (g)	Water (%)	Calories (kcal)	Pro-tein (g)	Total fat (g)	Fatty acids Satu-rated (g)	Mono-unsatu-rated (g)	Poly-unsatu-rated (g)

Beverages (continued)

Fruit drinks, noncarbonated, canned or bottled, with added ascorbic acid

32	Cranberry juice cocktail	8 fl oz	253	86	144	0	Tr	Tr	Tr	0.1
33	Fruit punch drink	8 fl oz	248	88	117	0	0	Tr	Tr	Tr
34	Grape drink	8 fl oz	250	88	113	0	0	Tr	0.0	Tr
35	Pineapple grapefruit juice drink	8 fl oz	250	88	118	1	Tr	Tr	Tr	0.1
36	Pineapple orange juice drink	8 fl oz	250	87	125	3	0	0.0	0.0	0.0
	Lemonade									
37	Frozen concentrate, prepared	8 fl oz	248	89	99	Tr	0	Tr	Tr	Tr
	Powder, prepared with water									
38	Regular	8 fl oz	266	89	112	0	0	Tr	Tr	Tr
39	Low calorie, sweetened with aspartame	8 fl oz	237	99	5	0	0	0.0	0.0	0.0
	Malted milk, with added nutrients									
	Chocolate									
40	Powder	3 heaping tsp	21	3	75	1	1	0.4	0.2	0.1
41	Prepared	1 cup	265	81	225	9	9	5.5	2.6	0.4
	Natural									
42	Powder	4-5 heaping tsp	21	3	80	2	1	0.3	0.2	0.1
43	Prepared	1 cup	265	81	231	10	9	5.4	2.5	0.4
	Milk and milk beverages. See Dairy Products.									
44	Rice beverage, canned (RICE DREAM)	1 cup	245	89	120	Tr	2	0.2	1.3	0.3
	Soy milk. See Legumes, Nuts, and Seeds.									
	Tea									
	Brewed									
45	Black	6 fl oz	178	100	2	0	0	Tr	Tr	Tr
	Herb									
46	Chamomile	6 fl oz	178	100	2	0	0	Tr	Tr	Tr
47	Other than chamomile	6 fl oz	178	100	2	0	0	Tr	Tr	Tr
	Instant, powder, prepared									
48	Unsweetened	8 fl oz	237	100	2	0	0	0.0	0.0	0.0
49	Sweetened, lemon flavor	8 fl oz	259	91	88	Tr	0	Tr	Tr	Tr
50	Sweetened with saccharin, lemon flavor	8 fl oz	237	99	5	0	0	0.0	0.0	Tr
51	Water, tap	8 fl oz	237	100	0	0	0	0.0	0.0	0.0

Dairy Products

Butter. See Fats and Oils.
Cheese
Natural

52	Blue	1 oz	28	42	100	6	8	5.3	2.2	0.2
53	Camembert (3 wedges per 4-oz container)	1 wedge	38	52	114	8	9	5.8	2.7	0.3
	Cheddar									
54	Cut pieces	1 oz	28	37	114	7	9	6.0	2.7	0.3
55		1 cubic inch	17	37	68	4	6	3.6	1.6	0.2
56	Shredded	1 cup	113	37	455	28	37	23.8	10.6	1.1

| Choles-terol (mg) | Carbo-hydrate (g) | Total dietary fiber (g) | Calcium (mg) | Iron (mg) | Potas-sium (mg) | Sodium (mg) | Vitamin A | | Thiamin (mg) | Ribo-flavin (mg) | Niacin (mg) | Ascor-bic acid (mg) | Food No. |
							(IU)	(RE)					
0	36	0.3	8	0.4	46	5	10	0	0.02	0.02	0.1	90	32
0	30	0.2	20	0.5	62	55	35	2	0.05	0.06	0.1	73	33
0	29	0.0	8	0.4	13	15	3	0	0.01	0.01	0.1	85	34
0	29	0.3	18	0.8	153	35	88	10	0.08	0.04	0.7	115	35
0	30	0.3	13	0.7	115	8	1,328	133	0.08	0.05	0.5	56	36
0	26	0.2	7	0.4	37	7	52	5	0.01	0.05	Tr	10	37
0	29	0.0	29	0.1	3	19	0	0	0.00	Tr	0.0	34	38
0	1	0.0	50	0.1	0	7	0	0	0.00	0.00	0.0	6	39
1	18	0.2	93	3.6	251	125	2,751	824	0.64	0.86	10.7	32	40
34	29	0.3	384	3.8	620	244	3,058	901	0.73	1.26	10.9	34	41
4	17	0.1	79	3.5	203	85	2,222	668	0.62	0.75	10.2	27	42
34	28	0.0	371	3.6	572	204	2,531	742	0.71	1.14	10.4	29	43
0	25	0.0	20	0.2	69	86	5	0	0.08	0.01	1.9	1	44
0	1	0.0	0	Tr	66	5	0	0	0.00	0.02	0.0	0	45
0	Tr	0.0	4	0.1	16	2	36	4	0.02	0.01	0.0	0	46
0	Tr	0.0	4	0.1	16	2	0	0	0.02	0.01	0.0	0	47
0	Tr	0.0	5	Tr	47	7	0	0	0.00	Tr	0.1	0	48
0	22	0.0	5	0.1	49	8	0	0	0.00	0.05	0.1	0	49
0	1	0.0	5	0.1	40	24	0	0	0.00	0.01	0.1	0	50
0	0	0.0	5	Tr	0	7	0	0	0.00	0.00	0.0	0	51
21	1	0.0	150	0.1	73	396	204	65	0.01	0.11	0.3	0	52
27	Tr	0.0	147	0.1	71	320	351	96	0.01	0.19	0.2	0	53
30	Tr	0.0	204	0.2	28	176	300	79	0.01	0.11	Tr	0	54
18	Tr	0.0	123	0.1	17	105	180	47	Tr	0.06	Tr	0	55
119	1	0.0	815	0.8	111	701	1,197	314	0.03	0.42	0.1	0	56

Table 9.   Nutritive Value of the Edible Part of Food

Food No.	Food Description	Measure of edible portion	Weight (g)	Water (%)	Calories (kcal)	Protein (g)	Total fat (g)	Fatty acids Saturated (g)	Mono-unsaturated (g)	Poly-unsaturated (g)

Dairy Products (continued)

Cheese (continued)
Natural (continued)
Cottage
Creamed (4% fat)

No.	Food Description	Measure	Weight	Water	Calories	Protein	Total fat	Saturated	Mono	Poly
57	Large curd	1 cup ...225		79	233	28	10	6.4	2.9	0.3
58	Small curd	1 cup ...210		79	217	26	9	6.0	2.7	0.3
59	With fruit	1 cup ...226		72	279	22	8	4.9	2.2	0.2
60	Low fat (2%)	1 cup ...226		79	203	31	4	2.8	1.2	0.1
61	Low fat (1%)	1 cup ...226		82	164	28	2	1.5	0.7	0.1
62	Uncreamed (dry curd, less than ½% fat)	1 cup ...145		80	123	25	1	0.4	0.2	Tr
	Cream									
63	Regular	1 oz ...28		54	99	2	10	6.2	2.8	0.4
64		1 tbsp ...15		54	51	1	5	3.2	1.4	0.2
65	Low fat	1 tbsp ...15		64	35	2	3	1.7	0.7	0.1
66	Fat free	1 tbsp ...16		76	15	2	Tr	0.1	0.1	Tr
67	Feta	1 oz ...28		55	75	4	6	4.2	1.3	0.2
68	Low fat, cheddar or colby	1 oz ...28		63	49	7	2	1.2	0.6	0.1
	Mozzarella, made with									
69	Whole milk	1 oz ...28		54	80	6	6	3.7	1.9	0.2
70	Part skim milk (low moisture)	1 oz ...28		49	79	8	5	3.1	1.4	0.1
71	Muenster	1 oz ...28		42	104	7	9	5.4	2.5	0.2
72	Neufchatel	1 oz ...28		62	74	3	7	4.2	1.9	0.2
73	Parmesan, grated	1 cup ...100		18	456	42	30	19.1	8.7	0.7
74		1 tbsp ...5		18	23	2	2	1.0	0.4	Tr
75		1 oz ...28		18	129	12	9	5.4	2.5	0.2
76	Provolone	1 oz ...28		41	100	7	8	4.8	2.1	0.2
	Ricotta, made with									
77	Whole milk	1 cup ...246		72	428	28	32	20.4	8.9	0.9
78	Part skim milk	1 cup ...246		74	340	28	19	12.1	5.7	0.6
79	Swiss	1 oz ...28		37	107	8	8	5.0	2.1	0.3
	Pasteurized process cheese American									
80	Regular	1 oz ...28		39	106	6	9	5.6	2.5	0.3
81	Fat free	1 slice ...21		57	31	5	Tr	0.1	Tr	Tr
82	Swiss	1 oz ...28		42	95	7	7	4.5	2.0	0.2
83	Pasteurized process cheese food, American	1 oz ...28		43	93	6	7	4.4	2.0	0.2
84	Pasteurized process cheese spread, American	1 oz ...28		48	82	5	6	3.8	1.8	0.2
	Cream, sweet									
85	Half and half (cream and milk)	1 cup ...242		81	315	7	28	17.3	8.0	1.0
86		1 tbsp ...15		81	20	Tr	2	1.1	0.5	0.1
87	Light, coffee, or table	1 cup ...240		74	469	6	46	28.8	13.4	1.7
88		1 tbsp ...15		74	29	Tr	3	1.8	0.8	0.1
	Whipping, unwhipped (volume about double when whipped)									
89	Light	1 cup ...239		64	699	5	74	46.2	21.7	2.1
90		1 tbsp ...15		64	44	Tr	5	2.9	1.4	0.1
91	Heavy	1 cup ...238		58	821	5	88	54.8	25.4	3.3
92		1 tbsp ...15		58	52	Tr	6	3.5	1.6	0.2
93	Whipped topping (pressurized)	1 cup ...60		61	154	2	13	8.3	3.9	0.5
94		1 tbsp ...3		61	8	Tr	1	0.4	0.2	Tr

Choles-terol (mg)	Carbo-hydrate (g)	Total dietary fiber (g)	Calcium (mg)	Iron (mg)	Potas-sium (mg)	Sodium (mg)	Vitamin A (IU)	(RE)	Thiamin (mg)	Ribo-flavin (mg)	Niacin (mg)	Ascor-bic acid (mg)	Food No.
34	6	0.0	135	0.3	190	911	367	108	0.05	0.37	0.3	0	57
31	6	0.0	126	0.3	177	850	342	101	0.04	0.34	0.3	0	58
25	30	0.0	108	0.2	151	915	278	81	0.04	0.29	0.2	0	59
19	8	0.0	155	0.4	217	918	158	45	0.05	0.42	0.3	0	60
10	6	0.0	138	0.3	193	918	84	25	0.05	0.37	0.3	0	61
10	3	0.0	46	0.3	47	19	44	12	0.04	0.21	0.2	0	62
31	1	0.0	23	0.3	34	84	405	108	Tr	0.06	Tr	0	63
16	Tr	0.0	12	0.2	17	43	207	55	Tr	0.03	Tr	0	64
8	1	0.0	17	0.3	25	44	108	33	Tr	0.04	Tr	0	65
1	1	0.0	29	Tr	25	85	145	44	0.01	0.03	Tr	0	66
25	1	0.0	140	0.2	18	316	127	36	0.04	0.24	0.3	0	67
6	1	0.0	118	0.1	19	174	66	18	Tr	0.06	Tr	0	68
22	1	0.0	147	0.1	19	106	225	68	Tr	0.07	Tr	0	69
15	1	0.0	207	0.1	27	150	199	54	0.01	0.10	Tr	0	70
27	Tr	0.0	203	0.1	38	178	318	90	Tr	0.09	Tr	0	71
22	1	0.0	21	0.1	32	113	321	85	Tr	0.06	Tr	0	72
79	4	0.0	1,376	1.0	107	1,862	701	173	0.05	0.39	0.3	0	73
4	Tr	0.0	69	Tr	5	93	35	9	Tr	0.02	Tr	0	74
22	1	0.0	390	0.3	30	528	199	49	0.01	0.11	0.1	0	75
20	1	0.0	214	0.1	39	248	231	75	0.01	0.09	Tr	0	76
124	7	0.0	509	0.9	257	207	1,205	330	0.03	0.48	0.3	0	77
76	13	0.0	669	1.1	308	307	1,063	278	0.05	0.46	0.2	0	78
26	1	0.0	272	Tr	31	74	240	72	0.01	0.10	Tr	0	79
27	Tr	0.0	174	0.1	46	406	343	82	0.01	0.10	Tr	0	80
2	3	0.0	145	0.1	60	321	308	92	0.01	0.10	Tr	0	81
24	1	0.0	219	0.2	61	388	229	65	Tr	0.08	Tr	0	82
18	2	0.0	163	0.2	79	337	259	62	0.01	0.13	Tr	0	83
16	2	0.0	159	0.1	69	381	223	54	0.01	0.12	Tr	0	84
89	10	0.0	254	0.2	314	98	1,050	259	0.08	0.36	0.2	2	85
6	1	0.0	16	Tr	19	6	65	16	0.01	0.02	Tr	Tr	86
159	9	0.0	231	0.1	292	95	1,519	437	0.08	0.36	0.1	2	87
10	1	0.0	14	Tr	18	6	95	27	Tr	0.02	Tr	Tr	88
265	7	0.0	166	0.1	231	82	2,694	705	0.06	0.30	0.1	1	89
17	Tr	0.0	10	Tr	15	5	169	44	Tr	0.02	Tr	Tr	90
326	7	0.0	154	0.1	179	89	3,499	1,002	0.05	0.26	0.1	1	91
21	Tr	0.0	10	Tr	11	6	221	63	Tr	0.02	Tr	Tr	92
46	7	0.0	61	Tr	88	78	506	124	0.02	0.04	Tr	0	93
2	Tr	0.0	3	Tr	4	4	25	6	Tr	Tr	Tr	0	94

Table 9. Nutritive Value of the Edible Part of Food

Food No.	Food Description	Measure of edible portion	Weight (g)	Water (%)	Calories (kcal)	Protein (g)	Total fat (g)	Fatty acids Saturated (g)	Mono-unsaturated (g)	Poly-unsaturated (g)

Dairy Products (continued)

	Cream, sour									
95	Regular	1 cup	230	71	493	7	48	30.0	13.9	1.8
96		1 tbsp	12	71	26	Tr	3	1.6	0.7	0.1
97	Reduced fat	1 tbsp	15	80	20	Tr	2	1.1	0.5	0.1
98	Fat free	1 tbsp	16	81	12	Tr	0	0.0	0.0	0.0
	Cream product, imitation (made with vegetable fat)									
	Sweet									
	Creamer									
99	Liquid (frozen)	1 tbsp	15	77	20	Tr	1	0.3	1.1	Tr
100	Powdered	1 tsp	2	2	11	Tr	1	0.7	Tr	Tr
	Whipped topping									
101	Frozen	1 cup	75	50	239	1	19	16.3	1.2	0.4
102		1 tbsp	4	50	13	Tr	1	0.9	0.1	Tr
103	Powdered, prepared with whole milk	1 cup	80	67	151	3	10	8.5	0.7	0.2
104		1 tbsp	4	67	8	Tr	Tr	0.4	Tr	Tr
105	Pressurized	1 cup	70	60	184	1	16	13.2	1.3	0.2
106		1 tbsp	4	60	11	Tr	1	0.8	0.1	Tr
107	Sour dressing (filled cream type, nonbutterfat)	1 cup	235	75	417	8	39	31.2	4.6	1.1
108		1 tbsp	12	75	21	Tr	2	1.6	0.2	0.1
	Frozen dessert									
	Frozen yogurt, soft serve									
109	Chocolate	½ cup.................	72	64	115	3	4	2.6	1.3	0.2
110	Vanilla	½ cup.................	72	65	114	3	4	2.5	1.1	0.2
	Ice cream									
	Regular									
111	Chocolate..............................	½ cup.................	66	56	143	3	7	4.5	2.1	0.3
112	Vanilla..................................	½ cup.................	66	61	133	2	7	4.5	2.1	0.3
113	Light (50% reduced fat), vanilla..................	½ cup.................	66	68	92	3	3	1.7	0.8	0.1
114	Premium low fat, chocolate	½ cup.................	72	61	113	3	2	1.0	0.6	0.1
115	Rich, vanilla	½ cup.................	74	57	178	3	12	7.4	3.4	0.4
116	Soft serve, french vanilla.....	½ cup.................	86	60	185	4	11	6.4	3.0	0.4
117	Sherbet, orange	½ cup.................	74	66	102	1	1	0.9	0.4	0.1
	Milk									
	Fluid, no milk solids added									
118	Whole (3.3% fat)	1 cup	244	88	150	8	8	5.1	2.4	0.3
119	Reduced fat (2%)	1 cup	244	89	121	8	5	2.9	1.4	0.2
120	Lowfat (1%)	1 cup	244	90	102	8	3	1.6	0.7	0.1
121	Nonfat (skim)	1 cup	245	91	86	8	Tr	0.3	0.1	Tr
122	Buttermilk	1 cup	245	90	99	8	2	1.3	0.6	0.1
	Canned									
123	Condensed, sweetened.........	1 cup	306	27	982	24	27	16.8	7.4	1.0
	Evaporated									
124	Whole milk..........................	1 cup	252	74	339	17	19	11.6	5.9	0.6
125	Skim milk	1 cup	256	79	199	19	1	0.3	0.2	Tr
	Dried									
126	Buttermilk	1 cup	120	3	464	41	7	4.3	2.0	0.3
127	Nonfat, instant, with added vitamin A	1 cup	68	4	244	24	Tr	0.3	0.1	Tr
	Milk beverage									
	Chocolate milk (commercial)									
128	Whole	1 cup	250	82	208	8	8	5.3	2.5	0.3
129	Reduced fat (2%)	1 cup	250	84	179	8	5	3.1	1.5	0.2
130	Lowfat (1%)	1 cup	250	85	158	8	3	1.5	0.8	0.1

*The vitamin A values listed for imitation sweet cream products are mostly from beta-carotene added for coloring.

Choles-terol (mg)	Carbo-hydrate (g)	Total dietary fiber (g)	Calcium (mg)	Iron (mg)	Potas-sium (mg)	Sodium (mg)	Vitamin A		Thiamin (mg)	Ribo-flavin (mg)	Niacin (mg)	Ascor-bic acid (mg)	Food No.
							(IU)	(RE)					
102	10	0.0	268	0.1	331	123	1,817	449	0.08	0.34	0.2	2	95
5	1	0.0	14	Tr	17	6	95	23	Tr	0.02	Tr	Tr	96
6	1	0.0	16	Tr	19	6	68	17	0.01	0.02	Tr	Tr	97
1	2	0.0	20	0.0	21	23	100	13	0.01	0.02	Tr	0	98
0	2	0.0	1	Tr	29	12	13*	1*	0.00	0.00	0.0	0	99
0	1	0.0	Tr	Tr	16	4	4	Tr	0.00	Tr	0.0	0	100
0	17	0.0	5	0.1	14	19	646*	65*	0.00	0.00	0.0	0	101
0	1	0.0	Tr	Tr	1	1	34*	3*	0.00	0.00	0.0	0	102
8	13	0.0	72	Tr	121	53	289*	39*	0.02	0.09	Tr	1	103
Tr	1	0.0	4	Tr	6	3	14*	2*	Tr	Tr	Tr	Tr	104
0	11	0.0	4	Tr	13	43	331*	33*	0.00	0.00	0.0	0	105
0	1	0.0	Tr	Tr	1	2	19*	2*	0.00	0.00	0.0	0	106
13	11	0.0	266	0.1	380	113	24	5	0.09	0.38	0.2	2	107
1	1	0.0	14	Tr	19	6	1	Tr	Tr	0.02	Tr	Tr	108
4	18	1.6	106	0.9	188	71	115	31	0.03	0.15	0.2	Tr	109
1	17	0.0	103	0.2	152	63	153	41	0.03	0.16	0.2	1	110
22	19	0.8	72	0.6	164	50	275	79	0.03	0.13	0.1	Tr	111
29	16	0.0	84	0.1	131	53	270	77	0.03	0.16	0.1	Tr	112
9	15	0.0	92	0.1	139	56	109	31	0.04	0.17	0.1	1	113
7	22	0.7	107	0.4	179	50	163	47	0.02	0.13	0.1	1	114
45	17	0.0	87	Tr	118	41	476	136	0.03	0.12	0.1	1	115
78	19	0.0	113	0.2	152	52	464	132	0.04	0.16	0.1	1	116
4	22	0.0	40	0.1	71	34	56	10	0.02	0.06	Tr	2	117
33	11	0.0	291	0.1	370	120	307	76	0.09	0.40	0.2	2	118
18	12	0.0	297	0.1	377	122	500	139	0.10	0.40	0.2	2	119
10	12	0.0	300	0.1	381	123	500	144	0.10	0.41	0.2	2	120
4	12	0.0	302	0.1	406	126	500	149	0.09	0.34	0.2	2	121
9	12	0.0	285	0.1	371	257	81	20	0.08	0.38	0.1	2	122
104	166	0.0	868	0.6	1,136	389	1,004	248	0.28	1.27	0.6	8	123
74	25	0.0	657	0.5	764	267	612	136	0.12	0.80	0.5	5	124
9	29	0.0	741	0.7	849	294	1,004	300	0.12	0.79	0.4	3	125
83	59	0.0	1,421	0.4	1,910	621	262	65	0.47	1.89	1.1	7	126
12	35	0.0	837	0.2	1,160	373	1,612	483	0.28	1.19	0.6	4	127
31	26	2.0	280	0.6	417	149	303	73	0.09	0.41	0.3	2	128
17	26	1.3	284	0.6	422	151	500	143	0.09	0.41	0.3	2	129
7	26	1.3	287	0.6	426	152	500	148	0.10	0.42	0.3	2	130

Table 9. Nutritive Value of the Edible Part of Food

Food No.	Food Description	Measure of edible portion	Weight (g)	Water (%)	Calories (kcal)	Pro-tein (g)	Total fat (g)	Fatty acids Satu-rated (g)	Mono-unsatu-rated (g)	Poly-unsatu-rated (g)
	Dairy Products (continued)									
	Milk beverage (continued)									
131	Eggnog (commercial)	1 cup 254		74	342	10	19	11.3	5.7	0.9
	Milk shake, thick									
132	Chocolate	10.6 fl oz 300		72	356	9	8	5.0	2.3	0.3
133	Vanilla	11 fl oz 313		74	350	12	9	5.9	2.7	0.4
	Sherbet. See Dairy Products, frozen dessert.									
	Yogurt									
	With added milk solids									
	Made with lowfat milk									
134	Fruit flavored....................	8-oz container ...227		74	231	10	2	1.6	0.7	0.1
135	Plain.................................	8-oz container ...227		85	144	12	4	2.3	1.0	0.1
	Made with nonfat milk									
136	Fruit flavored....................	8-oz container ...227		75	213	10	Tr	0.3	0.1	Tr
137	Plain.................................	8-oz container ...227		85	127	13	Tr	0.3	0.1	Tr
	Without added milk solids									
138	Made with whole milk, plain	8-oz container ...227		88	139	8	7	4.8	2.0	0.2
139	Made with nonfat milk, low calorie sweetener, vanilla or lemon flavor ...	8-oz container ...227		87	98	9	Tr	0.3	0.1	Tr
	Eggs									
	Egg									
	Raw									
140	Whole	1 medium 44		75	66	5	4	1.4	1.7	0.6
141		1 large.................50		75	75	6	5	1.6	1.9	0.7
142		1 extra large........58		75	86	7	6	1.8	2.2	0.8
143	White	1 large.................33		88	17	4	0	0.0	0.0	0.0
144	Yolk	1 large.................17		49	59	3	5	1.6	1.9	0.7
	Cooked, whole									
145	Fried, in margarine, with salt...........................	1 large.................46		69	92	6	7	1.9	2.7	1.3
146	Hard cooked, shell removed........................	1 large.................50		75	78	6	5	1.6	2.0	0.7
147		1 cup, chopped 136		75	211	17	14	4.4	5.5	1.9
148	Poached, with salt...............	1 large.................50		75	75	6	5	1.5	1.9	0.7
149	Scrambled, in margarine, with whole milk, salt......	1 large.................61		73	101	7	7	2.2	2.9	1.3
150	Egg substitute, liquid	¼ cup.....................63		83	53	8	2	0.4	0.6	1.0
	Fats and Oils									
	Butter (4 sticks per lb)									
151	Salted	1 stick 113		16	813	1	92	57.3	26.6	3.4
152		1 tbsp 14		16	102	Tr	12	7.2	3.3	0.4
153		1 tsp 5		16	36	Tr	4	2.5	1.2	0.2
154	Unsalted	1 stick 113		18	813	1	92	57.3	26.6	3.4
155	Lard	1 cup 205		0	1,849	0	205	80.4	92.5	23.0
156		1 tbsp 13		0	115	0	13	5.0	5.8	1.4
	Margarine, vitamin A-fortified, salt added									
	Regular (about 80% fat)									
157	Hard (4 sticks per lb)	1 stick 113		16	815	1	91	17.9	40.6	28.8
158		1 tbsp 14		16	101	Tr	11	2.2	5.0	3.6
159		1 tsp 5		16	34	Tr	4	0.7	1.7	1.2
160	Soft	1 cup 227		16	1,626	2	183	31.3	64.7	78.5
161		1 tsp 5		16	34	Tr	4	0.6	1.3	1.6

Choles-terol (mg)	Carbo-hydrate (g)	Total dietary fiber (g)	Calcium (mg)	Iron (mg)	Potas-sium (mg)	Sodium (mg)	Vitamin A		Thiamin (mg)	Ribo-flavin (mg)	Niacin (mg)	Ascor-bic acid (mg)	Food No.
							(IU)	(RE)					
149	34	0.0	330	0.5	420	138	894	203	0.09	0.48	0.3	4	131
32	63	0.9	396	0.9	672	333	258	63	0.14	0.67	0.4	0	132
37	56	0.0	457	0.3	572	299	357	88	0.09	0.61	0.5	0	133
10	43	0.0	345	0.2	442	133	104	25	0.08	0.40	0.2	1	134
14	16	0.0	415	0.2	531	159	150	36	0.10	0.49	0.3	2	135
5	43	0.0	345	0.2	440	132	16	5	0.09	0.41	0.2	2	136
4	17	0.0	452	0.2	579	174	16	5	0.11	0.53	0.3	2	137
29	11	0.0	274	0.1	351	105	279	68	0.07	0.32	0.2	1	138
5	17	0.0	325	0.3	402	134	0	0	0.08	0.37	0.2	2	139
187	1	0.0	22	0.6	53	55	279	84	0.03	0.22	Tr	0	140
213	1	0.0	25	0.7	61	63	318	96	0.03	0.25	Tr	0	141
247	1	0.0	28	0.8	70	73	368	111	0.04	0.29	Tr	0	142
0	Tr	0.0	2	Tr	48	55	0	0	Tr	0.15	Tr	0	143
213	Tr	0.0	23	0.6	16	7	323	97	0.03	0.11	Tr	0	144
211	1	0.0	25	0.7	61	162	394	114	0.03	0.24	Tr	0	145
212	1	0.0	25	0.6	63	62	280	84	0.03	0.26	Tr	0	146
577	2	0.0	68	1.6	171	169	762	228	0.09	0.70	0.1	0	147
212	1	0.0	25	0.7	60	140	316	95	0.02	0.22	Tr	0	148
215	1	0.0	43	0.7	84	171	416	119	0.03	0.27	Tr	Tr	149
1	Tr	0.0	33	1.3	208	112	1,361	136	0.07	0.19	0.1	0	150
248	Tr	0.0	27	0.2	29	937	3,468	855	0.01	0.04	Tr	0	151
31	Tr	0.0	3	Tr	4	117	434	107	Tr	Tr	Tr	0	152
11	Tr	0.0	1	Tr	1	41	153	38	Tr	Tr	Tr	0	153
248	Tr	0.0	27	0.2	29	12	3,468	855	0.01	0.04	Tr	0	154
195	0	0.0	Tr	0.0	Tr	Tr	0	0	0.00	0.00	0.0	0	155
12	0	0.0	Tr	0.0	Tr	Tr	0	0	0.00	0.00	0.0	0	156
0	1	0.0	34	0.1	48	1,070	4,050	906	0.01	0.04	Tr	Tr	157
0	Tr	0.0	4	Tr	6	132	500	112	Tr	0.01	Tr	Tr	158
0	Tr	0.0	1	Tr	2	44	168	38	Tr	Tr	Tr	Tr	159
0	1	0.0	60	0.0	86	2,449	8,106	1,814	0.02	0.07	Tr	Tr	160
0	Tr	0.0	1	0.0	2	51	168	38	Tr	Tr	Tr	Tr	161

Table 9. Nutritive Value of the Edible Part of Food

Food No.	Food Description	Measure of edible portion	Weight (g)	Water (%)	Calories (kcal)	Pro-tein (g)	Total fat (g)	Fatty acids Satu-rated (g)	Mono-unsatu-rated (g)	Poly-unsatu-rated (g)
	Fats and Oils (continued)									
	Margarine, vitamin A-fortified, salt added (continued)									
	Spread (about 60% fat)									
162	Hard (4 sticks per lb)	1 stick	115	37	621	1	70	16.2	29.9	20.8
163		1 tbsp	14	37	76	Tr	9	2.0	3.6	2.5
164		1 tsp	5	37	26	Tr	3	0.7	1.2	0.9
165	Soft	1 cup	229	37	1,236	1	139	29.3	72.1	31.6
166		1 tsp	5	37	26	Tr	3	0.6	1.5	0.7
167	Spread (about 40% fat)	1 cup	232	58	801	1	90	17.9	36.4	32.0
168		1 tsp	5	58	17	Tr	2	0.4	0.8	0.7
169	Margarine butter blend	1 stick	113	16	811	1	91	32.1	37.0	18.0
170		1 tbsp	14	16	102	Tr	11	4.0	4.7	2.3
	Oils, salad or cooking									
171	Canola	1 cup	218	0	1,927	0	218	15.5	128.4	64.5
172		1 tbsp	14	0	124	0	14	1.0	8.2	4.1
173	Corn	1 cup	218	0	1,927	0	218	27.7	52.8	128.0
174		1 tbsp	14	0	120	0	14	1.7	3.3	8.0
175	Olive	1 cup	216	0	1,909	0	216	29.2	159.2	18.1
176		1 tbsp	14	0	119	0	14	1.8	9.9	1.1
177	Peanut	1 cup	216	0	1,909	0	216	36.5	99.8	69.1
178		1 tbsp	14	0	119	0	14	2.3	6.2	4.3
179	Safflower, high oleic	1 cup	218	0	1,927	0	218	13.5	162.7	31.3
180		1 tbsp	14	0	120	0	14	0.8	10.2	2.0
181	Sesame	1 cup	218	0	1,927	0	218	31.0	86.5	90.9
182		1 tbsp	14	0	120	0	14	1.9	5.4	5.7
183	Soybean, hydrogenated	1 cup	218	0	1,927	0	218	32.5	93.7	82.0
184		1 tbsp	14	0	120	0	14	2.0	5.8	5.1
185	Soybean, hydrogenated and cottonseed oil blend	1 cup	218	0	1,927	0	218	39.2	64.3	104.9
186		1 tbsp	14	0	120	0	14	2.4	4.0	6.5
187	Sunflower	1 cup	218	0	1,927	0	218	22.5	42.5	143.2
188		1 tbsp	14	0	120	0	14	1.4	2.7	8.9
	Salad dressings									
	Commercial									
	Blue cheese									
189	Regular	1 tbsp	15	32	77	1	8	1.5	1.9	4.3
190	Low calorie	1 tbsp	15	80	15	1	1	0.4	0.3	0.4
	Caesar									
191	Regular	1 tbsp	15	34	78	Tr	8	1.3	2.0	4.8
192	Low calorie	1 tbsp	15	73	17	Tr	1	0.1	0.2	0.4
	French									
193	Regular	1 tbsp	16	38	67	Tr	6	1.5	1.2	3.4
194	Low calorie	1 tbsp	16	69	22	Tr	1	0.1	0.2	0.6
	Italian									
195	Regular	1 tbsp	15	38	69	Tr	7	1.0	1.6	4.1
196	Low calorie	1 tbsp	15	82	16	Tr	1	0.2	0.3	0.9
	Mayonnaise									
197	Regular	1 tbsp	14	15	99	Tr	11	1.6	3.1	5.7
198	Light, cholesterol free	1 tbsp	15	56	49	Tr	5	0.7	1.1	2.8
199	Fat free	1 tbsp	16	84	12	0	Tr	0.1	0.1	0.2
	Russian									
200	Regular	1 tbsp	15	35	76	Tr	8	1.1	1.8	4.5
201	Low calorie	1 tbsp	16	65	23	Tr	1	0.1	0.1	0.4
	Thousand island									
202	Regular	1 tbsp	16	46	59	Tr	6	0.9	1.3	3.1
203	Low calorie	1 tbsp	15	69	24	Tr	2	0.2	0.4	0.9

Choles-terol (mg)	Carbo-hydrate (g)	Total dietary fiber (g)	Calcium (mg)	Iron (mg)	Potas-sium (mg)	Sodium (mg)	Vitamin A (IU)	Vitamin A (RE)	Thiamin (mg)	Ribo-flavin (mg)	Niacin (mg)	Ascor-bic acid (mg)	Food No.
0	0	0.0	24	0.0	34	1,143	4,107	919	0.01	0.03	Tr	Tr	162
0	0	0.0	3	0.0	4	139	500	112	Tr	Tr	Tr	Tr	163
0	0	0.0	1	0.0	1	48	171	38	Tr	Tr	Tr	Tr	164
0	0	0.0	48	0.0	68	2,276	8,178	1,830	0.02	0.06	Tr	Tr	165
0	0	0.0	1	0.0	1	48	171	38	Tr	Tr	Tr	Tr	166
0	1	0.0	41	0.0	59	2,226	8,285	1,854	0.01	0.05	Tr	Tr	167
0	Tr	0.0	1	0.0	1	46	171	38	Tr	Tr	Tr	Tr	168
99	1	0.0	32	0.1	41	1,014	4,035	903	0.01	0.04	Tr	Tr	169
12	Tr	0.0	4	Tr	5	127	507	113	Tr	Tr	Tr	Tr	170
0	0	0.0	0	0.0	0	0	0	0	0.00	0.00	0.0	0	171
0	0	0.0	0	0.0	0	0	0	0	0.00	0.00	0.0	0	172
0	0	0.0	0	0.0	0	0	0	0	0.00	0.00	0.0	0	173
0	0	0.0	0	0.0	0	0	0	0	0.00	0.00	0.0	0	174
0	0	0.0	Tr	0.8	0	Tr	0	0	0.00	0.00	0.0	0	175
0	0	0.0	Tr	0.1	0	Tr	0	0	0.00	0.00	0.0	0	176
0	0	0.0	Tr	0.1	Tr	Tr	0	0	0.00	0.00	0.0	0	177
0	0	0.0	Tr	Tr	Tr	Tr	0	0	0.00	0.00	0.0	0	178
0	0	0.0	0	0.0	0	0	0	0	0.00	0.00	0.0	0	179
0	0	0.0	0	0.0	0	0	0	0	0.00	0.00	0.0	0	180
0	0	0.0	0	0.0	0	0	0	0	0.00	0.00	0.0	0	181
0	0	0.0	0	0.0	0	0	0	0	0.00	0.00	0.0	0	182
0	0	0.0	0	0.0	0	0	0	0	0.00	0.00	0.0	0	183
0	0	0.0	0	0.0	0	0	0	0	0.00	0.00	0.0	0	184
0	0	0.0	0	0.0	0	0	0	0	0.00	0.00	0.0	0	185
0	0	0.0	0	0.0	0	0	0	0	0.00	0.00	0.0	0	186
0	0	0.0	0	0.0	0	0	0	0	0.00	0.00	0.0	0	187
0	0	0.0	0	0.0	0	0	0	0	0.00	0.00	0.0	0	188
3	1	0.0	12	Tr	6	167	32	10	Tr	0.02	Tr	Tr	189
Tr	Tr	0.0	14	0.1	1	184	2	Tr	Tr	0.02	Tr	Tr	190
Tr	Tr	Tr	4	Tr	4	158	3	Tr	Tr	Tr	Tr	0	191
Tr	3	Tr	4	Tr	4	162	3	Tr	Tr	Tr	Tr	0	192
0	3	0.0	2	0.1	12	214	203	20	Tr	Tr	Tr	0	193
0	4	0.0	2	0.1	13	128	212	21	0.00	0.00	0.0	0	194
0	1	0.0	1	Tr	2	116	11	4	Tr	Tr	Tr	0	195
1	1	Tr	Tr	Tr	2	118	0	0	0.00	0.00	0.0	0	196
8	Tr	0.0	2	0.1	5	78	39	12	0.00	0.00	Tr	0	197
0	1	0.0	0	0.0	10	107	18	2	0.00	0.00	0.0	0	198
0	2	0.6	0	0.0	15	190	0	0	0.00	0.00	0.0	0	199
3	2	0.0	3	0.1	24	133	106	32	0.01	0.01	0.1	1	200
1	4	Tr	3	0.1	26	141	9	3	Tr	Tr	Tr	1	201
4	2	0.0	2	0.1	18	109	50	15	Tr	Tr	Tr	0	202
2	2	0.2	2	0.1	17	153	49	15	Tr	Tr	Tr	0	203

Table 9.   Nutritive Value of the Edible Part of Food

Food No.	Food Description	Measure of edible portion	Weight (g)	Water (%)	Calories (kcal)	Pro-tein (g)	Total fat (g)	Satu-rated (g)	Mono-unsatu-rated (g)	Poly-unsatu-rated (g)
								Fatty acids		

Fats and Oils (continued)

Salad dressings (continued)
Prepared from home recipe

Food No.	Food Description	Measure of edible portion	Weight (g)	Water (%)	Calories (kcal)	Pro-tein (g)	Total fat (g)	Saturated (g)	Mono-unsaturated (g)	Poly-unsaturated (g)
204	Cooked, made with margarine	1 tbsp 16		69	25	1	2	0.5	0.6	0.3
205	French	1 tbsp 14		24	88	Tr	10	1.8	2.9	4.7
206	Vinegar and oil	1 tbsp 16		47	70	0	8	1.4	2.3	3.8
207	Shortening (hydrogenated soybean and cottonseed oils)	1 cup 205		0	1,812	0	205	51.3	91.2	53.5
208		1 tbsp 13		0	113	0	13	3.2	5.7	3.3

Fish and Shellfish

Food No.	Food Description	Measure of edible portion	Weight (g)	Water (%)	Calories (kcal)	Pro-tein (g)	Total fat (g)	Saturated (g)	Mono-unsaturated (g)	Poly-unsaturated (g)
209	Catfish, breaded, fried	3 oz 85		59	195	15	11	2.8	4.8	2.8
	Clam									
210	Raw, meat only	3 oz 85		82	63	11	1	0.1	0.1	0.2
211		1 medium 15		82	11	2	Tr	Tr	Tr	Tr
212	Breaded, fried	¾ cup 115		29	451	13	26	6.6	11.4	6.8
213	Canned, drained solids	3 oz 85		64	126	22	2	0.2	0.1	0.5
214		1 cup 160		64	237	41	3	0.3	0.3	0.9
	Cod									
215	Baked or broiled	3 oz 85		76	89	20	1	0.1	0.1	0.3
216		1 fillet 90		76	95	21	1	0.1	0.1	0.3
217	Canned, solids and liquid	3 oz 85		76	89	19	1	0.1	0.1	0.2
	Crab									
	Alaska king									
218	Steamed	1 leg 134		78	130	26	2	0.2	0.2	0.7
219		3 oz 85		78	82	16	1	0.1	0.2	0.5
220	Imitation, from surimi	3 oz 85		74	87	10	1	0.2	0.2	0.6
	Blue									
221	Steamed	3 oz 85		77	87	17	2	0.2	0.2	0.6
222	Canned crabmeat	1 cup 135		76	134	28	2	0.3	0.3	0.6
223	Crab cake, with egg, onion, fried in margarine	1 cake 60		71	93	12	5	0.9	1.7	1.4
224	Fish fillet, battered or breaded, fried	1 fillet 91		54	211	13	11	2.6	2.3	5.7
225	Fish stick and portion, breaded, frozen, reheated	1 stick (4" x 1" x ½") 28		46	76	4	3	0.9	1.4	0.9
226		1 portion (4" x 2" x ½") 57		46	155	9	7	1.8	2.9	1.8
227	Flounder or sole, baked or broiled	3 oz 85		73	99	21	1	0.3	0.2	0.5
228		1 fillet 127		73	149	31	2	0.5	0.3	0.8
229	Haddock, baked or broiled	3 oz 85		74	95	21	1	0.1	0.1	0.3
230		1 fillet 150		74	168	36	1	0.3	0.2	0.5
231	Halibut, baked or broiled	3 oz 85		72	119	23	2	0.4	0.8	0.8
232		½ fillet 159		72	223	42	5	0.7	1.5	1.5
233	Herring, pickled	3 oz 85		55	223	12	15	2.0	10.2	1.4
234	Lobster, steamed	3 oz 85		76	83	17	1	0.1	0.1	0.1
235	Ocean perch, baked or broiled	3 oz 85		73	103	20	2	0.3	0.7	0.5
236		1 fillet 50		73	61	12	1	0.2	0.4	0.3
	Oyster									
237	Raw, meat only	1 cup 248		85	169	17	6	1.9	0.8	2.4
238		6 medium 84		85	57	6	2	0.6	0.3	0.8
239	Breaded, fried	3 oz 85		65	167	7	11	2.7	4.0	2.8
240	Pollock, baked or broiled	3 oz 85		74	96	20	1	0.2	0.1	0.4
241		1 fillet 60		74	68	14	1	0.1	0.1	0.3
242	Rockfish, baked or broiled	3 oz 85		73	103	20	2	0.4	0.4	0.5
243		1 fillet 149		73	180	36	3	0.7	0.7	0.9

Choles-terol (mg)	Carbo-hydrate (g)	Total dietary fiber (g)	Calcium (mg)	Iron (mg)	Potas-sium (mg)	Sodium (mg)	Vitamin A		Thiamin (mg)	Ribo-flavin (mg)	Niacin (mg)	Ascor-bic acid (mg)	Food No.
							(IU)	(RE)					
9	2	0.0	13	0.1	19	117	66	20	0.01	0.02	Tr	Tr	204
0	Tr	0.0	1	Tr	3	92	72	22	Tr	Tr	Tr	Tr	205
0	Tr	0.0	0	0.0	1	Tr	0	0	0.00	0.00	0.0	0	206
0	0	0.0	0	0.0	0	0	0	0	0.00	0.00	0.0	0	207
0	0	0.0	0	0.0	0	0	0	0	0.00	0.00	0.0	0	208
69	7	0.6	37	1.2	289	238	24	7	0.06	0.11	1.9	0	209
29	2	0.0	39	11.9	267	48	255	77	0.07	0.18	1.5	11	210
5	Tr	0.0	7	2.0	46	8	44	13	0.01	0.03	0.3	2	211
87	39	0.3	21	3.0	266	834	122	37	0.21	0.26	2.9	0	212
57	4	0.0	78	23.8	534	95	485	145	0.13	0.36	2.9	19	213
107	8	0.0	147	44.7	1,005	179	912	274	0.24	0.68	5.4	35	214
40	0	0.0	8	0.3	439	77	27	9	0.02	0.04	2.1	3	215
42	0	0.0	8	0.3	465	82	29	9	0.02	0.05	2.2	3	216
47	0	0.0	18	0.4	449	185	39	12	0.07	0.07	2.1	1	217
71	0	0.0	79	1.0	351	1,436	39	12	0.07	0.07	1.8	10	218
45	0	0.0	50	0.6	223	911	25	8	0.05	0.05	1.1	6	219
17	9	0.0	11	0.3	77	715	56	17	0.03	0.02	0.2	0	220
85	0	0.0	88	0.8	275	237	5	2	0.09	0.04	2.8	3	221
120	0	0.0	136	1.1	505	450	7	3	0.11	0.11	1.8	4	222
90	Tr	0.0	63	0.6	194	198	151	49	0.05	0.05	1.7	2	223
31	15	0.5	16	1.9	291	484	35	11	0.10	0.10	1.9	0	224
31	7	0.0	6	0.2	73	163	30	9	0.04	0.05	0.6	0	225
64	14	0.0	11	0.4	149	332	60	18	0.07	0.10	1.2	0	226
58	0	0.0	15	0.3	292	89	32	9	0.07	0.10	1.9	0	227
86	0	0.0	23	0.4	437	133	48	14	0.10	0.14	2.8	0	228
63	0	0.0	36	1.1	339	74	54	16	0.03	0.04	3.9	0	229
111	0	0.0	63	2.0	599	131	95	29	0.06	0.07	6.9	0	230
35	0	0.0	51	0.9	490	59	152	46	0.06	0.08	6.1	0	231
65	0	0.0	95	1.7	916	110	285	86	0.11	0.14	11.3	0	232
11	8	0.0	65	1.0	59	740	732	219	0.03	0.12	2.8	0	233
61	1	0.0	52	0.3	299	323	74	22	0.01	0.06	0.9	0	234
46	0	0.0	116	1.0	298	82	39	12	0.11	0.11	2.1	1	235
27	0	0.0	69	0.6	175	48	23	7	0.07	0.07	1.2	Tr	236
131	10	0.0	112	16.5	387	523	248	74	0.25	0.24	3.4	9	237
45	3	0.0	38	5.6	131	177	84	25	0.08	0.08	1.2	3	238
69	10	0.2	53	5.9	207	354	257	77	0.13	0.17	1.4	3	239
82	0	0.0	5	0.2	329	99	65	20	0.06	0.06	1.4	0	240
58	0	0.0	4	0.2	232	70	46	14	0.04	0.05	1.0	0	241
37	0	0.0	10	0.5	442	65	186	56	0.04	0.07	3.3	0	242
66	0	0.0	18	0.8	775	115	326	98	0.07	0.13	5.8	0	243

Table 9.   Nutritive Value of the Edible Part of Food

Food No.	Food Description	Measure of edible portion	Weight (g)	Water (%)	Calories (kcal)	Pro-tein (g)	Total fat (g)	Fatty acids Satu-rated (g)	Mono-unsatu-rated (g)	Poly-unsatu-rated (g)
	Fish and Shellfish (continued)									
244	Roughy, orange, baked or broiled	3 oz	85	69	76	16	1	Tr	0.5	Tr
	Salmon									
245	Baked or broiled (red)	3 oz	85	62	184	23	9	1.6	4.5	2.0
246		½ fillet	155	62	335	42	17	3.0	8.2	3.7
247	Canned (pink), solids and liquid (includes bones)	3 oz	85	69	118	17	5	1.3	1.5	1.7
248	Smoked (chinook)	3 oz	85	72	99	16	4	0.8	1.7	0.8
249	Sardine, Atlantic, canned in oil, drained solids (includes bones)	3 oz	85	60	177	21	10	1.3	3.3	4.4
	Scallop, cooked									
250	Breaded, fried	6 large	93	58	200	17	10	2.5	4.2	2.7
251	Steamed	3 oz	85	73	95	20	1	0.1	0.1	0.4
	Shrimp									
252	Breaded, fried	3 oz	85	53	206	18	10	1.8	3.2	4.3
253		6 large	45	53	109	10	6	0.9	1.7	2.3
254	Canned, drained solids	3 oz	85	73	102	20	2	0.3	0.2	0.6
255	Swordfish, baked or broiled	3 oz	85	69	132	22	4	1.2	1.7	1.0
256		1 piece	106	69	164	27	5	1.5	2.1	1.3
257	Trout, baked or broiled	3 oz	85	68	144	21	6	1.8	1.8	2.0
258		1 fillet	71	68	120	17	5	1.5	1.5	1.7
	Tuna									
259	Baked or broiled	3 oz	85	63	118	25	1	0.3	0.2	0.3
	Canned, drained solids									
260	Oil pack, chunk light	3 oz	85	60	168	25	7	1.3	2.5	2.5
261	Water pack, chunk light	3 oz	85	75	99	22	1	0.2	0.1	0.3
262	Water pack, solid white	3 oz	85	73	109	20	3	0.7	0.7	0.9
263	Tuna salad: light tuna in oil, pickle relish, mayo type salad dressing	1 cup	205	63	383	33	19	3.2	5.9	8.5
	Fruits and Fruit Juices									
	Apples									
	Raw									
264	Unpeeled, 2¾" dia (about 3 per lb)	1 apple	138	84	81	Tr	Tr	0.1	Tr	0.1
265	Peeled, sliced	1 cup	110	84	63	Tr	Tr	0.1	Tr	0.1
266	Dried (sodium bisulfite used to preserve color)	5 rings	32	32	78	Tr	Tr	Tr	Tr	Tr
267	Apple juice, bottled or canned	1 cup	248	88	117	Tr	Tr	Tr	Tr	0.1
268	Apple pie filling, canned	⅛ of 21-oz can	74	73	75	Tr	Tr	Tr	0.0	Tr
	Applesauce, canned									
269	Sweetened	1 cup	255	80	194	Tr	Tr	0.1	Tr	0.1
270	Unsweetened	1 cup	244	88	105	Tr	Tr	Tr	Tr	Tr
	Apricots									
271	Raw, without pits (about 12 per lb with pits)	1 apricot	35	86	17	Tr	Tr	Tr	0.1	Tr
	Canned, halves, fruit and liquid									
272	Heavy syrup pack	1 cup	258	78	214	1	Tr	Tr	0.1	Tr
273	Juice pack	1 cup	244	87	117	2	Tr	Tr	Tr	Tr
274	Dried, sulfured	10 halves	35	31	83	1	Tr	Tr	0.1	Tr
275	Apricot nectar, canned, with added ascorbic acid	1 cup	251	85	141	1	Tr	Tr	0.1	Tr
	Asian pear, raw									
276	2¼" high x 2½" dia	1 pear	122	88	51	1	Tr	Tr	0.1	0.1
277	3⅜" high x 3" dia	1 pear	275	88	116	1	1	Tr	0.1	0.2

Choles-terol (mg)	Carbo-hydrate (g)	Total dietary fiber (g)	Calcium (mg)	Iron (mg)	Potas-sium (mg)	Sodium (mg)	Vitamin A		Thiamin (mg)	Ribo-flavin (mg)	Niacin (mg)	Ascor-bic acid (mg)	Food No.
							(IU)	(RE)					
22	0	0.0	32	0.2	327	69	69	20	0.10	0.16	3.1	0	244
74	0	0.0	6	0.5	319	56	178	54	0.18	0.15	5.7	0	245
135	0	0.0	11	0.9	581	102	324	98	0.33	0.27	10.3	0	246
47	0	0.0	181	0.7	277	471	47	14	0.02	0.16	5.6	0	247
20	0	0.0	9	0.7	149	666	75	22	0.02	0.09	4.0	0	248
121	0	0.0	325	2.5	337	429	190	57	0.07	0.19	4.5	0	249
57	9	0.2	39	0.8	310	432	70	20	0.04	0.10	1.4	2	250
45	3	0.0	98	2.6	405	225	85	26	0.09	0.05	1.1	0	251
150	10	0.3	57	1.1	191	292	161	48	0.11	0.12	2.6	1	252
80	5	0.2	30	0.6	101	155	85	25	0.06	0.06	1.4	1	253
147	1	0.0	50	2.3	179	144	51	15	0.02	0.03	2.3	2	254
43	0	0.0	5	0.9	314	98	116	35	0.04	0.10	10.0	1	255
53	0	0.0	6	1.1	391	122	145	43	0.05	0.12	12.5	1	256
58	0	0.0	73	0.3	375	36	244	73	0.20	0.07	7.5	3	257
48	0	0.0	61	0.2	313	30	204	61	0.17	0.06	6.2	2	258
49	0	0.0	18	0.8	484	40	58	17	0.43	0.05	10.1	1	259
15	0	0.0	11	1.2	176	301	66	20	0.03	0.10	10.5	0	260
26	0	0.0	9	1.3	201	287	48	14	0.03	0.06	11.3	0	261
36	0	0.0	12	0.8	201	320	16	5	0.01	0.04	4.9	0	262
27	19	0.0	35	2.1	365	824	199	55	0.06	0.14	13.7	5	263
0	21	3.7	10	0.2	159	0	73	7	0.02	0.02	0.1	8	264
0	16	2.1	4	0.1	124	0	48	4	0.02	0.01	0.1	4	265
0	21	2.8	4	0.4	144	28	0	0	0.00	0.05	0.3	1	266
0	29	0.2	17	0.9	295	7	2	0	0.05	0.04	0.2	2	267
0	19	0.7	3	0.2	33	33	10	1	0.01	0.01	Tr	1	268
0	51	3.1	10	0.9	156	8	28	3	0.03	0.07	0.5	4	269
0	28	2.9	7	0.3	183	5	71	7	0.03	0.06	0.5	3	270
0	4	0.8	5	0.2	104	Tr	914	91	0.01	0.01	0.2	4	271
0	55	4.1	23	0.8	361	10	3,173	317	0.05	0.06	1.0	8	272
0	30	3.9	29	0.7	403	10	4,126	412	0.04	0.05	0.8	12	273
0	22	3.2	16	1.6	482	4	2,534	253	Tr	0.05	1.0	1	274
0	36	1.5	18	1.0	286	8	3,303	331	0.02	0.04	0.7	137	275
0	13	4.4	5	0.0	148	0	0	0	0.01	0.01	0.3	5	276
0	29	9.9	11	0.0	333	0	0	0	0.02	0.03	0.6	10	277

Table 9. Nutritive Value of the Edible Part of Food

Food No.	Food Description	Measure of edible portion	Weight (g)	Water (%)	Calories (kcal)	Pro-tein (g)	Total fat (g)	Fatty acids Satu-rated (g)	Mono-unsatu-rated (g)	Poly-unsatu-rated (g)

Fruits and Fruit Juices (continued)

	Avocados, raw, without skin and seed									
278	California (about ⅕ whole)....	1 oz 28		73	50	1	5	0.7	3.2	0.6
279	Florida (about ⅒ whole)	1 oz 28		80	32	Tr	3	0.5	1.4	0.4
	Bananas, raw									
280	Whole, medium (7" to 7⅞" long)..................	1 banana 118		74	109	1	1	0.2	Tr	0.1
281	Sliced	1 cup 150		74	138	2	1	0.3	0.1	0.1
282	Blackberries, raw	1 cup 144		86	75	1	1	Tr	0.1	0.3
	Blueberries									
283	Raw	1 cup 145		85	81	1	1	Tr	0.1	0.2
284	Frozen, sweetened, thawed	1 cup 230		77	186	1	Tr	Tr	Tr	0.1
	Cantaloupe. See Melons.									
	Carambola (starfruit), raw									
285	Whole (3⅝" long)..................	1 fruit................91		91	30	Tr	Tr	Tr	Tr	0.2
286	Sliced	1 cup 108		91	36	1	Tr	Tr	Tr	0.2
	Cherries									
287	Sour, red, pitted, canned, water pack.........................	1 cup 244		90	88	2	Tr	0.1	0.1	0.1
288	Sweet, raw, without pits and stems.................	10 cherries...........68		81	49	1	1	0.1	0.2	0.2
289	Cherry pie filling, canned	⅛ of 21-oz can 74		71	85	Tr	Tr	Tr	Tr	Tr
290	Cranberries, dried, sweetened...	¼ cup...................28		12	92	Tr	Tr	Tr	Tr	0.1
291	Cranberry sauce, sweetened, canned (about 8 slices per can).................	1 slice 57		61	86	Tr	Tr	Tr	Tr	Tr
	Dates, without pits									
292	Whole.......................	5 dates 42		23	116	1	Tr	0.1	0.1	Tr
293	Chopped	1 cup 178		23	490	4	1	0.3	0.3	0.1
294	Figs, dried...................	2 figs..............38		28	97	1	Tr	0.1	0.1	0.2
	Fruit cocktail, canned, fruit and liquid									
295	Heavy syrup pack	1 cup 248		80	181	1	Tr	Tr	Tr	0.1
296	Juice pack	1 cup 237		87	109	1	Tr	Tr	Tr	Tr
	Grapefruit									
	Raw, without peel, membrane and seeds (3¾" dia)									
297	Pink or red...........................	½ grapefruit 123		91	37	1	Tr	Tr	Tr	Tr
298	White	½ grapefruit 118		90	39	1	Tr	Tr	Tr	Tr
299	Canned, sections with light syrup..................	1 cup 254		84	152	1	Tr	Tr	Tr	0.1
	Grapefruit juice									
	Raw									
300	Pink	1 cup 247		90	96	1	Tr	Tr	Tr	0.1
301	White	1 cup 247		90	96	1	Tr	Tr	Tr	0.1
	Canned									
302	Unsweetened	1 cup 247		90	94	1	Tr	Tr	Tr	0.1
303	Sweetened	1 cup 250		87	115	1	Tr	Tr	Tr	0.1
	Frozen concentrate, unsweetened									
304	Undiluted.............................	6-fl-oz can 207		62	302	4	1	0.1	0.1	0.2
305	Diluted with 3 parts water by volume...........................	1 cup 247		89	101	1	Tr	Tr	Tr	0.1
306	Grapes, seedless, raw	10 grapes 50		81	36	Tr	Tr	0.1	Tr	0.1
307		1 cup 160		81	114	1	1	0.3	Tr	0.3

Choles-terol (mg)	Carbo-hydrate (g)	Total dietary fiber (g)	Calcium (mg)	Iron (mg)	Potas-sium (mg)	Sodium (mg)	Vitamin A		Thiamin (mg)	Ribo-flavin (mg)	Niacin (mg)	Ascor-bic acid (mg)	Food No.
							(IU)	(RE)					
0	2	1.4	3	0.3	180	3	174	17	0.03	0.03	0.5	2	278
0	3	1.5	3	0.2	138	1	174	17	0.03	0.03	0.5	2	279
0	28	2.8	7	0.4	467	1	96	9	0.05	0.12	0.6	11	280
0	35	3.6	9	0.5	594	2	122	12	0.07	0.15	0.8	14	281
0	18	7.6	46	0.8	282	0	238	23	0.04	0.06	0.6	30	282
0	20	3.9	9	0.2	129	9	145	15	0.07	0.07	0.5	19	283
0	50	4.8	14	0.9	138	2	101	9	0.05	0.12	0.6	2	284
0	7	2.5	4	0.2	148	2	449	45	0.03	0.02	0.4	19	285
0	8	2.9	4	0.3	176	2	532	53	0.03	0.03	0.4	23	286
0	22	2.7	27	3.3	239	17	1,840	183	0.04	0.10	0.4	5	287
0	11	1.6	10	0.3	152	0	146	14	0.03	0.04	0.3	5	288
0	21	0.4	8	0.2	78	13	152	16	0.02	0.01	0.1	3	289
0	24	2.5	5	0.1	24	1	0	0	0.01	0.03	Tr	Tr	290
0	22	0.6	2	0.1	15	17	11	1	0.01	0.01	0.1	1	291
0	31	3.2	13	0.5	274	1	21	2	0.04	0.04	0.9	0	292
0	131	13.4	57	2.0	1,161	5	89	9	0.16	0.18	3.9	0	293
0	25	4.6	55	0.8	271	4	51	5	0.03	0.03	0.3	Tr	294
0	47	2.5	15	0.7	218	15	508	50	0.04	0.05	0.9	5	295
0	28	2.4	19	0.5	225	9	723	73	0.03	0.04	1.0	6	296
0	9	1.4	14	0.1	159	0	319	32	0.04	0.02	0.2	47	297
0	10	1.3	14	0.1	175	0	12	1	0.04	0.02	0.3	39	298
0	39	1.0	36	1.0	328	5	0	0	0.10	0.05	0.6	54	299
0	23	0.2	22	0.5	400	2	1,087	109	0.10	0.05	0.5	94	300
0	23	0.2	22	0.5	400	2	25	2	0.10	0.05	0.5	94	301
0	22	0.2	17	0.5	378	2	17	2	0.10	0.05	0.6	72	302
0	28	0.3	20	0.9	405	5	0	0	0.10	0.06	0.8	67	303
0	72	0.8	56	1.0	1,002	6	64	6	0.30	0.16	1.6	248	304
0	24	0.2	20	0.3	336	2	22	2	0.10	0.05	0.5	83	305
0	9	0.5	6	0.1	93	1	37	4	0.05	0.03	0.2	5	306
0	28	1.6	18	0.4	296	3	117	11	0.15	0.09	0.5	17	307

Table 9.   Nutritive Value of the Edible Part of Food

Food No.	Food Description	Measure of edible portion	Weight (g)	Water (%)	Calories (kcal)	Protein (g)	Total fat (g)	Fatty acids Saturated (g)	Mono-unsaturated (g)	Poly-unsaturated (g)

Fruits and Fruit Juices (continued)

	Grape juice									
308	Canned or bottled	1 cup	253	84	154	1	Tr	0.1	Tr	0.1
	Frozen concentrate, sweetened, with added vitamin C									
309	Undiluted	6-fl-oz can	216	54	387	1	1	0.2	Tr	0.2
310	Diluted with 3 parts water by volume	1 cup	250	87	128	Tr	Tr	0.1	Tr	0.1
311	Kiwi fruit, raw, without skin (about 5 per lb with skin)	1 medium	76	83	46	1	Tr	Tr	Tr	0.2
312	Lemons, raw, without peel (2⅛" dia with peel)	1 lemon	58	89	17	1	Tr	Tr	Tr	0.1
	Lemon juice									
313	Raw (from 2⅛"-dia lemon)	juice of 1 lemon	47	91	12	Tr	0	0.0	0.0	0.0
314	Canned or bottled, unsweetened	1 cup	244	92	51	1	1	0.1	Tr	0.2
315		1 tbsp	15	92	3	Tr	Tr	Tr	Tr	Tr
	Lime juice									
316	Raw (from 2"-dia lime)	juice of 1 lime	38	90	10	Tr	Tr	Tr	Tr	Tr
317	Canned, unsweetened	1 cup	246	93	52	1	1	0.1	0.1	0.2
318		1 tbsp	15	93	3	Tr	Tr	Tr	Tr	Tr
	Mangos, raw, without skin and seed (about 1½ per lb with skin and seed)									
319	Whole	1 mango	207	82	135	1	1	0.1	0.2	0.1
320	Sliced	1 cup	165	82	107	1	Tr	0.1	0.2	0.1
	Melons, raw, without rind and cavity contents									
	Cantaloupe (5" dia)									
321	Wedge	⅛ melon	69	90	24	1	Tr	Tr	Tr	0.1
322	Cubes	1 cup	160	90	56	1	Tr	0.1	Tr	0.2
	Honeydew (6"-7" dia)									
323	Wedge	⅛ melon	160	90	56	1	Tr	Tr	Tr	0.1
324	Diced (about 20 pieces per cup)	1 cup	170	90	60	1	Tr	Tr	Tr	0.1
325	Mixed fruit, frozen, sweetened, thawed (peach, cherry, raspberry, grape and boysenberry)	1 cup	250	74	245	4	Tr	0.1	0.1	0.2
326	Nectarines, raw (2½" dia)	1 nectarine	136	86	67	1	1	0.1	0.2	0.3
	Oranges, raw									
327	Whole, without peel and seeds (2⅝" dia)	1 orange	131	87	62	1	Tr	Tr	Tr	Tr
328	Sections without membranes	1 cup	180	87	85	2	Tr	Tr	Tr	Tr
	Orange juice									
329	Raw, all varieties	1 cup	248	88	112	2	Tr	0.1	0.1	0.1
330		juice from 1 orange	86	88	39	1	Tr	Tr	Tr	Tr
331	Canned, unsweetened	1 cup	249	89	105	1	Tr	Tr	0.1	0.1
332	Chilled (refrigerator case)	1 cup	249	88	110	2	1	0.1	0.1	0.2
	Frozen concentrate									
333	Undiluted	6-fl-oz can	213	58	339	5	Tr	0.1	0.1	0.1
334	Diluted with 3 parts water by volume	1 cup	249	88	112	2	Tr	Tr	Tr	Tr
	Papayas, raw									
335	½" cubes	1 cup	140	89	55	1	Tr	0.1	0.1	Tr
336	Whole (5⅛" long x 3" dia)	1 papaya	304	89	119	2	Tr	0.1	0.1	0.1

*Sodium benzoate and sodium bisulfite added as preservatives.

Choles-terol (mg)	Carbo-hydrate (g)	Total dietary fiber (g)	Calcium (mg)	Iron (mg)	Potas-sium (mg)	Sodium (mg)	Vitamin A		Thiamin (mg)	Ribo-flavin (mg)	Niacin (mg)	Ascor-bic acid (mg)	Food No.
							(IU)	(RE)					
0	38	0.3	23	0.6	334	8	20	3	0.07	0.09	0.7	Tr	308
0	96	0.6	28	0.8	160	15	58	6	0.11	0.20	0.9	179	309
0	32	0.3	10	0.3	53	5	20	3	0.04	0.07	0.3	60	310
0	11	2.6	20	0.3	252	4	133	14	0.02	0.04	0.4	74	311
0	5	1.6	15	0.3	80	1	17	2	0.02	0.01	0.1	31	312
0	4	0.2	3	Tr	58	Tr	9	1	0.01	Tr	Tr	22	313
0	16	1.0	27	0.3	249	51*	37	5	0.10	0.02	0.5	61	314
0	1	0.1	2	Tr	16	3*	2	Tr	0.01	Tr	Tr	4	315
0	3	0.2	3	Tr	41	Tr	4	Tr	0.01	Tr	Tr	11	316
0	16	1.0	30	0.6	185	39*	39	5	0.08	0.01	0.4	16	317
0	1	0.1	2	Tr	11	2*	2	Tr	Tr	Tr	Tr	1	318
0	35	3.7	21	0.3	323	4	8,061	805	0.12	0.12	1.2	57	319
0	28	3.0	17	0.2	257	3	6,425	642	0.10	0.09	1.0	46	320
0	6	0.6	8	0.1	213	6	2,225	222	0.02	0.01	0.4	29	321
0	13	1.3	18	0.3	494	14	5,158	515	0.06	0.03	0.9	68	322
0	15	1.0	10	0.1	434	16	64	6	0.12	0.03	1.0	40	323
0	16	1.0	10	0.1	461	17	68	7	0.13	0.03	1.0	42	324
0	61	4.8	18	0.7	328	8	805	80	0.04	0.09	1.0	188	325
0	16	2.2	7	0.2	288	0	1,001	101	0.02	0.06	1.3	7	326
0	15	3.1	52	0.1	237	0	269	28	0.11	0.05	0.4	70	327
0	21	4.3	72	0.2	326	0	369	38	0.16	0.07	0.5	96	328
0	26	0.5	27	0.5	496	2	496	50	0.22	0.07	1.0	124	329
0	9	0.2	9	0.2	172	1	172	17	0.08	0.03	0.3	43	330
0	25	0.5	20	1.1	436	5	436	45	0.15	0.07	0.8	86	331
0	25	0.5	25	0.4	473	2	194	20	0.28	0.05	0.7	82	332
0	81	1.7	68	0.7	1,436	6	588	60	0.60	0.14	1.5	294	333
0	27	0.5	22	0.2	473	2	194	20	0.20	0.04	0.5	97	334
0	14	2.5	34	0.1	360	4	398	39	0.04	0.04	0.5	87	335
0	30	5.5	73	0.3	781	9	863	85	0.08	0.10	1.0	188	336

Table 9.   Nutritive Value of the Edible Part of Food

Food No.	Food Description	Measure of edible portion	Weight (g)	Water (%)	Calories (kcal)	Pro-tein (g)	Total fat (g)	Fatty acids Satu-rated (g)	Mono-unsatu-rated (g)	Poly-unsatu-rated (g)

Fruits and Fruit Juices (continued)

	Peaches									
	Raw									
337	Whole, 2½" dia, pitted (about 4 per lb)	1 peach	98	88	42	1	Tr	Tr	Tr	Tr
338	Sliced	1 cup	170	88	73	1	Tr	Tr	0.1	0.1
	Canned, fruit and liquid									
339	Heavy syrup pack	1 cup	262	79	194	1	Tr	Tr	0.1	0.1
340		1 half	98	79	73	Tr	Tr	Tr	Tr	Tr
341	Juice pack	1 cup	248	87	109	2	Tr	Tr	Tr	Tr
342		1 half	98	87	43	1	Tr	Tr	Tr	Tr
343	Dried, sulfured	3 halves	39	32	93	1	Tr	Tr	0.1	0.1
344	Frozen, sliced, sweetened, with added ascorbic acid, thawed	1 cup	250	75	235	2	Tr	Tr	0.1	0.2
	Pears									
345	Raw, with skin, cored, 2½" dia	1 pear	166	84	98	1	1	Tr	0.1	0.2
	Canned, fruit and liquid									
346	Heavy syrup pack	1 cup	266	80	197	1	Tr	Tr	0.1	0.1
347		1 half	76	80	56	Tr	Tr	Tr	Tr	Tr
348	Juice pack	1 cup	248	86	124	1	Tr	Tr	Tr	Tr
349		1 half	76	86	38	Tr	Tr	Tr	Tr	Tr
	Pineapple									
350	Raw, diced	1 cup	155	87	76	1	1	Tr	0.1	0.2
	Canned, fruit and liquid									
	Heavy syrup pack									
351	Crushed, sliced, or chunks	1 cup	254	79	198	1	Tr	Tr	Tr	0.1
352	Slices (3" dia)	1 slice	49	79	38	Tr	Tr	Tr	Tr	Tr
	Juice pack									
353	Crushed, sliced, or chunks	1 cup	249	84	149	1	Tr	Tr	Tr	0.1
354	Slice (3" dia)	1 slice	47	84	28	Tr	Tr	Tr	Tr	Tr
355	Pineapple juice, unsweetened, canned	1 cup	250	86	140	1	Tr	Tr	Tr	0.1
	Plantain, without peel									
356	Raw	1 medium	179	65	218	2	1	0.3	0.1	0.1
357	Cooked, slices	1 cup	154	67	179	1	Tr	0.1	Tr	0.1
	Plums									
358	Raw (2⅛" dia)	1 plum	66	85	36	1	Tr	Tr	0.3	0.1
	Canned, purple, fruit and liquid									
359	Heavy syrup pack	1 cup	258	76	230	1	Tr	Tr	0.2	0.1
360		1 plum	46	76	41	Tr	Tr	Tr	Tr	Tr
361	Juice pack	1 cup	252	84	146	1	Tr	Tr	Tr	Tr
362		1 plum	46	84	27	Tr	Tr	Tr	Tr	Tr
	Prunes, dried, pitted									
363	Uncooked	5 prunes	42	32	100	1	Tr	Tr	0.1	Tr
364	Stewed, unsweetened, fruit and liquid	1 cup	248	70	265	3	1	Tr	0.4	0.1
365	Prune juice, canned or bottled	1 cup	256	81	182	2	Tr	Tr	0.1	Tr
	Raisins, seedless									
366	Cup, not packed	1 cup	145	15	435	5	1	0.2	Tr	0.2
367	Packet, ½ oz (1½ tbsp)	1 packet	14	15	42	Tr	Tr	Tr	Tr	Tr
	Raspberries									
368	Raw	1 cup	123	87	60	1	1	Tr	0.1	0.4
369	Frozen, sweetened, thawed	1 cup	250	73	258	2	Tr	Tr	Tr	0.2
370	Rhubarb, frozen, cooked, with sugar	1 cup	240	68	278	1	Tr	Tr	Tr	0.1

| Choles-terol (mg) | Carbo-hydrate (g) | Total dietary fiber (g) | Calcium (mg) | Iron (mg) | Potas-sium (mg) | Sodium (mg) | Vitamin A | | Thiamin (mg) | Ribo-flavin (mg) | Niacin (mg) | Ascor-bic acid (mg) | Food No. |
							(IU)	(RE)					
0	11	2.0	5	0.1	193	0	524	53	0.02	0.04	1.0	6	337
0	19	3.4	9	0.2	335	0	910	92	0.03	0.07	1.7	11	338
0	52	3.4	8	0.7	241	16	870	86	0.03	0.06	1.6	7	339
0	20	1.3	3	0.3	90	6	325	32	0.01	0.02	0.6	3	340
0	29	3.2	15	0.7	317	10	945	94	0.02	0.04	1.4	9	341
0	11	1.3	6	0.3	125	4	373	37	0.01	0.02	0.6	4	342
0	24	3.2	11	1.6	388	3	844	84	Tr	0.08	1.7	2	343
0	60	4.5	8	0.9	325	15	710	70	0.03	0.09	1.6	236	344
0	25	4.0	18	0.4	208	0	33	3	0.03	0.07	0.2	7	345
0	51	4.3	13	0.6	173	13	0	0	0.03	0.06	0.6	3	346
0	15	1.2	4	0.2	49	4	0	0	0.01	0.02	0.2	1	347
0	32	4.0	22	0.7	238	10	15	2	0.03	0.03	0.5	4	348
0	10	1.2	7	0.2	73	3	5	1	0.01	0.01	0.2	1	349
0	19	1.9	11	0.6	175	2	36	3	0.14	0.06	0.7	24	350
0	51	2.0	36	1.0	264	3	36	3	0.23	0.06	0.7	19	351
0	10	0.4	7	0.2	51	Tr	7	Tr	0.04	0.01	0.1	4	352
0	39	2.0	35	0.7	304	2	95	10	0.24	0.05	0.7	24	353
0	7	0.4	7	0.1	57	Tr	18	2	0.04	0.01	0.1	4	354
0	34	0.5	43	0.7	335	3	13	0	0.14	0.06	0.6	27	355
0	57	4.1	5	1.1	893	7	2,017	202	0.09	0.10	1.2	33	356
0	48	3.5	3	0.9	716	8	1,400	140	0.07	0.08	1.2	17	357
0	9	1.0	3	0.1	114	0	213	21	0.03	0.06	0.3	6	358
0	60	2.6	23	2.2	235	49	668	67	0.04	0.10	0.8	1	359
0	11	0.5	4	0.4	42	9	119	12	0.01	0.02	0.1	Tr	360
0	38	2.5	25	0.9	388	3	2,543	255	0.06	0.15	1.2	7	361
0	7	0.5	5	0.2	71	Tr	464	46	0.01	0.03	0.2	1	362
0	26	3.0	21	1.0	313	2	835	84	0.03	0.07	0.8	1	363
0	70	16.4	57	2.8	828	5	759	77	0.06	0.25	1.8	7	364
0	45	2.6	31	3.0	707	10	8	0	0.04	0.18	2.0	10	365
0	115	5.8	71	3.0	1,089	17	12	1	0.23	0.13	1.2	5	366
0	11	0.6	7	0.3	105	2	1	Tr	0.02	0.01	0.1	Tr	367
0	14	8.4	27	0.7	187	0	160	16	0.04	0.11	1.1	31	368
0	65	11.0	38	1.6	285	3	150	15	0.05	0.11	0.6	41	369
0	75	4.8	348	0.5	230	2	166	17	0.04	0.06	0.5	8	370

Table 9.   Nutritive Value of the Edible Part of Food

Food No.	Food Description	Measure of edible portion	Weight (g)	Water (%)	Calories (kcal)	Pro-tein (g)	Total fat (g)	Fatty acids Satu-rated (g)	Fatty acids Mono-unsatu-rated (g)	Fatty acids Poly-unsatu-rated (g)
Fruits and Fruit Juices (continued)										
	Strawberries									
	Raw, capped									
371	Large (1⅛" dia)	1 strawberry 18		92	5	Tr	Tr	Tr	Tr	Tr
372	Medium (1¼" dia)	1 strawberry 12		92	4	Tr	Tr	Tr	Tr	Tr
373	Sliced	1 cup 166		92	50	1	1	Tr	0.1	0.3
374	Frozen, sweetened, sliced, thawed	1 cup 255		73	245	1	Tr	Tr	Tr	0.2
	Tangerines									
375	Raw, without peel and seeds (2⅜" dia)	1 tangerine..........84		88	37	1	Tr	Tr	Tr	Tr
376	Canned (mandarin oranges), light syrup, fruit and liquid	1 cup 252		83	154	1	Tr	Tr	Tr	0.1
377	Tangerine juice, canned, sweetened	1 cup 249		87	125	1	Tr	Tr	Tr	0.1
	Watermelon, raw (15" long x 7½" dia)									
378	Wedge (about 1/16 of melon)	1 wedge 286		92	92	2	1	0.1	0.3	0.4
379	Diced	1 cup 152		92	49	1	1	0.1	0.2	0.2
Grain Products										
	Bagels, enriched									
380	Plain	3½" bagel............71		33	195	7	1	0.2	0.1	0.5
381		4" bagel 89		33	245	9	1	0.2	0.1	0.6
382	Cinnamon raisin	3½" bagel............71		32	195	7	1	0.2	0.1	0.5
383		4" bagel 89		32	244	9	2	0.2	0.2	0.6
384	Egg	3½" bagel............71		33	197	8	1	0.3	0.3	0.5
385		4" bagel 89		33	247	9	2	0.4	0.4	0.6
386	Banana bread, prepared from recipe, with margarine	1 slice 60		29	196	3	6	1.3	2.7	1.9
	Barley, pearled									
387	Uncooked	1 cup 200		10	704	20	2	0.5	0.3	1.1
388	Cooked	1 cup 157		69	193	4	1	0.1	0.1	0.3
	Biscuits, plain or buttermilk, enriched									
389	Prepared from recipe, with 2% milk	2½" biscuit..........60		29	212	4	10	2.6	4.2	2.5
390		4" biscuit 101		29	358	7	16	4.4	7.0	4.2
	Refrigerated dough, baked									
391	Regular	2½" biscuit..........27		28	93	2	4	1.0	2.2	0.5
392	Lower fat	2¼" biscuit..........21		28	63	2	1	0.3	0.6	0.2
	Breads, enriched									
393	Cracked wheat	1 slice 25		36	65	2	1	0.2	0.5	0.2
394	Egg bread (challah)	½" slice 40		35	115	4	2	0.6	0.9	0.4
395	French or vienna (includes sourdough)	½" slice 25		34	69	2	1	0.2	0.3	0.2
396	Indian fry (navajo) bread	5" bread 90		27	296	6	9	2.1	3.6	2.3
397		10½" bread........160		27	526	11	15	3.7	6.4	4.1
398	Italian	1 slice 20		36	54	2	1	0.2	0.2	0.3
	Mixed grain									
399	Untoasted	1 slice 26		38	65	3	1	0.2	0.4	0.2
400	Toasted	1 slice 24		32	65	3	1	0.2	0.4	0.2
	Oatmeal									
401	Untoasted	1 slice 27		37	73	2	1	0.2	0.4	0.5
402	Toasted	1 slice 25		31	73	2	1	0.2	0.4	0.5
403	Pita	4" pita 28		32	77	3	Tr	Tr	Tr	0.1
404		6½" pita..............60		32	165	5	1	0.1	0.1	0.3

Choles-terol (mg)	Carbo-hydrate (g)	Total dietary fiber (g)	Calcium (mg)	Iron (mg)	Potas-sium (mg)	Sodium (mg)	Vitamin A		Thiamin (mg)	Ribo-flavin (mg)	Niacin (mg)	Ascor-bic acid (mg)	Food No.
							(IU)	(RE)					
0	1	0.4	3	0.1	30	Tr	5	1	Tr	0.01	Tr	10	371
0	1	0.3	2	Tr	20	Tr	3	Tr	Tr	0.01	Tr	7	372
0	12	3.8	23	0.6	276	2	45	5	0.03	0.11	0.4	94	373
0	66	4.8	28	1.5	250	8	61	5	0.04	0.13	1.0	106	374
0	9	1.9	12	0.1	132	1	773	77	0.09	0.02	0.1	26	375
0	41	1.8	18	0.9	197	15	2,117	212	0.13	0.11	1.1	50	376
0	30	0.5	45	0.5	443	2	1,046	105	0.15	0.05	0.2	55	377
0	21	1.4	23	0.5	332	6	1,047	106	0.23	0.06	0.6	27	378
0	11	0.8	12	0.3	176	3	556	56	0.12	0.03	0.3	15	379
0	38	1.6	53	2.5	72	379	0	0	0.38	0.22	3.2	0	380
0	48	2.0	66	3.2	90	475	0	0	0.48	0.28	4.1	0	381
0	39	1.6	13	2.7	105	229	52	0	0.27	0.20	2.2	Tr	382
0	49	2.0	17	3.4	132	287	65	0	0.34	0.25	2.7	1	383
17	38	1.6	9	2.8	48	359	77	23	0.38	0.17	2.4	Tr	384
21	47	2.0	12	3.5	61	449	97	29	0.48	0.21	3.1	1	385
26	33	0.7	13	0.8	80	181	278	72	0.10	0.12	0.9	1	386
0	155	31.2	58	5.0	560	18	44	4	0.38	0.23	9.2	0	387
0	44	6.0	17	2.1	146	5	11	2	0.13	0.10	3.2	0	388
2	27	0.9	141	1.7	73	348	49	14	0.21	0.19	1.8	Tr	389
3	45	1.5	237	2.9	122	586	83	23	0.36	0.31	3.0	Tr	390
0	13	0.4	5	0.7	42	325	0	0	0.09	0.06	0.8	0	391
0	12	0.4	4	0.6	39	305	0	0	0.09	0.05	0.7	0	392
0	12	1.4	11	0.7	44	135	0	0	0.09	0.06	0.9	0	393
20	19	0.9	37	1.2	46	197	30	9	0.18	0.17	1.9	0	394
0	13	0.8	19	0.6	28	152	0	0	0.13	0.08	1.2	0	395
0	48	1.6	210	3.2	67	626	0	0	0.39	0.27	3.3	0	396
0	85	2.9	373	5.8	118	1,112	0	0	0.69	0.49	5.8	0	397
0	10	0.5	16	0.6	22	117	0	0	0.09	0.06	0.9	0	398
0	12	1.7	24	0.9	53	127	0	0	0.11	0.09	1.1	Tr	399
0	12	1.6	24	0.9	53	127	0	0	0.08	0.08	1.0	Tr	400
0	13	1.1	18	0.7	38	162	4	1	0.11	0.06	0.8	0	401
0	13	1.1	18	0.7	39	163	4	1	0.09	0.06	0.8	Tr	402
0	16	0.6	24	0.7	34	150	0	0	0.17	0.09	1.3	0	403
0	33	1.3	52	1.6	72	322	0	0	0.36	0.20	2.8	0	404

Table 9. Nutritive Value of the Edible Part of Food

Food No.	Food Description	Measure of edible portion	Weight (g)	Water (%)	Calories (kcal)	Pro-tein (g)	Total fat (g)	Satu-rated (g)	Mono-unsatu-rated (g)	Poly-unsatu-rated (g)
									Fatty acids	

Grain Products (continued)

Breads, enriched (continued)

Pumpernickel

| 405 | Untoasted | 1 slice | 32 | 38 | 80 | 3 | 1 | 0.1 | 0.3 | 0.4 |
| 406 | Toasted | 1 slice | 29 | 32 | 80 | 3 | 1 | 0.1 | 0.3 | 0.4 |

Raisin

| 407 | Untoasted | 1 slice | 26 | 34 | 71 | 2 | 1 | 0.3 | 0.6 | 0.2 |
| 408 | Toasted | 1 slice | 24 | 28 | 71 | 2 | 1 | 0.3 | 0.6 | 0.2 |

Rye

409	Untoasted	1 slice	32	37	83	3	1	0.2	0.4	0.3
410	Toasted	1 slice	24	31	68	2	1	0.2	0.3	0.2
411	Rye, reduced calorie	1 slice	23	46	47	2	1	0.1	0.2	0.2

Wheat

412	Untoasted	1 slice	25	37	65	2	1	0.2	0.4	0.2
413	Toasted	1 slice	23	32	65	2	1	0.2	0.4	0.2
414	Wheat, reduced calorie	1 slice	23	43	46	2	1	0.1	0.1	0.2

White

415	Untoasted	1 slice	25	37	67	2	1	0.1	0.2	0.5
416	Toasted	1 slice	22	30	64	2	1	0.1	0.2	0.5
417	Soft crumbs	1 cup	45	37	120	4	2	0.2	0.3	0.9
418	White, reduced calorie	1 slice	23	43	48	2	1	0.1	0.2	0.1

Bread, whole wheat

| 419 | Untoasted | 1 slice | 28 | 38 | 69 | 3 | 1 | 0.3 | 0.5 | 0.3 |
| 420 | Toasted | 1 slice | 25 | 30 | 69 | 3 | 1 | 0.3 | 0.5 | 0.3 |

Bread crumbs, dry, grated

421	Plain, enriched	1 cup	108	6	427	14	6	1.3	2.6	1.2
422		1 oz	28	6	112	4	2	0.3	0.7	0.3
423	Seasoned, unenriched	1 cup	120	6	440	17	3	0.9	1.2	0.8

Bread crumbs, soft. See White bread.

| 424 | Bread stuffing, prepared from dry mix | ½ cup | 100 | 65 | 178 | 3 | 9 | 1.7 | 3.8 | 2.6 |
| 425 | Breakfast bar, cereal crust withfruit filling, fat free | 1 bar | 37 | 14 | 121 | 2 | Tr | Tr | Tr | 0.1 |

Breakfast Cereals

Hot type, cooked

Corn (hominy) grits

Regular or quick, enriched

426	White	1 cup	242	85	145	3	Tr	0.1	0.1	0.2
427	Yellow	1 cup	242	85	145	3	Tr	0.1	0.1	0.2
428	Instant, plain	1 packet	137	82	89	2	Tr	Tr	Tr	0.1

CREAM OF WHEAT

429	Regular	1 cup	251	87	133	4	1	0.1	0.1	0.3
430	Quick	1 cup	239	87	129	4	Tr	0.1	0.1	0.3
431	Mix'n Eat, plain	1 packet	142	82	102	3	Tr	Tr	Tr	0.2
432	MALT O MEAL	1 cup	240	88	122	4	Tr	0.1	0.1	Tr

Oatmeal

| 433 | Regular, quick or instant, plain, nonfortified | 1 cup | 234 | 85 | 145 | 6 | 2 | 0.4 | 0.7 | 0.9 |
| 434 | Instant, fortified, plain | 1 packet | 177 | 86 | 104 | 4 | 2 | 0.3 | 0.6 | 0.7 |

QUAKER instant

435	Apples and cinnamon	1 packet	149	79	125	3	1	0.3	0.5	0.6
436	Maple and brown sugar	1 packet	155	75	153	4	2	0.4	0.6	0.7
437	WHEATENA	1 cup	243	85	136	5	1	0.2	0.2	0.6

Ready to eat

438	ALL BRAN	½ cup	30	3	79	4	1	0.2	0.2	0.5
439	APPLE CINNAMON CHEERIOS	¾ cup	30	3	118	2	2	0.3	0.6	0.2
440	APPLE JACKS	1 cup	30	3	116	1	Tr	0.1	0.1	0.2

Choles-terol (mg)	Carbo-hydrate (g)	Total dietary fiber (g)	Calcium (mg)	Iron (mg)	Potas-sium (mg)	Sodium (mg)	Vitamin A		Thiamin (mg)	Ribo-flavin (mg)	Niacin (mg)	Ascor-bic acid (mg)	Food No.
							(IU)	(RE)					
0	15	2.1	22	0.9	67	215	0	0	0.10	0.10	1.0	0	405
0	15	2.1	21	0.9	66	214	0	0	0.08	0.09	0.9	0	406
0	14	1.1	17	0.8	59	101	0	0	0.09	0.10	0.9	Tr	407
0	14	1.1	17	0.8	59	102	Tr	0	0.07	0.09	0.8	Tr	408
0	15	1.9	23	0.9	53	211	2	Tr	0.14	0.11	1.2	Tr	409
0	13	1.5	19	0.7	44	174	1	0	0.09	0.08	0.9	Tr	410
0	9	2.8	17	0.7	23	93	1	0	0.08	0.06	0.6	Tr	411
0	12	1.1	26	0.8	50	133	0	0	0.10	0.07	1.0	0	412
0	12	1.2	26	0.8	50	132	0	0	0.08	0.06	0.9	0	413
0	10	2.8	18	0.7	28	118	0	0	0.10	0.07	0.9	Tr	414
Tr	12	0.6	27	0.8	30	135	0	0	0.12	0.09	1.0	0	415
Tr	12	0.6	26	0.7	29	130	0	0	0.09	0.07	0.9	0	416
Tr	22	1.0	49	1.4	54	242	0	0	0.21	0.15	1.8	0	417
0	10	2.2	22	0.7	17	104	1	Tr	0.09	0.07	0.8	Tr	418
0	13	1.9	20	0.9	71	148	0	0	0.10	0.06	1.1	0	419
0	13	1.9	20	0.9	71	148	0	0	0.08	0.05	1.0	0	420
0	78	2.6	245	6.6	239	931	1	0	0.83	0.47	7.4	0	421
0	21	0.7	64	1.7	63	244	Tr	0	0.22	0.12	1.9	0	422
1	84	5.0	119	3.8	324	3,180	16	4	0.19	0.20	3.3	Tr	423
0	22	2.9	32	1.1	74	543	313	81	0.14	0.11	1.5	0	424
Tr	28	0.8	49	4.5	92	203	1,249	125	1.01	0.42	5.0	1	425
0	31	0.5	0	1.5	53	0	0	0	0.24	0.15	2.0	0	426
0	31	0.5	0	1.5	53	0	145	15	0.24	0.15	2.0	0	427
0	21	1.2	8	8.2	38	289	0	0	0.15	0.08	1.4	0	428
0	28	1.8	50	10.3	43	3	0	0	0.25	0.00	1.5	0	429
0	27	1.2	50	10.3	45	139	0	0	0.24	0.00	1.4	0	430
0	21	0.4	20	8.1	38	241	1,252	376	0.43	0.28	5.0	0	431
0	26	1.0	5	9.6	31	2	0	0	0.48	0.24	5.8	0	432
0	25	4.0	19	1.6	131	2	37	5	0.26	0.05	0.3	0	433
0	18	3.0	163	6.3	99	285	1,510	453	0.53	0.28	5.5	0	434
0	26	2.5	104	3.9	106	121	1,019	305	0.30	0.35	4.1	Tr	435
0	31	2.6	105	3.9	112	234	1,008	302	0.30	0.34	4.0	0	436
0	29	6.6	10	1.4	187	5	0	0	0.02	0.05	1.3	0	437
0	23	9.7	106	4.5	342	61	750	225	0.39	0.42	5.0	15	438
0	25	1.6	35	4.5	60	150	750	225	0.38	0.43	5.0	15	439
0	27	0.6	3	4.5	32	134	750	225	0.39	0.42	5.0	15	440

Table 9.   Nutritive Value of the Edible Part of Food

Food No.	Food Description	Measure of edible portion	Weight (g)	Water (%)	Calories (kcal)	Pro-tein (g)	Total fat (g)	Fatty acids Satu-rated (g)	Fatty acids Mono-unsatu-rated (g)	Fatty acids Poly-unsatu-rated (g)

Grain Products (continued)

Breakfast Cereals (continued)

Ready to eat (continued)

441	BASIC 4	1 cup	55	7	201	4	3	0.4	1.0	1.1
442	BERRY BERRY KIX	¾ cup	30	2	120	1	1	0.2	0.5	0.1
443	CAP'N CRUNCH	¾ cup	27	2	107	1	1	0.4	0.3	0.2
444	CAP'N CRUNCH'S CRUNCHBERRIES	¾ cup	26	2	104	1	1	0.3	0.3	0.2
445	CAP'N CRUNCH'S PEANUT BUTTER CRUNCH	¾ cup	27	2	112	2	2	0.5	0.8	0.5
446	CHEERIOS	1 cup	30	3	110	3	2	0.4	0.6	0.2
	CHEX									
447	Corn	1 cup	30	3	113	2	Tr	0.1	0.1	0.2
448	Honey nut	¾ cup	30	2	117	2	1	0.1	0.4	0.2
449	Multi bran	1 cup	49	3	165	4	1	0.2	0.3	0.5
450	Rice	1¼ cup	31	3	117	2	Tr	Tr	Tr	Tr
451	Wheat	1 cup	30	3	104	3	1	0.1	0.1	0.3
452	CINNAMON LIFE	1 cup	50	4	190	4	2	0.3	0.6	0.8
453	CINNAMON TOAST CRUNCH	¾ cup	30	2	124	2	3	0.5	0.9	0.5
454	COCOA KRISPIES	¾ cup	31	2	120	2	1	0.6	0.1	0.1
455	COCOA PUFFS	1 cup	30	2	119	1	1	0.2	0.3	Tr
	Corn Flakes									
456	GENERAL MILLS, TOTAL	1⅓ cup	30	3	112	2	Tr	0.2	0.1	Tr
457	KELLOGG'S	1 cup	28	3	102	2	Tr	0.1	Tr	0.1
458	CORN POPS	1 cup	31	3	118	1	Tr	0.1	0.1	Tr
459	CRISPIX	1 cup	29	3	108	2	Tr	0.1	0.1	0.1
460	Complete Wheat Bran Flakes	¾ cup	29	4	95	3	1	0.1	0.1	0.4
461	FROOT LOOPS	1 cup	30	2	117	1	1	0.4	0.2	0.3
462	FROSTED FLAKES	¾ cup	31	3	119	1	Tr	0.1	Tr	0.1
	FROSTED MINI WHEATS									
463	Regular	1 cup	51	5	173	5	1	0.2	0.1	0.6
464	Bite size	1 cup	55	5	187	5	1	0.2	0.2	0.6
465	GOLDEN GRAHAMS	¾ cup	30	3	116	2	1	0.2	0.3	0.2
466	HONEY FROSTED WHEATIES	¾ cup	30	3	110	2	Tr	0.1	Tr	Tr
467	HONEY NUT CHEERIOS	1 cup	30	2	115	3	1	0.2	0.5	0.2
468	HONEY NUT CLUSTERS	1 cup	55	3	213	5	3	0.4	1.8	0.4
469	KIX	1⅓ cup	30	2	114	2	1	0.2	0.1	Tr
470	LIFE	¾ cup	32	4	121	3	1	0.2	0.4	0.6
471	LUCKY CHARMS	1 cup	30	2	116	2	1	0.2	0.4	0.2
472	NATURE VALLEY Granola	¾ cup	55	4	248	6	10	1.3	6.5	1.9
	100% Natural Cereal									
473	With oats, honey, and raisins	½ cup	51	4	218	5	7	3.2	3.2	0.8
474	With raisins, low fat	½ cup	50	4	195	4	3	0.8	1.3	0.5
475	PRODUCT 19	1 cup	30	3	110	3	Tr	Tr	0.2	0.2
476	Puffed Rice	1 cup	14	3	56	1	Tr	Tr	Tr	Tr
477	Puffed Wheat	1 cup	12	3	44	2	Tr	Tr	Tr	Tr
	Raisin Bran									
478	GENERAL MILLS, TOTAL	1 cup	55	9	178	4	1	0.2	0.2	0.2
479	KELLOGG'S	1 cup	61	8	186	6	1	0.0	0.2	0.8
480	RAISIN NUT BRAN	1 cup	55	5	209	5	4	0.7	1.9	0.5
481	REESE'S PEANUT BUTTER PUFFS	¾ cup	30	2	129	3	3	0.6	1.4	0.6
482	RICE KRISPIES	1¼ cup	33	3	124	2	Tr	0.1	0.1	0.2

Choles-terol (mg)	Carbo-hydrate (g)	Total dietary fiber (g)	Calcium (mg)	Iron (mg)	Potas-sium (mg)	Sodium (mg)	Vitamin A		Thiamin (mg)	Ribo-flavin (mg)	Niacin (mg)	Ascor-bic acid (mg)	Food No.
							(IU)	(RE)					
0	42	3.4	310	4.5	162	323	1,250	375	0.37	0.42	5.0	15	441
0	26	0.2	66	4.5	24	185	750	225	0.38	0.43	5.0	15	442
0	23	0.9	5	4.5	35	208	36	4	0.38	0.42	5.0	0	443
0	22	0.6	7	4.5	37	190	33	5	0.37	0.42	5.0	Tr	444
0	22	0.8	3	4.5	62	204	37	4	0.38	0.42	5.0	0	445
0	23	2.6	55	8.1	89	284	1,250	375	0.38	0.43	5.0	15	446
0	26	0.5	100	9.0	32	289	0	0	0.38	0.00	5.0	6	447
0	26	0.4	102	9.0	27	224	0	0	0.38	0.44	5.0	6	448
0	41	6.4	95	13.7	191	325	0	0	0.32	0.00	4.4	5	449
0	27	0.3	104	9.0	36	291	0	0	0.38	0.02	5.0	6	450
0	24	3.3	60	9.0	116	269	0	0	0.23	0.04	3.0	4	451
0	40	3.0	135	7.5	113	220	16	2	0.63	0.71	8.4	Tr	452
0	24	1.5	42	4.5	44	210	750	225	0.38	0.43	5.0	15	453
0	27	0.4	4	1.8	60	210	750	225	0.37	0.43	5.0	15	454
0	27	0.2	33	4.5	52	181	0	0	0.38	0.43	5.0	15	455
0	26	0.8	237	18.0	34	203	1,250	375	1.50	1.70	20.1	60	456
0	24	0.8	1	8.7	25	298	700	210	0.36	0.39	4.7	14	457
0	28	0.4	2	1.9	23	123	775	233	0.40	0.43	5.2	16	458
0	25	0.6	3	1.8	35	240	750	225	0.38	0.44	5.0	15	459
0	23	4.6	14	8.1	175	226	1,208	363	0.38	0.44	5.0	15	460
0	26	0.6	3	4.2	32	141	703	211	0.39	0.42	5.0	14	461
0	28	0.6	1	4.5	20	200	750	225	0.37	0.43	5.0	15	462
0	42	5.5	18	14.3	170	2	0	0	0.36	0.41	5.0	0	463
0	45	5.9	0	15.4	186	2	0	0	0.33	0.39	4.7	0	464
0	26	0.9	14	4.5	53	275	750	225	0.38	0.43	5.0	15	465
0	26	1.5	8	4.5	56	211	750	225	0.38	0.43	5.0	15	466
0	24	1.6	20	4.5	85	259	750	225	0.38	0.43	5.0	15	467
0	43	4.2	72	4.5	171	239	0	0	0.37	0.42	5.0	9	468
0	26	0.8	44	8.1	41	263	1,250	375	0.38	0.43	5.0	15	469
0	25	2.0	98	9.0	79	174	12	1	0.40	0.45	5.3	0	470
0	25	1.2	32	4.5	54	203	750	225	0.38	0.43	5.0	15	471
0	36	3.5	41	1.7	183	89	0	0	0.17	0.06	0.6	0	472
1	36	3.7	39	1.7	214	11	4	1	0.14	0.09	0.8	Tr	473
1	40	3.0	30	1.3	169	129	9	1	0.15	0.06	0.9	Tr	474
0	25	1.0	3	18.0	41	216	750	225	1.50	1.71	20.0	60	475
0	13	0.2	1	4.4	16	Tr	0	0	0.36	0.25	4.9	0	476
0	10	0.5	3	3.8	42	Tr	0	0	0.31	0.22	4.2	0	477
0	43	5.0	238	18.0	287	240	1,250	375	1.50	1.70	20.0	0	478
0	47	8.2	35	5.0	437	354	832	250	0.43	0.49	5.6	0	479
0	41	5.1	74	4.5	218	246	0	0	0.37	0.42	5.0	0	480
0	23	0.4	21	4.5	62	177	750	225	0.38	0.43	5.0	15	481
0	29	0.4	3	2.0	42	354	825	248	0.43	0.46	5.5	17	482

Table 9.   Nutritive Value of the Edible Part of Food

Food No.	Food Description	Measure of edible portion	Weight (g)	Water (%)	Calories (kcal)	Pro-tein (g)	Total fat (g)	Fatty acids Satu-rated (g)	Mono-unsatu-rated (g)	Poly-unsatu-rated (g)
	Grain Products (continued)									
	Breakfast Cereals (continued)									
	Ready to eat (continued)									
483	RICE KRISPIES									
	TREATS cereal	¾ cup	30	4	120	1	2	0.4	1.0	0.2
484	SHREDDED WHEAT	2 biscuits	46	4	156	5	1	0.1	NA	NA
485	SMACKS	¾ cup	27	3	103	2	1	0.3	0.1	0.2
486	SPECIAL K	1 cup	31	3	115	6	Tr	0.0	0.0	0.2
487	QUAKER Toasted Oatmeal,									
	Honey Nut	1 cup	49	3	191	5	3	0.5	1.2	0.7
488	TOTAL, Whole Grain	¾ cup	30	3	105	3	1	0.2	0.1	0.1
489	TRIX	1 cup	30	2	122	1	2	0.4	0.9	0.3
490	WHEATIES	1 cup	30	3	110	3	1	0.2	0.2	0.2
	Brownies, without icing									
	Commercially prepared									
491	Regular, large									
	(2¾" sq x ⅞")	1 brownie	56	14	227	3	9	2.4	5.0	1.3
492	Fat free, 2" sq	1 brownie	28	12	89	1	Tr	0.2	0.1	Tr
493	Prepared from dry mix,									
	reduced calorie, 2" sq	1 brownie	22	13	84	1	2	1.1	1.0	0.2
494	Buckwheat flour, whole groat	1 cup	120	11	402	15	4	0.8	1.1	1.1
495	Buckwheat groats, roasted									
	(kasha), cooked	1 cup	168	76	155	6	1	0.2	0.3	0.3
	Bulgur									
496	Uncooked	1 cup	140	9	479	17	2	0.3	0.2	0.8
497	Cooked	1 cup	182	78	151	6	Tr	0.1	0.1	0.2
	Cakes, prepared from dry mix									
498	Angelfood (1/12 of 10" dia)	1 piece	50	33	129	3	Tr	Tr	Tr	0.1
499	Yellow, light, with water, egg									
	whites, no frosting									
	(1/12 of 9" dia)	1 piece	69	37	181	3	2	1.1	0.9	0.2
	Cakes, prepared from recipe									
500	Chocolate, without frosting									
	(1/12 of 9" dia)	1 piece	95	24	340	5	14	5.2	5.7	2.6
501	Gingerbread (1/9 of									
	8" square)	1 piece	74	28	263	3	12	3.1	5.3	3.1
502	Pineapple upside down (1/9									
	of 8" square)	1 piece	115	32	367	4	14	3.4	6.0	3.8
503	Shortcake, biscuit type (about									
	3" dia)	1 shortcake	65	28	225	4	9	2.5	3.9	2.4
504	Sponge (1/12 of 16-oz cake)	1 piece	63	29	187	5	3	0.8	1.0	0.4
	White									
505	With coconut frosting (1/12									
	of 9" dia)	1 piece	112	21	399	5	12	4.4	4.1	2.4
506	Without frosting (1/12 of 9"									
	dia)	1 piece	74	23	264	4	9	2.4	3.9	2.3
	Cakes, commercially prepared									
507	Angelfood (1/12 of									
	12-oz cake)	1 piece	28	33	72	2	Tr	Tr	Tr	0.1
508	Boston cream (1/6 of pie)	1 piece	92	45	232	2	8	2.2	4.2	0.9
509	Chocolate with chocolate									
	frosting (1/8 of									
	18-oz cake)	1 piece	64	23	235	3	10	3.1	5.6	1.2
510	Coffeecake, crumb (1/9 of									
	20-oz cake)	1 piece	63	22	263	4	15	3.7	8.2	2.0
511	Fruitcake	1 piece	43	25	139	1	4	0.5	1.8	1.4
	Pound									
512	Butter (1/12 of 12-oz cake)	1 piece	28	25	109	2	6	3.2	1.7	0.3
513	Fat free (3¼" x 2¾" x									
	⅝" slice)	1 slice	28	31	79	2	Tr	0.1	Tr	0.1

Choles-terol (mg)	Carbo-hydrate (g)	Total dietary fiber (g)	Calcium (mg)	Iron (mg)	Potas-sium (mg)	Sodium (mg)	Vitamin A		Thiamin (mg)	Ribo-flavin (mg)	Niacin (mg)	Ascor-bic acid (mg)	Food No.
							(IU)	(RE)					
0	26	0.3	2	1.8	19	190	750	225	0.39	0.42	5.0	15	483
0	38	5.3	20	1.4	196	3	0	NA	0.12	0.05	2.6	0	484
0	24	0.9	3	1.8	42	51	750	225	0.38	0.43	5.0	15	485
0	22	1.0	5	8.7	55	250	750	225	0.53	0.59	7.0	15	486
Tr	39	3.3	27	4.5	185	166	500	150	0.37	0.42	5.0	6	487
0	24	2.6	258	18.0	97	199	1,250	375	1.50	1.70	20.1	60	488
0	26	0.7	32	4.5	18	197	750	225	0.38	0.43	5.0	15	489
0	24	2.1	55	8.1	104	222	750	225	0.38	0.43	5.0	15	490
10	36	1.2	16	1.3	83	175	39	3	0.14	0.12	1.0	0	491
0	22	1.0	17	0.7	89	90	1	Tr	0.03	0.04	0.3	Tr	492
0	16	0.8	3	0.3	69	21	0	0	0.02	0.03	0.2	0	493
0	85	12.0	49	4.9	692	13	0	0	0.50	0.23	7.4	0	494
0	33	4.5	12	1.3	148	7	0	0	0.07	0.07	1.6	0	495
0	106	25.6	49	3.4	574	24	0	0	0.32	0.16	7.2	0	496
0	34	8.2	18	1.7	124	9	0	0	0.10	0.05	1.8	0	497
0	29	0.1	42	0.1	68	255	0	0	0.05	0.10	0.1	0	498
0	37	0.6	69	0.6	41	279	6	1	0.06	0.12	0.6	0	499
55	51	1.5	57	1.5	133	299	133	38	0.13	0.20	1.1	Tr	500
24	36	0.7	53	2.1	325	242	36	10	0.14	0.12	1.3	Tr	501
25	58	0.9	138	1.7	129	367	291	75	0.18	0.18	1.4	1	502
2	32	0.8	133	1.7	69	329	47	12	0.20	0.18	1.7	Tr	503
107	36	0.4	26	1.0	89	144	163	49	0.10	0.19	0.8	0	504
1	71	1.1	101	1.3	111	318	43	12	0.14	0.21	1.2	Tr	505
1	42	0.6	96	1.1	70	242	41	12	0.14	0.18	1.1	Tr	506
0	16	0.4	39	0.1	26	210	0	0	0.03	0.14	0.2	0	507
34	39	1.3	21	0.3	36	132	74	21	0.38	0.25	0.2	Tr	508
27	35	1.8	28	1.4	128	214	54	16	0.02	0.09	0.4	Tr	509
20	29	1.3	34	1.2	77	221	70	21	0.13	0.14	1.1	Tr	510
2	26	1.6	14	0.9	66	116	9	2	0.02	0.04	0.3	Tr	511
62	14	0.1	10	0.4	33	111	170	44	0.04	0.06	0.4	0	512
0	17	0.3	12	0.6	31	95	27	8	0.04	0.08	0.2	0	513

Table 9.　Nutritive Value of the Edible Part of Food

Food No.	Food Description	Measure of edible portion	Weight (g)	Water (%)	Calories (kcal)	Pro- tein (g)	Total fat (g)	Satu- rated (g)	Mono- unsatu- rated (g)	Poly- unsatu- rated (g)
									Fatty acids	

Grain Products (continued)

Cakes, commercially prepared (continued)
　Snack cakes

Food No.	Food Description	Measure of edible portion	Weight (g)	Water (%)	Calories (kcal)	Pro- tein (g)	Total fat (g)	Satu- rated (g)	Mono- unsatu- rated (g)	Poly- unsatu- rated (g)
514	Chocolate, creme filled, with frosting	1 cupcake	50	20	188	2	7	1.4	2.8	2.6
515	Chocolate, with frosting, low fat	1 cupcake	43	23	131	2	2	0.5	0.8	0.2
516	Sponge, creme filled	1 cake	43	20	155	1	5	1.1	1.7	1.4
517	Sponge, individual shortcake	1 shortcake	30	30	87	2	1	0.2	0.3	0.1
	Yellow									
518	With chocolate frosting	1 piece	64	22	243	2	11	3.0	6.1	1.4
519	With vanilla frosting	1 piece	64	22	239	2	9	1.5	3.9	3.3
520	Cheesecake (⅙ of 17-oz cake)	1 piece	80	46	257	4	18	7.9	6.9	1.3
521	Cheese flavor puffs or twists	1 oz	28	2	157	2	10	1.9	5.7	1.3
522	CHEX mix	1 oz (about ⅔ cup)	28	4	120	3	5	1.6	NA	NA
	Cookies									
523	Butter, commercially prepared	1 cookie	5	5	23	Tr	1	0.6	0.3	Tr
	Chocolate chip, medium (2¼"-2½" dia)									
	Commercially prepared									
524	Regular	1 cookie	10	4	48	1	2	0.7	1.2	0.2
525	Reduced fat	1 cookie	10	4	45	1	2	0.4	0.6	0.5
526	From refrigerated dough (spooned from roll)	1 cookie	26	3	128	1	6	2.0	2.9	0.6
527	Prepared from recipe, with margarine	1 cookie	16	6	78	1	5	1.3	1.7	1.3
528	Devil's food, commercially prepared, fat free	1 cookie	16	18	49	1	Tr	0.1	Tr	Tr
529	Fig bar	1 cookie	16	17	56	1	1	0.2	0.5	0.4
	Molasses									
530	Medium	1 cookie	15	6	65	1	2	0.5	1.1	0.3
531	Large (3½"-4" dia)	1 cookie	32	6	138	2	4	1.0	2.3	0.6
	Oatmeal									
	Commercially prepared, with or without raisins									
532	Regular, large	1 cookie	25	6	113	2	5	1.1	2.5	0.6
533	Soft type	1 cookie	15	11	61	1	2	0.5	1.2	0.3
534	Fat free	1 cookie	11	13	36	1	Tr	Tr	Tr	0.1
535	Prepared from recipe, with raisins (2⅝" dia)	1 cookie	15	6	65	1	2	0.5	1.0	0.8
	Peanut butter									
536	Commercially prepared	1 cookie	15	6	72	1	4	0.7	1.9	0.8
537	Prepared from recipe, with margarine (3" dia)	1 cookie	20	6	95	2	5	0.9	2.2	1.4
	Sandwich type, with creme filling									
538	Chocolate cookie	1 cookie	10	2	47	Tr	2	0.4	0.9	0.7
	Vanilla cookie									
539	Oval	1 cookie	15	2	72	1	3	0.4	1.3	1.1
540	Round	1 cookie	10	2	48	Tr	2	0.3	0.8	0.8
	Shortbread, commercially prepared									
541	Plain (1⅝" sq)	1 cookie	8	4	40	Tr	2	0.5	1.1	0.3
	Pecan									
542	Regular (2" dia)	1 cookie	14	3	76	1	5	1.1	2.6	0.6
543	Reduced fat	1 cookie	16	5	73	1	3	0.6	1.6	0.4

Choles-terol (mg)	Carbo-hydrate (g)	Total dietary fiber (g)	Calcium (mg)	Iron (mg)	Potas-sium (mg)	Sodium (mg)	Vitamin A		Thiamin (mg)	Ribo-flavin (mg)	Niacin (mg)	Ascor-bic acid (mg)	Food No.
							(IU)	(RE)					
9	30	0.4	37	1.7	61	213	9	3	0.11	0.15	1.2	0	514
0	29	1.8	15	0.7	96	178	0	0	0.02	0.06	0.3	0	515
7	27	0.2	19	0.5	37	155	7	2	0.07	0.06	0.5	Tr	516
31	18	0.2	21	0.8	30	73	46	14	0.07	0.08	0.6	0	517
35	35	1.2	24	1.3	114	216	70	21	0.08	0.10	0.8	0	518
35	38	0.2	40	0.7	34	220	40	12	0.06	0.04	0.3	0	519
44	20	0.3	41	0.5	72	166	438	117	0.02	0.15	0.2	Tr	520
1	15	0.3	16	0.7	47	298	75	10	0.07	0.10	0.9	Tr	521
0	18	1.6	10	7.0	76	288	41	4	0.44	0.14	4.8	13	522
6	3	Tr	1	0.1	6	18	34	8	0.02	0.02	0.2	0	523
0	7	0.3	3	0.3	14	32	Tr	0	0.02	0.03	0.3	0	524
0	7	0.4	2	0.3	12	38	Tr	0	0.03	0.03	0.3	0	525
7	18	0.4	7	0.7	52	60	15	4	0.04	0.05	0.5	0	526
5	9	0.4	6	0.4	36	58	102	26	0.03	0.03	0.2	Tr	527
0	12	0.3	5	0.4	18	28	Tr	NA	0.01	0.03	0.2	Tr	528
0	11	0.7	10	0.5	33	56	5	1	0.03	0.03	0.3	Tr	529
0	11	0.1	11	1.0	52	69	0	0	0.05	0.04	0.5	0	530
0	24	0.3	24	2.1	111	147	0	0	0.11	0.08	1.0	0	531
0	17	0.7	9	0.6	36	96	5	1	0.07	0.06	0.6	Tr	532
1	10	0.4	14	0.4	20	52	5	1	0.03	0.03	0.3	Tr	533
0	9	0.8	4	0.2	23	33	0	0	0.02	0.03	0.1	0	534
5	10	0.5	15	0.4	36	81	96	25	0.04	0.02	0.2	Tr	535
Tr	9	0.3	5	0.4	25	62	1	Tr	0.03	0.03	0.6	0	536
6	12	0.4	8	0.4	46	104	120	31	0.04	0.04	0.7	Tr	537
0	7	0.3	3	0.4	18	60	Tr	0	0.01	0.02	0.2	0	538
0	11	0.2	4	0.3	14	52	0	0	0.04	0.04	0.4	0	539
0	7	0.2	3	0.2	9	35	0	0	0.03	0.02	0.3	0	540
2	5	0.1	3	0.2	8	36	7	1	0.03	0.03	0.3	0	541
5	8	0.3	4	0.3	10	39	Tr	Tr	0.04	0.03	0.3	0	542
0	11	0.2	8	0.5	15	55	1	Tr	0.05	0.03	0.4	Tr	543

Table 9.   Nutritive Value of the Edible Part of Food

Food No.	Food Description	Measure of edible portion	Weight (g)	Water (%)	Calories (kcal)	Protein (g)	Total fat (g)	Saturated (g)	Mono-unsaturated (g)	Poly-unsaturated (g)
								Fatty acids		

Grain Products (continued)

Cookies (continued)

Sugar

544	Commercially prepared	1 cookie	15	5	72	1	3	0.8	1.8	0.4
545	From refrigerated dough	1 cookie	15	5	73	1	3	0.9	2.0	0.4
546	Prepared from recipe, with margarine (3" dia)	1 cookie	14	9	66	1	3	0.7	1.4	1.0
547	Vanilla wafer, lower fat, medium size	1 cookie	4	5	18	Tr	1	0.2	0.3	0.2

Corn chips

| 548 | Plain | 1 oz | 28 | 1 | 153 | 2 | 9 | 1.3 | 2.7 | 4.7 |
| 549 | Barbecue flavor | 1 oz | 28 | 1 | 148 | 2 | 9 | 1.3 | 2.7 | 4.6 |

Cornbread

| 550 | Prepared from mix, piece 3¾" x 2½" x ¾" | 1 piece | 60 | 32 | 188 | 4 | 6 | 1.6 | 3.1 | 0.7 |
| 551 | Prepared from recipe, with 2% milk, piece 2½" sq x 1½" | 1 piece | 65 | 39 | 173 | 4 | 5 | 1.0 | 1.2 | 2.1 |

Cornmeal, yellow, dry form

552	Whole grain	1 cup	122	10	442	10	4	0.6	1.2	2.0
553	Degermed, enriched	1 cup	138	12	505	12	2	0.3	0.6	1.0
554	Self rising, degermed, enriched	1 cup	138	10	490	12	2	0.3	0.6	1.0
555	Cornstarch	1 tbsp	8	8	30	Tr	Tr	Tr	Tr	Tr

Couscous

| 556 | Uncooked | 1 cup | 173 | 9 | 650 | 22 | 1 | 0.2 | 0.2 | 0.4 |
| 557 | Cooked | 1 cup | 157 | 73 | 176 | 6 | Tr | Tr | Tr | 0.1 |

Crackers

| 558 | Cheese, 1" sq | 10 crackers | 10 | 3 | 50 | 1 | 3 | 0.9 | 1.2 | 0.2 |

Graham, plain

559	2½" sq	2 squares	14	4	59	1	1	0.2	0.6	0.5
560	Crushed	1 cup	84	4	355	6	8	1.3	3.4	3.2
561	Melba toast, plain	4 pieces	20	5	78	2	1	0.1	0.2	0.3
562	Rye wafer, whole grain, plain	1 wafer	11	5	37	1	Tr	Tr	Tr	Tr

Saltine

| 563 | Square | 4 crackers | 12 | 4 | 52 | 1 | 1 | 0.4 | 0.8 | 0.2 |
| 564 | Oyster type | 1 cup | 45 | 4 | 195 | 4 | 5 | 1.3 | 2.9 | 0.8 |

Sandwich type

| 565 | Wheat with cheese | 1 sandwich | 7 | 4 | 33 | 1 | 1 | 0.4 | 0.8 | 0.2 |
| 566 | Cheese with peanut butter | 1 sandwich | 7 | 4 | 34 | 1 | 2 | 0.4 | 0.8 | 0.3 |

Standard snack type

567	Bite size	1 cup	62	4	311	5	16	2.3	6.6	5.9
568	Round	4 crackers	12	4	60	1	3	0.5	1.3	1.1
569	Wheat, thin square	4 crackers	8	3	38	1	2	0.4	0.9	0.2
570	Whole wheat	4 crackers	16	3	71	1	3	0.5	0.9	1.1
571	Croissant, butter	1 croissant	57	23	231	5	12	6.6	3.1	0.6
572	Croutons, seasoned	1 cup	40	4	186	4	7	2.1	3.8	0.9

Danish pastry, enriched

| 573 | Cheese filled | 1 danish | 71 | 31 | 266 | 6 | 16 | 4.8 | 8.0 | 1.8 |
| 574 | Fruit filled | 1 danish | 71 | 27 | 263 | 4 | 13 | 3.5 | 7.1 | 1.7 |

Doughnuts

575	Cake type	1 hole	14	21	59	1	3	0.5	1.3	1.1
576		1 medium	47	21	198	2	11	1.7	4.4	3.7
577	Yeast leavened, glazed	1 hole	13	25	52	1	3	0.8	1.7	0.4
578		1 medium	60	25	242	4	14	3.5	7.7	1.7
579	Eclair, prepared from recipe, 5" x 2" x 1¾"	1 eclair	100	52	262	6	16	4.1	6.5	3.9

English muffin, plain, enriched

| 580 | Untoasted | 1 muffin | 57 | 42 | 134 | 4 | 1 | 0.1 | 0.2 | 0.5 |
| 581 | Toasted | 1 muffin | 52 | 37 | 133 | 4 | 1 | 0.1 | 0.2 | 0.5 |

Choles-terol (mg)	Carbo-hydrate (g)	Total dietary fiber (g)	Calcium (mg)	Iron (mg)	Potas-sium (mg)	Sodium (mg)	Vitamin A		Thiamin (mg)	Ribo-flavin (mg)	Niacin (mg)	Ascor-bic acid (mg)	Food No.
							(IU)	(RE)					
8	10	0.1	3	0.3	9	54	14	4	0.03	0.03	0.4	Tr	544
5	10	0.1	14	0.3	24	70	6	2	0.03	0.02	0.4	0	545
4	8	0.2	10	0.3	11	69	135	35	0.04	0.04	0.3	Tr	546
2	3	0.1	2	0.1	4	12	1	Tr	0.01	0.01	0.1	0	547
0	16	1.4	36	0.4	40	179	27	3	0.01	0.04	0.3	0	548
0	16	1.5	37	0.4	67	216	173	17	0.02	0.06	0.5	Tr	549
37	29	1.4	44	1.1	77	467	123	26	0.15	0.16	1.2	Tr	550
26	28	1.9	162	1.6	96	428	180	35	0.19	0.19	1.5	Tr	551
0	94	8.9	7	4.2	350	43	572	57	0.47	0.25	4.4	0	552
0	107	10.2	7	5.7	224	4	570	57	0.99	0.56	6.9	0	553
0	103	9.8	483	6.5	235	1,860	570	57	0.94	0.53	6.3	0	554
0	7	0.1	Tr	Tr	Tr	1	0	0	0.00	0.00	0.0	0	555
0	134	8.7	42	1.9	287	17	0	0	0.28	0.13	6.0	0	556
0	36	2.2	13	0.6	91	8	0	0	0.10	0.04	1.5	0	557
1	6	0.2	15	0.5	15	100	16	3	0.06	0.04	0.5	0	558
0	11	0.4	3	0.5	19	85	0	0	0.03	0.04	0.6	0	559
0	65	2.4	20	3.1	113	508	0	0	0.19	0.26	3.5	0	560
0	15	1.3	19	0.7	40	166	0	0	0.08	0.05	0.8	0	561
0	9	2.5	4	0.7	54	87	1	0	0.05	0.03	0.2	Tr	562
0	9	0.4	14	0.6	15	156	0	0	0.07	0.06	0.6	0	563
0	32	1.4	54	2.4	58	586	0	0	0.25	0.21	2.4	0	564
Tr	4	0.1	18	0.2	30	98	5	1	0.03	0.05	0.3	Tr	565
Tr	4	0.2	6	0.2	17	69	22	2	0.03	0.02	0.5	Tr	566
0	38	1.0	74	2.2	82	525	0	0	0.25	0.21	2.5	0	567
0	7	0.2	14	0.4	16	102	0	0	0.05	0.04	0.5	0	568
0	5	0.4	4	0.4	15	64	0	0	0.04	0.03	0.4	0	569
0	11	1.7	8	0.5	48	105	0	0	0.03	0.02	0.7	0	570
38	26	1.5	21	1.2	67	424	424	106	0.22	0.14	1.2	Tr	571
3	25	2.0	38	1.1	72	495	16	4	0.20	0.17	1.9	0	572
11	26	0.7	25	1.1	70	320	104	32	0.13	0.18	1.4	Tr	573
81	34	1.3	33	1.3	59	251	53	16	0.19	0.16	1.4	3	574
5	7	0.2	6	0.3	18	76	8	2	0.03	0.03	0.3	Tr	575
17	23	0.7	21	0.9	60	257	27	8	0.10	0.11	0.9	Tr	576
1	6	0.2	6	0.3	14	44	2	1	0.05	0.03	0.4	Tr	577
4	27	0.7	26	1.2	65	205	8	2	0.22	0.13	1.7	Tr	578
127	24	0.6	63	1.2	117	337	718	191	0.12	0.27	0.8	Tr	579
0	26	1.5	99	1.4	75	264	0	0	0.25	0.16	2.2	0	580
0	26	1.5	98	1.4	74	262	0	0	0.20	0.14	2.0	Tr	581

Table 9.   Nutritive Value of the Edible Part of Food

Food No.	Food Description	Measure of edible portion	Weight (g)	Water (%)	Calories (kcal)	Pro-tein (g)	Total fat (g)	Fatty acids		
								Satu-rated (g)	Mono-unsatu-rated (g)	Poly-unsatu-rated (g)

Grain Products (continued)

	French toast									
582	Prepared from recipe, with 2% milk, fried in margarine	1 slice	65	55	149	5	7	1.8	2.9	1.7
583	Frozen, ready to heat	1 slice	59	53	126	4	4	0.9	1.2	0.7
	Granola bar									
584	Hard, plain	1 bar	28	4	134	3	6	0.7	1.2	3.4
	Soft, uncoated									
585	Chocolate chip	1 bar	28	5	119	2	5	2.9	1.0	0.6
586	Raisin	1 bar	28	6	127	2	5	2.7	0.8	0.9
587	Soft, chocolate-coated, peanut butter	1 bar	28	3	144	3	9	4.8	1.9	0.5
588	Macaroni (elbows), enriched, cooked	1 cup	140	66	197	7	1	0.1	0.1	0.4
589	Matzo, plain	1 matzo	28	4	112	3	Tr	0.1	Tr	0.2
	Muffins									
	Blueberry									
590	Commercially prepared (2¾" dia x 2")	1 muffin	57	38	158	3	4	0.8	1.1	1.4
591	Prepared from mix (2¼" dia x 1¾")	1 muffin	50	36	150	3	4	0.7	1.8	1.5
592	Prepared from recipe, with 2% milk	1 muffin	57	40	162	4	6	1.2	1.5	3.1
593	Bran with raisins, toaster type, toasted	1 muffin	34	27	106	2	3	0.5	0.8	1.7
	Corn									
594	Commercially prepared (2½" dia x 2¼")	1 muffin	57	33	174	3	5	0.8	1.2	1.8
595	Prepared from mix (2¼" dia x 1½")	1 muffin	50	31	161	4	5	1.4	2.6	0.6
596	Oat bran, commercially prepared (2½" dia x 2¼")	1 muffin	57	35	154	4	4	0.6	1.0	2.4
597	Noodles, chow mein, canned	1 cup	45	1	237	4	14	2.0	3.5	7.8
	Noodles (egg noodles), enriched, cooked									
598	Regular	1 cup	160	69	213	8	2	0.5	0.7	0.7
599	Spinach	1 cup	160	69	211	8	3	0.6	0.8	0.6
600	NUTRI GRAIN Cereal Bar, fruit filled	1 bar	37	15	136	2	3	0.6	1.9	0.3
	Oat bran									
601	Uncooked	1 cup	94	7	231	16	7	1.2	2.2	2.6
602	Cooked	1 cup	219	84	88	7	2	0.4	0.6	0.7
603	Oriental snack mix	1 oz (about ¼ cup)	28	3	156	5	7	1.1	2.8	3.0
	Pancakes, plain (4" dia)									
604	Frozen, ready to heat	1 pancake	36	45	82	2	1	0.3	0.4	0.3
605	Prepared from complete mix	1 pancake	38	53	74	2	1	0.2	0.3	0.3
606	Prepared from incomplete mix, with 2% milk, egg and oil	1 pancake	38	53	83	3	3	0.8	0.8	1.1
	Pie crust, baked									
	Standard type									
607	From recipe	1 pie shell	180	10	949	12	62	15.5	27.3	16.4
608	From frozen	1 pie shell	126	11	648	6	41	13.3	19.8	5.1
609	Graham cracker	1 pie shell	239	4	1,181	10	60	12.4	27.2	16.5

Choles-terol (mg)	Carbo-hydrate (g)	Total dietary fiber (g)	Calcium (mg)	Iron (mg)	Potas-sium (mg)	Sodium (mg)	Vitamin A		Thiamin (mg)	Ribo-flavin (mg)	Niacin (mg)	Ascor-bic acid (mg)	Food No.
							(IU)	(RE)					
75	16	0.7	65	1.1	87	311	315	86	0.13	0.21	1.1	Tr	582
48	19	0.7	63	1.3	79	292	110	32	0.16	0.22	1.6	Tr	583
0	18	1.5	17	0.8	95	83	43	4	0.07	0.03	0.4	Tr	584
Tr	20	1.4	26	0.7	96	77	12	1	0.06	0.04	0.3	0	585
Tr	19	1.2	29	0.7	103	80	0	0	0.07	0.05	0.3	0	586
3	15	0.8	31	0.4	96	55	37	10	0.03	0.06	0.9	Tr	587
0	40	1.8	10	2.0	43	1	0	0	0.29	0.14	2.3	0	588
0	24	0.9	4	0.9	32	1	0	0	0.11	0.08	1.1	0	589
17	27	1.5	32	0.9	70	255	19	5	0.08	0.07	0.6	1	590
23	24	0.6	13	0.6	39	219	39	11	0.07	0.16	1.1	1	591
21	23	1.1	108	1.3	70	251	80	22	0.16	0.16	1.3	1	592
3	19	2.8	13	1.0	60	179	58	16	0.07	0.10	0.8	0	593
15	29	1.9	42	1.6	39	297	119	21	0.16	0.19	1.2	0	594
31	25	1.2	38	1.0	66	398	105	23	0.12	0.14	1.1	Tr	595
0	28	2.6	36	2.4	289	224	0	0	0.15	0.05	0.2	0	596
0	26	1.8	9	2.1	54	198	38	4	0.26	0.19	2.7	0	597
53	40	1.8	19	2.5	45	11	32	10	0.30	0.13	2.4	0	598
53	39	3.7	30	1.7	59	19	165	22	0.39	0.20	2.4	0	599
0	27	0.8	15	1.8	73	110	750	227	0.37	0.41	5.0	0	600
0	62	14.5	55	5.1	532	4	0	0	1.10	0.21	0.9	0	601
0	25	5.7	22	1.9	201	2	0	0	0.35	0.07	0.3	0	602
0	15	3.7	15	0.7	93	117	1	0	0.09	0.04	0.9	Tr	603
3	16	0.6	22	1.3	26	183	36	10	0.14	0.17	1.4	Tr	604
5	14	0.5	48	0.6	67	239	12	3	0.08	0.08	0.7	Tr	605
27	11	0.7	82	0.5	76	192	95	27	0.08	0.12	0.5	Tr	606
0	86	3.0	18	5.2	121	976	0	0	0.70	0.50	6.0	0	607
0	62	1.3	26	2.8	139	815	0	0	0.35	0.48	3.1	0	608
0	156	3.6	50	5.2	210	1,365	1,876	483	0.25	0.42	5.1	0	609

Table 9.   Nutritive Value of the Edible Part of Food

Food No.	Food Description	Measure of edible portion	Weight (g)	Water (%)	Calories (kcal)	Protein (g)	Total fat (g)	Fatty acids Saturated (g)	Mono-unsaturated (g)	Poly-unsaturated (g)

Grain Products (continued)

Pies
Commercially prepared (⅙ of 8" dia)

610	Apple	1 piece	117	52	277	2	13	4.4	5.1	2.6
611	Blueberry	1 piece	117	53	271	2	12	2.0	5.0	4.1
612	Cherry	1 piece	117	46	304	2	13	3.0	6.8	2.4
613	Chocolate creme	1 piece	113	44	344	3	22	5.6	12.6	2.7
614	Coconut custard	1 piece	104	49	270	6	14	6.1	5.7	1.2
615	Lemon meringue	1 piece	113	42	303	2	10	2.0	3.0	4.1
616	Pecan	1 piece	113	19	452	5	21	4.0	12.1	3.6
617	Pumpkin	1 piece	109	58	229	4	10	1.9	4.4	3.4

Prepared from recipe (⅛ of 9" dia)

618	Apple	1 piece	155	47	411	4	19	4.7	8.4	5.2
619	Blueberry	1 piece	147	51	360	4	17	4.3	7.5	4.5
620	Cherry	1 piece	180	46	486	5	22	5.4	9.6	5.8
621	Lemon meringue	1 piece	127	43	362	5	16	4.0	7.1	4.2
622	Pecan	1 piece	122	20	503	6	27	4.9	13.6	7.0
623	Pumpkin	1 piece	155	59	316	7	14	4.9	5.7	2.8
624	Fried, cherry	1 pie	128	38	404	4	21	3.1	9.5	6.9

Popcorn

| 625 | Air popped, unsalted | 1 cup | 8 | 4 | 31 | 1 | Tr | Tr | 0.1 | 0.2 |
| 626 | Oil popped, salted | 1 cup | 11 | 3 | 55 | 1 | 3 | 0.5 | 0.9 | 1.5 |

Caramel coated

627	With peanuts	1 cup	42	3	168	3	3	0.4	1.1	1.4
628	Without peanuts	1 cup	35	3	152	1	5	1.3	1.0	1.6
629	Cheese flavor	1 cup	11	3	58	1	4	0.7	1.1	1.7
630	Popcorn cake	1 cake	10	5	38	1	Tr	Tr	0.1	0.1

Pretzels, made with enriched flour

631	Stick, 2¼" long	10 pretzels	3	3	11	Tr	Tr	Tr	Tr	Tr
632	Twisted, regular	10 pretzels	60	3	229	5	2	0.5	0.8	0.7
633	Twisted, dutch, 2¾" x 2⅝"	1 pretzel	16	3	61	1	1	0.1	0.2	0.2

Rice

| 634 | Brown, long grain, cooked | 1 cup | 195 | 73 | 216 | 5 | 2 | 0.4 | 0.6 | 0.6 |

White, long grain, enriched
Regular

635	Raw	1 cup	185	12	675	13	1	0.3	0.4	0.3
636	Cooked	1 cup	158	68	205	4	Tr	0.1	0.1	0.1
637	Instant, prepared	1 cup	165	76	162	3	Tr	0.1	0.1	0.1

Parboiled

638	Raw	1 cup	185	10	686	13	1	0.3	0.3	0.3
639	Cooked	1 cup	175	72	200	4	Tr	0.1	0.1	0.1
640	Wild, cooked	1 cup	164	74	166	7	1	0.1	0.1	0.3
641	Rice cake, brown rice, plain	1 cake	9	6	35	1	Tr	0.1	0.1	0.1
642	RICE KRISPIES Treat Squares	1 bar	22	6	91	1	2	0.3	0.6	1.1

Rolls

643	Dinner	1 roll	28	32	84	2	2	0.5	1.0	0.3
644	Hamburger or hotdog	1 roll	43	34	123	4	2	0.5	0.4	1.1
645	Hard, kaiser	1 roll	57	31	167	6	2	0.3	0.6	1.0

Spaghetti, cooked

| 646 | Enriched | 1 cup | 140 | 66 | 197 | 7 | 1 | 0.1 | 0.1 | 0.4 |
| 647 | Whole wheat | 1 cup | 140 | 67 | 174 | 7 | 1 | 0.1 | 0.1 | 0.3 |

Sweet rolls, cinnamon

| 648 | Commercial, with raisins | 1 roll | 60 | 25 | 223 | 4 | 10 | 1.8 | 2.9 | 4.5 |
| 649 | Refrigerated dough, baked, with frosting | 1 roll | 30 | 23 | 109 | 2 | 4 | 1.0 | 2.2 | 0.5 |

Choles-terol (mg)	Carbo-hydrate (g)	Total dietary fiber (g)	Calcium (mg)	Iron (mg)	Potas-sium (mg)	Sodium (mg)	Vitamin A		Thiamin (mg)	Ribo-flavin (mg)	Niacin (mg)	Ascor-bic acid (mg)	Food No.
							(IU)	(RE)					
0	40	1.9	13	0.5	76	311	145	35	0.03	0.03	0.3	4	610
0	41	1.2	9	0.4	59	380	164	40	0.01	0.04	0.4	3	611
0	47	0.9	14	0.6	95	288	329	63	0.03	0.03	0.2	1	612
6	38	2.3	41	1.2	144	154	0	0	0.04	0.12	0.8	0	613
36	31	1.9	84	0.8	182	348	114	28	0.09	0.15	0.4	1	614
51	53	1.4	63	0.7	101	165	198	59	0.07	0.24	0.7	4	615
36	65	4.0	19	1.2	84	479	198	53	0.10	0.14	0.3	1	616
22	30	2.9	65	0.9	168	307	3,743	405	0.06	0.17	0.2	1	617
0	58	3.6	11	1.7	122	327	90	19	0.23	0.17	1.9	3	618
0	49	3.6	10	1.8	74	272	62	6	0.22	0.19	1.8	1	619
0	69	3.5	18	3.3	139	344	736	86	0.27	0.23	2.3	2	620
67	50	0.7	15	1.3	83	307	203	56	0.15	0.20	1.2	4	621
106	64	2.2	39	1.8	162	320	410	109	0.23	0.22	1.0	Tr	622
65	41	2.9	146	2.0	288	349	11,833	1,212	0.14	0.31	1.2	3	623
0	55	3.3	28	1.6	83	479	220	22	0.18	0.14	1.8	2	624
0	6	1.2	1	0.2	24	Tr	16	2	0.02	0.02	0.2	0	625
0	6	1.1	1	0.3	25	97	17	2	0.01	0.01	0.2	Tr	626
0	34	1.6	28	1.6	149	124	27	3	0.02	0.05	0.8	0	627
2	28	1.8	15	0.6	38	73	18	4	0.02	0.02	0.8	0	628
1	6	1.1	12	0.2	29	98	27	5	0.01	0.03	0.2	Tr	629
0	8	0.3	1	0.2	33	29	7	1	0.01	0.02	0.6	0	630
0	2	0.1	1	0.1	4	51	0	0	0.01	0.02	0.2	0	631
0	48	1.9	22	2.6	88	1,029	0	0	0.28	0.37	3.2	0	632
0	13	0.5	6	0.7	23	274	0	0	0.07	0.10	0.8	0	633
0	45	3.5	20	0.8	84	10	0	0	0.19	0.05	3.0	0	634
0	148	2.4	52	8.0	213	9	0	0	1.07	0.09	7.8	0	635
0	45	0.6	16	1.9	55	2	0	0	0.26	0.02	2.3	0	636
0	35	1.0	13	1.0	7	5	0	0	0.12	0.08	1.5	0	637
0	151	3.1	111	6.6	222	9	0	0	1.10	0.13	6.7	0	638
0	43	0.7	33	2.0	65	5	0	0	0.44	0.03	2.5	0	639
0	35	3.0	5	1.0	166	5	0	0	0.09	0.14	2.1	0	640
0	7	0.4	1	0.1	26	29	4	Tr	0.01	0.01	0.7	0	641
0	18	0.1	1	0.5	9	77	200	60	0.15	0.18	2.0	0	642
Tr	14	0.8	33	0.9	37	146	0	0	0.14	0.09	1.1	Tr	643
0	22	1.2	60	1.4	61	241	0	0	0.21	0.13	1.7	Tr	644
0	30	1.3	54	1.9	62	310	0	0	0.27	0.19	2.4	0	645
0	40	2.4	10	2.0	43	1	0	0	0.29	0.14	2.3	0	646
0	37	6.3	21	1.5	62	4	0	0	0.15	0.06	1.0	0	647
40	31	1.4	43	1.0	67	230	129	38	0.19	0.16	1.4	1	648
0	17	0.6	10	0.8	19	250	1	0	0.12	0.07	1.1	Tr	649

Table 9.   Nutritive Value of the Edible Part of Food

Food No.	Food Description	Measure of edible portion	Weight (g)	Water (%)	Calories (kcal)	Pro-tein (g)	Total fat (g)	Fatty acids Satu-rated (g)	Mono-unsatu-rated (g)	Poly-unsatu-rated (g)
Grain Products (continued)										
650	Taco shell, baked...................... 1 medium 13			6	62	1	3	0.4	1.2	1.1
651	Tapioca, pearl, dry.................... 1 cup 152			11	544	Tr	Tr	Tr	Tr	Tr
	Toaster pastries									
652	Brown sugar cinnamon.......... 1 pastry...............50			11	206	3	7	1.8	4.0	0.9
653	Chocolate with frosting .... 1 pastry...............52			13	201	3	5	1.0	2.7	1.1
654	Fruit filled................................ 1 pastry...............52			12	204	2	5	0.8	2.2	2.0
655	Low fat .... 1 pastry...............52			12	193	2	3	0.7	1.7	0.5
	Tortilla chips									
	Plain									
656	Regular .... 1 oz 28			2	142	2	7	1.4	4.4	1.0
657	Low fat, baked...................... 10 chips 14			2	54	2	1	0.1	0.2	0.4
	Nacho flavor									
658	Regular .... 1 oz 28			2	141	2	7	1.4	4.3	1.0
659	Light, reduced fat................. 1 oz 28			1	126	2	4	0.8	2.5	0.6
	Tortillas, ready to cook (about 6" dia)									
660	Corn .... 1 tortilla...............26			44	58	1	1	0.1	0.2	0.3
661	Flour .... 1 tortilla...............32			27	104	3	2	0.6	1.2	0.3
	Waffles, plain									
662	Prepared from recipe, 7" dia .. 1 waffle...............75			42	218	6	11	2.1	2.6	5.1
663	Frozen, toasted, 4" dia........... 1 waffle...............33			42	87	2	3	0.5	1.1	0.9
664	Low fat, 4" dia .... 1 waffle...............35			43	83	2	1	0.3	0.4	0.4
	Wheat flours									
	All purpose, enriched									
665	Sifted, spooned.................... 1 cup 115			12	419	12	1	0.2	0.1	0.5
666	Unsifted, spooned .... 1 cup 125			12	455	13	1	0.2	0.1	0.5
667	Bread, enriched...................... 1 cup 137			13	495	16	2	0.3	0.2	1.0
668	Cake or pastry flour, enriched, unsifted, spooned........................... 1 cup 137			13	496	11	1	0.2	0.1	0.5
669	Self rising, enriched, unsifted, spooned .... 1 cup 125			11	443	12	1	0.2	0.1	0.5
670	Whole wheat, from hard wheats, stirred, spooned.... 1 cup 120			10	407	16	2	0.4	0.3	0.9
671	Wheat germ, toasted, plain .... 1 tbsp 7			6	27	2	1	0.1	0.1	0.5
Legumes, Nuts, and Seeds										
	Almonds, shelled									
672	Sliced .... 1 cup 95			5	549	20	48	3.7	30.5	11.6
673	Whole...................................... 1 oz (24 nuts) 28			5	164	6	14	1.1	9.1	3.5
	Beans, dry									
	Cooked									
674	Black .... 1 cup 172			66	227	15	1	0.2	0.1	0.4
675	Great Northern .... 1 cup 177			69	209	15	1	0.2	Tr	0.3
676	Kidney, red .... 1 cup 177			67	225	15	1	0.1	0.1	0.5
677	Lima, large .... 1 cup 188			70	216	15	1	0.2	0.1	0.3
678	Pea (navy) .... 1 cup 182			63	258	16	1	0.3	0.1	0.4
679	Pinto .... 1 cup 171			64	234	14	1	0.2	0.2	0.3
	Canned, solids and liquid									
	Baked beans									
680	Plain or vegetarian .... 1 cup 254			73	236	12	1	0.3	0.1	0.5
681	With frankfurters............... 1 cup 259			69	368	17	17	6.1	7.3	2.2
682	With pork in tomato sauce .... 1 cup 253			73	248	13	3	1.0	1.1	0.3
683	With pork in sweet sauce ... 1 cup 253			71	281	13	4	1.4	1.6	0.5
684	Kidney, red .... 1 cup 256			77	218	13	1	0.1	0.1	0.5
685	Lima, large .... 1 cup 241			77	190	12	Tr	0.1	Tr	0.2
686	White .... 1 cup 262			70	307	19	1	0.2	0.1	0.3

Choles-terol (mg)	Carbo-hydrate (g)	Total dietary fiber (g)	Calcium (mg)	Iron (mg)	Potas-sium (mg)	Sodium (mg)	Vitamin A		Thiamin (mg)	Ribo-flavin (mg)	Niacin (mg)	Ascor-bic acid (mg)	Food No.
							(IU)	(RE)					
0	8	1.0	21	0.3	24	49	0	0	0.03	0.01	0.2	0	650
0	135	1.4	30	2.4	17	2	0	0	0.01	0.00	0.0	0	651
0	34	0.5	17	2.0	57	212	493	112	0.19	0.29	2.3	Tr	652
0	37	0.6	20	1.8	82	203	500	NA	0.16	0.16	2.0	0	653
0	37	1.1	14	1.8	58	218	501	2	0.15	0.19	2.0	Tr	654
0	40	0.8	23	1.8	34	131	494	49	0.15	0.29	2.0	2	655
0	18	1.8	44	0.4	56	150	56	6	0.02	0.05	0.4	0	656
0	11	0.7	22	0.2	37	57	52	6	0.03	0.04	0.1	Tr	657
1	18	1.5	42	0.4	61	201	105	12	0.04	0.05	0.4	1	658
1	20	1.4	45	0.5	77	284	108	12	0.06	0.08	0.1	Tr	659
0	12	1.4	46	0.4	40	42	0	0	0.03	0.02	0.4	0	660
0	18	1.1	40	1.1	42	153	0	0	0.17	0.09	1.1	0	661
52	25	0.7	191	1.7	119	383	171	49	0.20	0.26	1.6	Tr	662
8	13	0.8	77	1.5	42	260	400	120	0.13	0.16	1.5	0	663
9	15	0.4	20	1.9	50	155	506	NA	0.31	0.26	2.6	0	664
0	88	3.1	17	5.3	123	2	0	0	0.90	0.57	6.8	0	665
0	95	3.4	19	5.8	134	3	0	0	0.98	0.62	7.4	0	666
0	99	3.3	21	6.0	137	3	0	0	1.11	0.70	10.3	0	667
0	107	2.3	19	10.0	144	3	0	0	1.22	0.59	9.3	0	668
0	93	3.4	423	5.8	155	1,588	0	0	0.84	0.52	7.3	0	669
0	87	14.6	41	4.7	486	6	0	0	0.54	0.26	7.6	0	670
0	3	0.9	3	0.6	66	Tr	0	0	0.12	0.06	0.4	Tr	671
0	19	11.2	236	4.1	692	1	10	1	0.23	0.77	3.7	0	672
0	6	3.3	70	1.2	206	Tr	3	Tr	0.07	0.23	1.1	0	673
0	41	15.0	46	3.6	611	2	10	2	0.42	0.10	0.9	0	674
0	37	12.4	120	3.8	692	4	2	0	0.28	0.10	1.2	2	675
0	40	13.1	50	5.2	713	4	0	0	0.28	0.10	1.0	2	676
0	39	13.2	32	4.5	955	4	0	0	0.30	0.10	0.8	0	677
0	48	11.6	127	4.5	670	2	4	0	0.37	0.11	1.0	2	678
0	44	14.7	82	4.5	800	3	3	0	0.32	0.16	0.7	4	679
0	52	12.7	127	0.7	752	1,008	434	43	0.39	0.15	1.1	8	680
16	40	17.9	124	4.5	609	1,114	399	39	0.15	0.15	2.3	6	681
18	49	12.1	142	8.3	759	1,113	314	30	0.13	0.12	1.3	8	682
18	53	13.2	154	4.2	673	850	288	28	0.12	0.15	0.9	8	683
0	40	16.4	61	3.2	658	873	0	0	0.27	0.23	1.2	3	684
0	36	11.6	51	4.4	530	810	0	0	0.13	0.08	0.6	0	685
0	57	12.6	191	7.8	1,189	13	0	0	0.25	0.10	0.3	0	686

Table 9.   Nutritive Value of the Edible Part of Food

Food No.	Food Description	Measure of edible portion	Weight (g)	Water (%)	Calories (kcal)	Protein (g)	Total fat (g)	Fatty acids Saturated (g)	Mono-unsaturated (g)	Poly-unsaturated (g)

Legumes, Nuts, and Seeds (continued)

	Black eyed peas, dry									
687	Cooked	1 cup	172	70	200	13	1	0.2	0.1	0.4
688	Canned, solids and liquid	1 cup	240	80	185	11	1	0.3	0.1	0.6
689	Brazil nuts, shelled	1 oz (6-8 nuts)	28	3	186	4	19	4.6	6.5	6.8
690	Carob flour	1 cup	103	4	229	5	1	0.1	0.2	0.2
	Cashews, salted									
691	Dry roasted	1 oz	28	2	163	4	13	2.6	7.7	2.2
692	Oil roasted	1 cup	130	4	749	21	63	12.4	36.9	10.6
693		1 oz (18 nuts)	28	4	163	5	14	2.7	8.1	2.3
694	Chestnuts, European, roasted, shelled	1 cup	143	40	350	5	3	0.6	1.1	1.2
	Chickpeas, dry									
695	Cooked	1 cup	164	60	269	15	4	0.4	1.0	1.9
696	Canned, solids and liquid	1 cup	240	70	286	12	3	0.3	0.6	1.2
	Coconut Raw									
697	Piece, about 2" x 2" x ½"	1 piece	45	47	159	1	15	13.4	0.6	0.2
698	Shredded, not packed	1 cup	80	47	283	3	27	23.8	1.1	0.3
699	Dried, sweetened, shredded	1 cup	93	13	466	3	33	29.3	1.4	0.4
700	Hazelnuts (filberts), chopped	1 cup	115	5	722	17	70	5.1	52.5	9.1
701		1 oz	28	5	178	4	17	1.3	12.9	2.2
702	Hummus, commercial	1 tbsp	14	67	23	1	1	0.2	0.6	0.5
703	Lentils, dry, cooked	1 cup	198	70	230	18	1	0.1	0.1	0.3
704	Macadamia nuts, dry roasted, salted	1 cup	134	2	959	10	102	16.0	79.4	2.0
705		1 oz (10-12 nuts)	28	2	203	2	22	3.4	16.8	0.4
	Mixed nuts, with peanuts, salted									
706	Dry roasted	1 oz	28	2	168	5	15	2.0	8.9	3.1
707	Oil roasted	1 oz	28	2	175	5	16	2.5	9.0	3.8
	Peanuts Dry roasted									
708	Salted	1 oz (about 28)	28	2	166	7	14	2.0	7.0	4.4
709	Unsalted	1 cup	146	2	854	35	73	10.1	36.0	22.9
710		1 oz (about 28)	28	2	166	7	14	2.0	7.0	4.4
711	Oil roasted, salted	1 cup	144	2	837	38	71	9.9	35.2	22.4
712		1 oz	28	2	165	7	14	1.9	6.9	4.4
	Peanut butter Regular									
713	Smooth style	1 tbsp	16	1	95	4	8	1.7	3.9	2.2
714	Chunk style	1 tbsp	16	1	94	4	8	1.5	3.8	2.3
715	Reduced fat, smooth	1 tbsp	18	1	94	5	6	1.3	2.9	1.8
716	Peas, split, dry, cooked	1 cup	196	69	231	16	1	0.1	0.2	0.3
717	Pecans, halves	1 cup	108	4	746	10	78	6.7	44.0	23.3
718		1 oz (20 halves)	28	4	196	3	20	1.8	11.6	6.1
719	Pine nuts (pignolia), shelled	1 oz	28	7	160	7	14	2.2	5.4	6.1
720		1 tbsp	9	7	49	2	4	0.7	1.6	1.8
721	Pistachio nuts, dry roasted, with salt, shelled	1 oz (47 nuts)	28	2	161	6	13	1.6	6.8	3.9
722	Pumpkin and squash kernels, roasted, with salt	1 oz (142 seeds)	28	7	148	9	12	2.3	3.7	5.4
723	Refried beans, canned	1 cup	252	76	237	14	3	1.2	1.4	0.4
724	Sesame seeds	1 tbsp	8	5	47	2	4	0.6	1.7	1.9
725	Soybeans, dry, cooked	1 cup	172	63	298	29	15	2.2	3.4	8.7
	Soy products									
726	Miso	1 cup	275	41	567	32	17	2.4	3.7	9.4
727	Soy milk	1 cup	245	93	81	7	5	0.5	0.8	2.0

Choles-terol (mg)	Carbo-hydrate (g)	Total dietary fiber (g)	Calcium (mg)	Iron (mg)	Potas-sium (mg)	Sodium (mg)	Vitamin A		Thiamin (mg)	Ribo-flavin (mg)	Niacin (mg)	Ascor-bic acid (mg)	Food No.
							(IU)	(RE)					
0	36	11.2	41	4.3	478	7	26	3	0.35	0.09	0.9	1	687
0	33	7.9	48	2.3	413	718	31	2	0.18	0.18	0.8	6	688
0	4	1.5	50	1.0	170	1	0	0	0.28	0.03	0.5	Tr	689
0	92	41.0	358	3.0	852	36	14	1	0.05	0.47	2.0	Tr	690
0	9	0.9	13	1.7	160	181	0	0	0.06	0.06	0.4	0	691
0	37	4.9	53	5.3	689	814	0	0	0.55	0.23	2.3	0	692
0	8	1.1	12	1.2	150	177	0	0	0.12	0.05	0.5	0	693
0	76	7.3	41	1.3	847	3	34	3	0.35	0.25	1.9	37	694
0	45	12.5	80	4.7	477	11	44	5	0.19	0.10	0.9	2	695
0	54	10.6	77	3.2	413	718	58	5	0.07	0.08	0.3	9	696
0	7	4.1	6	1.1	160	9	0	0	0.03	0.01	0.2	1	697
0	12	7.2	11	1.9	285	16	0	0	0.05	0.02	0.4	3	698
0	44	4.2	14	1.8	313	244	0	0	0.03	0.02	0.4	1	699
0	19	11.2	131	5.4	782	0	46	5	0.74	0.13	2.1	7	700
0	5	2.7	32	1.3	193	0	11	1	0.18	0.03	0.5	2	701
0	2	0.8	5	0.3	32	53	4	Tr	0.03	0.01	0.1	0	702
0	40	15.6	38	6.6	731	4	16	2	0.33	0.14	2.1	3	703
0	17	10.7	94	3.6	486	355	0	0	0.95	0.12	3.0	1	704
0	4	2.3	20	0.8	103	75	0	0	0.20	0.02	0.6	Tr	705
0	7	2.6	20	1.0	169	190	4	Tr	0.06	0.06	1.3	Tr	706
0	6	2.6	31	0.9	165	185	5	1	0.14	0.06	1.4	Tr	707
0	6	2.3	15	0.6	187	230	0	0	0.12	0.03	3.8	0	708
0	31	11.7	79	3.3	961	9	0	0	0.64	0.14	19.7	0	709
0	6	2.3	15	0.6	187	2	0	0	0.12	0.03	3.8	0	710
0	27	13.2	127	2.6	982	624	0	0	0.36	0.16	20.6	0	711
0	5	2.6	25	0.5	193	123	0	0	0.07	0.03	4.0	0	712
0	3	0.9	6	0.3	107	75	0	0	0.01	0.02	2.1	0	713
0	3	1.1	7	0.3	120	78	0	0	0.02	0.02	2.2	0	714
0	6	0.9	6	0.3	120	97	0	0	0.05	0.01	2.6	0	715
0	41	16.3	27	2.5	710	4	14	2	0.37	0.11	1.7	1	716
0	15	10.4	76	2.7	443	0	83	9	0.71	0.14	1.3	1	717
0	4	2.7	20	0.7	116	0	22	2	0.19	0.04	0.3	Tr	718
0	4	1.3	7	2.6	170	1	8	1	0.23	0.05	1.0	1	719
0	1	0.4	2	0.8	52	Tr	2	Tr	0.07	0.02	0.3	Tr	720
0	8	2.9	31	1.2	293	121	151	15	0.24	0.04	0.4	1	721
0	4	1.1	12	4.2	229	163	108	11	0.06	0.09	0.5	1	722
20	39	13.4	88	4.2	673	753	0	0	0.07	0.04	0.8	15	723
0	1	0.9	10	0.6	33	3	5	1	0.06	0.01	0.4	0	724
0	17	10.3	175	8.8	886	2	15	2	0.27	0.49	0.7	3	725
0	77	14.9	182	7.5	451	10,029	239	25	0.27	0.69	2.4	0	726
0	4	3.2	10	1.4	345	29	78	7	0.39	0.17	0.4	0	727

Table 9.   Nutritive Value of the Edible Part of Food

Food No.	Food Description	Measure of edible portion	Weight (g)	Water (%)	Calories (kcal)	Pro-tein (g)	Total fat (g)	Fatty acids Satu-rated (g)	Fatty acids Mono-unsatu-rated (g)	Fatty acids Poly-unsatu-rated (g)

Legumes, Nuts, and Seeds (continued)

Soy products (continued)
  Tofu

Food No.	Food Description	Measure of edible portion	Weight (g)	Water (%)	Calories (kcal)	Pro-tein (g)	Total fat (g)	Satu-rated (g)	Mono-unsatu-rated (g)	Poly-unsatu-rated (g)
728	Firm	¼ block	81	84	62	7	4	0.5	0.8	2.0
729	Soft, piece 2½" x 2¾" x 1"	1 piece	120	87	73	8	4	0.6	1.0	2.5
730	Sunflower seed kernels, dry roasted, with salt	¼ cup	32	1	186	6	16	1.7	3.0	10.5
731		1 oz	28	1	165	5	14	1.5	2.7	9.3
732	Tahini	1 tbsp	15	3	89	3	8	1.1	3.0	3.5
733	Walnuts, English	1 cup, chopped	120	4	785	18	78	7.4	10.7	56.6
734		1 oz (14 halves)	28	4	185	4	18	1.7	2.5	13.4

Meat and Meat Products

Beef, cooked
  Cuts braised, simmered, or pot roasted
    Relatively fat, such as chuck blade, piece, 2½" x 2½" x ¾"

Food No.	Food Description	Measure of edible portion	Weight (g)	Water (%)	Calories (kcal)	Pro-tein (g)	Total fat (g)	Satu-rated (g)	Mono-unsatu-rated (g)	Poly-unsatu-rated (g)
735	Lean and fat	3 oz	85	47	293	23	22	8.7	9.4	0.8
736	Lean only	3 oz	85	55	213	26	11	4.3	4.8	0.4

Relatively lean, such as bottom round, piece, 4⅛" x 2¼" x ½"

| 737 | Lean and fat | 3 oz | 85 | 52 | 234 | 24 | 14 | 5.4 | 6.2 | 0.5 |
| 738 | Lean only | 3 oz | 85 | 58 | 178 | 27 | 7 | 2.4 | 3.1 | 0.3 |

Ground beef, broiled

739	83% lean	3 oz	85	57	218	22	14	5.5	6.1	0.5
740	79% lean	3 oz	85	56	231	21	16	6.2	6.9	0.6
741	73% lean	3 oz	85	54	246	20	18	6.9	7.7	0.7
742	Liver, fried, slice, 6½" x 2⅜" x ⅜"	3 oz	85	56	184	23	7	2.3	1.4	1.5

Roast, oven cooked, no liquid added
  Relatively fat, such as rib, 2 pieces, 4⅛" x 2¼" x ¼"

| 743 | Lean and fat | 3 oz | 85 | 47 | 304 | 19 | 25 | 9.9 | 10.6 | 0.9 |
| 744 | Lean only | 3 oz | 85 | 59 | 195 | 23 | 11 | 4.2 | 4.5 | 0.3 |

Relatively lean, such as eye of round, 2 pieces, 2½" x 2½" x ⅜"

| 745 | Lean and fat | 3 oz | 85 | 59 | 195 | 23 | 11 | 4.2 | 4.7 | 0.4 |
| 746 | Lean only | 3 oz | 85 | 65 | 143 | 25 | 4 | 1.5 | 1.8 | 0.1 |

Steak, sirloin, broiled, piece, 2½" x 2½" x ¾"

747	Lean and fat	3 oz	85	57	219	24	13	5.2	5.6	0.5
748	Lean only	3 oz	85	62	166	26	6	2.4	2.6	0.2
749	Beef, canned, corned	3 oz	85	58	213	23	13	5.3	5.1	0.5
750	Beef, dried, chipped	1 oz	28	57	47	8	1	0.5	0.5	0.1

Lamb, cooked
  Chops
    Arm, braised

| 751 | Lean and fat | 3 oz | 85 | 44 | 294 | 26 | 20 | 8.4 | 8.7 | 1.5 |
| 752 | Lean only | 3 oz | 85 | 49 | 237 | 30 | 12 | 4.3 | 5.2 | 0.8 |

Loin, broiled

| 753 | Lean and fat | 3 oz | 85 | 52 | 269 | 21 | 20 | 8.4 | 8.2 | 1.4 |
| 754 | Lean only | 3 oz | 85 | 61 | 184 | 25 | 8 | 3.0 | 3.6 | 0.5 |

Choles-terol (mg)	Carbo-hydrate (g)	Total dietary fiber (g)	Calcium (mg)	Iron (mg)	Potas-sium (mg)	Sodium (mg)	Vitamin A		Thiamin (mg)	Ribo-flavin (mg)	Niacin (mg)	Ascor-bic acid (mg)	Food No.
							(IU)	(RE)					
0	2	0.3	131	1.2	143	6	6	1	0.08	0.08	Tr	Tr	728
0	2	0.2	133	1.3	144	10	8	1	0.06	0.04	0.6	Tr	729
0	8	2.9	22	1.2	272	250	0	0	0.03	0.08	2.3	Tr	730
0	7	2.6	20	1.1	241	221	0	0	0.03	0.07	2.0	Tr	731
0	3	1.4	64	1.3	62	17	10	1	0.18	0.07	0.8	0	732
0	16	8.0	125	3.5	529	2	49	5	0.41	0.18	2.3	2	733
0	4	1.9	29	0.8	125	1	12	1	0.10	0.04	0.5	Tr	734
88	0	0.0	11	2.6	196	54	0	0	0.06	0.20	2.1	0	735
90	0	0.0	11	3.1	224	60	0	0	0.07	0.24	2.3	0	736
82	0	0.0	5	2.7	240	43	0	0	0.06	0.20	3.2	0	737
82	0	0.0	4	2.9	262	43	0	0	0.06	0.22	3.5	0	738
71	0	0.0	6	2.0	266	60	0	0	0.05	0.23	4.2	0	739
74	0	0.0	9	1.8	256	65	0	0	0.04	0.18	4.4	0	740
77	0	0.0	9	2.1	248	71	0	0	0.03	0.16	4.9	0	741
410	7	0.0	9	5.3	309	90	30,689	9,120	0.18	3.52	12.3	20	742
71	0	0.0	9	2.0	256	54	0	0	0.06	0.14	2.9	0	743
68	0	0.0	9	2.4	318	61	0	0	0.07	0.18	3.5	0	744
61	0	0.0	5	1.6	308	50	0	0	0.07	0.14	3.0	0	745
59	0	0.0	4	1.7	336	53	0	0	0.08	0.14	3.2	0	746
77	0	0.0	9	2.6	311	54	0	0	0.09	0.23	3.3	0	747
76	0	0.0	9	2.9	343	56	0	0	0.11	0.25	3.6	0	748
73	0	0.0	10	1.8	116	855	0	0	0.02	0.12	2.1	0	749
12	Tr	0.0	2	1.3	126	984	0	0	0.02	0.06	1.5	0	750
102	0	0.0	21	2.0	260	61	0	0	0.06	0.21	5.7	0	751
103	0	0.0	22	2.3	287	65	0	0	0.06	0.23	5.4	0	752
85	0	0.0	17	1.5	278	65	0	0	0.09	0.21	6.0	0	753
81	0	0.0	16	1.7	320	71	0	0	0.09	0.24	5.8	0	754

Table 9. Nutritive Value of the Edible Part of Food

Food No.	Food Description	Measure of edible portion	Weight (g)	Water (%)	Calories (kcal)	Protein (g)	Total fat (g)	Fatty acids Saturated (g)	Fatty acids Monounsaturated (g)	Fatty acids Polyunsaturated (g)
Meat and Meat Products (continued)										
	Lamb (continued)									
	Leg, roasted, 2 pieces, 4⅛" x 2¼" x ¼"									
755	Lean and fat	3 oz	85	57	219	22	14	5.9	5.9	1.0
756	Lean only	3 oz	85	64	162	24	7	2.3	2.9	0.4
	Rib, roasted, 3 pieces, 2½" x 2½" x ¼"									
757	Lean and fat	3 oz	85	48	305	18	25	10.9	10.6	1.8
758	Lean only	3 oz	85	60	197	22	11	4.0	5.0	0.7
	Pork, cured, cooked									
	Bacon									
759	Regular	3 medium slices	19	13	109	6	9	3.3	4.5	1.1
760	Canadian style (6 slices per 6-oz pkg)	2 slices	47	62	86	11	4	1.3	1.9	0.4
	Ham, light cure, roasted, 2 pieces, 4⅛" x 2¼" x ¼"									
761	Lean and fat	3 oz	85	58	207	18	14	5.1	6.7	1.5
762	Lean only	3 oz	85	66	133	21	5	1.6	2.2	0.5
763	Ham, canned, roasted, 2 pieces, 4⅛" x 2¼" x ¼"	3 oz	85	67	142	18	7	2.4	3.5	0.8
	Pork, fresh, cooked									
	Chop, loin (cut 3 per lb with bone)									
	Broiled									
764	Lean and fat	3 oz	85	58	204	24	11	4.1	5.0	0.8
765	Lean only	3 oz	85	61	172	26	7	2.5	3.1	0.5
	Pan fried									
766	Lean and fat	3 oz	85	53	235	25	14	5.1	6.0	1.6
767	Lean only	3 oz	85	57	197	27	9	3.1	3.8	1.1
	Ham (leg), roasted, piece, 2½" x 2½" x ¾"									
768	Lean and fat	3 oz	85	55	232	23	15	5.5	6.7	1.4
769	Lean only	3 oz	85	61	179	25	8	2.8	3.8	0.7
	Rib roast, piece, 2½" x 2½" x ¾"									
770	Lean and fat	3 oz	85	56	217	23	13	5.0	5.9	1.1
771	Lean only	3 oz	85	59	190	24	9	3.7	4.5	0.7
	Ribs, lean and fat, cooked									
772	Backribs, roasted	3 oz	85	45	315	21	25	9.3	11.4	2.0
773	Country style, braised	3 oz	85	54	252	20	18	6.8	7.9	1.6
774	Spareribs, braised	3 oz	85	40	337	25	26	9.5	11.5	2.3
	Shoulder cut, braised, 3 pieces, 2½" x 2½" x ¼"									
775	Lean and fat	3 oz	85	48	280	24	20	7.2	8.8	1.9
776	Lean only	3 oz	85	54	211	27	10	3.5	4.9	1.0
	Sausages and luncheon meats									
777	Bologna, beef and pork (8 slices per 8-oz pkg)	2 slices	57	54	180	7	16	6.1	7.6	1.4
778	Braunschweiger (6 slices per 6-oz pkg)	2 slices	57	48	205	8	18	6.2	8.5	2.1
779	Brown and serve, cooked, link, 4" x ⅞" raw	2 links	26	45	103	4	9	3.4	4.5	1.0
	Canned, minced luncheon meat									
780	Pork, ham, and chicken, reduced sodium (7 slices per 7-oz can)	2 slices	57	56	172	7	15	5.1	7.1	1.5
781	Pork with ham (12 slices per 12-oz can)	2 slices	57	52	188	8	17	5.7	7.7	1.2
782	Pork and chicken (12 slices per 12-oz can)	2 slices	57	64	117	9	8	2.7	3.8	0.8

Choles-terol (mg)	Carbo-hydrate (g)	Total dietary fiber (g)	Calcium (mg)	Iron (mg)	Potas-sium (mg)	Sodium (mg)	Vitamin A		Thiamin (mg)	Ribo-flavin (mg)	Niacin (mg)	Ascor-bic acid (mg)	Food No.
							(IU)	(RE)					
79	0	0.0	9	1.7	266	56	0	0	0.09	0.23	5.6	0	755
76	0	0.0	7	1.8	287	58	0	0	0.09	0.25	5.4	0	756
82	0	0.0	19	1.4	230	62	0	0	0.08	0.18	5.7	0	757
75	0	0.0	18	1.5	268	69	0	0	0.08	0.20	5.2	0	758
16	Tr	0.0	2	0.3	92	303	0	0	0.13	0.05	1.4	0	759
27	1	0.0	5	0.4	181	719	0	0	0.38	0.09	3.2	0	760
53	0	0.0	6	0.7	243	1,009	0	0	0.51	0.19	3.8	0	761
47	0	0.0	6	0.8	269	1,128	0	0	0.58	0.22	4.3	0	762
35	Tr	0.0	6	0.9	298	908	0	0	0.82	0.21	4.3	0	763
70	0	0.0	28	0.7	304	49	8	3	0.91	0.24	4.5	Tr	764
70	0	0.0	26	0.7	319	51	7	2	0.98	0.26	4.7	Tr	765
78	0	0.0	23	0.8	361	68	7	2	0.97	0.26	4.8	1	766
78	0	0.0	20	0.8	382	73	7	2	1.06	0.28	5.1	1	767
80	0	0.0	12	0.9	299	51	9	3	0.54	0.27	3.9	Tr	768
80	0	0.0	6	1.0	317	54	8	3	0.59	0.30	4.2	Tr	769
62	0	0.0	24	0.8	358	39	5	2	0.62	0.26	5.2	Tr	770
60	0	0.0	22	0.8	371	40	5	2	0.64	0.27	5.5	Tr	771
100	0	0.0	38	1.2	268	86	8	3	0.36	0.17	3.0	Tr	772
74	0	0.0	25	1.0	279	50	7	2	0.43	0.22	3.3	1	773
103	0	0.0	40	1.6	272	79	9	3	0.35	0.32	4.7	0	774
93	0	0.0	15	1.4	314	75	8	3	0.46	0.26	4.4	Tr	775
97	0	0.0	7	1.7	344	87	7	2	0.51	0.31	5.0	Tr	776
31	2	0.0	7	0.9	103	581	0	0	0.10	0.08	1.5	0	777
89	2	0.0	5	5.3	113	652	8,009	2,405	0.14	0.87	4.8	0	778
18	1	0.0	3	0.3	49	209	0	0	0.09	0.04	0.9	0	779
43	1	0.0	0	0.4	321	539	0	0	0.15	0.10	1.8	18	780
40	1	0.0	0	0.4	233	758	0	0	0.18	0.10	2.0	0	781
43	1	0.0	0	0.7	352	539	0	0	0.10	0.12	2.0	18	782

Table 9.   Nutritive Value of the Edible Part of Food

Food No.	Food Description	Measure of edible portion	Weight (g)	Water (%)	Calories (kcal)	Protein (g)	Total fat (g)	Fatty acids Saturated (g)	Mono-unsaturated (g)	Poly-unsaturated (g)

Meat and Meat Products (continued)

Sausages and luncheon meats (continued)

783	Chopped ham (8 slices per 6-oz pkg)	2 slices	21	64	48	4	4	1.2	1.7	0.4
	Cooked ham (8 slices per 8-oz pkg)									
784	Regular	2 slices	57	65	104	10	6	1.9	2.8	0.7
785	Extra lean	2 slices	57	71	75	11	3	0.9	1.3	0.3
	Frankfurter (10 per 1-lb pkg), heated									
786	Beef and pork	1 frank	45	54	144	5	13	4.8	6.2	1.2
787	Beef	1 frank	45	55	142	5	13	5.4	6.1	0.6
	Pork sausage, fresh, cooked									
788	Link (4" x ⅞" raw)	2 links	26	45	96	5	8	2.8	3.6	1.0
789	Patty (3⅞" x ¼" raw)	1 patty	27	45	100	5	8	2.9	3.8	1.0
	Salami, beef and pork									
790	Cooked type (8 slices per 8-oz pkg)	2 slices	57	60	143	8	11	4.6	5.2	1.2
791	Dry type, slice, 3⅛" x ¹⁄₁₆"	2 slices	20	35	84	5	7	2.4	3.4	0.6
792	Sandwich spread (pork, beef)	1 tbsp	15	60	35	1	3	0.9	1.1	0.4
793	Vienna sausage (7 per 4-oz can)	1 sausage	16	60	45	2	4	1.5	2.0	0.3
	Veal, lean and fat, cooked									
794	Cutlet, braised, 4⅛" x 2¼" x ½"	3 oz	85	55	179	31	5	2.2	2.0	0.4
795	Rib, roasted, 2 pieces, 4⅛" x 2¼" x ¼"	3 oz	85	60	194	20	12	4.6	4.6	0.8

Mixed Dishes and Fast Foods

Mixed dishes

796	Beef macaroni, frozen, HEALTHY CHOICE	1 package	240	78	211	14	2	0.7	1.2	0.3
797	Beef stew, canned	1 cup	232	82	218	11	12	5.2	5.5	0.5
798	Chicken pot pie, frozen	1 small pie	217	60	484	13	29	9.7	12.5	4.5
799	Chili con carne with beans, canned	1 cup	222	74	255	20	8	2.1	2.2	1.4
800	Macaroni and cheese, canned, made with corn oil	1 cup	252	82	199	8	6	3.0	NA	1.3
801	Meatless burger crumbles, MORNINGSTAR FARMS	1 cup	110	60	231	22	13	3.3	4.6	4.9
802	Meatless burger patty, frozen, MORNINGSTAR FARMS	1 patty	85	71	91	14	1	0.1	0.3	0.2
803	Pasta with meatballs in tomato sauce, canned	1 cup	252	78	260	11	10	4.0	4.2	0.6
804	Spaghetti bolognese (meat sauce), frozen, HEALTHY CHOICE	1 package	283	78	255	14	3	1.0	0.9	0.9
805	Spaghetti in tomato sauce with cheese, canned	1 cup	252	80	192	6	2	0.7	0.3	0.3
806	Spinach souffle, home-prepared	1 cup	136	74	219	11	18	7.1	6.8	3.1
807	Tortellini, pasta with cheese filling, frozen	¾ cup (yields 1 cup cooked)	81	31	249	11	6	2.9	1.7	0.4

| Choles-terol (mg) | Carbo-hydrate (g) | Total dietary fiber (g) | Calcium (mg) | Iron (mg) | Potas-sium (mg) | Sodium (mg) | Vitamin A | | Thiamin (mg) | Ribo-flavin (mg) | Niacin (mg) | Ascor-bic acid (mg) | Food No. |
							(IU)	(RE)					
11	0	0.0	1	0.2	67	288	0	0	0.13	0.04	0.8	0	783
32	2	0.0	4	0.6	189	751	0	0	0.49	0.14	3.0	0	784
27	1	0.0	4	0.4	200	815	0	0	0.53	0.13	2.8	0	785
23	1	0.0	5	0.5	75	504	0	0	0.09	0.05	1.2	0	786
27	1	0.0	9	0.6	75	462	0	0	0.02	0.05	1.1	0	787
22	Tr	0.0	8	0.3	94	336	0	0	0.19	0.07	1.2	1	788
22	Tr	0.0	9	0.3	97	349	0	0	0.20	0.07	1.2	1	789
37	1	0.0	7	1.5	113	607	0	0	0.14	0.21	2.0	0	790
16	1	0.0	2	0.3	76	372	0	0	0.12	0.06	1.0	0	791
6	2	Tr	2	0.1	17	152	13	1	0.03	0.02	0.3	0	792
8	Tr	0.0	2	0.1	16	152	0	0	0.01	0.02	0.3	0	793
114	0	0.0	7	1.1	326	57	0	0	0.05	0.30	9.0	0	794
94	0	0.0	9	0.8	251	78	0	0	0.04	0.23	5.9	0	795
14	33	4.6	46	2.7	365	444	514	50	0.28	0.16	3.1	58	796
37	16	3.5	28	1.6	404	947	3,860	494	0.17	0.14	2.9	10	797
41	43	1.7	33	2.1	256	857	2,285	343	0.25	0.36	4.1	2	798
24	24	8.2	67	3.3	608	1,032	884	93	0.15	0.15	2.1	1	799
8	29	3.0	113	2.0	123	1,058	713	NA	0.28	0.25	2.5	0	800
0	7	5.1	79	6.4	178	476	0	0	9.92	0.35	3.0	0	801
0	8	4.3	87	2.9	434	383	0	0	0.26	0.55	4.1	0	802
20	31	6.8	28	2.3	416	1,053	920	93	0.19	0.16	3.3	8	803
17	43	5.1	51	3.5	408	473	492	48	0.35	3.77	0.5	15	804
8	39	7.8	40	2.8	305	963	932	58	0.35	0.28	4.5	10	805
184	3	NA	230	1.3	201	763	3,461	675	0.09	0.30	0.5	3	806
34	38	1.5	123	1.2	72	279	50	13	0.25	0.25	2.2	0	807

Table 9.   Nutritive Value of the Edible Part of Food

Food No.	Food Description	Measure of edible portion	Weight (g)	Water (%)	Calories (kcal)	Protein (g)	Total fat (g)	Fatty acids Saturated (g)	Fatty acids Mono-unsaturated (g)	Fatty acids Poly-unsaturated (g)

Mixed Dishes and Fast Foods (continued)

Fast foods
  Breakfast items

Food No.	Food Description	Measure of edible portion	Weight (g)	Water (%)	Calories (kcal)	Protein (g)	Total fat (g)	Saturated (g)	Mono-unsaturated (g)	Poly-unsaturated (g)
808	Biscuit with egg and sausage	1 biscuit	180	43	581	19	39	15.0	16.4	4.4
809	Croissant with egg, cheese, bacon	1 croissant	129	44	413	16	28	15.4	9.2	1.8
	Danish pastry									
810	Cheese filled	1 pastry	91	34	353	6	25	5.1	15.6	2.4
811	Fruit filled	1 pastry	94	29	335	5	16	3.3	10.1	1.6
812	English muffin with egg, cheese, Canadian bacon	1 muffin	137	57	289	17	13	4.7	4.7	1.6
813	French toast with butter	2 slices	135	51	356	10	19	7.7	7.1	2.4
814	French toast sticks	5 sticks	141	30	513	8	29	4.7	12.6	9.9
815	Hashed brown potatoes	½ cup	72	60	151	2	9	4.3	3.9	0.5
816	Pancakes with butter, syrup	2 pancakes	232	50	520	8	14	5.9	5.3	2.0
	Burrito									
817	With beans and cheese	1 burrito	93	54	189	8	6	3.4	1.2	0.9
818	With beans and meat	1 burrito	116	52	255	11	9	4.2	3.5	0.6
	Cheeseburger									
	Regular size, with condiments									
819	Double patty with mayo type dressing, vegetables	1 sandwich	166	51	417	21	21	8.7	7.8	2.7
820	Single patty	1 sandwich	113	48	295	16	14	6.3	5.3	1.1
	Regular size, plain									
821	Double patty	1 sandwich	155	42	457	28	28	13.0	11.0	1.9
822	Double patty with 3-piece bun	1 sandwich	160	43	461	22	22	9.5	8.3	1.8
823	Single patty	1 sandwich	102	37	319	15	15	6.5	5.8	1.5
	Large, with condiments									
824	Single patty with mayo type dressing, vegetables	1 sandwich	219	53	563	28	33	15.0	12.6	2.0
825	Single patty with bacon	1 sandwich	195	44	608	32	37	16.2	14.5	2.7
826	Chicken fillet (breaded and fried) sandwich, plain	1 sandwich	182	47	515	24	29	8.5	10.4	8.4
	Chicken, fried. See Poultry and Poultry Products.									
827	Chicken pieces, boneless, breaded and fried, plain	6 pieces	106	47	319	18	21	4.7	10.5	4.6
828	Chili con carne	1 cup	253	77	256	25	8	3.4	3.4	0.5
829	Chimichanga with beef	1 chimichanga	174	51	425	20	20	8.5	8.1	1.1
830	Coleslaw	¾ cup	99	74	147	1	11	1.6	2.4	6.4
	Desserts									
831	Ice milk, soft, vanilla, in cone	1 cone	103	65	164	4	6	3.5	1.8	0.4
832	Pie, fried, with fruit filling (5" x 3¾")	1 pie	128	38	404	4	21	3.1	9.5	6.9
833	Sundae, hot fudge	1 sundae	158	60	284	6	9	5.0	2.3	0.8
834	Enchilada with cheese	1 enchilada	163	63	319	10	19	10.6	6.3	0.8
835	Fish sandwich, with tartar sauce and cheese	1 sandwich	183	45	523	21	29	8.1	8.9	9.4
836	French fries	1 small	85	35	291	4	16	3.3	9.0	2.7
837		1 medium	134	35	458	6	25	5.2	14.3	4.2
838		1 large	169	35	578	7	31	6.5	18.0	5.3
839	Frijoles (refried beans, chili sauce, cheese)	1 cup	167	69	225	11	8	4.1	2.6	0.7

Choles-terol (mg)	Carbo-hydrate (g)	Total dietary fiber (g)	Calcium (mg)	Iron (mg)	Potas-sium (mg)	Sodium (mg)	Vitamin A		Thiamin (mg)	Ribo-flavin (mg)	Niacin (mg)	Ascor-bic acid (mg)	Food No.
							(IU)	(RE)					
302	41	0.9	155	4.0	320	1,141	635	164	0.50	0.45	3.6	0	808
215	24	NA	151	2.2	201	889	472	120	0.35	0.34	2.2	2	809
20	29	NA	70	1.8	116	319	155	43	0.26	0.21	2.5	3	810
19	45	NA	22	1.4	110	333	86	24	0.29	0.21	1.8	2	811
234	27	1.5	151	2.4	199	729	586	156	0.49	0.45	3.3	2	812
116	36	NA	73	1.9	177	513	473	146	0.58	0.50	3.9	Tr	813
75	58	2.7	78	3.0	127	499	45	13	0.23	0.25	3.0	0	814
9	16	NA	7	0.5	267	290	18	3	0.08	0.01	1.1	5	815
58	91	NA	128	2.6	251	1,104	281	70	0.39	0.56	3.4	3	816
14	27	NA	107	1.1	248	583	625	119	0.11	0.35	1.8	1	817
24	33	NA	53	2.5	329	670	319	32	0.27	0.42	2.7	1	818
60	35	NA	171	3.4	335	1,051	398	65	0.35	0.28	8.1	2	819
37	27	NA	111	2.4	223	616	462	94	0.25	0.23	3.7	2	820
110	22	NA	233	3.4	308	636	332	79	0.25	0.37	6.0	0	821
80	44	NA	224	3.7	285	891	277	66	0.34	0.38	6.0	0	822
50	32	NA	141	2.4	164	500	153	37	0.40	0.40	3.7	0	823
88	38	NA	206	4.7	445	1,108	613	129	0.39	0.46	7.4	8	824
111	37	NA	162	4.7	332	1,043	406	80	0.31	0.41	6.6	2	825
60	39	NA	60	4.7	353	957	100	31	0.33	0.24	6.8	9	826
61	15	0.0	14	0.9	305	513	0	0	0.12	0.16	7.5	0	827
134	22	NA	68	5.2	691	1,007	1,662	167	0.13	1.14	2.5	2	828
9	43	NA	63	4.5	586	910	146	16	0.49	0.64	5.8	5	829
5	13	NA	34	0.7	177	267	338	50	0.04	0.03	0.1	8	830
28	24	0.1	153	0.2	169	92	211	52	0.05	0.26	0.3	1	831
0	55	3.3	28	1.6	83	479	35	4	0.18	0.14	1.8	2	832
21	48	0.0	207	0.6	395	182	221	57	0.06	0.30	1.1	2	833
44	29	NA	324	1.3	240	784	1,161	186	0.08	0.42	1.9	1	834
68	48	NA	185	3.5	353	939	432	97	0.46	0.42	4.2	3	835
0	34	3.0	12	0.7	586	168	0	0	0.07	0.03	2.4	10	836
0	53	4.7	19	1.0	923	265	0	0	0.11	0.05	3.8	16	837
0	67	5.9	24	1.3	1,164	335	0	0	0.14	0.07	4.8	20	838
37	29	NA	189	2.2	605	882	456	70	0.13	0.33	1.5	2	839

Table 9.   Nutritive Value of the Edible Part of Food

Food No.	Food Description	Measure of edible portion	Weight (g)	Water (%)	Calories (kcal)	Protein (g)	Total fat (g)	Fatty acids Saturated (g)	Mono-unsaturated (g)	Poly-unsaturated (g)
	Mixed Dishes and Fast Foods (continued)									
	Fast foods (continued)									
	Hamburger									
	Regular size, with condiments									
840	Double patty	1 sandwich	215	51	576	32	32	12.0	14.1	2.8
841	Single patty	1 sandwich	106	45	272	12	10	3.6	3.4	1.0
	Large, with condiments, mayo type dressing, and vegetables									
842	Double patty	1 sandwich	226	54	540	34	27	10.5	10.3	2.8
843	Single patty	1 sandwich	218	56	512	26	27	10.4	11.4	2.2
	Hot dog									
844	Plain	1 sandwich	98	54	242	10	15	5.1	6.9	1.7
845	With chili	1 sandwich	114	48	296	14	13	4.9	6.6	1.2
846	With corn flour coating (corndog)	1 corndog	175	47	460	17	19	5.2	9.1	3.5
847	Hush puppies	5 pieces	78	32	257	5	12	2.7	7.8	0.4
848	Mashed potatoes	⅓ cup	80	79	66	2	1	0.4	0.3	0.2
849	Nachos, with cheese sauce	6-8 nachos	113	40	346	9	19	7.8	8.0	2.2
850	Onion rings, breaded and fried	8-9 rings	83	37	276	4	16	7.0	6.7	0.7
	Pizza (slice = ⅛ of 12" pizza)									
851	Cheese	1 slice	63	48	140	8	3	1.5	1.0	0.5
852	Meat and vegetables	1 slice	79	48	184	13	5	1.5	2.5	0.9
853	Pepperoni	1 slice	71	47	181	10	7	2.2	3.1	1.2
854	Roast beef sandwich, plain	1 sandwich	139	49	346	22	14	3.6	6.8	1.7
855	Salad, tossed, with chicken, no dressing	1½ cups	218	87	105	17	2	0.6	0.7	0.6
856	Salad, tossed, with egg, cheese, no dressing	1½ cups	217	90	102	9	6	3.0	1.8	0.5
	Shake									
857	Chocolate	16 fl oz	333	72	423	11	12	7.7	3.6	0.5
858	Vanilla	16 fl oz	333	75	370	12	10	6.2	2.9	0.4
859	Shrimp, breaded and fried	6-8 shrimp	164	48	454	19	25	5.4	17.4	0.6
	Submarine sandwich (6" long), with oil and vinegar									
860	Cold cuts (with lettuce, cheese, salami, ham, tomato, onion)	1 sandwich	228	58	456	22	19	6.8	8.2	2.3
861	Roast beef (with tomato, lettuce, mayo)	1 sandwich	216	59	410	29	13	7.1	1.8	2.6
862	Tuna salad (with mayo, lettuce)	1 sandwich	256	54	584	30	28	5.3	13.4	7.3
863	Taco, beef	1 small	171	58	369	21	21	11.4	6.6	1.0
864		1 large	263	58	568	32	32	17.5	10.1	1.5
865	Taco salad (with ground beef, cheese, taco shell)	1½ cups	198	72	279	13	15	6.8	5.2	1.7
	Tostada (with cheese, tomato, lettuce)									
866	With beans and beef	1 tostada	225	70	333	16	17	11.5	3.5	0.6
867	With guacamole	1 tostada	131	73	181	6	12	5.0	4.3	1.5

Choles-terol (mg)	Carbo-hydrate (g)	Total dietary fiber (g)	Calcium (mg)	Iron (mg)	Potas-sium (mg)	Sodium (mg)	Vitamin A (IU)	Vitamin A (RE)	Thiamin (mg)	Ribo-flavin (mg)	Niacin (mg)	Ascor-bic acid (mg)	Food No.
103	39	NA	92	5.5	527	742	54	4	0.34	0.41	6.7	1	840
30	34	2.3	126	2.7	251	534	74	10	0.29	0.24	3.9	2	841
122	40	NA	102	5.9	570	791	102	11	0.36	0.38	7.6	1	842
87	40	NA	96	4.9	480	824	312	33	0.41	0.37	7.3	3	843
44	18	NA	24	2.3	143	670	0	0	0.24	0.27	3.6	Tr	844
51	31	NA	19	3.3	166	480	58	6	0.22	0.40	3.7	3	845
79	56	NA	102	6.2	263	973	207	37	0.28	0.70	4.2	0	846
135	35	NA	69	1.4	188	965	94	27	0.00	0.02	2.0	0	847
2	13	NA	17	0.4	235	182	33	8	0.07	0.04	1.0	Tr	848
18	36	NA	272	1.3	172	816	559	92	0.19	0.37	1.5	1	849
14	31	NA	73	0.8	129	430	8	1	0.08	0.10	0.9	1	850
9	21	NA	117	0.6	110	336	382	74	0.18	0.16	2.5	1	851
21	21	NA	101	1.5	179	382	524	101	0.21	0.17	2.0	2	852
14	20	NA	65	0.9	153	267	282	55	0.13	0.23	3.0	2	853
51	33	NA	54	4.2	316	792	210	21	0.38	0.31	5.9	2	854
72	4	NA	37	1.1	447	209	935	96	0.11	0.13	5.9	17	855
98	5	NA	100	0.7	371	119	822	115	0.09	0.17	1.0	10	856
43	68	2.7	376	1.0	666	323	310	77	0.19	0.82	0.5	1	857
37	60	1.3	406	0.3	579	273	433	107	0.15	0.61	0.6	3	858
200	40	NA	84	3.0	184	1,446	120	36	0.21	0.90	0.0	0	859
36	51	NA	189	2.5	394	1,651	424	80	1.00	0.80	5.5	12	860
73	44	NA	41	2.8	330	845	413	50	0.41	0.41	6.0	6	861
49	55	NA	74	2.6	335	1,293	187	41	0.46	0.33	11.3	4	862
56	27	NA	221	2.4	474	802	855	147	0.15	0.44	3.2	2	863
87	41	NA	339	3.7	729	1,233	1,315	226	0.24	0.68	4.9	3	864
44	24	NA	192	2.3	416	762	588	77	0.10	0.36	2.5	4	865
74	30	NA	189	2.5	491	871	1,276	173	0.09	0.50	2.9	4	866
20	16	NA	212	0.8	326	401	879	109	0.07	0.29	1.0	2	867

Table 9.   Nutritive Value of the Edible Part of Food

Food No.	Food Description	Measure of edible portion	Weight (g)	Water (%)	Calories (kcal)	Pro-tein (g)	Total fat (g)	Fatty acids Satu-rated (g)	Mono-unsatu-rated (g)	Poly-unsatu-rated (g)
Poultry and Poultry Products										
	Chicken									
	Fried in vegetable shortening, meat with skin									
	Batter dipped									
868	Breast, ½ breast (5.6 oz with bones)	½ breast	140	52	364	35	18	4.9	7.6	4.3
869	Drumstick (3.4 oz with bones)	1 drumstick	72	53	193	16	11	3.0	4.6	2.7
870	Thigh	1 thigh	86	52	238	19	14	3.8	5.8	3.4
871	Wing	1 wing	49	46	159	10	11	2.9	4.4	2.5
	Flour coated									
872	Breast, ½ breast (4.2 oz with bones)	½ breast	98	57	218	31	9	2.4	3.4	1.9
873	Drumstick (2.6 oz with bones)	1 drumstick	49	57	120	13	7	1.8	2.7	1.6
	Fried, meat only									
874	Dark meat	3 oz	85	56	203	25	10	2.7	3.7	2.4
875	Light meat	3 oz	85	60	163	28	5	1.3	1.7	1.1
	Roasted, meat only									
876	Breast, ½ breast (4.2 oz with bone and skin)	½ breast	86	65	142	27	3	0.9	1.1	0.7
877	Drumstick (2.9 oz with bone and skin)	1 drumstick	44	67	76	12	2	0.7	0.8	0.6
878	Thigh	1 thigh	52	63	109	13	6	1.6	2.2	1.3
879	Stewed, meat only, light and dark meat, chopped or diced	1 cup	140	56	332	43	17	4.3	5.7	4.0
880	Chicken giblets, simmered, chopped	1 cup	145	68	228	37	7	2.2	1.7	1.6
881	Chicken liver, simmered	1 liver	20	68	31	5	1	0.4	0.3	0.2
882	Chicken neck, meat only, simmered	1 neck	18	67	32	4	1	0.4	0.5	0.4
883	Duck, roasted, flesh only	½ duck	221	64	444	52	25	9.2	8.2	3.2
	Turkey									
	Roasted, meat only									
884	Dark meat	3 oz	85	63	159	24	6	2.1	1.4	1.8
885	Light meat	3 oz	85	66	133	25	3	0.9	0.5	0.7
886	Light and dark meat, chopped or diced	1 cup	140	65	238	41	7	2.3	1.4	2.0
	Ground, cooked									
887	Patty, from 4 oz raw	1 patty	82	59	193	22	11	2.8	4.0	2.6
888	Crumbled	1 cup	127	59	298	35	17	4.3	6.2	4.1
889	Turkey giblets, simmered, chopped	1 cup	145	65	242	39	7	2.2	1.7	1.7
890	Turkey neck, meat only, simmered	1 neck	152	65	274	41	11	3.7	2.5	3.3
	Poultry food products									
	Chicken									
891	Canned, boneless	5 oz	142	69	234	31	11	3.1	4.5	2.5
892	Frankfurter (10 per 1 lb pkg)	1 frank	45	58	116	6	9	2.5	3.8	1.8
893	Roll, light meat (6 slices per 6-oz pkg)	2 slices	57	69	90	11	4	1.1	1.7	0.9

Choles- terol (mg)	Carbo- hydrate (g)	Total dietary fiber (g)	Calcium (mg)	Iron (mg)	Potas- sium (mg)	Sodium (mg)	Vitamin A		Thiamin (mg)	Ribo- flavin (mg)	Niacin (mg)	Ascor- bic acid (mg)	Food No.
							(IU)	(RE)					
119	13	0.4	28	1.8	281	385	94	28	0.16	0.20	14.7	0	868
62	6	0.2	12	1.0	134	194	62	19	0.08	0.15	3.7	0	869
80	8	0.3	15	1.2	165	248	82	25	0.10	0.20	4.9	0	870
39	5	0.1	10	0.6	68	157	55	17	0.05	0.07	2.6	0	871
87	2	0.1	16	1.2	254	74	49	15	0.08	0.13	13.5	0	872
44	1	Tr	6	0.7	112	44	41	12	0.04	0.11	3.0	0	873
82	2	0.0	15	1.3	215	82	67	20	0.08	0.21	6.0	0	874
77	Tr	0.0	14	1.0	224	69	26	8	0.06	0.11	11.4	0	875
73	0	0.0	13	0.9	220	64	18	5	0.06	0.10	11.8	0	876
41	0	0.0	5	0.6	108	42	26	8	0.03	0.10	2.7	0	877
49	0	0.0	6	0.7	124	46	34	10	0.04	0.12	3.4	0	878
116	0	0.0	18	2.0	283	109	157	46	0.16	0.39	9.0	0	879
570	1	0.0	17	9.3	229	84	10,775	3,232	0.13	1.38	5.9	12	880
126	Tr	0.0	3	1.7	28	10	3,275	983	0.03	0.35	0.9	3	881
14	0	0.0	8	0.5	25	12	22	6	0.01	0.05	0.7	0	882
197	0	0.0	27	6.0	557	144	170	51	0.57	1.04	11.3	0	883
72	0	0.0	27	2.0	247	67	0	0	0.05	0.21	3.1	0	884
59	0	0.0	16	1.1	259	54	0	0	0.05	0.11	5.8	0	885
106	0	0.0	35	2.5	417	98	0	0	0.09	0.25	7.6	0	886
84	0	0.0	21	1.6	221	88	0	0	0.04	0.14	4.0	0	887
130	0	0.0	32	2.5	343	136	0	0	0.07	0.21	6.1	0	888
606	3	0.0	19	9.7	290	86	8,752	2,603	0.07	1.31	6.5	2	889
185	0	0.0	56	3.5	226	85	0	0	0.05	0.29	2.6	0	890
88	0	0.0	20	2.2	196	714	166	48	0.02	0.18	9.0	3	891
45	3	0.0	43	0.9	38	617	59	17	0.03	0.05	1.4	0	892
28	1	0.0	24	0.5	129	331	46	14	0.04	0.07	3.0	0	893

Table 9.   Nutritive Value of the Edible Part of Food

Food No.	Food Description	Measure of edible portion	Weight (g)	Water (%)	Calories (kcal)	Protein (g)	Total fat (g)	Fatty acids		
								Saturated (g)	Mono-unsaturated (g)	Poly-unsaturated (g)

Poultry and Poultry Products (continued)

Poultry food products (continued)
Turkey

894	Gravy and turkey, frozen ..... 5-oz package 142			85	95	8	4	1.2	1.4	0.7
895	Patties, breaded or battered, fried (2.25 oz) .... 1 patty.................64			50	181	9	12	3.0	4.8	3.0
896	Roast, boneless, frozen, seasoned, light and dark meat, cooked.................. 3 oz 85			68	132	18	5	1.6	1.0	1.4

Soups, Sauces, and Gravies

Soups
Canned, condensed
Prepared with equal volume
of whole milk

897	Clam chowder, New England................ 1 cup 248			85	164	9	7	3.0	2.3	1.1
898	Cream of chicken .... 1 cup 248			85	191	7	11	4.6	4.5	1.6
899	Cream of mushroom .... 1 cup 248			85	203	6	14	5.1	3.0	4.6
900	Tomato .... 1 cup 248			85	161	6	6	2.9	1.6	1.1
	Prepared with equal volume of water									
901	Bean with pork .... 1 cup 253			84	172	8	6	1.5	2.2	1.8
902	Beef broth, bouillon, consomme .... 1 cup 241			96	29	5	0	0.0	0.0	0.0
903	Beef noodle .... 1 cup 244			92	83	5	3	1.1	1.2	0.5
904	Chicken noodle................ 1 cup 241			92	75	4	2	0.7	1.1	0.6
905	Chicken and rice................ 1 cup 241			94	60	4	2	0.5	0.9	0.4
906	Clam chowder, Manhattan .... 1 cup 244			92	78	2	2	0.4	0.4	1.3
907	Cream of chicken .... 1 cup 244			91	117	3	7	2.1	3.3	1.5
908	Cream of mushroom .... 1 cup 244			90	129	2	9	2.4	1.7	4.2
909	Minestrone........................ 1 cup 241			91	82	4	3	0.6	0.7	1.1
910	Pea, green .... 1 cup 250			83	165	9	3	1.4	1.0	0.4
911	Tomato .... 1 cup 244			90	85	2	2	0.4	0.4	1.0
912	Vegetable beef .... 1 cup 244			92	78	6	2	0.9	0.8	0.1
913	Vegetarian vegetable .... 1 cup 241			92	72	2	2	0.3	0.8	0.7
	Canned, ready to serve, chunky									
914	Bean with ham .... 1 cup 243			79	231	13	9	3.3	3.8	0.9
915	Chicken noodle .... 1 cup 240			84	175	13	6	1.4	2.7	1.5
916	Chicken and vegetable .... 1 cup 240			83	166	12	5	1.4	2.2	1.0
917	Vegetable .... 1 cup 240			88	122	4	4	0.6	1.6	1.4
	Canned, ready to serve, low fat, reduced sodium									
918	Chicken broth..................... 1 cup 240			97	17	3	0	0.0	0.0	0.0
919	Chicken noodle .... 1 cup 237			92	76	6	2	0.4	0.6	0.4
920	Chicken and rice .... 1 cup 241			88	116	7	3	0.9	1.3	0.7
921	Chicken and rice with vegetables .... 1 cup 239			91	88	6	1	0.4	0.5	0.5
922	Clam chowder, New England.................. 1 cup 244			89	117	5	2	0.5	0.7	0.4
923	Lentil .... 1 cup 242			88	126	8	2	0.3	0.8	0.2
924	Minestrone .... 1 cup 241			87	123	5	3	0.4	0.9	1.0
925	Vegetable .... 1 cup 238			91	81	4	1	0.3	0.4	0.3

Choles-terol (mg)	Carbo-hydrate (g)	Total dietary fiber (g)	Calcium (mg)	Iron (mg)	Potas-sium (mg)	Sodium (mg)	Vitamin A (IU)	Vitamin A (RE)	Thiamin (mg)	Ribo-flavin (mg)	Niacin (mg)	Ascor-bic acid (mg)	Food No.
26	7	0.0	20	1.3	87	787	60	18	0.03	0.18	2.6	0	894
40	10	0.3	9	1.4	176	512	24	7	0.06	0.12	1.5	0	895
45	3	0.0	4	1.4	253	578	0	0	0.04	0.14	5.3	0	896
22	17	1.5	186	1.5	300	992	164	40	0.07	0.24	1.0	3	897
27	15	0.2	181	0.7	273	1,047	714	94	0.07	0.26	0.9	1	898
20	15	0.5	179	0.6	270	918	154	37	0.08	0.28	0.9	2	899
17	22	2.7	159	1.8	449	744	848	109	0.13	0.25	1.5	68	900
3	23	8.6	81	2.0	402	951	888	89	0.09	0.03	0.6	2	901
0	2	0.0	10	0.5	154	636	0	0	0.02	0.03	0.7	1	902
5	9	0.7	15	1.1	100	952	630	63	0.07	0.06	1.1	Tr	903
7	9	0.7	17	0.8	55	1,106	711	72	0.05	0.06	1.4	Tr	904
7	7	0.7	17	0.7	101	815	660	65	0.02	0.02	1.1	Tr	905
2	12	1.5	27	1.6	188	578	964	98	0.03	0.04	0.8	4	906
10	9	0.2	34	0.6	88	986	561	56	0.03	0.06	0.8	Tr	907
2	9	0.5	46	0.5	100	881	0	0	0.05	0.09	0.7	1	908
2	11	1.0	34	0.9	313	911	2,338	234	0.05	0.04	0.9	1	909
0	27	2.8	28	2.0	190	918	203	20	0.11	0.07	1.2	2	910
0	17	0.5	12	1.8	264	695	688	68	0.09	0.05	1.4	66	911
5	10	0.5	17	1.1	173	791	1,891	190	0.04	0.05	1.0	2	912
0	12	0.5	22	1.1	210	822	3,005	301	0.05	0.05	0.9	1	913
22	27	11.2	78	3.2	425	972	3,951	396	0.15	0.15	1.7	4	914
19	17	3.8	24	1.4	108	850	1,222	122	0.07	0.17	4.3	0	915
17	19	NA	26	1.5	367	1,068	5,990	600	0.04	0.17	3.3	6	916
0	19	1.2	55	1.6	396	1,010	5,878	588	0.07	0.06	1.2	6	917
0	1	0.0	19	0.6	204	554	0	0	Tr	0.03	1.6	1	918
19	9	1.2	19	1.1	209	460	920	95	0.11	0.11	3.4	1	919
14	14	0.7	22	1.0	422	482	2,010	202	0.05	0.13	5.0	2	920
17	12	0.7	24	1.2	275	459	1,644	165	0.12	0.07	2.6	1	921
5	20	1.2	17	0.9	283	529	244	59	0.05	0.09	0.9	5	922
0	20	5.6	41	2.7	336	443	951	94	0.11	0.09	0.7	1	923
0	20	1.2	39	1.7	306	470	1,357	135	0.15	0.08	1.0	1	924
5	13	1.4	31	1.5	290	466	3,196	319	0.08	0.07	1.8	1	925

Table 9.   Nutritive Value of the Edible Part of Food

Food No.	Food Description	Measure of edible portion	Weight (g)	Water (%)	Calories (kcal)	Protein (g)	Total fat (g)	Fatty acids Saturated (g)	Mono-unsaturated (g)	Poly-unsaturated (g)

Soups, Sauces, and Gravies (continued)

Soups (continued)
Dehydrated
Unprepared

No.	Description	Measure	Wt	Water	Cal	Prot	Fat	Sat	Mono	Poly
926	Beef bouillon	1 packet	6	3	14	1	1	0.3	0.2	Tr
927	Onion	1 packet	39	4	115	5	2	0.5	1.4	0.3

Prepared with water

| 928 | Chicken noodle | 1 cup | 252 | 94 | 58 | 2 | 1 | 0.3 | 0.5 | 0.4 |
| 929 | Onion | 1 cup | 246 | 96 | 27 | 1 | 1 | 0.1 | 0.3 | 0.1 |

Home prepared, stock

930	Beef	1 cup	240	96	31	5	Tr	0.1	0.1	Tr
931	Chicken	1 cup	240	92	86	6	3	0.8	1.4	0.5
932	Fish	1 cup	233	97	40	5	2	0.5	0.5	0.3

Sauces
Home recipe

| 933 | Cheese | 1 cup | 243 | 67 | 479 | 25 | 36 | 19.5 | 11.5 | 3.4 |
| 934 | White, medium, made with whole milk | 1 cup | 250 | 75 | 368 | 10 | 27 | 7.1 | 11.1 | 7.2 |

Ready to serve

935	Barbecue	1 tbsp	16	81	12	Tr	Tr	Tr	0.1	0.1
936	Cheese	¼ cup	63	71	110	4	8	3.8	2.4	1.6
937	Hoisin	1 tbsp	16	44	35	1	1	0.1	0.2	0.3
938	Nacho cheese	¼ cup	63	70	119	5	10	4.2	3.1	2.1
939	Pepper or hot	1 tsp	5	90	1	Tr	Tr	Tr	Tr	Tr
940	Salsa	1 tbsp	16	90	4	Tr	Tr	Tr	Tr	Tr
941	Soy	1 tbsp	16	69	9	1	Tr	Tr	Tr	Tr
942	Spaghetti/marinara/pasta	1 cup	250	87	143	4	5	0.7	2.2	1.8
943	Teriyaki	1 tbsp	18	68	15	1	0	0.0	0.0	0.0
944	Tomato chili	¼ cup	68	68	71	2	Tr	Tr	Tr	0.1
945	Worcestershire	1 tbsp	17	70	11	0	0	0.0	0.0	0.0

Gravies, canned

946	Beef	¼ cup	58	87	31	2	1	0.7	0.6	Tr
947	Chicken	¼ cup	60	85	47	1	3	0.8	1.5	0.9
948	Country sausage	¼ cup	62	75	96	3	8	2.0	2.9	2.2
949	Mushroom	¼ cup	60	89	30	1	2	0.2	0.7	0.6
950	Turkey	¼ cup	60	89	31	2	1	0.4	0.5	0.3

Sugars and Sweets

Candy

| 951 | BUTTERFINGER (NESTLE) | 1 fun size bar | 7 | 2 | 34 | 1 | 1 | 0.7 | 0.4 | 0.2 |

Caramel

952	Plain	1 piece	10	9	39	Tr	1	0.7	0.1	Tr
953	Chocolate flavored roll	1 piece	7	7	25	Tr	Tr	Tr	0.1	0.1
954	Carob	1 oz	28	2	153	2	9	8.2	0.1	0.1

Chocolate, milk

955	Plain	1 bar (1.55 oz)	44	1	226	3	14	8.1	4.4	0.5
956	With almonds	1 bar (1.45 oz)	41	2	216	4	14	7.0	5.5	0.9
957	With peanuts, MR. GOODBAR (HERSHEY)	1 bar (1.75 oz)	49	1	267	5	17	7.3	5.7	2.4
958	With rice cereal, NESTLE CRUNCH	1 bar (1.55 oz)	44	1	230	3	12	6.7	3.8	0.4

Chocolate chips

959	Milk	1 cup	168	1	862	12	52	31.0	16.7	1.8
960	Semisweet	1 cup	168	1	805	7	50	29.8	16.7	1.6
961	White	1 cup	170	1	916	10	55	33.0	15.5	1.7
962	Chocolate coated peanuts	10 pieces	40	2	208	5	13	5.8	5.2	1.7
963	Chocolate coated raisins	10 pieces	10	11	39	Tr	1	0.9	0.5	0.1
964	Fruit leather, pieces	1 oz	28	12	97	Tr	2	0.3	0.9	0.8

Choles-terol (mg)	Carbo-hydrate (g)	Total dietary fiber (g)	Calcium (mg)	Iron (mg)	Potas-sium (mg)	Sodium (mg)	Vitamin A		Thiamin (mg)	Ribo-flavin (mg)	Niacin (mg)	Ascor-bic acid (mg)	Food No.
							(IU)	(RE)					
1	1	0.0	4	0.1	27	1,019	3	Tr	Tr	0.01	0.3	0	926
2	21	4.1	55	0.6	260	3,493	8	1	0.11	0.24	2.0	1	927
10	9	0.3	5	0.5	33	578	15	5	0.20	0.08	1.1	0	928
0	5	1.0	12	0.1	64	849	2	0	0.03	0.06	0.5	Tr	929
0	3	0.0	19	0.6	444	475	0	0	0.08	0.22	2.1	0	930
7	8	0.0	7	0.5	252	343	0	0	0.08	0.20	3.8	Tr	931
2	0	0.0	7	Tr	336	363	0	0	0.08	0.18	2.8	Tr	932
92	13	0.2	756	0.9	345	1,198	1,473	389	0.11	0.59	0.5	1	933
18	23	0.5	295	0.8	390	885	1,383	138	0.17	0.46	1.0	2	934
0	2	0.2	3	0.1	28	130	139	14	Tr	Tr	0.1	1	935
18	4	0.3	116	0.1	19	522	199	40	Tr	0.07	Tr	Tr	936
Tr	7	0.4	5	0.2	19	258	2	Tr	Tr	0.03	0.2	Tr	937
20	3	0.5	118	0.2	20	492	128	32	Tr	0.08	Tr	Tr	938
0	Tr	0.1	Tr	Tr	7	124	14	1	Tr	Tr	Tr	4	939
0	1	0.3	5	0.2	34	69	96	10	0.01	0.01	0.1	2	940
0	1	0.1	3	0.3	64	871	0	0	0.01	0.03	0.4	0	941
0	21	4.0	55	1.8	738	1,030	938	95	0.14	0.10	2.7	20	942
0	3	Tr	5	0.3	41	690	0	0	0.01	0.01	0.2	0	943
0	17	4.0	14	0.5	252	910	462	46	0.06	0.05	1.1	11	944
0	3	0.0	18	0.9	136	167	18	2	0.01	0.02	0.1	2	945
2	3	0.2	3	0.4	47	325	0	0	0.02	0.02	0.4	0	946
1	3	0.2	12	0.3	65	346	221	67	0.01	0.03	0.3	0	947
13	4	0.4	4	0.3	48	236	0	0	0.10	0.04	0.7	Tr	948
0	3	0.2	4	0.4	64	342	0	0	0.02	0.04	0.4	0	949
1	3	0.2	2	0.4	65	346	0	0	0.01	0.05	0.8	0	950
Tr	5	0.2	2	0.1	27	14	0	0	0.01	Tr	0.2	0	951
1	8	0.1	14	Tr	22	25	3	1	Tr	0.02	Tr	Tr	952
0	6	Tr	2	Tr	7	6	1	Tr	Tr	0.01	Tr	Tr	953
1	16	1.1	86	0.4	179	30	7	2	0.03	0.05	0.3	Tr	954
10	26	1.5	84	0.6	169	36	81	24	0.03	0.13	0.1	Tr	955
8	22	2.5	92	0.7	182	30	30	6	0.02	0.18	0.3	Tr	956
4	25	1.7	53	0.6	219	73	70	18	0.08	0.12	1.6	Tr	957
6	29	1.1	74	0.2	151	59	30	9	0.15	0.25	1.7	Tr	958
37	99	5.7	321	2.3	647	138	311	92	0.13	0.51	0.5	1	959
0	106	9.9	54	5.3	613	18	35	3	0.09	0.15	0.7	0	960
36	101	0.0	338	0.4	486	153	60	2	0.11	0.48	1.3	1	961
4	20	1.9	42	0.5	201	16	0	0	0.05	0.07	1.7	0	962
Tr	7	0.4	9	0.2	51	4	4	1	0.01	0.02	Tr	Tr	963
0	22	1.0	5	0.2	46	114	33	3	0.01	0.03	Tr	16	964

Table 9.   Nutritive Value of the Edible Part of Food

Sugars and Sweets (continued)

Food No.	Food Description	Measure of edible portion	Weight (g)	Water (%)	Calories (kcal)	Pro-tein (g)	Total fat (g)	Fatty acids Satu-rated (g)	Mono-unsatu-rated (g)	Poly-unsatu-rated (g)
	Candy (continued)									
965	Fruit leather, rolls	1 large................21		11	74	Tr	1	0.1	0.3	0.1
966		1 small................14		11	49	Tr	Tr	0.1	0.2	0.1
	Fudge, prepared from recipe									
	Chocolate									
967	Plain...................................	1 piece 17		10	65	Tr	1	0.9	0.4	0.1
968	With nuts	1 piece 19		7	81	1	3	1.1	0.8	1.0
	Vanilla									
969	Plain...................................	1 piece 16		11	59	Tr	1	0.5	0.2	Tr
970	With nuts	1 piece 15		8	62	Tr	2	0.6	0.5	0.8
	Gumdrops/gummy candies									
971	Gumdrops (¾" dia)	1 cup 182		1	703	0	0	0.0	0.0	0.0
972		1 medium 4		1	16	0	0	0.0	0.0	0.0
973	Gummy bears	10 bears 22		1	85	0	0	0.0	0.0	0.0
974	Gummy worms.....................	10 worms............74		1	286	0	0	0.0	0.0	0.0
975	Hard candy............................	1 piece 6		1	24	0	Tr	0.0	0.0	0.0
976		1 small piece 3		1	12	0	Tr	0.0	0.0	0.0
977	Jelly beans............................	10 large................28		6	104	0	Tr	Tr	0.1	Tr
978		10 small...............11		6	40	0	Tr	Tr	Tr	Tr
979	KIT KAT (HERSHEY)	1 bar (1.5 oz).......42		2	216	3	11	6.8	3.1	0.3
	Marshmallows									
980	Miniature............................	1 cup 50		16	159	1	Tr	Tr	Tr	Tr
981	Regular	1 regular 7		16	23	Tr	Tr	Tr	Tr	Tr
	M&M's (M&M MARS)									
982	Peanut...................................	¼ cup...................43		2	222	4	11	4.4	4.7	1.8
983		10 pieces..............20		2	103	2	5	2.1	2.2	0.8
984	Plain.....................................	¼ cup...................52		2	256	2	11	6.8	3.6	0.3
985		10 pieces...............7		2	34	Tr	1	0.9	0.5	Tr
986	MILKY WAY (M&M MARS).................	1 fun size bar.......18		6	76	1	3	1.4	1.1	0.1
987		1 bar (2.15 oz).....61		6	258	3	10	4.8	3.7	0.4
988	REESE'S Peanut butter cup (HERSHEY)	1 miniature cup 7		2	38	1	2	0.8	0.9	0.4
989		1 package (contains 2) 45		2	243	5	14	5.0	5.9	2.5
990	SNICKERS bar (M&M MARS).................	1 fun size bar.......15		5	72	1	4	1.3	1.6	0.7
991		1 king size bar (4 oz) 113		5	541	9	28	10.2	11.8	5.6
992		1 bar (2 oz) 57		5	273	5	14	5.1	6.0	2.8
993	SPECIAL DARK sweet chocolate (HERSHEY)	1 miniature 8		1	46	Tr	3	1.7	0.9	0.1
994	STARBURST fruit chews (M&M MARS).................	1 piece 5		7	20	Tr	Tr	0.1	0.2	0.2
995		1 package (2.07 oz) 59		7	234	Tr	5	0.7	2.1	1.8
	Frosting, ready to eat									
996	Chocolate	¹⁄₁₂ package..........38		17	151	Tr	7	2.1	3.4	0.8
997	Vanilla	¹⁄₁₂ package..........38		13	159	Tr	6	1.9	3.3	0.9
	Frozen desserts (nondairy)									
998	Fruit and juice bar	1 bar (2.5 fl oz) ...77		78	63	1	Tr	0.0	0.0	Tr
999	Ice pop...................................	1 bar (2 fl oz) 59		80	42	0	0	0.0	0.0	0.0
1000	Italian ices.............................	½ cup.................116		86	61	Tr	Tr	0.0	0.0	0.0
1001	Fruit butter, apple	1 tbsp 17		56	29	Tr	0	0.0	0.0	0.0
	Gelatin dessert, prepared with gelatin dessert powder and water									
1002	Regular	½ cup.................135		85	80	2	0	0.0	0.0	0.0
1003	Reduced calorie (with aspartame).................	½ cup.................117		98	8	1	0	0.0	0.0	0.0

Choles-terol (mg)	Carbo-hydrate (g)	Total dietary fiber (g)	Calcium (mg)	Iron (mg)	Potas-sium (mg)	Sodium (mg)	Vitamin A (IU)	Vitamin A (RE)	Thiamin (mg)	Ribo-flavin (mg)	Niacin (mg)	Ascor-bic acid (mg)	Food No.
0	18	0.8	7	0.2	62	13	24	3	0.01	Tr	Tr	1	965
0	12	0.5	4	0.1	41	9	16	2	0.01	Tr	Tr	1	966
2	14	0.1	7	0.1	18	11	32	8	Tr	0.01	Tr	Tr	967
3	14	0.2	10	0.1	30	11	38	9	0.01	0.02	Tr	Tr	968
3	13	0.0	6	Tr	8	11	33	8	Tr	0.01	Tr	Tr	969
2	11	0.1	7	0.1	17	9	30	7	0.01	0.01	Tr	Tr	970
0	180	0.0	5	0.7	9	80	0	0	0.00	Tr	Tr	0	971
0	4	0.0	Tr	Tr	Tr	2	0	0	0.00	Tr	Tr	0	972
0	22	0.0	1	0.1	1	10	0	0	0.00	Tr	Tr	0	973
0	73	0.0	2	0.3	4	33	0	0	0.00	Tr	Tr	0	974
0	6	0.0	Tr	Tr	Tr	2	0	0	Tr	Tr	Tr	0	975
0	3	0.0	Tr	Tr	Tr	1	0	0	Tr	Tr	Tr	0	976
0	26	0.0	1	0.3	10	7	0	0	0.00	0.00	0.0	0	977
0	10	0.0	Tr	0.1	4	3	0	0	0.00	0.00	0.0	0	978
3	27	0.8	69	0.4	122	32	68	20	0.07	0.23	1.1	Tr	979
0	41	0.1	2	0.1	3	24	1	0	Tr	Tr	Tr	0	980
0	6	Tr	Tr	Tr	Tr	3	Tr	0	Tr	Tr	Tr	0	981
4	26	1.5	43	0.5	149	21	40	10	0.04	0.07	1.6	Tr	982
2	12	0.7	20	0.2	69	10	19	5	0.02	0.03	0.7	Tr	983
7	37	1.3	55	0.6	138	32	106	28	0.03	0.11	0.1	Tr	984
1	5	0.2	7	0.1	19	4	14	4	Tr	0.01	Tr	Tr	985
3	13	0.3	23	0.1	43	43	19	6	0.01	0.04	0.1	Tr	986
9	44	1.0	79	0.5	147	146	66	20	0.02	0.14	0.2	1	987
Tr	4	0.2	5	0.1	25	22	5	1	0.02	0.01	0.3	Tr	988
2	25	1.4	35	0.5	158	143	33	9	0.11	0.08	2.1	Tr	989
2	9	0.4	14	0.1	49	40	23	6	0.01	0.02	0.6	Tr	990
15	67	2.8	106	0.9	366	301	172	44	0.11	0.17	4.7	1	991
7	34	1.4	54	0.4	185	152	87	22	0.06	0.09	2.4	Tr	992
Tr	5	0.4	2	0.2	25	1	3	Tr	Tr	0.01	Tr	0	993
0	4	0.0	Tr	Tr	Tr	3	0	0	Tr	Tr	Tr	3	994
0	50	0.0	2	0.1	1	33	0	0	Tr	Tr	Tr	31	995
0	24	0.2	3	0.5	74	70	249	75	Tr	0.01	Tr	0	996
0	26	Tr	1	Tr	14	34	283	86	0.00	Tr	Tr	0	997
0	16	0.0	4	0.1	41	3	22	2	0.01	0.01	0.1	7	998
0	11	0.0	0	0.0	2	7	0	0	0.00	0.00	0.0	0	999
0	16	0.0	1	0.1	7	5	194	0	0.01	0.01	0.8	1	1000
0	7	0.3	2	0.1	15	1	20	2	Tr	Tr	Tr	Tr	1001
0	19	0.0	3	Tr	1	57	0	0	0.00	Tr	Tr	0	1002
0	1	0.0	2	Tr	0	56	0	0	0.00	Tr	Tr	0	1003

Table 9.   Nutritive Value of the Edible Part of Food

Food No.	Food Description	Measure of edible portion	Weight (g)	Water (%)	Calories (kcal)	Pro-tein (g)	Total fat (g)	Fatty acids Satu-rated (g)	Mono-unsatu-rated (g)	Poly-unsatu-rated (g)
	Sugars and Sweets (continued)									
1004	Honey, strained or extracted	1 tbsp 21		17	64	Tr	0	0.0	0.0	0.0
1005		1 cup 339		17	1,031	1	0	0.0	0.0	0.0
1006	Jams and preserves...................	1 tbsp 20		30	56	Tr	Tr	Tr	Tr	0.0
1007		1 packet (0.5 oz) 14		30	39	Tr	Tr	Tr	Tr	0.0
1008	Jellies	1 tbsp 19		29	54	Tr	Tr	Tr	Tr	Tr
1009		1 packet (0.5 oz) 14		29	40	Tr	Tr	Tr	Tr	Tr
	Puddings									
	Prepared with dry mix and 2% milk									
	Chocolate									
1010	Instant	½ cup...............147		75	150	5	3	1.6	0.9	0.2
1011	Regular (cooked)	½ cup...............142		74	151	5	3	1.8	0.8	0.1
	Vanilla									
1012	Instant	½ cup...............142		75	148	4	2	1.4	0.7	0.1
1013	Regular (cooked)	½ cup...............140		76	141	4	2	1.5	0.7	0.1
	Ready to eat									
	Regular									
1014	Chocolate...........................	4 oz 113		69	150	3	5	0.8	1.9	1.6
1015	Rice............................	4 oz 113		68	184	2	8	1.3	3.6	3.2
1016	Tapioca...........................	4 oz 113		74	134	2	4	0.7	1.8	1.5
1017	Vanilla...........................	4 oz 113		71	147	3	4	0.6	1.7	1.5
	Fat free									
1018	Chocolate...........................	4 oz 113		76	107	3	Tr	0.3	0.1	Tr
1019	Tapioca...........................	4 oz 113		77	98	2	Tr	0.1	Tr	Tr
1020	Vanilla...........................	4 oz 113		76	105	2	Tr	0.1	Tr	Tr
	Sugar									
	Brown									
1021	Packed	1 cup 220		2	827	0	0	0.0	0.0	0.0
1022	Unpacked...........................	1 cup 145		2	545	0	0	0.0	0.0	0.0
1023		1 tbsp 9		2	34	0	0	0.0	0.0	0.0
	White									
1024	Granulated...........................	1 packet 6		0	23	0	0	0.0	0.0	0.0
1025		1 tsp 4		0	16	0	0	0.0	0.0	0.0
1026		1 cup 200		0	774	0	0	0.0	0.0	0.0
1027	Powdered, unsifted...............	1 tbsp 8		Tr	31	0	Tr	Tr	Tr	Tr
1028		1 cup 120		Tr	467	0	Tr	Tr	Tr	0.1
	Syrup									
	Chocolate flavored syrup or topping									
1029	Thin type	1 tbsp 19		31	53	Tr	Tr	0.1	0.1	Tr
1030	Fudge type...........................	1 tbsp 19		22	67	1	2	0.8	0.7	0.1
1031	Corn, light...........................	1 tbsp 20		23	56	0	0	0.0	0.0	0.0
1032	Maple	1 tbsp 20		32	52	0	Tr	Tr	Tr	Tr
1033	Molasses, blackstrap	1 tbsp 20		29	47	0	0	0.0	0.0	0.0
1034		1 cup 328		29	771	0	0	0.0	0.0	0.0
	Table blend, pancake									
1035	Regular	1 tbsp 20		24	57	0	0	0.0	0.0	0.0
1036	Reduced calorie...................	1 tbsp 15		55	25	0	0	0.0	0.0	0.0

Choles-terol (mg)	Carbo-hydrate (g)	Total dietary fiber (g)	Calcium (mg)	Iron (mg)	Potas-sium (mg)	Sodium (mg)	Vitamin A (IU)	Vitamin A (RE)	Thiamin (mg)	Ribo-flavin (mg)	Niacin (mg)	Ascor-bic acid (mg)	Food No.
0	17	Tr	1	0.1	11	1	0	0	0.00	0.01	Tr	Tr	1004
0	279	0.7	20	1.4	176	14	0	0	0.00	0.13	0.4	2	1005
0	14	0.2	4	0.1	15	6	2	Tr	0.00	Tr	Tr	2	1006
0	10	0.2	3	0.1	11	4	2	Tr	0.00	Tr	Tr	1	1007
0	13	0.2	2	Tr	12	5	3	Tr	Tr	Tr	Tr	Tr	1008
0	10	0.1	1	Tr	9	4	2	Tr	Tr	Tr	Tr	Tr	1009
9	28	0.6	153	0.4	247	417	253	56	0.05	0.21	0.1	1	1010
10	28	0.4	160	0.5	240	149	253	68	0.05	0.21	0.2	1	1011
9	28	0.0	146	0.1	185	406	241	64	0.05	0.20	0.1	1	1012
10	26	0.0	153	0.1	193	224	252	70	0.04	0.20	0.1	1	1013
3	26	1.1	102	0.6	203	146	41	12	0.03	0.18	0.4	2	1014
1	25	0.1	59	0.3	68	96	129	40	0.02	0.08	0.2	1	1015
1	22	0.1	95	0.3	110	180	0	0	0.02	0.11	0.4	1	1016
8	25	0.1	99	0.1	128	153	24	7	0.02	0.16	0.3	0	1017
2	23	0.9	89	0.6	235	192	174	52	0.02	0.12	0.1	Tr	1018
1	23	0.1	76	0.2	99	251	121	36	0.02	0.09	0.1	Tr	1019
1	24	0.1	86	Tr	123	241	174	52	0.02	0.10	0.1	Tr	1020
0	214	0.0	187	4.2	761	86	0	0	0.02	0.02	0.2	0	1021
0	141	0.0	123	2.8	502	57	0	0	0.01	0.01	0.1	0	1022
0	9	0.0	8	0.2	31	4	0	0	Tr	Tr	Tr	0	1023
0	6	0.0	Tr	Tr	Tr	Tr	0	0	0.00	Tr	0.0	0	1024
0	4	0.0	Tr	Tr	Tr	Tr	0	0	0.00	Tr	0.0	0	1025
0	200	0.0	2	0.1	4	2	0	0	0.00	0.04	0.0	0	1026
0	8	0.0	Tr	Tr	Tr	Tr	0	0	0.00	0.00	0.0	0	1027
0	119	0.0	1	0.1	2	1	0	0	0.00	0.00	0.0	0	1028
0	12	0.3	3	0.4	43	14	6	1	Tr	0.01	0.1	Tr	1029
Tr	12	0.5	15	0.2	69	66	3	1	0.01	0.04	0.1	Tr	1030
0	15	0.0	1	Tr	1	24	0	0	Tr	Tr	Tr	0	1031
0	13	0.0	13	0.2	41	2	0	0	Tr	Tr	Tr	0	1032
0	12	0.0	172	3.5	498	11	0	0	0.01	0.01	0.2	0	1033
0	199	0.0	2,821	57.4	8,174	180	0	0	0.11	0.17	3.5	0	1034
0	15	0.0	Tr	Tr	Tr	17	0	0	Tr	Tr	Tr	0	1035
0	7	0.0	Tr	Tr	Tr	30	0	0	Tr	Tr	Tr	0	1036

Table 9. Nutritive Value of the Edible Part of Food

Food No.	Food Description	Measure of edible portion	Weight (g)	Water (%)	Calories (kcal)	Pro-tein (g)	Total fat (g)	Fatty acids		
								Satu-rated (g)	Mono-unsatu-rated (g)	Poly-unsatu-rated (g)

Vegetables and Vegetable Products

1037	Alfalfa sprouts, raw	1 cup	33	91	10	1	Tr	Tr	Tr	0.1
1038	Artichokes, globe or French, cooked, drained	1 cup	168	84	84	6	Tr	0.1	Tr	0.1
1039		1 medium	120	84	60	4	Tr	Tr	Tr	0.1
	Asparagus, green Cooked, drained									
1040	From raw	1 cup	180	92	43	5	1	0.1	Tr	0.2
1041		4 spears	60	92	14	2	Tr	Tr	Tr	0.1
1042	From frozen	1 cup	180	91	50	5	1	0.2	Tr	0.3
1043		4 spears	60	91	17	2	Tr	0.1	Tr	0.1
1044	Canned, spears, about 5" long, drained	1 cup	242	94	46	5	2	0.4	0.1	0.7
1045		4 spears	72	94	14	2	Tr	0.1	Tr	0.2
1046	Bamboo shoots, canned, drained	1 cup	131	94	25	2	1	0.1	Tr	0.2
	Beans Lima, immature seeds, frozen, cooked, drained									
1047	Ford hooks	1 cup	170	74	170	10	1	0.1	Tr	0.3
1048	Baby limas	1 cup	180	72	189	12	1	0.1	Tr	0.3
	Snap, cut Cooked, drained From raw									
1049	Green	1 cup	125	89	44	2	Tr	0.1	Tr	0.2
1050	Yellow	1 cup	125	89	44	2	Tr	0.1	Tr	0.2
	From frozen									
1051	Green	1 cup	135	91	38	2	Tr	0.1	Tr	0.1
1052	Yellow	1 cup	135	91	38	2	Tr	0.1	Tr	0.1
	Canned, drained									
1053	Green	1 cup	135	93	27	2	Tr	Tr	Tr	0.1
1054	Yellow	1 cup	135	93	27	2	Tr	Tr	Tr	0.1
	Beans, dry. See Legumes. Bean sprouts (mung)									
1055	Raw	1 cup	104	90	31	3	Tr	Tr	Tr	0.1
1056	Cooked, drained	1 cup	124	93	26	3	Tr	Tr	Tr	Tr
	Beets Cooked, drained									
1057	Slices	1 cup	170	87	75	3	Tr	Tr	0.1	0.1
1058	Whole beet, 2" dia	1 beet	50	87	22	1	Tr	Tr	Tr	Tr
	Canned, drained									
1059	Slices	1 cup	170	91	53	2	Tr	Tr	Tr	0.1
1060	Whole beet	1 beet	24	91	7	Tr	Tr	Tr	Tr	Tr
1061	Beet greens, leaves and stems, cooked, drained, 1" pieces	1 cup	144	89	39	4	Tr	Tr	0.1	0.1
	Black eyed peas, immature seeds, cooked, drained									
1062	From raw	1 cup	165	75	160	5	1	0.2	0.1	0.3
1063	From frozen	1 cup	170	66	224	14	1	0.3	0.1	0.5
	Broccoli Raw									
1064	Chopped or diced	1 cup	88	91	25	3	Tr	Tr	Tr	0.1
1065	Spear, about 5" long	1 spear	31	91	9	1	Tr	Tr	Tr	0.1
1066	Flower cluster	1 floweret	11	91	3	Tr	Tr	Tr	Tr	Tr
	Cooked, drained From raw									
1067	Chopped	1 cup	156	91	44	5	1	0.1	Tr	0.3
1068	Spear, about 5" long	1 spear	37	91	10	1	Tr	Tr	Tr	0.1
1069	From frozen, chopped	1 cup	184	91	52	6	Tr	Tr	Tr	0.1

Choles-terol (mg)	Carbo-hydrate (g)	Total dietary fiber (g)	Calcium (mg)	Iron (mg)	Potas-sium (mg)	Sodium (mg)	Vitamin A		Thiamin (mg)	Ribo-flavin (mg)	Niacin (mg)	Ascor-bic acid (mg)	Food No.
							(IU)	(RE)					
0	1	0.8	11	0.3	26	2	51	5	0.03	0.04	0.2	3	1037
0	19	9.1	76	2.2	595	160	297	30	0.11	0.11	1.7	17	1038
0	13	6.5	54	1.5	425	114	212	22	0.08	0.08	1.2	12	1039
0	8	2.9	36	1.3	288	20	970	97	0.22	0.23	1.9	19	1040
0	3	1.0	12	0.4	96	7	323	32	0.07	0.08	0.6	6	1041
0	9	2.9	41	1.2	392	7	1,472	148	0.12	0.19	1.9	44	1042
0	3	1.0	14	0.4	131	2	491	49	0.04	0.06	0.6	15	1043
0	6	3.9	39	4.4	416	695	1,285	128	0.15	0.24	2.3	45	1044
0	2	1.2	12	1.3	124	207	382	38	0.04	0.07	0.7	13	1045
0	4	1.8	10	0.4	105	9	10	1	0.03	0.03	0.2	1	1046
0	32	9.9	37	2.3	694	90	323	32	0.13	0.10	1.8	22	1047
0	35	10.8	50	3.5	740	52	301	31	0.13	0.10	1.4	10	1048
0	10	4.0	58	1.6	374	4	833	84	0.09	0.12	0.8	12	1049
0	10	4.1	58	1.6	374	4	101	10	0.09	0.12	0.8	12	1050
0	9	4.1	66	1.2	170	12	541	54	0.05	0.12	0.5	6	1051
0	9	4.1	66	1.2	170	12	151	15	0.05	0.12	0.5	6	1052
0	6	2.6	35	1.2	147	354	471	47	0.02	0.08	0.3	6	1053
0	6	1.8	35	1.2	147	339	142	15	0.02	0.08	0.3	6	1054
0	6	1.9	14	0.9	155	6	22	2	0.09	0.13	0.8	14	1055
0	5	1.5	15	0.8	125	12	17	1	0.06	0.13	1.0	14	1056
0	17	3.4	27	1.3	519	131	60	7	0.05	0.07	0.6	6	1057
0	5	1.0	8	0.4	153	39	18	2	0.01	0.02	0.2	2	1058
0	12	2.9	26	3.1	252	330	19	2	0.02	0.07	0.3	7	1059
0	2	0.4	4	0.4	36	47	3	Tr	Tr	0.01	Tr	1	1060
0	8	4.2	164	2.7	1,309	347	7,344	734	0.17	0.42	0.7	36	1061
0	34	8.3	211	1.8	690	7	1,305	130	0.17	0.24	2.3	4	1062
0	40	10.9	39	3.6	638	9	128	14	0.44	0.11	1.2	4	1063
0	5	2.6	42	0.8	286	24	1,357	136	0.06	0.10	0.6	82	1064
0	2	0.9	15	0.3	101	8	478	48	0.02	0.04	0.2	29	1065
0	1	0.3	5	0.1	36	3	330	33	0.01	0.01	0.1	10	1066
0	8	4.5	72	1.3	456	41	2,165	217	0.09	0.18	0.9	116	1067
0	2	1.1	17	0.3	108	10	514	51	0.02	0.04	0.2	28	1068
0	10	5.5	94	1.1	331	44	3,481	348	0.10	0.15	0.8	74	1069

Table 9. Nutritive Value of the Edible Part of Food

Food No.	Food Description	Measure of edible portion	Weight (g)	Water (%)	Calories (kcal)	Pro-tein (g)	Total fat (g)	Fatty acids Satu-rated (g)	Mono-unsatu-rated (g)	Poly-unsatu-rated (g)

Vegetables and Vegetable Products (continued)

	Brussels sprouts, cooked, drained									
1070	From raw	1 cup	156	87	61	4	1	0.2	0.1	0.4
1071	From frozen	1 cup	155	87	65	6	1	0.1	Tr	0.3
	Cabbage, common varieties, shredded									
1072	Raw	1 cup	70	92	18	1	Tr	Tr	Tr	0.1
1073	Cooked, drained	1 cup	150	94	33	2	1	0.1	Tr	0.3
	Cabbage, Chinese, shredded, cooked, drained									
1074	Pak choi or bok choy	1 cup	170	96	20	3	Tr	Tr	Tr	0.1
1075	Pe tsai	1 cup	119	95	17	2	Tr	Tr	Tr	0.1
1076	Cabbage, red, raw, shredded	1 cup	70	92	19	1	Tr	Tr	Tr	0.1
1077	Cabbage, savoy, raw, shredded	1 cup	70	91	19	1	Tr	Tr	Tr	Tr
1078	Carrot juice, canned	1 cup	236	89	94	2	Tr	0.1	Tr	0.2
	Carrots									
	Raw									
1079	Whole, 7½" long	1 carrot	72	88	31	1	Tr	Tr	Tr	0.1
1080	Grated	1 cup	110	88	47	1	Tr	Tr	Tr	0.1
1081	Baby	1 medium	10	90	4	Tr	Tr	Tr	Tr	Tr
	Cooked, sliced, drained									
1082	From raw	1 cup	156	87	70	2	Tr	0.1	Tr	0.1
1083	From frozen	1 cup	146	90	53	2	Tr	Tr	Tr	0.1
1084	Canned, sliced, drained	1 cup	146	93	37	1	Tr	0.1	Tr	0.1
	Cauliflower									
1085	Raw	1 floweret	13	92	3	Tr	Tr	Tr	Tr	Tr
1086		1 cup	100	92	25	2	Tr	Tr	Tr	0.1
	Cooked, drained, 1" pieces									
1087	From raw	1 cup	124	93	29	2	1	0.1	Tr	0.3
1088		3 flowerets	54	93	12	1	Tr	Tr	Tr	0.1
1089	From frozen	1 cup	180	94	34	3	Tr	0.1	Tr	0.2
	Celery									
	Raw									
1090	Stalk, 7½ to 8" long	1 stalk	40	95	6	Tr	Tr	Tr	Tr	Tr
1091	Pieces, diced	1 cup	120	95	19	1	Tr	Tr	Tr	0.1
	Cooked, drained									
1092	Stalk, medium	1 stalk	38	94	7	Tr	Tr	Tr	Tr	Tr
1093	Pieces, diced	1 cup	150	94	27	1	Tr	0.1	Tr	0.1
1094	Chives, raw, chopped	1 tbsp	3	91	1	Tr	Tr	Tr	Tr	Tr
1095	Cilantro, raw	1 tsp	2	92	Tr	Tr	Tr	Tr	Tr	Tr
1096	Coleslaw, home prepared	1 cup	120	82	83	2	3	0.5	0.8	1.6
	Collards, cooked, drained, chopped									
1097	From raw	1 cup	190	92	49	4	1	0.1	Tr	0.3
1098	From frozen	1 cup	170	88	61	5	1	0.1	Tr	0.4
	Corn, sweet, yellow									
	Cooked, drained									
1099	From raw, kernels on cob	1 ear	77	70	83	3	1	0.2	0.3	0.5
	From frozen									
1100	Kernels on cob	1 ear	63	73	59	2	Tr	0.1	0.1	0.2
1101	Kernels	1 cup	164	77	131	5	1	0.1	0.2	0.3
	Canned									
1102	Cream style	1 cup	256	79	184	4	1	0.2	0.3	0.5
1103	Whole kernel, vacuum pack	1 cup	210	77	166	5	1	0.2	0.3	0.5
1104	Corn, sweet, white, cooked, drained	1 ear	77	70	83	3	1	0.2	0.3	0.5

*White varieties contain only a trace amount of vitamin A; other nutrients are the same.

Choles- terol (mg)	Carbo- hydrate (g)	Total dietary fiber (g)	Calcium (mg)	Iron (mg)	Potas- sium (mg)	Sodium (mg)	Vitamin A		Thiamin (mg)	Ribo- flavin (mg)	Niacin (mg)	Ascor- bic acid (mg)	Food No.
							(IU)	(RE)					
0	14	4.1	56	1.9	495	33	1,122	112	0.17	0.12	0.9	97	1070
0	13	6.4	37	1.1	504	36	913	91	0.16	0.18	0.8	71	1071
0	4	1.6	33	0.4	172	13	93	9	0.04	0.03	0.2	23	1072
0	7	3.5	47	0.3	146	12	198	20	0.09	0.08	0.4	30	1073
0	3	2.7	158	1.8	631	58	4,366	437	0.05	0.11	0.7	44	1074
0	3	3.2	38	0.4	268	11	1,151	115	0.05	0.05	0.6	19	1075
0	4	1.4	36	0.3	144	8	28	3	0.04	0.02	0.2	40	1076
0	4	2.2	25	0.3	161	20	700	70	0.05	0.02	0.2	22	1077
0	22	1.9	57	1.1	689	68	25,833	2,584	0.22	0.13	0.9	20	1078
0	7	2.2	19	0.4	233	25	20,253	2,025	0.07	0.04	0.7	7	1079
0	11	3.3	30	0.6	355	39	30,942	3,094	0.11	0.06	1.0	10	1080
0	1	0.2	2	0.1	28	4	1,501	150	Tr	0.01	0.1	1	1081
0	16	5.1	48	1.0	354	103	38,304	3,830	0.05	0.09	0.8	4	1082
0	12	5.1	41	0.7	231	86	25,845	2,584	0.04	0.05	0.6	4	1083
0	8	2.2	37	0.9	261	353	20,110	2,010	0.03	0.04	0.8	4	1084
0	1	0.3	3	0.1	39	4	2	Tr	0.01	0.01	0.1	6	1085
0	5	2.5	22	0.4	303	30	19	2	0.06	0.06	0.5	46	1086
0	5	3.3	20	0.4	176	19	21	2	0.05	0.06	0.5	55	1087
0	2	1.5	9	0.2	77	8	9	1	0.02	0.03	0.2	24	1088
0	7	4.9	31	0.7	250	32	40	4	0.07	0.10	0.6	56	1089
0	1	0.7	16	0.2	115	35	54	5	0.02	0.02	0.1	3	1090
0	4	2.0	48	0.5	344	104	161	16	0.06	0.05	0.4	8	1091
0	2	0.6	16	0.2	108	35	50	5	0.02	0.02	0.1	2	1092
0	6	2.4	63	0.6	426	137	198	20	0.06	0.07	0.5	9	1093
0	Tr	0.1	3	Tr	9	Tr	131	13	Tr	Tr	Tr	2	1094
0	Tr	Tr	1	Tr	8	1	98	10	Tr	Tr	Tr	1	1095
10	15	1.8	54	0.7	217	28	762	98	0.08	0.07	0.3	39	1096
0	9	5.3	226	0.9	494	17	5,945	595	0.08	0.20	1.1	35	1097
0	12	4.8	357	1.9	427	85	10,168	1,017	0.08	0.20	1.1	45	1098
0	19	2.2	2	0.5	192	13	167	17	0.17	0.06	1.2	5	1099
0	14	1.8	2	0.4	158	3	133*	13*	0.11	0.04	1.0	3	1100
0	32	3.9	7	0.6	241	8	361*	36*	0.14	0.12	2.1	5	1101
0	46	3.1	8	1.0	343	730	248*	26*	0.06	0.14	2.5	12	1102
0	41	4.2	11	0.9	391	571	506*	50*	0.09	0.15	2.5	17	1103
0	19	2.1	2	0.5	192	13	0	0	0.17	0.06	1.2	5	1104

Table 9. Nutritive Value of the Edible Part of Food

Food No.	Food Description	Measure of edible portion	Weight (g)	Water (%)	Calories (kcal)	Protein (g)	Total fat (g)	Fatty acids Saturated (g)	Mono-unsaturated (g)	Poly-unsaturated (g)

Vegetables and Vegetable Products (continued)

	Cucumber									
	Peeled									
1105	Sliced	1 cup	119	96	14	1	Tr	Tr	Tr	0.1
1106	Whole, 8¼" long	1 large	280	96	34	2	Tr	0.1	Tr	0.2
	Unpeeled									
1107	Sliced	1 cup	104	96	14	1	Tr	Tr	Tr	0.1
1108	Whole, 8¼" long	1 large	301	96	39	2	Tr	0.1	Tr	0.2
1109	Dandelion greens, cooked, drained	1 cup	105	90	35	2	1	0.2	Tr	0.3
1110	Dill weed, raw	5 sprigs	1	86	Tr	Tr	Tr	Tr	Tr	Tr
1111	Eggplant, cooked, drained	1 cup	99	92	28	1	Tr	Tr	Tr	0.1
1112	Endive, curly (including escarole), raw, small pieces	1 cup	50	94	9	1	Tr	Tr	Tr	Tr
1113	Garlic, raw	1 clove	3	59	4	Tr	Tr	Tr	Tr	Tr
1114	Hearts of palm, canned	1 piece	33	90	9	1	Tr	Tr	Tr	0.1
1115	Jerusalem artichoke, raw, sliced	1 cup	150	78	114	3	Tr	0.0	Tr	Tr
	Kale, cooked, drained, chopped									
1116	From raw	1 cup	130	91	36	2	1	0.1	Tr	0.3
1117	From frozen	1 cup	130	91	39	4	1	0.1	Tr	0.3
1118	Kohlrabi, cooked, drained, slices	1 cup	165	90	48	3	Tr	Tr	Tr	0.1
1119	Leeks, bulb and lower leaf portion, chopped or diced, cooked, drained	1 cup	104	91	32	1	Tr	Tr	Tr	0.1
	Lettuce, raw									
	Butterhead, as Boston types									
1120	Leaf	1 medium leaf	8	96	1	Tr	Tr	Tr	Tr	Tr
1121	Head, 5" dia	1 head	163	96	21	2	Tr	Tr	Tr	0.2
	Crisphead, as iceberg									
1122	Leaf	1 medium	8	96	1	Tr	Tr	Tr	Tr	Tr
1123	Head, 6" dia	1 head	539	96	65	5	1	0.1	Tr	0.5
1124	Pieces, shredded or chopped	1 cup	55	96	7	1	Tr	Tr	Tr	0.1
	Looseleaf									
1125	Leaf	1 leaf	10	94	2	Tr	Tr	Tr	Tr	Tr
1126	Pieces, shredded	1 cup	56	94	10	1	Tr	Tr	Tr	0.1
	Romaine or cos									
1127	Innerleaf	1 leaf	10	95	1	Tr	Tr	Tr	Tr	Tr
1128	Pieces, shredded	1 cup	56	95	8	1	Tr	Tr	Tr	0.1
	Mushrooms									
1129	Raw, pieces or slices	1 cup	70	92	18	2	Tr	Tr	Tr	0.1
1130	Cooked, drained, pieces	1 cup	156	91	42	3	1	0.1	Tr	0.3
1131	Canned, drained, pieces	1 cup	156	91	37	3	Tr	0.1	Tr	0.2
	Mushrooms, shiitake									
1132	Cooked pieces	1 cup	145	83	80	2	Tr	0.1	0.1	Tr
1133	Dried	1 mushroom	4	10	11	Tr	Tr	Tr	Tr	Tr
1134	Mustard greens, cooked, drained	1 cup	140	94	21	3	Tr	Tr	0.2	0.1
	Okra, sliced, cooked, drained									
1135	From raw	1 cup	160	90	51	3	Tr	0.1	Tr	0.1
1136	From frozen	1 cup	184	91	52	4	1	0.1	0.1	0.1
	Onions									
	Raw									
1137	Chopped	1 cup	160	90	61	2	Tr	Tr	Tr	0.1
1138	Whole, medium, 2½" dia	1 whole	110	90	42	1	Tr	Tr	Tr	0.1
1139	Slice, ⅛" thick	1 slice	14	90	5	Tr	Tr	Tr	Tr	Tr

Choles-terol (mg)	Carbo-hydrate (g)	Total dietary fiber (g)	Calcium (mg)	Iron (mg)	Potas-sium (mg)	Sodium (mg)	Vitamin A (IU)	Vitamin A (RE)	Thiamin (mg)	Ribo-flavin (mg)	Niacin (mg)	Ascor-bic acid (mg)	Food No.
0	3	0.8	17	0.2	176	2	88	8	0.02	0.01	0.1	3	1105
0	7	2.0	39	0.4	414	6	207	20	0.06	0.03	0.3	8	1106
0	3	0.8	15	0.3	150	2	224	22	0.02	0.02	0.2	6	1107
0	8	2.4	42	0.8	433	6	647	63	0.07	0.07	0.7	16	1108
0	7	3.0	147	1.9	244	46	12,285	1,229	0.14	0.18	0.5	19	1109
0	Tr	Tr	2	0.1	7	1	77	8	Tr	Tr	Tr	1	1110
0	7	2.5	6	0.3	246	3	63	6	0.08	0.02	0.6	1	1111
0	2	1.6	26	0.4	157	11	1,025	103	0.04	0.04	0.2	3	1112
0	1	0.1	5	0.1	12	1	0	0	0.01	Tr	Tr	1	1113
0	2	0.8	19	1.0	58	141	0	0	Tr	0.02	0.1	3	1114
0	26	2.4	21	5.1	644	6	30	3	0.30	0.09	2.0	6	1115
0	7	2.6	94	1.2	296	30	9,620	962	0.07	0.09	0.7	53	1116
0	7	2.6	179	1.2	417	20	8,260	826	0.06	0.15	0.9	33	1117
0	11	1.8	41	0.7	561	35	58	7	0.07	0.03	0.6	89	1118
0	8	1.0	31	1.1	90	10	48	5	0.03	0.02	0.2	4	1119
0	Tr	0.1	2	Tr	19	Tr	73	7	Tr	Tr	Tr	1	1120
0	4	1.6	52	0.5	419	8	1,581	158	0.10	0.10	0.5	13	1121
0	Tr	0.1	2	Tr	13	1	26	3	Tr	Tr	Tr	Tr	1122
0	11	7.5	102	2.7	852	49	1,779	178	0.25	0.16	1.0	21	1123
0	1	0.8	10	0.3	87	5	182	18	0.03	0.02	0.1	2	1124
0	Tr	0.2	7	0.1	26	1	190	19	0.01	0.01	Tr	2	1125
0	2	1.1	38	0.8	148	5	1,064	106	0.03	0.04	0.2	10	1126
0	Tr	0.2	4	0.1	29	1	260	26	0.01	0.01	0.1	2	1127
0	1	1.0	20	0.6	162	4	1,456	146	0.06	0.06	0.3	13	1128
0	3	0.8	4	0.7	259	3	0	0	0.06	0.30	2.8	2	1129
0	8	3.4	9	2.7	555	3	0	0	0.11	0.47	7.0	6	1130
0	8	3.7	17	1.2	201	663	0	0	0.13	0.03	2.5	0	1131
0	21	3.0	4	0.6	170	6	0	0	0.05	0.25	2.2	Tr	1132
0	3	0.4	Tr	0.1	55	Tr	0	0	0.01	0.05	0.5	Tr	1133
0	3	2.8	104	1.0	283	22	4,243	424	0.06	0.09	0.6	35	1134
0	12	4.0	101	0.7	515	8	920	93	0.21	0.09	1.4	26	1135
0	11	5.2	177	1.2	431	6	946	94	0.18	0.23	1.4	22	1136
0	14	2.9	32	0.4	251	5	0	0	0.07	0.03	0.2	10	1137
0	9	2.0	22	0.2	173	3	0	0	0.05	0.02	0.2	7	1138
0	1	0.3	3	Tr	22	Tr	0	0	0.01	Tr	Tr	1	1139

Table 9. Nutritive Value of the Edible Part of Food

Food No.	Food Description	Measure of edible portion	Weight (g)	Water (%)	Calories (kcal)	Pro-tein (g)	Total fat (g)	Fatty acids Satu-rated (g)	Mono-unsatu-rated (g)	Poly-unsatu-rated (g)

Vegetables and Vegetable Products (continued)

Food No.	Food Description	Measure of edible portion	Weight (g)	Water (%)	Calories (kcal)	Pro-tein (g)	Total fat (g)	Satu-rated (g)	Mono-unsatu-rated (g)	Poly-unsatu-rated (g)
1140	Cooked (whole or sliced), drained	1 cup	210	88	92	3	Tr	0.1	0.1	0.2
1141		1 medium	94	88	41	1	Tr	Tr	Tr	0.1
1142	Dehydrated flakes	1 tbsp	5	4	17	Tr	Tr	Tr	Tr	Tr
	Onions, spring, raw, top and bulb									
1143	Chopped	1 cup	100	90	32	2	Tr	Tr	Tr	0.1
1144	Whole, medium, 4⅛" long	1 whole	15	90	5	Tr	Tr	Tr	Tr	Tr
1145	Onion rings, 2"-3" dia, breaded, par fried, frozen, oven heated	10 rings	60	29	244	3	16	5.2	6.5	3.1
1146	Parsley, raw	10 sprigs	10	88	4	Tr	Tr	Tr	Tr	Tr
1147	Parsnips, sliced, cooked, drained	1 cup	156	78	126	2	Tr	0.1	0.2	0.1
	Peas, edible pod, cooked, drained									
1148	From raw	1 cup	160	89	67	5	Tr	0.1	Tr	0.2
1149	From frozen	1 cup	160	87	83	6	1	0.1	0.1	0.3
	Peas, green									
1150	Canned, drained	1 cup	170	82	117	8	1	0.1	0.1	0.3
1151	Frozen, boiled, drained	1 cup	160	80	125	8	Tr	0.1	Tr	0.2
	Peppers									
	Hot chili, raw									
1152	Green	1 pepper	45	88	18	1	Tr	Tr	Tr	Tr
1153	Red	1 pepper	45	88	18	1	Tr	Tr	Tr	Tr
1154	Jalapeno, canned, sliced, solids and liquids	¼ cup	26	89	7	Tr	Tr	Tr	Tr	0.1
	Sweet (2¾" long, 2½" dia)									
	Raw									
	Green									
1155	Chopped	1 cup	149	92	40	1	Tr	Tr	Tr	0.2
1156	Ring (¼" thick)	1 ring	10	92	3	Tr	Tr	Tr	Tr	Tr
1157	Whole (2¾" x 2½")	1 pepper	119	92	32	1	Tr	Tr	Tr	0.1
	Red									
1158	Chopped	1 cup	149	92	40	1	Tr	Tr	Tr	0.2
1159	Whole (2¾" x 2½")	1 pepper	119	92	32	1	Tr	Tr	Tr	0.1
	Cooked, drained, chopped									
1160	Green	1 cup	136	92	38	1	Tr	Tr	Tr	0.1
1161	Red	1 cup	136	92	38	1	Tr	Tr	Tr	0.1
1162	Pimento, canned	1 tbsp	12	93	3	Tr	Tr	Tr	Tr	Tr
	Potatoes									
	Baked (2⅓" x 4¾")									
1163	With skin	1 potato	202	71	220	5	Tr	0.1	Tr	0.1
1164	Flesh only	1 potato	156	75	145	3	Tr	Tr	Tr	0.1
1165	Skin only	1 skin	58	47	115	2	Tr	Tr	Tr	Tr
	Boiled (2½" dia)									
1166	Peeled after boiling	1 potato	136	77	118	3	Tr	Tr	Tr	0.1
1167	Peeled before boiling	1 potato	135	77	116	2	Tr	Tr	Tr	0.1
1168		1 cup	156	77	134	3	Tr	Tr	Tr	0.1
	Potato products, prepared									
	Au gratin									
1169	From dry mix, with whole milk, butter	1 cup	245	79	228	6	10	6.3	2.9	0.3
1170	From home recipe, with butter	1 cup	245	74	323	12	19	11.6	5.3	0.7
1171	French fried, frozen, oven heated	10 strips	50	57	100	2	4	0.6	2.4	0.4

Choles-terol (mg)	Carbo-hydrate (g)	Total dietary fiber (g)	Calcium (mg)	Iron (mg)	Potas-sium (mg)	Sodium (mg)	Vitamin A (IU)	Vitamin A (RE)	Thiamin (mg)	Ribo-flavin (mg)	Niacin (mg)	Ascor-bic acid (mg)	Food No.
0	21	2.9	46	0.5	349	6	0	0	0.09	0.05	0.3	11	1140
0	10	1.3	21	0.2	156	3	0	0	0.04	0.02	0.2	5	1141
0	4	0.5	13	0.1	81	1	0	0	0.03	0.01	Tr	4	1142
0	7	2.6	72	1.5	276	16	385	39	0.06	0.08	0.5	19	1143
0	1	0.4	11	0.2	41	2	58	6	0.01	0.01	0.1	3	1144
0	23	0.8	19	1.0	77	225	135	14	0.17	0.08	2.2	1	1145
0	1	0.3	14	0.6	55	6	520	52	0.01	0.01	0.1	13	1146
0	30	6.2	58	0.9	573	16	0	0	0.13	0.08	1.1	20	1147
0	11	4.5	67	3.2	384	6	210	21	0.20	0.12	0.9	77	1148
0	14	5.0	94	3.8	347	8	267	27	0.10	0.19	0.9	35	1149
0	21	7.0	34	1.6	294	428	1,306	131	0.21	0.13	1.2	16	1150
0	23	8.8	38	2.5	269	139	1,069	107	0.45	0.16	2.4	16	1151
0	4	0.7	8	0.5	153	3	347	35	0.04	0.04	0.4	109	1152
0	4	0.7	8	0.5	153	3	4,838	484	0.04	0.04	0.4	109	1153
0	1	0.7	6	0.5	50	434	442	44	0.01	0.01	0.1	3	1154
0	10	2.7	13	0.7	264	3	942	94	0.10	0.04	0.8	133	1155
0	1	0.2	1	Tr	18	Tr	63	6	0.01	Tr	0.1	9	1156
0	8	2.1	11	0.5	211	2	752	75	0.08	0.04	0.6	106	1157
0	10	3.0	13	0.7	264	3	8,493	849	0.10	0.04	0.8	283	1158
0	8	2.4	11	0.5	211	2	6,783	678	0.08	0.04	0.6	226	1159
0	9	1.6	12	0.6	226	3	805	80	0.08	0.04	0.6	101	1160
0	9	1.6	12	0.6	226	3	5,114	511	0.08	0.04	0.6	233	1161
0	1	0.2	1	0.2	19	2	319	32	Tr	0.01	0.1	10	1162
0	51	4.8	20	2.7	844	16	0	0	0.22	0.07	3.3	26	1163
0	34	2.3	8	0.5	610	8	0	0	0.16	0.03	2.2	20	1164
0	27	4.6	20	4.1	332	12	0	0	0.07	0.06	1.8	8	1165
0	27	2.4	7	0.4	515	5	0	0	0.14	0.03	2.0	18	1166
0	27	2.4	11	0.4	443	7	0	0	0.13	0.03	1.8	10	1167
0	31	2.8	12	0.5	512	8	0	0	0.15	0.03	2.0	12	2268
37	31	2.2	203	0.8	537	1,076	522	76	0.05	0.20	2.3	8	1169
56	28	4.4	292	1.6	970	1,061	647	93	0.16	0.28	2.4	24	1170
0	16	1.6	4	0.6	209	15	0	0	0.06	0.01	1.0	5	1171

Table 9.   Nutritive Value of the Edible Part of Food

Food No.	Food Description	Measure of edible portion	Weight (g)	Water (%)	Calories (kcal)	Protein (g)	Total fat (g)	Fatty acids Saturated (g)	Fatty acids Mono-unsaturated (g)	Fatty acids Poly-unsaturated (g)

Vegetables and Vegetable Products (continued)

Potato products, prepared (continued)
Hashed brown

No.	Food Description	Measure	Weight	Water	Calories	Protein	Fat	Sat	Mono	Poly
1172	From frozen (about 3" x 1½" x ½") .... 1 patty	29	56	63	1	3	1.3	1.5	0.4
1173	From home recipe .... 1 cup	156	62	326	4	22	8.5	9.7	2.5
	Mashed									
1174	From dehydrated flakes (without milk); whole milk, butter, and salt added .... 1 cup	210	76	237	4	12	7.2	3.3	0.5
	From home recipe									
1175	With whole milk .... 1 cup	210	78	162	4	1	0.7	0.3	0.1
1176	With whole milk and margarine .... 1 cup	210	76	223	4	9	2.2	3.7	2.5
1177	Potato pancakes, home prepared .... 1 pancake	76	47	207	5	12	2.3	3.5	5.0
1178	Potato puffs, from frozen .... 10 puffs	79	53	175	3	8	4.0	3.4	0.6
1179	Potato salad, home prepared .. 1 cup	250	76	358	7	21	3.6	6.2	9.3
	Scalloped									
1180	From dry mix, with whole milk, butter .... 1 cup	245	79	228	5	11	6.5	3.0	0.5
1181	From home recipe, with butter .... 1 cup	245	81	211	7	9	5.5	2.5	0.4
	Pumpkin									
1182	Cooked, mashed .... 1 cup	245	94	49	2	Tr	0.1	Tr	Tr
1183	Canned .... 1 cup	245	90	83	3	1	0.4	0.1	Tr
1184	Radishes, raw (¾" to 1" dia) .... 1 radish	5	95	1	Tr	Tr	Tr	Tr	Tr
1185	Rutabagas, cooked, drained, cubes .... 1 cup	170	89	66	2	Tr	Tr	Tr	0.2
1186	Sauerkraut, canned, solids and liquid .... 1 cup	236	93	45	2	Tr	0.1	Tr	0.1
	Seaweed									
1187	Kelp, raw .... 2 tbsp	10	82	4	Tr	Tr	Tr	Tr	Tr
1188	Spirulina, dried .... 1 tbsp	1	5	3	1	Tr	Tr	Tr	Tr
1189	Shallots, raw, chopped .... 1 tbsp	10	80	7	Tr	Tr	Tr	Tr	Tr
1190	Soybeans, green, cooked, drained .... 1 cup	180	69	254	22	12	1.3	2.2	5.4
	Spinach									
	Raw									
1191	Chopped .... 1 cup	30	92	7	1	Tr	Tr	Tr	Tr
1192	Leaf .... 1 leaf	10	92	2	Tr	Tr	Tr	Tr	Tr
	Cooked, drained									
1193	From raw .... 1 cup	180	91	41	5	Tr	0.1	Tr	0.2
1194	From frozen (chopped or leaf) .... 1 cup	190	90	53	6	Tr	0.1	Tr	0.2
1195	Canned, drained .... 1 cup	214	92	49	6	1	0.2	Tr	0.4
	Squash									
	Summer (all varieties), sliced									
1196	Raw .... 1 cup	113	94	23	1	Tr	Tr	Tr	0.1
1197	Cooked, drained .... 1 cup	180	94	36	2	1	0.1	Tr	0.2
1198	Winter (all varieties), baked, cubes .... 1 cup	205	89	80	2	1	0.3	0.1	0.5
1199	Winter, butternut, frozen, cooked, mashed .... 1 cup	240	88	94	3	Tr	Tr	Tr	0.1
	Sweetpotatoes									
	Cooked (2" dia, 5" long raw)									
1200	Baked, with skin .... 1 potato	146	73	150	3	Tr	Tr	Tr	0.1
1201	Boiled, without skin .... 1 potato	156	73	164	3	Tr	0.1	Tr	0.2

Choles-terol (mg)	Carbo-hydrate (g)	Total dietary fiber (g)	Calcium (mg)	Iron (mg)	Potas-sium (mg)	Sodium (mg)	Vitamin A		Thiamin (mg)	Ribo-flavin (mg)	Niacin (mg)	Ascor-bic acid (mg)	Food No.
							(IU)	(RE)					
0	8	0.6	4	0.4	126	10	0	0	0.03	0.01	0.7	2	1172
0	33	3.1	12	1.3	501	37	0	0	0.12	0.03	3.1	9	1173
29	32	4.8	103	0.5	489	697	378	44	0.23	0.11	1.4	20	1174
4	37	4.2	55	0.6	628	636	40	13	0.18	0.08	2.3	14	1175
4	35	4.2	55	0.5	607	620	355	42	0.18	0.08	2.3	13	1176
73	22	1.5	18	1.2	597	386	109	11	0.10	0.13	1.6	17	1177
0	24	2.5	24	1.2	300	589	13	2	0.15	0.06	1.7	5	1178
170	28	3.3	48	1.6	635	1,323	523	83	0.19	0.15	2.2	25	1179
27	31	2.7	88	0.9	497	835	363	51	0.05	0.14	2.5	8	1180
29	26	4.7	140	1.4	926	821	331	47	0.17	0.23	2.6	26	1181
0	12	2.7	37	1.4	564	2	2,651	265	0.08	0.19	1.0	12	1182
0	20	7.1	64	3.4	505	12	54,037	5,405	0.06	0.13	0.9	10	1183
0	Tr	0.1	1	Tr	10	1	Tr	Tr	Tr	Tr	Tr	1	1184
0	15	3.1	82	0.9	554	34	954	95	0.14	0.07	1.2	32	1185
0	10	5.9	71	3.5	401	1,560	42	5	0.05	0.05	0.3	35	1186
0	1	0.1	17	0.3	9	23	12	1	0.01	0.02	Tr	Tr	1187
0	Tr	Tr	1	0.3	14	10	6	1	0.02	0.04	0.1	Tr	1188
0	2	0.2	4	0.1	33	1	119	12	0.01	Tr	Tr	1	1189
0	20	7.6	261	4.5	970	25	281	29	0.47	0.28	2.3	31	1190
0	1	0.8	30	0.8	167	24	2,015	202	0.02	0.06	0.2	8	1191
0	Tr	0.3	10	0.3	56	8	672	67	0.01	0.02	0.1	3	1192
0	7	4.3	245	6.4	839	126	14,742	1,474	0.17	0.42	0.9	18	1193
0	10	5.7	277	2.9	566	163	14,790	1,478	0.11	0.32	0.8	23	1194
0	7	5.1	272	4.9	740	58	18,781	1,879	0.03	0.30	0.8	31	1195
0	5	2.1	23	0.5	220	2	221	23	0.07	0.04	0.6	17	1196
0	8	2.5	49	0.6	346	2	517	52	0.08	0.07	0.9	10	1197
0	18	5.7	29	0.7	896	2	7,292	730	0.17	0.05	1.4	20	1198
0	24	2.2	46	1.4	319	5	8,014	802	0.12	0.09	1.1	8	1199
0	35	4.4	41	0.7	508	15	31,860	3,186	0.11	0.19	0.9	36	1200
0	38	2.8	33	0.9	287	20	26,604	2,660	0.08	0.22	1.0	27	1201

Table 9.   Nutritive Value of the Edible Part of Food

Food No.	Food Description	Measure of edible portion	Weight (g)	Water (%)	Calories (kcal)	Pro-tein (g)	Total fat (g)	Fatty acids Satu-rated (g)	Mono-unsatu-rated (g)	Poly-unsatu-rated (g)
	Vegetables and Vegetable Products (continued)									
	Sweetpotatoes (continued)									
1202	Candied (2½" x 2" piece)	1 piece	105	67	144	1	3	1.4	0.7	0.2
	Canned									
1203	Syrup pack, drained	1 cup	196	72	212	3	1	0.1	Tr	0.3
1204	Vacuum pack, mashed	1 cup	255	76	232	4	1	0.1	Tr	0.2
1205	Tomatillos, raw	1 medium	34	92	11	Tr	Tr	Tr	0.1	0.1
	Tomatoes									
	Raw, year round average									
1206	Chopped or sliced	1 cup	180	94	38	2	1	0.1	0.1	0.2
1207	Slice, medium, ¼" thick	1 slice	20	94	4	Tr	Tr	Tr	Tr	Tr
	Whole									
1208	Cherry	1 cherry	17	94	4	Tr	Tr	Tr	Tr	Tr
1209	Medium, 2⅗" dia	1 tomato	123	94	26	1	Tr	0.1	0.1	0.2
1210	Canned, solids and liquid	1 cup	240	94	46	2	Tr	Tr	Tr	0.1
	Sun dried									
1211	Plain	1 piece	2	15	5	Tr	Tr	Tr	Tr	Tr
1212	Packed in oil, drained	1 piece	3	54	6	Tr	Tr	0.1	0.3	0.1
1213	Tomato juice, canned, with salt added	1 cup	243	94	41	2	Tr	Tr	Tr	0.1
	Tomato products, canned									
1214	Paste	1 cup	262	74	215	10	1	0.2	0.2	0.6
1215	Puree	1 cup	250	87	100	4	Tr	0.1	0.1	0.2
1216	Sauce	1 cup	245	89	74	3	Tr	0.1	0.1	0.2
	Spaghetti/marinara/pasta sauce. See Soups, Sauces, and Gravies.									
1217	Stewed	1 cup	255	91	71	2	Tr	Tr	0.1	0.1
1218	Turnips, cooked, cubes	1 cup	156	94	33	1	Tr	Tr	Tr	0.1
	Turnip greens, cooked, drained									
1219	From raw (leaves and stems)	1 cup	144	93	29	2	Tr	0.1	Tr	0.1
1220	From frozen (chopped)	1 cup	164	90	49	5	1	0.2	Tr	0.3
1221	Vegetable juice cocktail, canned	1 cup	242	94	46	2	Tr	Tr	Tr	0.1
	Vegetables, mixed									
1222	Canned, drained	1 cup	163	87	77	4	Tr	0.1	Tr	0.2
1223	Frozen, cooked, drained	1 cup	182	83	107	5	Tr	0.1	Tr	0.1
1224	Waterchestnuts, canned, slices, solids and liquids	1 cup	140	86	70	1	Tr	Tr	Tr	Tr
	Miscellaneous Items									
1225	Bacon bits, meatless	1 tbsp	7	8	31	2	2	0.3	0.4	0.9
	Baking powders for home use									
	Double acting									
1226	Sodium aluminum sulfate	1 tsp	5	5	2	0	0	0.0	0.0	0.0
1227	Straight phosphate	1 tsp	5	4	2	Tr	0	0.0	0.0	0.0
1228	Low sodium	1 tsp	5	6	5	Tr	Tr	Tr	Tr	Tr
1229	Baking soda	1 tsp	5	Tr	0	0	0	0.0	0.0	0.0
1230	Beef jerky	1 large piece	20	23	81	7	5	2.1	2.2	0.2
1231	Catsup	1 cup	240	67	250	4	1	0.1	0.1	0.4
1232		1 tbsp	15	67	16	Tr	Tr	Tr	Tr	Tr
1233		1 packet	6	67	6	Tr	Tr	Tr	Tr	Tr
1234	Celery seed	1 tsp	2	6	8	Tr	1	Tr	0.3	0.1
1235	Chili powder	1 tsp	3	8	8	Tr	Tr	0.1	0.1	0.2
	Chocolate, unsweetened, baking									
1236	Solid	1 square	28	1	148	3	16	9.2	5.2	0.5
1237	Liquid	1 oz	28	1	134	3	14	7.2	2.6	3.0

*For product with no salt added: If salt added, consult the nutrition label for sodium value.

Choles-terol (mg)	Carbo-hydrate (g)	Total dietary fiber (g)	Calcium (mg)	Iron (mg)	Potas-sium (mg)	Sodium (mg)	Vitamin A		Thiamin (mg)	Ribo-flavin (mg)	Niacin (mg)	Ascor-bic acid (mg)	Food No.
							(IU)	(RE)					
8	29	2.5	27	1.2	198	74	4,398	440	0.02	0.04	0.4	7	1202
0	50	5.9	33	1.9	378	76	14,028	1,403	0.05	0.07	0.7	21	1203
0	54	4.6	56	2.3	796	135	20,357	2,035	0.09	0.15	1.9	67	1204
0	2	0.6	2	0.2	91	Tr	39	4	0.01	0.01	0.6	4	1205
0	8	2.0	9	0.8	400	16	1,121	112	0.11	0.09	1.1	34	1206
0	1	0.2	1	0.1	44	2	125	12	0.01	0.01	0.1	4	1207
0	1	0.2	1	0.1	38	2	106	11	0.01	0.01	0.1	3	1208
0	6	1.4	6	0.6	273	11	766	76	0.07	0.06	0.8	23	1209
0	10	2.4	72	1.3	530	355	1,428	144	0.11	0.07	1.8	34	1210
0	1	0.2	2	0.2	69	42	17	2	0.01	0.01	0.2	1	1211
0	1	0.2	1	0.1	47	8	39	4	0.01	0.01	0.1	3	1212
0	10	1.0	22	1.4	535	877	1,351	136	0.11	0.08	1.6	44	1213
0	51	10.7	92	5.1	2,455	231	6,406	639	0.41	0.50	8.4	111	1214
0	24	5.0	43	3.1	1,065	85*	3,188	320	0.18	0.14	4.3	26	1215
0	18	3.4	34	1.9	909	1,482	2,399	240	0.16	0.14	2.8	32	1216
0	17	2.6	84	1.9	607	564	1,380	138	0.12	0.09	1.8	29	1217
0	8	3.1	34	0.3	211	78	0	0	0.04	0.04	0.5	18	1218
0	6	5.0	197	1.2	292	42	7,917	792	0.06	0.10	0.6	39	1219
0	8	5.6	249	3.2	367	25	13,079	1,309	0.09	0.12	0.8	36	1220
0	11	1.9	27	1.0	467	653	2,831	283	0.10	0.07	1.8	67	1221
0	15	4.9	44	1.7	474	243	18,985	1,899	0.07	0.08	0.9	8	1222
0	24	8.0	46	1.5	308	64	7,784	779	0.13	0.22	1.5	6	1223
0	17	3.5	6	1.2	165	11	6	0	0.02	0.03	0.5	2	1224
0	2	0.7	7	0.1	10	124	0	0	0.04	Tr	0.1	Tr	1225
0	1	Tr	270	0.5	1	488	0	0	0.00	0.00	0.0	0	1226
0	1	Tr	339	0.5	Tr	363	0	0	0.00	0.00	0.0	0	1227
0	2	0.1	217	0.4	505	5	0	0	0.00	0.00	0.0	0	1228
0	0	0.0	0	0.0	0	1,259	0	0	0.00	0.00	0.0	0	1229
10	2	0.4	4	1.1	118	438	0	0	0.03	0.03	0.3	0	1230
0	65	3.1	46	1.7	1,154	2,846	2,438	245	0.21	0.18	3.3	36	1231
0	4	0.2	3	0.1	72	178	152	15	0.01	0.01	0.2	2	1232
0	2	0.1	1	Tr	29	71	61	6	0.01	Tr	0.1	1	1233
0	1	0.2	35	0.9	28	3	1	Tr	0.01	0.01	0.1	Tr	1234
0	1	0.9	7	0.4	50	26	908	91	0.01	0.02	0.2	2	1235
0	8	4.4	21	1.8	236	4	28	3	0.02	0.05	0.3	0	1236
0	10	5.1	15	1.2	331	3	3	Tr	0.01	0.08	0.6	0	1237

Table 9.   Nutritive Value of the Edible Part of Food

Food No.	Food Description	Measure of edible portion	Weight (g)	Water (%)	Calories (kcal)	Pro-tein (g)	Total fat (g)	Fatty acids Satu-rated (g)	Mono-unsatu-rated (g)	Poly-unsatu-rated (g)

Miscellaneous Items (continued)

Food No.	Food Description	Measure	Weight	Water	Calories	Protein	Total fat	Saturated	Mono	Poly
1238	Cinnamon	1 tsp ...2	10	6	Tr	Tr	Tr	Tr	Tr
1239	Cocoa powder, unsweetened	1 cup ...86	3	197	17	12	6.9	3.9	0.4
1240		1 tbsp ...5	3	12	1	1	0.4	0.2	Tr
1241	Cream of tartar	1 tsp ...3	2	8	0	0	0.0	0.0	0.0
1242	Curry powder	1 tsp ...2	10	7	Tr	Tr	Tr	0.1	0.1
1243	Garlic powder	1 tsp ...3	6	9	Tr	Tr	Tr	Tr	Tr
1244	Horseradish, prepared	1 tsp ...5	85	2	Tr	Tr	Tr	Tr	Tr
1245	Mustard, prepared, yellow	1 tsp or 1 packet...5	82	3	Tr	Tr	Tr	0.1	Tr
	Olives, canned									
1246	Pickled, green	5 medium ...17	78	20	Tr	2	0.3	1.6	0.2
1247	Ripe, black	5 large...22	80	25	Tr	2	0.3	1.7	0.2
1248	Onion powder	1 tsp ...2	5	7	Tr	Tr	Tr	Tr	Tr
1249	Oregano, ground	1 tsp ...2	7	5	Tr	Tr	Tr	Tr	0.1
1250	Paprika	1 tsp ...2	10	6	Tr	Tr	Tr	Tr	0.2
1251	Parsley, dried	1 tbsp ...1	9	4	Tr	Tr	Tr	Tr	Tr
1252	Pepper, black	1 tsp ...2	11	5	Tr	Tr	Tr	Tr	Tr
	Pickles, cucumber									
1253	Dill, whole, medium (3¾" long)	1 pickle ...65	92	12	Tr	Tr	Tr	Tr	0.1
1254	Fresh (bread and butter pickles), slices 1½" dia, ¼" thick	3 slices...24	79	18	Tr	Tr	Tr	Tr	Tr
1255	Pickle relish, sweet	1 tbsp ...15	62	20	Tr	Tr	Tr	Tr	Tr
1256	Pork skins/rinds, plain	1 oz ...28	2	155	17	9	3.2	4.2	1.0
	Potato chips									
	Regular									
	Plain									
1257	Salted	1 oz ...28	2	152	2	10	3.1	2.8	3.5
1258	Unsalted	1 oz ...28	2	152	2	10	3.1	2.8	3.5
1259	Barbecue flavor	1 oz ...28	2	139	2	9	2.3	1.9	4.6
1260	Sour cream and onion flavor	1 oz ...28	2	151	2	10	2.5	1.7	4.9
1261	Reduced fat	1 oz ...28	1	134	2	6	1.2	1.4	3.1
1262	Fat free, made with olestra	1 oz ...28	2	75	2	Tr	Tr	0.1	0.1
	Made from dried potatoes									
1263	Plain	1 oz ...28	1	158	2	11	2.7	2.1	5.7
1264	Sour cream and onion flavor	1 oz ...28	2	155	2	10	2.7	2.0	5.3
1265	Reduced fat	1 oz ...28	1	142	2	7	1.5	1.7	3.8
1266	Salt	1 tsp ...6	Tr	0	0	0	0.0	0.0	0.0
	Trail mix									
1267	Regular, with raisins, chocolate chips, salted nuts and seeds	1 cup ...146	7	707	21	47	8.9	19.8	16.5
1268	Tropical	1 cup ...140	9	570	9	24	11.9	3.5	7.2
1269	Vanilla extract	1 tsp ...4	53	12	Tr	Tr	Tr	Tr	Tr
	Vinegar									
1270	Cider	1 tbsp ...15	94	2	0	0	0.0	0.0	0.0
1271	Distilled	1 tbsp ...17	95	2	0	0	0.0	0.0	0.0
	Yeast, baker's									
1272	Dry, active	1 pkg...7	8	21	3	Tr	Tr	0.2	Tr
1273		1 tsp ...4	8	12	2	Tr	Tr	0.1	Tr
1274	Compressed	1 cake ...17	69	18	1	Tr	Tr	0.2	Tr

Choles- terol (mg)	Carbo- hydrate (g)	Total dietary fiber (g)	Calcium (mg)	Iron (mg)	Potas- sium (mg)	Sodium (mg)	Vitamin A		Thiamin (mg)	Ribo- flavin (mg)	Niacin (mg)	Ascor- bic acid (mg)	Food No.
							(IU)	(RE)					
0	2	1.2	28	0.9	11	1	6	1	Tr	Tr	Tr	1	1238
0	47	28.6	110	11.9	1,311	18	17	2	0.07	0.21	1.9	0	1239
0	3	1.8	7	0.7	82	1	1	Tr	Tr	0.01	0.1	0	1240
0	2	Tr	Tr	0.1	495	2	0	0	0.00	0.00	0.0	0	1241
0	1	0.7	10	0.6	31	1	20	2	0.01	0.01	0.1	Tr	1242
0	2	0.3	2	0.1	31	1	0	0	0.01	Tr	Tr	1	1243
0	1	0.2	3	Tr	12	16	Tr	0	Tr	Tr	Tr	1	1244
0	Tr	0.2	4	0.1	8	56	7	1	Tr	Tr	Tr	Tr	1245
0	Tr	0.2	10	0.3	9	408	51	5	0.00	0.00	Tr	0	1246
0	1	0.7	19	0.7	2	192	89	9	Tr	0.00	Tr	Tr	1247
0	2	0.1	8	0.1	20	1	0	0	0.01	Tr	Tr	Tr	1248
0	1	0.6	24	0.7	25	Tr	104	10	0.01	Tr	0.1	1	1249
0	1	0.4	4	0.5	49	1	1,273	127	0.01	0.04	0.3	1	1250
0	1	0.4	19	1.3	49	6	303	30	Tr	0.02	0.1	2	1251
0	1	0.6	9	0.6	26	1	4	Tr	Tr	0.01	Tr	Tr	1252
0	3	0.8	6	0.3	75	833	214	21	0.01	0.02	Tr	1	1253
0	4	0.4	8	0.1	48	162	34	3	0.00	0.01	0.0	2	1254
0	5	0.2	Tr	0.1	4	122	23	2	0.00	Tr	Tr	Tr	1255
27	0	0.0	9	0.2	36	521	37	11	0.03	0.08	0.4	Tr	1256
0	15	1.3	7	0.5	361	168	0	0	0.05	0.06	1.1	9	1257
0	15	1.4	7	0.5	361	2	0	0	0.05	0.06	1.1	9	1258
0	15	1.2	14	0.5	357	213	62	6	0.06	0.06	1.3	10	1259
2	15	1.5	20	0.5	377	177	48	6	0.05	0.06	1.1	11	1260
0	19	1.7	6	0.4	494	139	0	0	0.06	0.08	2.0	7	1261
0	17	1.1	10	0.4	366	185	1,469	441	0.10	0.02	1.3	8	1262
0	14	1.0	7	0.4	286	186	0	0	0.06	0.03	0.9	2	1263
1	15	0.3	18	0.4	141	204	214	28	0.05	0.03	0.7	3	1264
0	18	1.0	10	0.4	285	121	0	0	0.05	0.02	1.2	3	1265
0	0	0.0	1	Tr	Tr	2,325	0	0	0.00	0.00	0.0	0	1266
6	66	8.8	159	4.9	946	177	64	7	0.60	0.33	6.4	2	1267
0	92	10.6	80	3.7	993	14	69	7	0.63	0.16	2.1	11	1268
0	1	0.0	Tr	Tr	6	Tr	0	0	Tr	Tr	Tr	0	1269
0	1	0.0	1	0.1	15	Tr	0	0	0.00	0.00	0.0	0	1270
0	1	0.0	0	0.0	2	Tr	0	0	0.00	0.00	0.0	0	1271
0	3	1.5	4	1.2	140	4	Tr	0	0.17	0.38	2.8	Tr	1272
0	2	0.8	3	0.7	80	2	Tr	0	0.09	0.22	1.6	Tr	1273
0	3	1.4	3	0.6	102	5	0	0	0.32	0.19	2.1	Tr	1274

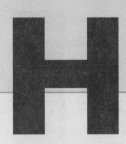

Dietary Reference Intakes

Literature Cited in This Appendix

Food and Nutrition Board, Institute of Medicine. *Dietary Reference Intakes for Calcium, Phosphorus, Magnesium, Vitamin D, and Fluoride.* Washington, DC: National Academies Press; 1997.

Food and Nutrition Board, Institute of Medicine. *Dietary Reference Intakes for Thiamin, Riboflavin, Niacin, Vitamin B_6, Folate, Vitamin B_{12}, Pantothenic Acid, Biotin, and Choline.* Washington, DC: National Academies Press; 1998

Food and Nutrition Board, Institute of Medicine. *Dietary Reference Intakes for Vitamin C, Vitamin E, Selenium, and Carotenoids.* Washington, DC: National Academies Press; 2000.

Food and Nutrition Board, Institute of Medicine. *Dietary Reference Intakes for Vitamin A, Vitamin K, Arsenic, Boron, Chromium, Copper, Iodine, Iron, Manganese, Molybdenum, Nickel, Silicon, Vanadium, and Zinc.* Washington, DC: National Academies Press; 2001.

Food and Nutrition Board, Institute of Medicine. *Dietary Reference Intakes for Energy, Carbohydrates, Fiber, Fat, Protein and Amino Acids (Macronutrients).* Washington, DC: National Academies Press; 2002.

Food and Nutrition Board, Institute of Medicine. *Dietary Reference Intakes for Energy, Carbohydrate, Fiber, Fat, Fatty Acids, Cholesterol, Protein, and Amino Acids.* Washington, DC: National Academies Press; 2002/2005.

Food and Nutrition Board, Institute of Medicine. *Dietary Reference Intakes for Calcium and Vitamin D.* Washington, DC: National Academies Press; 2011.

TABLE 1
Dietary Reference Intakes: Recommended Intakes for Individuals, Vitamins

Life Stage Group	Vitamin A (μg/d)[a]	Vitamin C (mg/d)	Vitamin D (μg/d)[b,c]	Vitamin E (mg/d)[d]	Vitamin K (μg/d)	Thiamin (mg/d)	Riboflavin (mg/d)	Niacin (mg/d)[e]	Vitamin B6 (mg/d)	Folate (μg/d)[f]	Vitamin B12 (μg/d)	Pantothenic Acid (mg/d)	Biotin (μg/d)	Choline[g] (mg/d)
Infants														
0–6 mo	400*	40*	5*	4*	2.0*	0.2*	0.3*	2*	0.1*	65*	0.4*	1.7*	5*	125*
7–12 mo	500*	50*	5*	5*	2.5*	0.3*	0.4*	4*	0.3*	80*	0.5*	1.8*	6*	150*
Children														
1–3 y	300	15	5	6	30	0.5	0.5	6	0.5	150	0.9	2	8	200
4–8 y	400	25	5	7	55	0.6	0.6	8	0.6	200	1.2	3	12	250
Males														
9–13 y	600	45	5	11	60	0.9	0.9	12	1.0	300	1.8	4	20	375
14–18 y	900	75	5	15	75	1.2	1.3	16	1.3	400	2.4	5	25	550
19–30 y	900	90	5	15	120	1.2	1.3	16	1.3	400	2.4	5	30	550
31–50 y	900	90	5	15	120	1.2	1.3	16	1.3	400	2.4	5	30	550
51–70 y	900	90	10	15	120	1.2	1.3	16	1.7	400	2.4[h]	5	30	550
>70 y	900	90	15	15	120	1.2	1.3	16	1.7	400	2.4[h]	5	30	550
Females														
9–13 y	600	45	5	11	60	0.9	0.9	12	1.0	300	1.8	4	20	375
14–18 y	700	65	5	15	75	1.0	1.0	14	1.2	400[i]	2.4	5	25	400
19–30 y	700	75	5	15	90	1.1	1.1	14	1.3	400[i]	2.4	5	30	425
31–50 y	700	75	5	15	90	1.1	1.1	14	1.3	400[i]	2.4	5	30	425
51–70 y	700	75	10	15	90	1.1	1.1	14	1.5	400	2.4[h]	5	30	425
>70 y	700	75	15	15	90	1.1	1.1	14	1.5	400	2.4[h]	5	30	425

Pregnancy													
≤18 y	**750**	**80**	**15**	5	75	**1.4**	**1.4**	**18**	**1.9**	**600**[j]	**2.6**	6	30	450
10–30 y	**770**	**85**	**15**	5	90	**1.4**	**1.4**	**18**	**1.9**	**600**[j]	**2.6**	6	30	450
31–50 y	**770**	**85**	**15**	5	90	**1.4**	**1.4**	**18**	**1.9**	**600**[j]	**2.6**	6	30	450
Lactation													
≤18 y	**1,200**	**115**	**19**	5	75	**1.4**	**1.6**	**17**	**2.0**	**500**	**2.8**	7	35	550
19–30 y	**1,300**	**120**	**19**	5	90	**1.4**	**1.6**	**17**	**2.0**	**500**	**2.8**	7	35	550
31–50 y	**1,300**	**120**	**19**	5	90	**1.4**	**1.6**	**17**	**2.0**	**500**	**2.8**	7	35	550

NOTE: This table (taken from the DRI reports, see www.nap.edu) presents Recommended Dietary Allowances (RDAs) in **bold type** and Adequate Intakes (AIs) in ordinary type followed by an asterisk (*). RDAs and AIs may both be used as goals for individual intake. RDAs are set to meet the needs of almost all (97 to 98 percent) individuals in a group. For healthy breastfed infants, the AI is the mean intake. The AI for other life stage and gender groups is believed to cover needs of all individuals in the group, but lack of data or uncertainty in the data prevent being able to specify with confidence the percentage of individuals covered by this intake.

[a] As retinol activity equivalents (RAEs). 1 RAE = 1 μg retinol, 12 μg β-carotene, 24 μg α-carotene, or 24 μg β-cryptoxanthin in foods. To calculate RAEs from REs of provitamin A carotenoids in foods, divide the REs by 2. For preformed vitamin A in foods or supplements and for provitamin A carotenoids in supplements, 1 RE = 1 RAE.

[b] Cholecalciferol. 1 μg cholecalciferol = 40 IU vitamin D.

[c] In the absence of adequate exposure to sunlight.

[d] As α-tocopherol. α-Tocopherol includes RRR-α-tocopherol, the only form of α-tocopherol that occurs naturally in foods, and the 2R-stereoisomeric forms of α-tocopherol (RRR-, RSR-, RSR-, RRS-, and RSS-α-tocopherol) that occur in fortified foods and supplements. It does not include the 2S-stereoisomeric forms of α-tocopherol (SRR-, SSR-, SRS-, and SSS-α-tocopherol), also found in fortified foods and supplements.

[e] As niacin equivalents (NE). 1 mg of niacin = 60 mg of tryptophan; 0–6 months = preformed niacin (not NE).

[f] As dietary folate equivalents (DFE). 1 DFE = 1 μg food folate = 0.6 μg of folic acid from fortified food or as a supplement consumed with food = 0.5 μg of a supplement taken on an empty stomach.

[g] Although AIs have been set for choline, there are few data to assess whether a dietary supply of choline is needed at all stages of the life cycle, and it may be that the choline requirement can be met by endogenous synthesis at some of these stages.

[h] Because 10 to 30 percent of older people may malabsorb food-bound B_{12}, it is advisable for those older than 50 years to meet their RDA mainly by consuming foods fortified with B_{12} or a supplement containing B_{12}.

[i] In view of evidence linking folate intake with neural tube defects in the fetus, it is recommended that all women capable of becoming pregnant consume 400 μg from supplements or fortified foods in addition to intake of food folate from a varied diet.

[j] It is assumed that women will continue consuming 400 μg from supplements or fortified food until their pregnancy is confirmed and they enter prenatal care, which ordinarily occurs after the end of the periconceptional period—the critical time for formation of the neural tube.

TABLE 2
Dietary Reference Intakes: Recommended Intakes for Individuals, Minerals

Life Stage Group	Calcium (mg/d)	Chromium (µg/d)	Copper (µg/d)	Fluoride (mg/d)	Iodine (µg/d)	Iron (mg/d)	Magnesium (mg/d)	Manganese (mg/d)	Molybdenum (µg/d)	Phosphorus (mg/d)	Selenium (µg/d)	Zinc (mg/d)
Infants												
0–6 mo	200*	0.2*	200*	0.01*	110*	0.27*	30*	0.003*	2*	100*	15*	2*
7–12 mo	260*	5.5*	220*	0.5*	130*	11	75*	0.6*	3*	275*	20*	3
Children												
1–3 y	700	11	340	0.7	90	7	80	1.2	17	460	20	3
4–8 y	1,000	15	440	1	90	10	130	1.5	22	500	30	5
Males												
9–13 y	1,300	25	700	2	120	8	240	1.9	34	1,250	40	8
14–18 y	1,300	35	890	3	150	11	410	2.2	43	1,250	55	11
19–30 y	1,000	35	900	4	150	8	400	2.3	45	700	55	11
31–50 y	1,000	35	900	4	150	8	420	2.3	45	700	55	11
51–70 y	1,000	30	900	4	150	8	420	2.3	45	700	55	11
>70 y	1,200	30	900	4	150	8	420	2.3	45	700	55	11
Females												
9–13 y	1,300	21	700	2	120	8	240	1.6	34	1,250	40	8
14–18 y	1,300	24	890	3	150	15	360	1.6	43	1,250	55	9
19–30 y	1,000	25	900	3	150	18	310	1.8	45	700	55	8
31–50 y	1,000	25	900	3	150	18	320	1.8	45	700	55	8
51–70 y	1,200	20	900	3	150	8	320	1.8	45	700	55	8
>70 y	1,200	20	900	3	150	8	320	1.8	45	700	55	8

Pregnancy											
≤18 y	**1,300**	29	**1,000**	3	**220**	**27**	**400**	2.0	50	1,250	60	13
10–30 y	**1,000**	30	**1,000**	3	**220**	**27**	**350**	2.0	50	700	60	11
31–50 y	**1,000**	30	**1,000**	3	**220**	**27**	**360**	2.0	50	700	60	11
Lactation											
≤18 y	**1,300**	44	**1,300**	3	**290**	**10**	**360**	2.6	50	1,250	70	14
19–30 y	**1,000**	45	**1,300**	3	**290**	**9**	**310**	2.6	50	700	70	12
31–50 y	**1,000**	45	**1,300**	3	**290**	**9**	**320**	2.6	60	700	70	12

NOTE: This table presents Recommended Dietary Allowances (RDAs) in **bold type** and Adequate Intakes (AIs) in ordinary type followed by an asterisk (*). RDAs and AIs may both be used as goals for individual intake. RDAs are set to meet the needs of almost all (97 to 98 percent) individuals in a group. For healthy breastfed infants, the AI is the mean intake. The AI for other life stage and gender groups is believed to cover needs of all individuals in the group, but lack of data or uncertainty in the data prevent being able to specify with confidence the percentage of individuals covered by this intake.

SOURCES: Dietary Reference Intakes for Calcium, Phosphorus, Magnesium, Vitamin D, and Fluoride (1997); Dietary Reference Intakes for Thiamin, Riboflavin, Niacin, Vitamin B₆, Folate, Vitamin B₁₂, Pantothenic Acid, Biotin, and Choline (1998); Dietary Reference Intakes for Vitamin C, Vitamin E, Selenium, and Carotenoids (2000); and Dietary Reference Intakes for Vitamin A, Vitamin K, Arsenic, Boron, Chromium, Copper, Iodine, Iron, Manganese, Molybdenum, Nickel, Silicon, Vanadium, and Zinc (2001). These reports may be accessed via www.nap.edu. Copyright 2001 by The National Academies of Sciences. All rights reserved.

TABLE 3
Dietary Reference Intakes (DRIs); Tolerable Upper Intake Levels (UL)[a], Vitamins

Life Stage Group	Vitamin A (μg/d)[b]	Vitamin C (mg/d)	Vitamin D (μg/d)	Vitamin E (mg/d)[c,d]	Vitamin K	Thiamin	Riboflavin	Niacin (mg/d)[d]	Vitamin B6 (mg/d)	Folate (μg/d)[d]	Vitamin B12	Pantothenic Acid	Biotin	Choline (g/d)	Carotenoids[e]
Infants															
0–6 mo	600	ND[f]	25	ND	ND	ND	ND	ND	ND	ND	ND	ND	ND	ND	ND
7–12 mo	600	ND	38	ND	ND	ND	ND	ND	ND	ND	ND	ND	ND	ND	ND
Children															
1–3 y	600	400	63	200	ND	ND	ND	10	30	300	ND	ND	ND	1.0	ND
4–8 y	900	650	75	300	ND	ND	ND	15	40	400	ND	ND	ND	1.0	ND
Males, Females															
9–13 y	1,700	1,200	100	600	ND	ND	ND	20	60	600	ND	ND	ND	2.0	ND
14–18 y	2,800	1,800	100	800	ND	ND	ND	30	80	800	ND	ND	ND	3.0	ND
19–70 y	3,000	2,000	100	1,000	ND	ND	ND	35	100	1,000	ND	ND	ND	3.5	ND
>70 y	3,000	2,000	100	1,000	ND	ND	ND	35	100	1,000	ND	ND	ND	3.5	ND
Pregnancy															
≤18 y	2,800	1,800	100	800	ND	ND	ND	30	80	800	ND	ND	ND	3.0	ND
19–50 y	3,000	2,000	100	1,000	ND	ND	ND	35	100	1,000	ND	ND	ND	3.5	ND
Lactation															
≤18 y	2,800	1,800	100	800	ND	ND	ND	30	80	800	ND	ND	ND	3.0	ND
19–50 y	3,000	2,000	100	1,000	ND	ND	ND	35	100	1,000	ND	ND	ND	3.5	ND

[a] UL = The maximum level of daily nutrient intake that is likely to pose no risk of adverse effects. Unless otherwise specified, the UL represents total intake from food, water, and supplements. Due to lack of suitable data, ULs could not be established for vitamin K, thiamin, riboflavin, vitamin B12 pantothenic acid, biotin, or carotenoids. In the absence of ULs, extra caution may be warranted in consuming levels above recommended intakes.

[b] As preformed vitamin A only.

[c] As α-tocopherol; applies to any form of supplemental α-tocopherol.

[d] The ULs for vitamin E, niacin, and folate apply to synthetic forms obtained from supplements, fortified foods, or a combination of the two.

[e] β-Carotene supplements are advised only to serve as a provitamin A source for individuals at risk of vitamin A deficiency.

[f] ND = Not determinable due to lack of data of adverse effects in this age group and concern with regard to lack of ability to handle excess amounts. Source of intake should be from food only to prevent high levels of intake.

SOURCES: Dietary Reference Intakes for Calcium, Phosphorus, Magnesium, Vitamin D, and Fluoride (1997); Dietary Reference intakes for Thiamin, Riboflavin, Niacin, Vitamin B6, Folate, Vitamin B12, Pantothenic Acid, Biotin, and Choline (1998); Dietary Reference Intakes for Vitamin C, Vitamin E, Selenium, and Carotenoids (2000); and Dietary Reference Intakes for Vitamin A, Vitamin K, Arsenic, Boron, Chromium, Copper, Iodine, Iron, Manganese, Molybdenum, Nickel, Silicon, Vanadium, and Zinc (2001). These reports may be accessed via www.nap.edu. Copyright 2001 by The National Academies of Sciences. All rights reserved.

TABLE 4
Dietary Reference Intakes (DRIs); Tolerable Upper Intake Levels (UL)[a], Elements

Life Stage Group	Arsenic[b]	Boron (mg/d)	Calcium (g/d)	Chromium	Copper (µg/d)	Fluoride (mg/d)	Iodine (µg/d)	Iron (mg/d)	Magnesium (mg/d)[e]	Manganese (mg/d)	Molybdenum (µg/d)	Nickel (mg/d)	Phosphorus (g/d)	Selenium (µg/d)	Silicon[d]	Vanadium (mg/d)[e]	Zinc (mg/d)
Infants																	
0–6 mo	ND	ND	1	ND	ND	0.7	ND	40	ND	ND	ND	ND	ND	45	ND	ND	4
7–12 mo	ND	ND	1.5	ND	ND	0.9	ND	40	ND	ND	ND	ND	ND	60	ND	ND	5
Children																	
1–3 y	ND	3	2.5	ND	1,000	1.3	200	40	65	2	300	0.2	3	90	ND	ND	7
4–8 y	ND	6	2.5	ND	3,000	2.2	300	40	110	3	600	0.3	3	150	ND	ND	12
Males, Females																	
9–13 y	ND	11	3.0	ND	5,000	10	600	40	350	6	1,100	0.6	4	280	ND	ND	23
14–18 y	ND	17	3.0	ND	8,000	10	900	45	350	9	1,700	1.0	4	400	ND	ND	34
19–70 y	ND	20	2.5	ND	10,000	10	1,100	45	350	11	2,000	1.0	4	400	ND	1.8	40
>70 y	ND	20	2.0	ND	10,000	10	1,100	45	350	11	2,000	1.0	3	400	ND	1.8	40
Pregnancy																	
≤18 y	ND	17	3.0	ND	8,000	10	900	45	350	9	1,700	1.0	3.5	400	ND	ND	34
19–50 y	ND	20	2.5	ND	10,000	10	1,100	45	350	11	2,000	1.0	3.5	400	ND	ND	40
Lactation																	
≤18 y	ND	17	3.0	ND	8,000	10	900	45	350	9	1,700	1.0	4	400	ND	ND	34
19–50 y	ND	20	2.5	ND	10,000	10	1,100	45	350	11	2,000	1.0	4	400	ND	ND	40

[a] UL = The maximum level of daily nutrient intake that is likely to pose no risk of adverse effects. Unless otherwise specified, the UL represents total intake from food, water, and supplements. Due to lack of suitable data, ULs could not be established for arsenic, chromium, and silicon. In the absence of ULs, extra caution may be warranted in consuming levels above recommended intakes.

[b] Although the UL was not determined for arsenic, there is no justification for adding arsenic to food or supplements.

[c] The ULs for magnesium represent intake from a pharmacological agent only and do not include intake from food and water.

[d] Although silicon has not been shown to cause adverse effects in humans, there is no justification for adding silicon to supplements.

[e] Although vanadium in food has not been shown to cause adverse effects in laboratory animals and these data could be used to set a UL for adults but not children and adolescents, there is no justification for adding vanadium to food and vanadium supplements should be used with caution. The UL is based on adverse effects in laboratory animals and these data could be used to set a UL for adults but not children and adolescents. Source of intake should be from food only to prevent high levels of intake.

[f] ND = Not determinable due to lack of data of adverse effects in this age group and concern with regard to lack of ability to handle excess amounts. Source of intake should be from food only to prevent high levels of intake.

SOURCES: Dietary Reference Intakes for Calcium, Phosphorus, Magnesium, Vitamin D, and Fluoride (1997); Dietary Reference Intakes for Thiamin, Riboflavin, Niacin, Vitamin B6, Folate, Vitamin B12, Pantothenic Acid, Biotin, and Choline (1998); Dietary Reference Intakes for Vitamin C, Vitamin E, Selenium, and Carotenoids (2000); and Dietary Reference Intakes for Vitamin A, Vitamin K, Arsenic, Boron, Chromium, Copper, Iodine, Iron, Manganese, Molybdenum, Nickel, Silicon, Vanadium, and Zinc (2001). These reports may be accessed via www.nap.edu.

TABLE 5

Criteria and Dietary Reference Intake Values for Energy by Active Individuals by Life Stage Group[a]

Life Stage Group	Criterion	Active PAL[b] EER (kcal/d)	
		Male	Female
0 through 6 mo	Energy expenditure plus energy deposition	570	520 (3 mo)
7 through 12 mo	Energy expenditure plus energy deposition	743	676 (9 mo)
1 through 2 y	Energy expenditure plus energy deposition	1,046	992 (24 mo)
3 through 8 y	Energy expenditure plus energy deposition	1,742	1,642 (6 y)
9 through 13 y	Energy expenditure plus energy deposition	2,279	2,071 (11 y)
14 through 18 y	Energy expenditure plus energy deposition	3,152	2,368 (16 y)
> 18 y	Energy expenditure	3,067[c]	2,403[c] (19 y)
Pregnancy			
14 through 18 y	Adolescent female HER plus change in TEE		
1st trimester	plus pregnancy energy deposition		2,368 (16 y)
2nd trimester			2,708 (16 y)
3rd trimester			2,820 (16 y)
19 through 50 y	Adult female EER plus change in TEE plus		
1st trimester	pregnancy energy deposition		2,403[c] (19 y)
2nd trimester			2,743[c] (19 y)
3rd trimester			2,855[c] (19 y)
Lactation			
14 through 18 y	Adolescent female EER plus milk energy		
1st 6 mo	output minus weight loss		2,698 (16 y)
2nd 6 mo			2,768 (16 y)
19 through 50 y	Adult female EER plus milk energy output		
1st 6 mo	minus weight loss		2,733[c] (19 y)
2nd 6 mo			2,803[c] (19 y)

[a] For healthy moderately active Americans and Canadians.
[b] PAL = physical activity level. EER = estimated energy requirement, TEE = total energy expenditure.
The intake that meets the average energy expenditure of individuals at the reference height, weight, and age.
[c] Subject 10 kcal/day for males and 7 kcal/day for females for each year of age above 19 years.

TABLE 6
Criteria and Dietary Reference Intake Values for Protein by Active Individuals by Life Stage Group

Life Stage Group	Criterion	AI or RDA for Reference Individual (g/day)		EAR (g/kg/d)[a]		RDA (g/kg/d)[b]		AI (g/kg/d)[c]
		Male	Female	Male	Female	Male	Female	
0 through 6 mo	Average consumption of protein from human milk	9.1 (AI)	9.1 (AI)					1.52
7 through 12 mo	Nitrogen equilibrium + protein deposition	13.5	13.5	1.1	1.1	1.5	1.5	
1 through 3 y	Nitrogen equilibrium + protein deposition	13	13	0.88	0.88	1.10	1.10	
4 through 8 y	Nitrogen equilibrium + protein deposition	19	19	0.76	0.76	0.95	0.95	
9 through 13 y	Nitrogen equilibrium + protein deposition	34	34	0.76	0.76	0.95	0.95	
14 through 18 y	Nitrogen equilibrium + protein deposition	52	46	0.73	0.71	0.85	0.85	
> 18 y	Nitrogen equilibrium	56	46	0.66	0.66	0.80	0.80	
Pregnancy								
14 through 18 y	Nitrogen equilibrium + protein deposition		71[d]		0.88		1.1	
19 through 50 y	Nitrogen equilibrium + protein deposition		71		0.88		1.1	
Lactation								
14 through 18 y	Nitrogen equilibrium + milk nitrogen		71		1.05		1.3	
19 through 50 y	Nitrogen equilibrium + milk nitrogen		71		1.05		1.3	

[a] EAR = Estimated Average Requirement. The intake that meets the estimated nutrient needs of half of the individuals in a group.

[b] RDA = Recommended Dietary Allowance. The intake that meets the nutrient needs of almost all (97–98 percent) of individuals in a group.

[c] AI = Adequate Intake. The observed average or experimentally determined intake by a defined population or subgroup that appears to sustain a defined nutrition status, such as growth rate, normal circulating nutrient values, or other functional indicators of health. The AI is used if sufficient scientific evidence is not available to derive an EAR. For healthy infants receiving human milk, the AI is the mean intake. **The AI is not equivalent to an RDA.**

[d] The EAR and RDA for pregnancy are only for the second half of pregnancy. For the first half of pregnancy the protein requirements are the same as those of the nonpregnant woman.

TABLE 7
Criteria and Dietary Reference Intake Values for *Total Fiber* by Life Stage Group

Life Stage Group	Criterion	AI (g/d)[a] Male	AI (g/d)[a] Female
0 through 6 mo		ND[b]	ND
7 through 12 mo		ND	ND
1 through 3 y	Intake level shown to provide the greatest protection against coronary heart disease (14 g/1,000 kcal) × median energy intake level (kcal/1,000 kcal/d)	19	19
4 through 8 y	Intake level shown to provide the greatest protection against coronary heart disease (14 g/1,000 kcal) × median energy intake level (kcal/1,000 kcal/d)	25	25
9 through 13 y	Intake level shown to provide the greatest protection against coronary heart disease (14 g/1,000 kcal) × median energy intake level (kcal/1,000 kcal/d)	31	26
14 through 18 y	Intake level shown to provide the greatest protection against coronary heart disease (14 g/1,000 kcal) × median energy intake level (kcal/1,000 kcal/d)	38	26
19 through 30 y	Intake level shown to provide the greatest protection against coronary heart disease (14 g/1,000 kcal) × median energy intake level (kcal/1,000 kcal/d)	38	25
31 through 50 y	Intake level shown to provide the greatest protection against coronary heart disease (14 g/1,000 kcal) × median energy intake level (kcal/1,000 kcal/d)	38	25
51 through 70 y	Intake level shown to provide the greatest protection against coronary heart disease (14 g/1,000 kcal) × median energy intake level (kcal/1,000 kcal/d)	30	21
> 70 y	Intake level shown to provide the greatest protection against coronary heart disease (14 g/1,000 kcal) × median energy intake level (kcal/1,000 kcal/d)	30	21
Pregnancy			
14 through 18 y	Intake level shown to provide the greatest protection against coronary heart disease (14 g/1,000 kcal) × median energy intake level (kcal/1,000 kcal/d)		28
19 through 50 y	Intake level shown to provide the greatest protection against coronary heart disease (14 g/1,000 kcal) × median energy intake level (kcal/1,000 kcal/d)		28
Lactation			
14 through 18 y	Intake level shown to provide the greatest protection against coronary heart disease (14 g/1,000 kcal) × median energy intake level (kcal/1,000 kcal/d)		29
19 through 50 y	Intake level shown to provide the greatest protection against coronary heart disease (14 g/1,000 kcal) × median energy intake level (kcal/1,000 kcal/d)		29

[a] AI = Adequate Intake. Based on 14 g/1,000 kcal of required energy.
[b] ND = not determined. The observed average or experimentally determined intake by a defined population or subgroup that appears to sustain a defined nutritional status, such as growth rate, normal circulating nutrient values, or other functional indicators of health. The AI is used if sufficient scientific evidence is not available to derive an Estimated Average Requirement (EAR). For healthy infants receiving human milk, the AI is the mean intake. **The AI is not equivalent to an RDA.**

TABLE 8
Criteria and Dietary Reference Intake Values[a] for Total Water[b]

Life Stage Group	Criterion	AI[c] (L/d)[a] Male From Foods	AI[c] (L/d)[a] Male From Beverages	AI[c] (L/d)[a] Male Total Water	AI[c] (L/d)[a] Female From Foods	AI[c] (L/d)[a] Female From Beverages	AI[c] (L/d)[a] Female Total Water
0 through 6 mo	Human milk[d]	0	0.7	0.7	0	0.7	0.7
7 through 12 mo	Milk and foods[e]	0.2	0.6	0.8	0.2	0.6	0.8
1 through 3 y	Median intake[f]	0.4	0.9	1.3	0.4	0.9	1.3
4 through 8 y	Median intake[f]	0.5	1.2	1.7	0.5	1.2	1.7
9 through 13 y	Median intake[f]	0.6	1.8	2.4	0.5	1.6	2.1
14 through 18 y	Median intake[f]	0.7	2.6	3.3	0.5	1.8	2.3
> 19 y	Median intake[f]	0.7	3.0	3.7	0.5	2.2	2.7
Pregnancy	Median intake[f]				0.7	2.3	3.0
14 through 50 y							
Lactation	Median intake[f]				0.7	3.1	3.8
14 through 50 y							

[a] No UL established; however, maximal capacity to excrete excess water in individuals with normal kidney function approximately 0.7 L/hour.
[b] Total water represents drinking water, other beverages, and water from food.
[c] AI = Adequate Intake. The observed or experimentally determined intake by a defined population or subgroup that appears to sustain a defined nutritional status, such as growth rate, normal circulating nutrient values, or other functional indicators of health. The AI is used if sufficient scientific evidence is not available to derive an EAR. **The AI is not equivalent to an RDA.**
[d] Average consumption of water from human milk.
[e] Average consumption of water from human milk and complementary foods.
[f] Median total water intake from NHANES III.

TABLE 9

Criteria and Dietary Reference Intake Values[a] for Potassium by Life Stage Group

Life Stage Group	Criterion	AI (g/day)[b] Male	AI (g/day)[b] Female
0 through 6 mo	Human milk[c]	0.4	0.4
7 through 12 mo	Milk and foods[d]	0.7	0.7
1 through 3 y	Extrapolation[e]	3.0	3.0
4 through 8 y	Extrapolation[e]	3.8	3.8
9 through 13 y	Extrapolation[e]	4.5	4.5
14 through 18 y	Extrapolation[e]	4.7	4.7
> 18 y	Normal function[f]	4.7	4.7
Pregnancy			
14 through 50 y	Normal function[f]		4.7
Lactation			
14 through 50 y	Normal function[g]		5.1

[a] No UL is established; however, caution is warranted given concerns about adverse effects when consuming excess amounts of potassium from potassium supplements while on drug therapy or in the presence of undiagnosed chronic disease.

[b] AI = Adequate Intake. The observed or experimentally determined intake by a defined population or subgroup that appears to sustain a defined nutritional status, such as growth rate, normal circulating nutrient values, or other functional indicators of health. The AI is used if sufficient scientific evidence is not available to derive an EAR. **The AI is not equivalent to an RDA.**

[c] Average consumption of potassium from human milk.

[d] Average consumption of potassium from human milk and complementary foods.

[e] Extrapolation of Adult AI based on energy intake.

[f] Intake level to lower blood pressure, reduce the extent of salt sensitivity, and to minimize the risk of kidney stones.

[g] Intake level to lower blood pressure, reduce the extent of salt sensitivity, and to minimize the risk of kidney stones plus the amount of potassium in breast milk (0.4 g/d).

TABLE 10
Criteria and Dietary Reference Intake Values for Sodium

Life Stage Group	Criterion for AI	AI[a] (g/d)		UL[b] (g/d)	
		Male	Female	Male	Female
0 through 6 mo	Human milk[d]	0.12	0.12	ND[c]	ND[c]
7 through 12 mo	Milk and foods[e]	0.37	0.37	ND	ND
1 through 3 y	Extrapolation[f]	1.0	1.0	1.5	1.5
4 through 8 y	Extrapolation[f]	1.2	1.2	1.9	1.9
9 through 13 y	Extrapolation[f]	1.5	1.5	2.2	2.2
14 through 18 y	Extrapolation[f]	1.5	1.5	2.3	2.3
19 through 50 y	Normal function[g]	1.5	1.5	2.3	2.3
51 through 70 y	Extrapolation[h]	1.3	1.3	2.3	2.3
>70 y	Extrapolation[h]	1.2	1.2	2.3	2.3
Pregnancy					
14 through 50 y	Same as nonpregnant		1.5		2.3
Lactation					
14 through 50 y	Same as nonlactating		1.5		2.3

[a] AI = Adequate Intake. The observed or experimentally determined intake by a defined population or subgroup that appears to sustain a defined nutritional status, such as growth rate, normal circulating nutrient values, or other functional indicators of health. The AI is used if sufficient scientific evidence is not available to derive an EAR. **The AI is not equivalent to an RDA.**

[b] UL = Tolerable Upper Intake Level. Based on prevention of increased blood pressure.

[c] ND = Not Determined. Intake should be from food or formula only.

[d] Average consumption of sodium from human milk.

[e] Average consumption of sodium from human milk and complementary foods.

[f] Extrapolation of Adult AI based on energy intake.

[g] Intake level to cover possible daily losses, provide adequate intakes of other nutrients, and maintain normal function.

[h] Extrapolated from younger adults based on energy intake.

TABLE 11

Criteria and Dietary Reference Intake Values for *n*-6 Polyunsaturated Fatty Acids (Linoleic Acid) by Life Stage Group

Life Stage Group	Criterion	AI (g/day)[a]	
		Male	Female
0 through 6 mo	Average consumption of total *n*-6 fatty acids from human milk	4.4	4.4
7 through 12 mo	Average consumption of total *n*-6 fatty acids from human milk and complementary foods	4.6	4.6
1 through 3 y	Median intake of linoleic acid from CFSII[b]	7	7
4 through 8 y	Median intake of linoleic acid from CFSII	10	10
9 through 13 y	Median intake of linoleic acid from CFSII	12	10
14 through 18 y	Median intake of linoleic acid from CFSII	16	11
19 through 30 y	Median intake of linoleic acid from CFSII	17	12
31 through 50 y	Median intake of linoleic acid from CFSII	17	12
51 through 70 y	Median intake of linoleic acid from CFSII	14	11
> 70 y	Median intake of linoleic acid from CFSII	14	11
Pregnancy			
14 through 18 y	Median intake of linoleic acid from CFSII		13
19 through 50 y	Median intake of linoleic acid from CFSII		13
Lactation			
14 through 18 y	Median intake of linoleic acid from CFSII		13
19 through 50 y	Median intake of linoleic acid from CFSII		13

[a] AI = Adequate Intake. The observed average or experimentally determined intake by a defined population or subgroup that appears to sustain a defined nutritional status, such as growth rate, normal circulating nutrient values, or other functional indicators of health. The AI is used if sufficient scientific evidence is not available to derive an Estimated Average Requirement (EAR). For healthy infants receiving human milk, the AI is the mean intake. **The AI is not equivalent to an RDA.**

[b] CSFII = Continuing Survey of Food Intake by Individuals.

TABLE 12
Criteria and Dietary Reference Intake Values for *n*-3 Polyunsaturated Fatty Acids (Linoleic Acid) by Life Stage Group

Life Stage Group	Criterion	AI (g/day)[a] Male	AI (g/day)[a] Female
0 through 6 mo	Average consumption of total *n*-3 fatty acids from human milk	0.5	0.5
7 through 12 mo	Average consumption of total *n*-3 fatty acids from human milk and complementary foods	0.5	0.5
1 through 3 y	Median intake of α-linolenic acid from CFSII[b]	0.7	0.7
4 through 8 y	Median intake of α-linolenic acid from CFSII	0.9	0.9
9 through 13 y	Median intake of α-linolenic acid from CFSII	1.2	1.0
14 through 18 y	Median intake of α-linolenic acid from CFSII	1.6	1.1
19 through 30 y	Median intake of α-linolenic acid from CFSII	1.6	1.1
31 through 50 y	Median intake of α-linolenic acid from CFSII	1.6	1.1
51 through 70 y	Median intake of α-linolenic acid from CFSII	1.6	1.1
> 70 y	Median intake of α-linolenic acid from CFSII	1.6	1.1
Pregnancy			
14 through 18 y	Median intake of α-linolenic acid from CFSII		1.4
19 through 50 y	Median intake of α-linolenic acid from CFSII		1.4
Lactation			
14 through 18 y	Median intake of α-linolenic acid from CFSII		1.3
19 through 50 y	Median intake of α-linolenic acid from CFSII		1.3

[a] AI = Adequate Intake. The observed average or experimentally determined intake by a defined population or subgroup that appears to sustain a defined nutritional status, such as growth rate, normal circulating nutrient values, or other functional indicators of health. The AI is used if sufficient scientific evidence is not available to derive an Estimated Average Requirement (EAR). For healthy infants receiving human milk, the AI is the mean intake. **The AI is not equivalent to an RDA.**
[b] CSFII = Continuing Survey of Food Intake by Individuals.

Dietary Fiber in Foods

Food Item	Moisture	Total Dietary Fiber (AOAC)[†]
	g per 100 g edible portion	
Baked Products		
Bagels, plain	31.6	2.1
Biscuit mix:		
Dry	8.7	1.3
Baked	29.4	1.8
Biscuits, made from refrigerated dough, baked	28.7	1.5
Breads:		
Boston brown	47.2	4.7
Bran	37.7	8.5
Cornbread mix:		
Dry	6.0	6.5
Baked	34.4	2.6
Cracked-wheat	35.9	5.3
French	33.9	2.3
Hollywood-type, light	37.8	4.8
Italian	34.1	2.7

Food Item	Moisture	Total Dietary Fiber (AOAC)[†]
	g per 100 g edible portion	
Baked Products (*continued*)		
Breads: (*continued*)		
Mixed-grain	38.2	6.3
Oatmeal	36.7	3.9
Pita:		
White	32.1	1.6
Whole-wheat	30.6	7.4
Pumpernickel	38.3	5.9
Reduced-calorie, high-fiber:		
Wheat	43.7	11.3
White	41.8	7.9
Rye	37.0	6.2
Vienna		3.2
Wheat	37.0	3.5
Toasted		5.2
White	37.1	1.9
Toasted		2.5

(*continues*)

Reproduced from U. S. Department of Agriculture, Human Nutrition Information Service, HNIS/PT-106, Provisional Table on the Dietary Fiber Content of Selected Foods.

TABLE 1
Provisional Table on The Dietary Fiber Content of Selected Foods (100 Grams Edible Portion) (*continued*)

Food Item	Moisture	Total Dietary Fiber (AOAC)[†]
	g per 100 g edible portion	
Baked Products (*continued*)		
Reduced-calorie, high-fiber: (*continued*)		
Whole-wheat	38.3	7.4
Toasted		8.9
Bread crumbs, plain or seasoned	5.7	4.2
Bread stuffing, flavored, from dry mix	65.1	2.9
Cake mix:		
Chocolate:		
Dry	3.8	2.4
Prepared	33.3	2.2
Yellow:		
Dry	4.1	1.1
Prepared	40	0.8
Cakes:		
Boston cream pie	47.6	1.4
Coffeecake:		
Crumb topping	22.3	3.3
Fruit	31.7	2.5
Fruitcake, commercial	22.0	3.7
Gingerbread, from dry mix	38.5	2.9
Cheesecake:		
Commercial	44.6	2.1
From no-bake mix	44.4	1.9
Cookies:		
Brownies	12.6	2.2
With nuts	12.6	2.8
Butter	4.7	2.4
Chocolate chip	4.0	2.7
Chocolate sandwich	2.2	2.9
Fig bars	16.7	4.6
Fortune	8.0	1.6
Oatmeal	5.7	2.9
Oatmeal soft-type		2.7
Peanut butter	6.7	1.8
Shortbread with pecans	3.3	1.8
Vanilla sandwich	2.1	1.5
Crackers:		
Cheese, sandwich with peanut butter filling	4.0	1.1

Food Item	Moisture	Total Dietary Fiber (AOAC)[†]
	g per 100 g edible portion	
Baked Products (*continued*)		
Crackers: (*continued*)		
Crisp bread, rye	6.1	16.2
Graham	4.1	3.2
Honey	4.1	1.7
Matzo:		
Plain	6.1	2.9
Egg/onion	8.0	5.0
Whole-wheat	3.0	11.8
Melba toast:		
Plain	5.6	6.3
Rye	6.7	7.9
Wheat	6.1	7.4
Rye	7.2	15.8
Saltines		2.6
Snack-type	4.2	1.2
Wheat	3.2	5.5
Whole-wheat	2.7	10.4
Croutons, plain or seasoned	5.6	4.7
Doughnuts:		
Cake	19.7	1.3
Yeast-leavened, glazed	26.7	2.2
English muffin, whole-wheat	45.7	6.7
French toast, commercial, ready-to-eat	48.1	3.1
Ice cream cones:		
Sugar, rolled type.	3.0	4.6
Water-type	5.3	4.1
Blueberry	37.3	3.6
Oat bran	35.0	7.5
Pancake/waffle mix:		
Regular:		
Dry	8.7	2.7
Prepared	50.4	1.4
Buckwheat, dry	9.1	2.3
Pastry, danish:		
Plain	19.3	1.3
Fruit	27.6	1.9
Pies commercial:		
Apple	51.7	1.6
Cherry	46.2	0.8
Chocolate cream.	43.5	2.0

TABLE 1
Provisional Table on The Dietary Fiber Content of Selected Foods (100 Grams Edible Portion) (*continued*)

Food Item	Moisture	Total Dietary Fiber (AOAC)[†]
	g per 100 g edible portion	
Baked Products		
Pies commercial: (*continued*)		
Egg custard	46.5	1.6
Fruit and coconut		0.9
Lemon meringue	41.7	1.2
Pecan	19.8	3.5
Pumpkin	58.1	2.7
Rolls, dinner, egg ,	30.4	3.8
Taco shells	6.0	8.0
Toaster pastries	8.9	1.0
Tortillas:		
Corn	43.6	5.2
Flour, wheat	26.2	2.9
Waffles, commercial, frozen, ready-to-eat	45.0	2.4
Breakfast Cereals, Ready-to-Eat		
Bran, high fiber	2.9	35.3
Extra fiber		45.9
Bran flakes	2.9	18.8
Bran flakes with raisins	8.3	13.4
Corn flakes;		
Plain	2.8	2.0
Frosted or sugar-sparkled	1.9	2.2
Fiber cereal with fruit		14.8
Granola	3.3	10.5
Oat cereal	5.0	10.6
Oat flakes, fortified	3.1	3.0
Puffed wheat, sugar-coated	1.5	1.5
Rice, crispy	2.4	1.2
Wheat and malted barley:		
Flakes	3.4	6.8
Nuggets	3.2	6.5
With raisins		6.0
Wheat flakes	4.3	9.0
Cereal Grains		
Amaranth	9.8	15.2
Amaranth flour, whole-grain	10.4	10.2
Arrowroot flour	11.4	3.4
Barley	9.4	17.3
Barley, pearled, raw ,	10.1	15.6

Food Item	Moisture	Total Dietary Fiber (AOAC)[†]
	g per 100 g edible portion	
Cereal Grains (*continued*)		
Bulgur, dry	8.0	18.3
Corn bran, crude	4.7	84.6
Corn flour, whole-grain	10.9	13.4
Cornmeal:		
Whole-grain	10.3	11
Degermed	11.6	5.2
Cornstarch	8.3	0.9
Farina, regular or instant:		
Dry	10.6	2.7
Cooked	85.8	1.4
Hominy, canned	79.8	2.5
Millet, hulled, raw		8.5
Oat. bran, raw	6.6	15.9
Oat flour	7.8	9.6
Oats, rolled or oatmeal, dry	8.8	10.3
Rice, brown, long-grain:		
Raw	11.1	3.5
Cooked	73.1	1.7
Rice white;		
Glutinous, raw	10.0	2.8
Long-grain:		
Raw	11.6	1.0
Parboiled:		
Dry	10.5	1.8
Cooked		0.5
Precooked or instant:		
Dry	8.1	1.6
Cooked	76.4	0.8
Medium-grain, raw	12.9	1.4
Rice bran, crude	6.1	21.7
Rice flour;		
Brown	12.0	1.1
White	11.9	2.4
Rye flour, medium or light	9.4	14.6
Semolina	12.7	3.9
Tapioca, pearl, dry	12.0	1.1
Triticale	10.5	18.1
Triticale flour whole-grain	10.0	14.6
Wheat bran, crude	9.9	42.4

(*continues*)

TABLE 1
Provisional Table on The Dietary Fiber Content of Selected Foods (100 Grams Edible Portion) (*continued*)

Food Item	Moisture	Total Dietary Fiber (AOAC)[†]
	g per 100 g edible portion	
Cereal Grains (*continued*)		
Wheat flour:		
White, all purpose	11.8	2.7
Whole-grain	10.9	12.9
Wheat germ:		
Crude	11.1	15.0
Toasted	2.9	12.9
Wild rice, raw	7.8	5.2
Fruits and Fruit Products		
Apples, raw:		
With skin	83.9	2.2
Without skin	84.5	1.9
Apple juice, unsweetened	87.9	0.1
Applesauce:		
Sweetened	79.6	1.2
Unsweetened	88.4	1.5
Apricots, dried	31.1	7.8
Apricot nectar	84.9	0.6
Bananas., raw	74.3	1.6
Blueberries, raw	84.6	2.3
Cantaloupe, raw	89.8	0.8
Figs, dried	28.4	9.3
Fruit cocktail, canned in heavy syrup, drained		1.5
Grapefruit, raw	90.9	0.6
Grapes, Thompson, seedless, raw	81.3	0.7
Kiwifruit, raw	83.0	3.4
Nectarines, raw	86.3	1.6
Olives:		
Green		2.6
Ripe		3.0
Oranges, raw	86.8	2.4
Orange juice, frozen concentrate:		
Undiluted	57.8	0.8
Prepared	88.1	0.2
Peaches:		
Raw	87.7	1.6
Canned in juice, Drained		1.0
Dried	31.8	8.2

Food Item	Moisture	Total Dietary Fiber (AOAC)[†]
	g per 100 g edible portion	
Fruits and Fruit Products (*continued*)		
Pears, raw	83.8	2.6
Pineapple:		
Raw	86.5	1.2
Canned in heavy syrup, chunks, drained	79.0	1.1
Prunes:		
Dried	32.4	7.2
Stewed		6.6
Prune juice	81.2	1.0
Raisins	15.4	5.3
Strawberries	91.6	2.6
Watermelon	91.5	0.4
Legumes, Nuts, and Seeds		
Almonds, oil-roasted	3.3	11.2
Baked beans, canned:		
Barbecue-style		5.8
Sweet or tomato sauce:		
Plain	72.6	7.7
With franks	69.3	6.9
With pork	71.7	5.5
Beans, Great Northern:		
Raw	10.7	40.0
Canned, drained	69.9	5.4
Cashews, oil-roasted	5.4	6.0
Chickpeas, canned, drained	68.2	5.8
Coconut raw	47.0	9.0
Cowpeas (black-eyed peas):		
Raw	12.0	27.0
Cooked, drained	70.0	9.5
Hazelnuts, oil-roasted	1.2	6.4
Lima beans:		
Raw	10.2	19.0
Cooked, drained	69.8	7.2
Miso	47.4	5.4
Mixed nuts, oil-roasted, with peanuts		9.0
Peanuts:		
Dry-roasted	1.6	8.0
oil-roasted	2.0	8.8

TABLE 1
Provisional Table on The Dietary Fiber Content of Selected Foods (100 Grams Edible Portion) (*continued*)

Food Item	Moisture	Total Dietary Fiber (AOAC)[†]
	g per 100 g edible portion	
Legumes, Nuts, and Seeds (continued)		
Peanut butter:		
Chunky	1.1	6.6
Smooth	1.4	6.0
Pecans, dried,	4.8	6.5
Pistachio nuts	3.9	10.8
Sunflower seeds, oil-roasted	2.6	6.8
Tahini	3.0	9.3
Tofu	84.6	1.2
Walnuts, dried		
Black	4.4	5.0
English	3.6	4.8
Miscellaneous		
Beer, regular	92.3	0.05
Candy:		
Caramels, vanilla	7.6	1.2
Chocolate, milk	0.8	2.8
Sugar-coated discs		3.1
Carob power, unsweetened	1.2	32.8
Chili powder	9.1	34.2
Chocolate, baking	0.7	15.4
Cocoa, baking	1.3	29.8
Cocoa mix, prepared	79.8	1.2
Curry powder	8.7	33.2
Gravy, beef, canned	89.1	0.4
Jelly apple	32.3	0.6
Milk, chocolate	82.3	1.5
Pepper, black	9.4	25.0
Pie filling:		
Apple	74.9	1.0
Cherry	69.7	0.6
Preserves:		
Peach	32.4	0.7
Strawberry	31.7	1.2
Soup, canned, condensed:		
Chicken with noodles or rice	86.5	0.6
Vegetable	84.9	1.3
Yeast active dry	6.8	31.6

Food Item	Moisture	Total Dietary Fiber (AOAC)[†]
	g per 100 g edible portion	
Pastas		
Macaroni (see spaghetti)		
Macaroni; protein-fortified, dry	10.2	4.3
Macaroni, tricolor dry	9.8	4.3
Noodles, Chinese, Chow mein	0.7	3.9
Noodles, egg, regular:		
Dry	9.7	2.7
Cooked	68.7	2.2
Noodles, Japanese, dry:		
Somen	9.2	4.3
Udon	8.7	5.4
Noodles, spinach, dry	8.5	6.8
Spaghetti and macaroni:		
Dry	10.5	2.4
Cooked	64.7	1.6
Spaghetti, dry		
Spinach	8.7	10.6
Whole-wheat	7.1	11.8
Snacks		
Cheese-flavored, corn-based puffs or twists		1.0
Corn, toasted		6.9
Corn chips		4.4
Barbecue-flavored		5.2
Granola bars crunchy:		
Chocolate chip		4.4
Cinnamon		5.0
Popcorn:		
Air-popped		15.1
Oil-popped		10
Potato chips	2.5	4.8
Flavored		4.5
Potato chips, formulated	1.6	3.6
Pretzels		2.8
Tortilla chips		6.5
Flavored		6.2
Vegetables and Vegetable Products		
Artichokes, raw	84.4	5.2

(*continues*)

TABLE 1
Provisional Table on The Dietary Fiber Content of Selected Foods (100 Grams Edible Portion) (*continued*)

Food Item	Moisture	Total Dietary Fiber (AOAC)[†]
	g per 100 g edible portion	
Vegetables and Vegetable Products (*continued*)		
Beans, snap:		
Raw	90.3	1.8
Canned:		
Drained solids	93.3	1.3
Solids and liquid	94.5	0.8
Beets, canned:		
Drained solids sliced	91.0	1.7
Solids and liquid	91.3	1.1
Broccoli:		
Raw	90.7	2.8
Cooked	90.2	2.6
Brussels sprouts, boiled	87.3	4.3
Cabbage, Chinese:		
Raw	94.9	1.0
Cooked	95.4	1.6
Cabbage, red:		
Raw	91.6	2.0
Cooked	93.6	2.0
Cabbage, white, raw	91.5	2.4
Carrots:		
Raw	87.8	3.2
Canned, deained solids	93.0	1.5
Cauliflower:		
Raw	92.3	2.4
Cooked	92.5	2.2
Celery, raw	94.7	1.6
Chives	92.0	3.2
Corn, sweet		
Raw	76.0	3.2
Cooked	69.6	3.7
Canned:		
Brine pack:		
Drained solids	76.9	1.4
Solids and liquid	81.9	0.8
Cream-style	78.7	1.2
Cucumbers, raw	96.0	1.0
Pared		5.0
Lettuce:		
Butterhead or iceberg	95.7	1.0
Romaine	94.9	1.7

Food Item	Moisture	Total Dietary Fiber (AOAC)[†]
	g per 100 g edible portion	
Vegetables and Vegetable Products (*continued*)		
Mushrooms:		
Raw	91.8	1.3
Boiled	91.1	2.2
Onions, raw	90.1	1.6
Onions, spring, raw	91.9	2.4
Parsley, raw	88.3	4.4
Peas, edible-podded:		
Raw	88.9	2.6
Cooked,	88.9	2.8
Peas, sweet, canned:		
Drained solids	81.7	3.4
Solids and liquid	86.5	2.0
Peppers, sweet, raw	92.8	1.6
Pickles:		
Dill.	93.8	1.2
Sweet	68.9	1.1
Potatoes:		
Raw:		
Flesh and skin	80.0	1.8
Flesh	79.0	1.6
Baked:		
Flesh	75.4	1.5
Skin	47.3	4.0
Boiled	77.0	1.5
French-fried, home-prepared from frozen	52.9	4.2
Hashed brown	56.1	2.0
Spinach:		
Raw	91.6	2.6
Boiled	91.2	2.2
Squash:		
Summer:		
Raw	93.7	1.2
Cooked	93.7	1.4
Winter:		
Raw	88.7	1.8
Cooked	89.0	2.8
Sweet potatoes:		
Raw	72.8	3.0
Cooked	72.8	3.0

TABLE 1
Provisional Table on The Dietary Fiber Content of Selected Foods (100 Grams Edible Portion) (*continued*)

Food Item	Moisture	Total Dietary Fiber (AOAC)[†]
	g per 100 g edible portion	
Vegetables and Vegetable Products (*continued*)		
Sweet potatoes: (*continued*)		
Canned, drained solids	72.5	1.8
Tomatoes, raw	94.0	1.3
Tomato products:		
Catsup		1.6
Paste	74.1	4.3
Puree	87.3	2.3
Sauce	89.1	1.5
Turnip greens:		
Raw	91.1	2.4
Boiled	33.2	3.1

Food Item	Moisture	Total Dietary Fiber (AOAC)[†]
	g per 100 g edible portion	
Vegetables and Vegetable Products (*continued*)		
Turnips:		
Raw	91.9	8.1
Boiled	93.6	2.0
Vegetables, mixed, frozen, cooked	83.2	3.8
Water chestnuts, canned, drained solids	87.9	2.2
Watercress	95.1	2.3

[†] AOAC = accepted methods of dietary fiber analysis of the Association of Official Analytical Chemists.

Fast Food
Composition Table

TABLE 1
Fast Food Composition

Food	Serving Size (g)	Calories	Calories from Fat	Total Fat (g)	Saturated Fat (g)	Trans Fat (g)	Cholesterol (mg)	Sodium (mg)	Total Carbs (g)	Dietary Fiber (g)	Total Sugar (g)	Protein (g)	Vitamin A, %DV	Vitamin C, %DV	Calcium %DV	Iron %DV
BURGER KING®																
Original WHOPPER® Sandwich	291	700	370	42	13	1	85	1020	52	4	8	31	20	15	10	30
Orig. WHOPPER® w/ Cheese Sand.	316	800	440	49	18	1.5	110	1450	53	4	9	35	25	15	25	30
Orig. DOUBLE WHOPPER® Sand.	374	970	550	61	22	2	160	1110	52	4	8	52	20	15	15	45
Orig. DBL WHOPPER® & Ch. Sand.	399	1060	620	69	27	3	185	1540	53	4	9	56	25	15	30	45
Original WHOPPER JR.® Sandwich	158	390	200	22	7	0.5	45	550	31	2	5	17	10	6	8	15
Orig. WHOPPER JR.® & Ch. Sand.	160	430	230	26	9	1	55	770	32	2	5	19	10	6	15	15
Chicken WHOPPER® Sandwich	272	570	230	25	4.5	0	75	1410	48	4	5	38	15	10	6	40
Original Chicken Sandwich	204	560	260	28	6	2	60	1270	52	3	5	25	8	0	6	15
CHICKEN TENDERS® 4 Pieces	62	170	90	9	2.5	2	25	420	10	0	0	11	0	0	0	2
CHICKEN TENDERS® 6 Pieces	92	250	130	14	4	2.5	35	630	15	<1	0	16	2	0	2	4
CHICKEN TENDERS® 8 Pieces	123	340	170	19	5	3.5	50	840	20	<1	0	22	2	0	2	4
BK FISH FILET™ Sandwich	185	520	270	30	8	0	55	840	44	2	4	18	6	2	15	15
BK Veggie® Burger	186	380	140	16	2.5	0	5	930	46	4	6	14	15	6	8	35
French Fries, Small	74	230	100	11	3	3	0	410	29	2	0	3	0	8	2	2
French Fries, Medium	117	360	160	18	5	4.5	0	640	46	4	1	4	0	15	2	4
French Fries, Large	160	500	220	25	7	6	0	880	63	5	1	6	0	20	2	6
French Fries, King	194	600	270	30	8	8	0	1070	76	6	1	7	0	20	2	6
Onion Rings, Small	51	180	80	9	2	2	0	260	22	2	3	2	0	0	6	0
Onion Rings, Medium	91	320	140	16	4	3.5	0	460	40	3	5	4	0	0	10	0
Onion Rings, Large	137	480	210	23	6	5	0	690	6	5	7	7	0	0	15	0
Onion Rings, King	159	550	240	27	7	6	5	800	70	5	8	8	0	0	20	8
Chili	216	190	70	8	3	0	25	1040	17	5	5	13	25	60	8	8
Barbecue Dipping Sauce	28	35	0	0	0	–	0	390	9	0	7	0	2	4	0	2

Honey Flavored Dipping Sauce	28	90	0	0	0	–	0	0	23	3	22	0	0	0	0
Honey Mustard Dipping Sauce	28	90	0	1	0	–	10	150	9	0	4	0	0	2	0
Sweet and Sour Dipping Sauce	28	40	0	0	0	–	0	65	10	0	5	0	2	0	4
Ranch Dipping Sauce	28	140	130	15	2.5	–	5	95	1	–	1	1	0	0	0
Zesty Onion Ring Dipping Sauce	28	150	140	15	2.5	0	15	210	3	<1	2	0	0	0	0
Ketchup (packet)	10	10	0	0	0	–	0	125	3	0	2	4	2	0	0
Side Garden Salad	106	20	0	0	0	0	15	15	4	<1	<1	1	20	1	2
Fire-Grilled Chicken Caesar Salad	286	190	60	7	3	0	50	900	9	1	1	25	40	85	15	8
Fire-Grilled Shrimp Caesar Salad	291	180	90	10	3	0.5	120	880	9	2	1	20	45	90	20	15
Fire-Grilled Chicken Garden Salad	340	210	60	7	3	0	50	910	12	2	3	26	45	130	20	10
Fire-Grilled Shrimp Garden Salad	349	200	90	10	3	0.5	120	900	13	3	6	21	45	90	25	20
Garden Ranch Dressing	57	120	90	10	1.5	0	20	610	7	0	2	<1	0	0	2	2
Creamy Garlic Caesar Dressing	57	130	100	11	2	0	20	710	7	0	2	2	0	2	6	2
Sweet Onion Vinaigrette	57	100	70	8	1	0	0	960	8	0	7	0	2	0	0	0
Tomato Balsamic Vinaigrette	57	110	80	9	1	0	0	760	9	0	8	0	2	2	2	2
Fat-Free Honey Mustard Dressing	57	70	0	0	0	–	0	230	18	0	15	0	0	0	0	0
Hidden Valley® Fat-Free Ranch	43	35	0	0	0	–	0	370	7	0	2	0	0	0	2	0
Dutch Apple Pie	113	340	130	14	3	3	0	470	52	1	23	2	2	2	0	8
Croissan'wich® w/Bacon, Egg & Ch.	119	360	200	22	8	2	195	950	25	<1	4	15	8	0	30	20
Croissan'wich® w/Ham, Egg & Ch.	146	360	180	20	8	2	200	1500	25	<1	3	18	8	2	30	25
Croissan'wich® w/Saus., Egg & Ch.	157	520	350	39	14	2.5	210	1090	24	1	4	19	10	0	30	25
Croissan'wich® w/Sausage & Ch.	107	420	280	31	11	2.5	45	840	23	<1	4	14	4	0	10	20
Croissan'wich® w/Egg & Cheese	112	320	170	19	7	2	185	730	24	<1	3	12	8	0	30	20
French Toast Sticks (5 sticks)	112	390	180	20	4.5	4.5	0	440	46	2	11	6	0	0	6	10

(continues)

TABLE 1
Fast Food Composition (*continued*)

Food	Serving Size (g)	Calories	Calories from Fat	Total Fat (g)	Saturated Fat (g)	Trans Fat (g)	Cholesterol (mg)	Sodium (mg)	Total Carbs (g)	Dietary Fiber (g)	Total Sugar (g)	Protein (g)	Vitamin A, %DV	Vitamin C, %DV	Calcium %DV	Iron %DV
Hash Brown Rounds, Small	75	230	130	15	4	5	0	450	23	2	0	20	0	2	0	2
Hash Brown Rounds, Large	128	390	230	25	7	8	0	760	38	4	0	3	0	2	2	4
Milk Shake, Vanilla, Small	298	400	130	15	9	0	60	240	57	0	56	8	10	4	35	0
Milk Shake, Vanilla, Medium	397	540	180	20	13	0.5	80	320	76	0	74	11	15	6	50	2
Milk Shake, Vanilla, Large	588	800	270	29	19	1	120	480	113	<1	110	16	20	10	70	2
KFC																
OR Chicken–Whole Wing	47	150	80	9	2.5	–	60	370	5	0	0	11	0	0	0	2
OR Chicken–Breast	161	380	170	19	6	–	145	1150	11	0	0	40	0	0	0	6
OR Chicken–Drum Stick	59	140	70	8	2	–	75	440	4	0	0	14	0	0	0	4
OR Chicken–Thigh	126	360	230	25	7	–	165	1060	12	0	0	22	0	0	0	6
EC Chicken–Whole Wing	52	190	110	12	4	–	55	390	10	0	0	10	0	0	0	2
EC Chicken–Breast	162	460	250	28	8	–	135	1230	19	0	0	34	0	0	0	8
EC Chicken–Drum Stick	60	160	90	10	2.5	–	70	420	5	0	0	12	0	0	0	4
EC Chicken–Thigh	114	370	230	26	7	–	120	710	12	0	0	21	0	0	0	6
Crispy Strips (3)	151	400	220	24	5	–	75	1250	17	0	0	29	0	6	0	10
Boneless Wings, HBBQ Sauced (7)	250	600	260	28	5	–	75	1950	49	2	7	35	0	0	4	8
Pop Corn Chicken–Kids	71	270	160	18	4	–	30	640	16	0	0	12	0	2	2	15
Pop Corn Chicken–Individual	114	450	270	30	7	–	50	1030	25	0	0	19	0	2	2	20
Pop Corn Chicken–Large	170	660	400	44	10	–	75	1530	37	0	0	29	0	4	4	35
Chicken Pot Pie	423	770	360	40	15	–	115	1680	70	5	2	33	200	0	0	20
HBBQ Wings Sauced (6)	157	540	300	33	7	–	150	1130	36	1	15	25	15	8	6	15
Hot Wings (6)	134	450	260	29	6	–	145	1120	23	1	1	24	6	6	8	10
Biscuit	57	190	90	10	2	–	1.5	580	23	0	1	2	0	0	0	4
Green Beans	113	50	15	1.5	0.5	–	5	460	5	2	2	5	15	2	0	4

Item																
Mashed Potatoes with Gravy	136	120	40	4.5	1	–	0	380	18	1	<1	2	2	4	0	2
Mac and Cheese	287	130	50	5	2	–	5	610	15	1	1	5	10	4	10	4
Potato Wedges (Small Size)	102	240	110	12	3	–	0	830	30	3	0	4	0	6	2	10
Corn on the Cob (5.5")	162	150	25	3	1	–	0	10	26	7	10	5	0	10	6	8
BBQ Beans	136	230	10	1	1	–	0	720	46	7	22	8	8	6	15	30
Potato Salad	128	180	80	9	1.5	–	5	470	22	1	5	2	0	10	0	2
Cole Slaw	130	190	100	11	2	–	5	300	22	3	13	1	25	40	4	0
OR Sandwich with sauce	260	450	240	27	6	–	65	1010	22	0	0	29	2	0	4	10
TC Sandwich with sauce	224	670	360	40	8	–	80	1640	42	1	3	36	0	8	6	20
Zinger Sandwich with sauce	224	680	370	41	8	–	90	1650	42	1	3	35	3	8	6	20
TR Sandwich with sauce	196	390	170	19	4	–	70	810	24	1	0	31	0	0	4	10
HBBQ Sandwich	147	300	50	6	1.5	–	50	640	41	4	16	21	2	4	6	15
Twister	252	670	340	38	7	–	60	1650	55	3	7	27	10	8	15	15
Double Choc. Chip Cake	76	400	260	29	5	–	45	230	31	2	27	4	0	0	4	8
Lil'Bucket Fudge Brownie	99	270	80	9	4	–	30	170	44	1	39	2	0	0	4	4
Lil'Bucket Lemon Creme	127	400	130	14	7	–	5	210	65	2	51	4	2	0	20	0
Lil'Bucket Chocolate Cream	113	270	120	13	8	–	0	180	37	2	28	2	2	0	2	6
Strawberry Creme Pie Slice	78	270	110	12	7	–	10	200	37	0	23	3	4	4	6	6
Lil'Bucket Strawberry Shortcake	99	200	50	6	4	–	20	110	34	0	34	2	0	0	2	0
Pecan Pie Slice	95	370	140	15	2.5	–	40	190	55	2	20	4	0	0	0	8
Apple Pie Slice	108	270	80	9	2	–	0	200	45	4	22	3	2	40	0	8
Lemon Meringue Pie	92	310	100	11	5	–	40	160	47	3	36	5	0	6	15	6
Cherry Cheesecake Parfait	120	300	100	11	5	–	4	130	46	2	37	3	4	0	2	2

(continues)

TABLE 1
Fast Food Composition (*continued*)

Food	Serving Size (g)	Calories	Calories from Fat	Total Fat (g)	Saturated Fat (g)	Trans Fat (g)	Cholesterol (mg)	Sodium (mg)	Total Carbs (g)	Dietary Fiber (g)	Total Sugar (g)	Protein (g)	Vitamin A, %DV	Vitamin C, %DV	Calcium, %DV	Iron %DV
MCDONALD'S																
Hamburger	105	280	90	10	4	–	30	550	23	2	7	12	0	4	15	15
Cheeseburger	119	330	130	14	6	–	45	790	36	2	7	15	6	4	20	15
Double Cheese Burger	173	490	240	26	12	–	85	1220	38	2	8	25	10	4	30	20
Quarter Pounder®	171	430	190	21	8	–	70	770	38	3	9	23	0	6	15	25
Quarter Pounder® with Cheese	199	540	260	29	13	–	95	1240	39	3	9	29	10	6	30	25
Double Quarter Pounder® with Cheese	280	770	430	47	20	–	165	1440	39	3	10	46	10	6	30	40
Big Mac®	219	600	300	33	11	–	85	1050	50	4	8	25	8	6	30	25
Filet-O-Fish®	141	410	180	20	4	–	45	660	41	1	5	15	4	0	15	10
Chicken McGrill®	213	400	140	16	3	–	70	1020	37	3	7	27	6	10	15	15
Crispy Chicken	219	510	2230	26	4.5	–	50	1090	47	3	7	22	6	10	15	15
McChicken®	147	430	200	23	4.5	–	45	830	41	3	6	14	2	0	15	15
Small French Fries	74	220	100	11	2	–	0	150	28	3	0	3	0	15	0	4
Medium French Fries	114	350	150	17	3	–	0	220	44	4	0	5	0	20	0	4
Large French Fries	171	520	230	25	4.5	–	0	340	66	6	0	7	0	35	2	8
Ketchup Packet	10	10	0	0	0	–	0	115	3	0	2	0	0	2	0	0
Chicken McNuggets® (4 pieces)	64	170	90	10	2	–	25	450	10	0	0	10	0	0	0	4
Chicken McNuggets® (6 pieces)	96	250	130	15	3	–	35	670	15	0	0	15	2	2	0	4
Chicken McNuggets® (10 pieces)	160	420	220	24	5	–	60	1120	26	0	0	25	4	2	2	6
Barbeque Sauce	28	45	0	0	0	–	0	250	10	0	10	0	0	6	0	0
Honey	14	45	0	0	0	–	0	0	12	0	11	0	0	0	0	0
Hot Mustard Sauce	28	60	30	3.5	0	–	5	240	7	<1	6	<1	0	0	0	4
Sweet 'N Sour Sauce	28	50	0	0	0	–	0	140	11	0	10	0	6	0	0	0
Grilled Chicken Bacon Ranch Salad	288	250	90	10	4.5	–	85	930	9	3	3	31	90	50	15	10

Item																
Crispy Chicken Bacon Ranch Salad	294	350	180	19	6	–	65	1000	20	3	4	26	90	50	15	10
Grilled Chicken Caesar Salad	278	200	50	6	3	–	70	820	9	3	3	29	90	50	20	10
Crispy Chicken Caesar Salad	284	310	140	16	4.5	–	50	890	20	3	4	23	90	50	20	10
Caesar Salad (with chicken)	190	90	35	4	2.5	–	10	170	7	3	3	7	90	50	20	8
Side Salad	87	15	0	0	0	–	0	10	3	1	1	1	40	25	2	4
Fiesta Salad (with Sour Cr. & Salsa)	297	450	250	27	13	–	95	920	28	5	3	24	110	45	30	20
Newman's Own® Cr. Caesar Dressing	59	190	170	18	3.5	–	20	500	4	0	2	2	0	0	6	0
Newman's Own® L. Fat Balsamic Vin.	44	40	25	3	0	–	0	730	4	0	3	0	0	4	0	0
Newman's Own® Ranch Dressing	59	170	130	15	2.5	–	20	530	9	0	4	1	0	0	4	0
Newman's Own® Salsa	89	30	0	0	0	–	0	290	7	1	0	1	6	15	2	6
Egg McMuffin®	138	300	110	12	5	–	235	850	28	2	2	18	10	4	30	15
Sausage McMuffin®	114	370	200	23	9	–	50	790	28	2	2	14	6	0	25	15
Sausage McMuffin® with Egg	164	450	250	28	10	–	260	940	29	2	2	20	10	0	30	20
Bacon, Egg & Cheese Biscuit	145	430	230	26	8	–	240	1230	31	1	3	18	10	0	15	15
Sausage Biscuit with Egg	162	490	300	33	10	–	245	1010	31	2	2	16	6	0	8	15
Sausage Biscuit	112	410	250	28	8	–	35	930	30	1	2	10	0	0	6	15
Bacon, Egg, and Cheese McGriddles	168	440	190	21	7	–	240	1270	43	1	16	19	10	0	20	15
Sausage, Egg and Cheese McGriddles	199	550	300	33	11	–	260	1290	43	1	16	20	10	0	20	15
Sausage McGriddles	135	420	210	23	7	–	35	970	42	1	15	11	0	0	8	10
Big Breakfast®	266	700	420	47	13	–	455	1430	45	3	3	24	10	4	10	20
Hotcakes and Sausage	271	780	300	33	9	–	50	1060	104	0	40	15	8	0	15	20
Hotcakes (margarine 2 pats & syrup)	228	600	150	17	3	–	20	770	104	0	40	9	8	0	10	25
Hash Browns	53	130	70	8	1.5	–	0	330	14	1	0	1	0	4	0	2

(continues)

TABLE 1
Fast Food Composition (*continued*)

Food	Serving Size (g)	Calories	Calories from Fat	Total Fat (g)	Saturated Fat (g)	Trans Fat (g)	Cholesterol (mg)	Sodium (mg)	Total Carbs (g)	Dietary Fiber (g)	Total Sugar (g)	Protein (g)	Vitamin A, %DV	Vitamin C, %DV	Calcium, %DV	Iron %DV
Chocolate Triple Thick® Shake (12 oz)	333 mL	430	110	12	8	–	50	210	70	1	61	11	20	2	35	2
Chocolate Triple Thick® Shake (16 oz)	444 mL	580	150	17	11	–	65	280	94	1	82	15	25	4	45	4
Chocolate Triple Thick® Shake (21 oz)	583 mL	750	200	22	14	–	90	360	123	2	107	19	30	6	60	4
Baked Apple Pie	77	260	120	13	3.5	–	0	200	34	<1	13	3	0	40	2	6
Subway																
6-Inch Sandwiches with 6 Grams of Fat or Less Values include Italian or wheat bread, lettuce, tomatoes, onions, green peppers, olives, and pickles.																
Veggie Delite® 6"	166	230	30	3	1	–	0	510	44	4	7	9	8	35	6	25
Savory Turkey Breast	223	280	40	4.5	1.5	–	20	1010	46	4	7	18	8	35	6	25
Savory Turkey Breast & Ham	232	290	45	5	1.5	–	25	1220	46	4	8	20	8	35	6	25
Ham Sandwich	223	290	45	5	1.5	–	25	1270	46	4	8	18	8	35	6	25
Roast Beef	223	290	45	5	2	–	20	910	45	4	8	19	8	35	8	35
Turkey Breast, Ham, & Roast Beef	256	320	50	6	2	–	35	1300	47	4	8	24	8	35	6	30
Oven Roasted Chicken Breast	237	330	50	6	1.5	–	45	1010	47	5	9	24	8	35	6	25
Sweet Onion Chicken Teriyaki	271	370	45	5	1.5	–	50	1090	59	5	19	26	8	40	8	25
Honey Mustard Ham	244	310	45	5	1.5	–	25	1410	54	5	14	19	8	35	6	25
6-Inch Hot Sandwiches Values based on standard formula and includes selected vegetables and cheese.																
Turkey Breast, Ham, & Bacon Melt	253	380	110	12	5	–	45	1610	47	4	8	25	10	35	15	25
Cheese Steak	248	360	90	10	4.5	–	36	1090	47	5	9	24	10	35	15	45
Chipotle Southwest Cheese Steak	258	440	170	19	6	–	45	1160	49	5	10	24	10	35	15	45
Dijon Turkey Breast, Ham & Bacon Melt	262	470	190	21	7	–	55	1620	48	5	8	26	10	35	15	25
Meatball Marinara	288	500	200	22	11	–	45	1180	52	5	9	23	10	40	15	35

6-Inch Cold Sandwiches																
Classic Tuna	240	430	170	19	5	–	45	1070	46	4	7	20	10	35	15	25
Cold Cut Combo	248	410	160	17	7	–	55	1570	46	4	7	21	10	35	15	30
Italian BMT®	241	450	190	21	8	–	55	1790	47	4	8	23	10	35	15	25
Subway® Seafood Sensation	248	380	120	13	4.5	–	25	1170	52	5	8	16	10	35	15	25
Deli-Style Sandwiches																
Savory Turkey Breast	152	210	35	3.5	1.5	–	15	730	36	3	4	13	4	20	6	25
Ham	142	210	35	4	1.5	–	10	770	35	3	4	11	4	20	6	25
Roast Beef	152	220	40	4.5	2	–	15	660	35	3	4	13	4	20	6	30
Classic Tuna	161	300	110	13	4.5	–	25	770	36	3	3	13	8	20	10	25
6-Inch Double Meat (DM)																
DM Turkey Breast	280	330	50	5	1.5	–	40	1510	48	4	8	28	8	35	8	25
DM Turkey Breast & Ham	298	360	60	7	2	–	45	1930	48	4	9	30	8	35	6	25
DM Ham	280	350	60	7	2.5	–	50	2030	49	4	9	28	8	35	6	30
DM Roast Beef	280	360	70	7	3.5	–	40	1310	46	4	9	29	8	35	6	40
DM Chicken	308	430	70	8	2.5	–	90	1510	50	5	11	38	8	35	6	25
DM Tuna Classic	319	580	290	32	7	–	75	1430	48	4	7	29	10	35	15	30
DM Seafood Sensation	319	490	180	20	5	–	35	1620	60	5	10	20	10	35	25	25
DM Italian BMT®	305	630	310	35	14	–	100	2860	49	4	10	34	10	35	15	30
DM Cold Cut Combo	319	550	250	28	10	–	105	2420	48	4	8	31	15	35	20	35
DM Cheese Steak	319	450	120	14	6	–	65	1460	50	6	11	37	10	35	15	60
Salads																
Garden Fresh	300	60	10	1	0	–	0	80	11	5	5	3	160	80	8	10
Mediterranean Chicken	385	170	40	4.5	2	–	55	520	11	5	5	22	160	80	10	10
Grilled Chicken and Spinach	284	420	240	26	10	–	215	970	10	5	2	38	220	60	40	35
Classic Club	430	390	190	21	10	–	210	1820	13	4	5	37	130	70	30	20

(continues)

TABLE 1
Fast Food Composition (*continued*)

Food	Serving Size (g)	Calories	Calories from fat	Total Fat (g)	Saturated Fat (g)	Trans Fat (g)	Cholesterol (mg)	Sodium (mg)	Total Carbs (g)	Dietary Fiber (g)	Total Sugar (g)	Protein (g)	Vitamin A, %DV	Vitamin C, %DV	Calcium %DV	Iron %DV
Salad Dressing (1 packet) and Salad Toppings																
Atkins Honey Mustard	57	200	200	22	3	–	0	510	1	0	0	1	0	0	0	0
Greek Vinaigrette	57	200	190	21	3	–	0	590	3	0	2	1	0	0	0	0
Kraft Fat Free Italian	57	35	0	0	0	–	0	720	7	0	4	1	0	0	2	0
Kraft Ranch	57	200	200	22	3.5	–	10	550	1	0.5	0	1	0	0	0	0
Red Wine Vinaigrette	57	80	10	1	0	–	0	910	17	0	7	1	0	0	0	0
Bacon Bits	14	60	40	4.5	1.5	–	20	260	0	0	0	5	0	0	0	0
Croutons	14	70	30	3	0	–	0	200	8	0	0	1	0	0	0	0
Diced Eggs	28	45	30	3	1	–	120	35	0	0	0	4	2	0	0	6
Garlic Almonds	14	80	70	7	0.5	–	0	65	3	2	1	3	0	0	4	6
Fruizle Express																
Berry Lishus	369	110	0	0	0	–	0	30	28	1	27	1	0	110	0	10
Sunrise Refresher	341	120	0	0	0	–	0	20	29	1	28	1	4	210	2	0
Pineapple Delight	369	130	0	0	0	–	0	25	33	1	33	1	0	150	0	0
Peach Pizzazz	341	100	0	0	0	–	0	25	26	0	26	0	2	110	0	0
Soups																
Roasted Chicken Noodle	240	60	15	1.5	0.5	–	10	940	7	1	1	6	15	2	0	0
Vegetable Beef	240	90	10	1	0.5	–	5	1050	15	3	3	5	15	0	2	4
Golden Broccoli & Cheese	240	180	100	11	4	–	15	1120	16	2	3	5	4	0	15	2
Cream of Broccoli	240	130	50	6	2	–	10	860	15	2	0	5	4	20	15	0
Cream of Potato with Bacon	240	200	100	11	4	–	15	840	21	2	3	4	6	0	8	2
Cheese with Ham and Bacon	240	240	140	15	6	–	20	1160	17	1	5	8	2	0	15	2
New England Style Clam Chowder	240	110	30	3.5	0.5	–	10	990	16	1	1	5	2	2	10	4
Minestrone	240	90	35	4	1	–	20	1180	7	1	1	7	40	6	2	4

Item																
Chicken and Dumpling	240	130	40	4.5	2.5	–	30	1030	16	1	2	7	20	0	2	4
Spanish Style Chicken with Rice	240	90	20	2	0.5	–	5	800	13	1	1	5	2	0	0	0
Brown and Wild Rice with Chicken	240	190	100	11	4.5	–	20	990	17	2	3	6	10	40	30	2
Chili Con Carne	240	240	90	10	5	–	15	860	23	8	14	15	15	0	6	10
Tomato Garden Vegetable w/ Rotini	240	100	5	0.5	0	–	0	2340	20	2	7	3	80	2	4	2

TACO BELL

15 "Fresco Style" Items Under 10 Grams of Fat

Item																
Crunchy Taco	92	150	70	7	2.5	–	20	360	14	3	2	7	6	6	2	6
Soft Taco, Beef	113	190	70	8	3	–	20	630	22	3	3	9	6	8	8	8
Ranchero Chicken Soft Taco	135	170	40	4.5	1	–	20	700	22	2	3	12	10	8	8	6
Grilled Steak Soft Taco	128	170	45	5	1.5	–	15	560	21	2	3	11	4	10	8	8
Gordita Baja®-Beef	153	250	90	9	3	–	20	640	30	4	7	12	10	10	8	15
Gordita Baja®-Chicken	153	230	50	6	1	–	25	570	29	2	7	15	6	10	6	10
Gordita Baja®-Steak	153	230	60	7	1.5	–	15	570	29	3	7	13	6	8	6	10
Bean Burrito	213	350	70	8	2	–	0	1220	56	9	4	13	10	10	15	15
Burrito Supreme®-Chicken	241	350	70	8	2	–	25	1270	50	6	5	19	10	15	15	15
Burrito Supreme®-Steak	241	350	80	9	2.5	–	15	1260	50	6	5	17	10	15	15	15
Fiesta Burrito-Chicken	198	350	80	9	2	–	25	1100	49	4	4	16	10	10	15	15
Tostado	177	200	50	6	1	–	0	670	30	8	2	8	10	10	6	8
Enchirito®-Beef	206	270	80	9	3	–	20	1300	35	7	3	13	20	15	10	10
Enchirito®-Chicken	206	250	50	5	1.5	–	25	1230	34	5	3	15	20	15	10	10
Enchirito®-Steak	206	250	60	7	2	–	15	1220	34	6	3	14	20	15	10	10

Big Bell Value Menu™

Item																
Grande Soft Taco	206	450	190	21	8	–	45	1400	44	5	5	20	10	8	20	15
Double Decker® Taco	156	340	120	14	5	–	25	800	39	6	3	15	6	4	15	20
½ lb Bean Burrito Especial	289	600	190	21	5	–	15	1760	82	12	6	21	10	8	30	20

(continues)

TABLE 1
Fast Food Composition (*continued*)

Food	Serving Size (g)	Calories	Calories from Fat	Total Fat (g)	Saturated Fat (g)	Trans Fat (g)	Cholesterol (mg)	Sodium (mg)	Total Carbs (g)	Dietary Fiber (g)	Total Sugar (g)	Protein (g)	Vitamin A %DV	Vitamin C %DV	Calcium %DV	Iron %DV
½ lb Beef Combo Burrito	241	470	170	19	5	–	45	1610	52	8	5	22	15	10	20	20
½ lb Beef & Potato Burrito	252	530	220	24	9	–	40	1670	65	6	5	15	15	10	20	20
Cheesy Fiesta Potatoes	138	280	160	18	6	–	20	800	27	2	2	4	6	0	6	6
Carmel Apple Empanada	85	290	130	15	4	–	<5	290	37	1	14	3	0	10	6	6
Tacos																
Crunchy Taco	78	170	90	10	4	–	25	350	13	3	1	8	6	4	6	6
Taco Supreme®	113	220	120	14	7	–	40	360	14	3	2	9	10	8	8	8
Soft Taco, Beef	99	210	90	10	4.5	–	25	620	21	2	2	10	6	4	10	10
Rancho Chicken Soft Taco	135	270	130	15	4	–	35	790	21	2	3	13	10	8	15	8
Soft Taco Supreme®-Beef	134	260	130	14	7	–	40	630	22	3	3	11	10	8	15	10
Soft Taco Supreme®-Chicken	134	230	90	10	5	–	45	570	21	1	3	15	8	8	15	6
Grilled Steak Soft Taco	127	280	150	17	4.5	–	30	650	21	1	3	12	4	6	10	8
Double Decker® Taco Supreme®	191	380	160	18	8	–	40	820	40	6	4	15	10	8	15	15
Gorditas																
Gordita Supreme®-Beef	153	310	140	16	7	–	35	590	30	3	7	14	10	8	15	15
Gordita Supreme®-Chicken	153	290	110	12	5	–	45	530	28	2	7	17	6	8	10	10
Gordita Supreme®-Steak	153	290	120	13	6	–	35	520	28	2	7	16	6	6	10	15
Gordita Baja®-Beef	153	350	170	19	5	–	30	750	31	4	7	14	8	8	15	15
Gordita Baja®-Chicken	153	320	140	15	3.5	–	40	690	29	2	7	17	6	6	10	10
Gordita Baja®-Steak	153	320	150	16	4	–	30	680	29	2	7	15	6	6	10	10
Gordita Nacho Cheese-Beef	153	300	120	13	4	–	20	740	32	3	7	13	6	10	10	15
Gordita Nacho Cheese-Chicken	153	270	90	10	2.5	–	25	670	30	2	7	16	2	8	8	10
Gordita Nacho Cheese-Steak	153	270	100	11	3	–	20	660	30	2	7	14	2	6	8	10

Chalupas

Chalupa Supreme-Beef	153	390	220	24	10	–	40	600	31	3	5	14	10	8	15	10
Chalupa Supreme-Chicken	153	370	180	20	8	–	45	530	30	1	4	17	6	8	10	6
Chalupa Supreme-Steak	153	370	190	22	8	–	35	520	29	2	4	15	6	6	10	8
Chalupa Baja-Beef	153	430	250	27	8	–	30	750	32	3	4	14	8	8	15	8
Chalupa Baja-Chicken	153	400	210	24	6	–	40	690	30	2	4	17	6	6	10	6
Chalupa Baja-Steak	153	400	220	25	7	–	30	680	30	2	4	15	6	6	10	8
Chalupa Nacho Cheese-Beef	153	380	200	22	7	–	20	740	33	3	5	12	6	10	10	8
Chalupa Nacho Cheese-Chicken	153	350	160	18	5	–	25	670	31	1	4	16	2	8	8	6
Chalupa Nacho Cheese-Steak	153	350	170	19	5	–	20	670	31	2	4	14	2	6	8	8

Burritos

Bean Burrito	198	370	90	10	3.5	–	10	1200	55	8	4	14	10	8	20	15
7–Layer Burrito	283	530	190	21	8	–	25	1350	66	10	6	18	15	8	30	20
Chili Cheese Burrito	156	390	160	18	9	–	40	1080	40	3	3	16	15	0	30	10
Burrito Supreme®-Beef	248	440	160	18	8	–	40	1330	51	7	6	18	20	15	20	15
Burrito Supreme®-Chicken	248	410	130	14	6	–	45	1270	50	5	5	21	15	15	20	15
Burrito Supreme®-Steak	248	420	140	16	7	–	35	1260	50	6	5	19	15	15	20	15
Fiesta Burrito-Beef	184	390	140	15	5	–	25	1150	50	5	4	14	10	8	20	15
Fiesta Burrito-Chicken	184	370	100	12	3.5	–	30	1090	48	3	4	18	10	6	20	15
Fiesta Burrito-Steak	184	370	110	13	4	–	25	1080	48	4	4	16	10	6	20	15
Grilled Stuft Burrito-Beef	325	730	300	33	11	–	55	2080	79'	10	7	28	20	10	35	25
Grilled Stuft Burrito-Chicken	325	680	230	26	7	–	70	1950	76	7	6	35	10	10	30	20
Grilled Stuft Burrito-Steak	325	380	250	28	8	–	55	1940	76	8	6	31	10	6	30	25

Specialties

Tostado	170	250	90	10	4	–	15	710	29	7	2	11	10	8	15	8
Mexian Pie	216	550	280	31	11	–	45	1030	46	7	3	21	15	10	35	20

(continues)

TABLE 1
Fast Food Composition (*continued*)

Food	Serving Size (g)	Calories	Calories from Fat	Total Fat (g)	Saturated Fat (g)	Trans Fat (g)	Cholesterol (mg)	Sodium (mg)	Total Carbs (g)	Dietary Fiber (g)	Total Sugar (g)	Protein (g)	Vitamin A, %DV	Vitamin C, %DV	Calcium %DV	Iron %DV
Enchirito®-Beef	213	380	160	18	9	–	45	1430	35	6	3	19	25	15	30	15
Enchirito®-Chicken	213	350	130	14	7	–	55	1360	33	5	3	23	25	15	25	10
Enchirito®-Steak	213	360	140	16	8	–	45	1350	33	5	3	21	25	10	25	10
MexiMelt®	128	290	140	16	8	–	45	880	23	8	3	15	10	6	25	10
Fiesta Taco Salad™	548	870	430	48	16	–	65	1770	80	15	11	32	25	25	40	35
Cheese Quesadilla	142	490	260	28	13	–	55	1150	39	3	4	19	10	0	50	8
Chicken Quesadilla	184	540	270	30	13	–	80	1380	40	3	4	28	15	4	50	10
Steak Quesadilla	184	540	280	31	14	–	70	1370	40	3	4	26	15	0	50	15
Zesty Chicken Border Bowl®	417	730	380	42	9	–	45	1640	65	12	5	23	20	15	15	20
Southwest Steak Bowl	443	700	290	32	8	–	55	2050	73	13	4	30	30	15	20	35
Nachos and Sides																
Nachos	99	320	170	19	4.5	–	<5	530	33	2	3	5	0	0	8	4
Nachos Supreme	195	450	230	26	9	–	35	800	42	7	4	13	8	10	10	10
Nachos BellGrande®	308	780	380	43	13	–	35	1300	80	12	6	20	10	10	20	15
Pintos 'n Cheese	128	180	60	7	3.5	–	15	700	20	6	1	10	10	6	15	6
Mexican Rice	131	210	90	10	4	–	15	740	23	3	<1	6	20	8	10	10
Cinnamon Twists	35	160	50	5	1	–	0	150	28	0	13	<1	0	0	0	2
WENDY'S																
Mandarin Chicken® Salad	348	190	25	3	1	0	50	740	17	3	11	22	–	–	–	–
Crispy Noodles	14	60	20	2	0	0.5	0	170	10	0	1	1	–	–	–	–
Roasted Almonds	21	130	100	11	1	0	0	70	4	2	1	5	–	–	–	–
Oriental Sesame Dressing	64	250	170	19	2.5	0	0	560	19	0	18	1	–	–	–	–
Spring Mix Salad	315	180	100	11	6	0.5	30	230	12	5	5	11	–	–	–	–
Honey Roasted Pecans	20	130	120	13	12	0	0	65	5	2	3	2	–	–	–	–

House Vinaigrette Dressing	64	190	160	18	2.5	0	0	750	8	0	0	7	0	—	—	—	—	—
Chicken BLT Salad	376	360	170	19	9	0.5	98	1140	10	4	4	4	34	—	—	·	—	—
Homestyle Garlic Croutons	14	70	25	2.5	0	0	0	120	9	0	0	0	1	—	—	—	—	—
Honey Mustard Dressing	64	280	230	26	4	0.5	25	350	11	0	0	10	1	—	—	—	—	—
Taco Supreme Salad	495	360	140	16	8	1	65	1090	29	8	8	8	27	—	—	—	—	—
Salsa	85	30	0	0	0	0	0	440	6	0	0	4	1	—	—	—	—	—
Sour Cream	28	60	45	3.5	2	0	20	20	2	0	2	1	1	—	—	—	—	—
Taco Chips	43	220	100	11	2	2	0	200	27	2	2	0	3	—	—	—	—	—
Homestyle Chicken Strips Salad	420	450	200	22	9	2.5	70	1190	34	5	5	6	29	—	—	—	—	—
Creamy Ranch Dressing	64	230	200	23	4	0.5	15	580	5	0	0	3	1	—	—	—	—	—
Fat Free French Style Dressing	64	80	0	0	0	0	0	210	19	0	0	16	0	—	—	—	—	—
Reduced Fat Creamy Ranch	64	100	70	8	1.5	0	15	550	6	1	1	3	1	—	—	—	—	—
Low Fat Honey Mustard	64	110	25	3	0	0.5	0	340	21	0	0	16	0	—	—	—	—	—
Side Salad	167	35	0	0	0	0	0	20	7	3	3	4	2	—	—	—	—	—
Caesar Side Salad	99	70	40	4.5	2	0	10	190	2	1	1	1	6	—	—	—	—	—
Caesar Dressing	28	150	16	2.5	0	20	240	1	0	0	0	1	—	—	—	—	—	—
Frosty™ Junior, 6 oz. cup	113	160	35	4	2.5	0	15	75	28	0	0	21	4	—	—	—	—	—
Frosty™ Small, 12 oz. cup	227	330	70	8	5	0	35	150	56	0	0	42	8	—	—	—	—	—
Frosty™ Medium, 16 oz cup	298	430	100	11	7	0	45	200	74	0	0	55	10	—	—	—	—	—
Baked Potato, Plain	284	270	0	0	0	0	0	25	61	7	7	3	7	—	—	—	—	—
Baked Potato, Sour Cream, & Chives	312	340	60	6	3.5	0	15	40	62	7	7	3	8	—	—	—	—	—
Baked Potato, Broccoli, & Cheese	411	440	130	15	3	0	10	540	70	9	9	6	10	—	—	—	—	—
Baked Potato, Bacon, & Cheese	380	560	220	25	7	0	35	910	67	7	7	6	16	—	—	—	—	—
Country Crock® Spread	14	60	60	7	1.5	0.5	0	115	0	0	0	0	0	—	—	—	—	—
Chili, Small	227	20	45	5	2	0	35	870	21	5	5	5	17	—	—	—	—	—
Chili, Large	340	300	70	7	3	0	50	1310	31	7	7	7	25	—	—	—	—	—

(continues)

TABLE 1
Fast Food Composition (continued)

Food	Serving Size (g)	Calories	Calories from Fat	Total Fat (g)	Saturated Fat (g)	Trans Fat (g)	Cholesterol (mg)	Sodium (mg)	Total Carbs (g)	Dietary Fiber (g)	Total Sugar (g)	Protein (g)	Vitamin A %DV	Vitamin C %DV	Calcium %DV	Iron %DV
Saltine Crackers	6	25	5	0.5	0	0	0	70	5	0	0	1	–	–	–	–
Cheddar Cheese, shredded	17	70	50	6	3.5	0	15	110	1	0	0	4	–	–	–	–
French Fries, Kid's Meal	91	250	100	11	2	3	0	220	36	4	0	3	–	–	–	–
French Fries, Medium	142	390	150	17	3	4.5	0	340	56	6	0	4	–	–	–	–
French Fries, Biggie®	159	440	170	19	3.5	5	0	380	63	7	0	5	–	–	–	–
French Fries, Great Biggie®	190	530	200	23	4.5	5.5	0	450	75	8	1	6	–	–	–	–
Homestyle Chicken Strips	159	410	160	18	3.5	3	60	1470	33	0	0	28	–	–	–	–
Deli Honey Mustard Sauce	35	170	140	16	2.5	0	15	190	6	0	4	0	–	–	–	–
Spicy Southwest Chipotle Sauce	35	140	120	13	2	0	20	170	5	0	1	0	–	–	–	–
Heartland Ranch Sauce	35	200	190	21	3.5	0	20	280	1	0	5	1	–	–	–	–
Nuggets, 4 piece Kid's Meal	60	180	100	11	2.5	1.5	25	390	10	0	0	8	–	–	–	–
Nuggets, 5 piece	75	220	130	14	3	1.5	35	490	13	0	0	10	–	–	–	–
Barbecue Sauce	28	40	0	0	0	0	0	160	10	0	5	1	–	–	–	–
Sweet & Sour Sauce	28	45	0	0	0	0	0	120	12	0	7	0	–	–	–	–
Honey Mustard Sauce	28	130	100	12	2	0	10	220	6	0	5	0	–	–	–	–
Jr. Hamburger	117	270	80	9	3.5	0.5	30	610	34	2	7	15	–	–	–	–
Jr. Cheeseburger	129	310	110	12	6	0.5	45	820	34	2	7	17	–	–	–	–
Jr. Cheeseburger Deluxe™	179	350	140	15	6	1	45	880	36	2	8	18	–	–	–	–
Jr. Bacon Cheeseburger	165	380	170	19	7	1	55	830	34	2	6	20	–	–	–	–
Hamburger, Kid's Meal	110	270	80	9	3.5	0.5	30	610	33	1	6	15	–	–	–	–
Cheeseburger, Kid's Meal	122	310	110	12	6	0.5	45	820	33	1	7	17	–	–	–	–
Classic Single® w/ Everything	218	410	170	19	7	1	70	910	37	2	8	25	–	–	–	–
Big Bacon Classic®	282	580	260	29	12	1.5	95	1430	45	3	11	33	–	–	–	–
Ultimate Chicken Grill Sandwich	225	360	60	7	1.5	0	75	1100	44	2	11	31	–	–	–	–

Item																
Spicy Chicken Fillet Sandwich	225	510	170	19	3.5	1.5	55	1480	57	2	8	29	–	–	–	–
Homestyle Chicken Fillet Sandwich	230	540	190	22	4	1.5	55	1320	57	2	8	29	–	–	–	–
PIZZA HUT																
12" Medium Pan Pizzas, slice																
Cheese Only	104	280	120	13	5	–	25	500	29	1	6	11	6	2	20	15
Pepperoni	102	290	130	15	5	–	25	560	29	2	6	11	6	4	15	15
Quartered Ham	103	260	100	11	4	–	20	540	29	1	6	11	6	10	15	15
Supreme	127	320	150	16	6	–	25	650	30	2	7	13	6	10	15	15
Super Supreme	139	340	160	18	6	–	35	760	30	2	7	14	6	15	15	15
Chicken Supreme	124	280	100	12	4	–	25	530	30	2	7	13	6	10	15	15
Meat Lover's®	123	340	170	19	7	–	35	750	29	2	6	15	6	10	15	15
Veggie Lover's®	119	260	100	12	4	–	15	470	30	2	7	10	8	15	15	15
Pepperoni Lover's	118	340	170	19	7	–	40	700	29	2	6	15	6	4	20	15
Sausage Lover's®	117	330	160	17	6	–	30	640	29	2	6	13	6	6	15	15
12" Medium Thin 'N Crispy Pizza, slice																
Cheese Only	79	200	80	8	4.5	–	25	490	21	1	4	10	6	2	20	6
Pepperoni	77	210	90	10	4.5	–	25	550	21	1	5	10	6	4	15	8
Quartered Ham	78	180	60	6	3	–	20	530	21	1	5	9	6	10	15	6
Supreme	106	240	100	11	5	–	25	640	22	2	5	11	6	15	15	10
Super Supreme	119	260	120	13	6	–	35	760	23	2	6	13	6	20	15	10
Chicken Supreme	103	200	60	7	3.5	–	25	520	22	1	5	12	6	15	15	8
Meat Lover's®	98	270	130	14	6	–	35	740	21	2	5	13	6	10	15	8
Veggie Lover's®	101	180	60	7	3	–	15	480	23	2	5	8	8	15	15	8
Pepperoni Lover's®	92	260	120	14	7	–	40	690	21	2	5	13	6	4	20	8
Sausage Lover's®	91	240	110	13	6	–	30	630	21	2	5	11	6	6	15	8

(continues)

TABLE 1
Fast Food Composition (*continued*)

Food	Serving Size (g)	Calories	Calories from Fat	Total Fat (g)	Saturated Fat (g)	Trans Fat (g)	Cholesterol (mg)	Sodium (mg)	Total Carbs (g)	Dietary Fiber (g)	Total Sugar (g)	Protein (g)	Vitamin A, %DV	Vitamin C, %DV	Calcium, %DV	Iron %DV
14" Large Pan Pizza, slice																
Cheese Only	102	270	120	13	5	—	25	470	27	1	6	11	6	2	20	10
Pepperoni	100	280	130	14	5	—	25	530	26	1	6	11	4	4	10	15
Quartered Ham	102	250	100	11	4	—	20	510	26	1	6	11	4	10	10	15
Supreme	124	300	140	16	6	—	25	600	27	2	6	12	6	10	15	15
Super Supreme	135	320	150	17	6	—	30	700	28	2	6	13	6	15	15	15
Chicken Supreme	113	260	100	11	4	—	20	490	27	1	6	12	6	10	10	15
Meat Lover's®	114	320	160	18	6	—	35	690	27	2	6	14	4	10	10	15
Veggie Lover's®	109	250	100	11	4	—	15	440	28	2	6	9	6	10	15	15
Pepperoni Lover's®	111	330	170	18	7	—	35	670	27	2	6	14	6	4	20	15
Sausage Lover's®	113	300	150	17	6	—	30	590	27	2	6	12	4	4	15	15
14" Large Thin 'N Crispy Pizza, slice																
Cheese Only	74	190	70	8	4.5	—	25	460	20	1	4	9	6	2	20	6
Pepperoni	72	200	90	9	4.5	—	25	520	19	1	4	9	4	4	10	6
Quartered Ham	73	170	60	6	3	—	20	500	19	1	4	9	4	10	10	6
Supreme	99	220	100	11	5	—	25	600	21	2	5	11	6	15	15	8
Super Supreme	111	240	110	12	5	—	30	710	21	2	5	12	6	15	15	10
Chicken Supreme	95	180	60	6	3	—	20	480	21	1	5	11	6	10	10	8
Meat Lover's®	92	250	120	13	6	—	35	700	20	2	5	12	4	10	15	8
Veggie Lover's®	94	170	60	7	3	—	15	450	21	2	5	8	8	15	15	8
Pepperoni Lover's®	88	250	120	14	6	—	35	660	20	1	5	12	6	4	20	8
Sausage Lover's®	84	230	100	12	5	—	30	580	20	1	4	10	4	4	15	8

16" Extra Large Pizza, slice

Cheese Only	175	420	140	15	8	—	45	1080	51	3	11	20	8	6	35	15
Pepperoni	168	430	150	17	8	—	45	1130	50	3	11	19	6	8	25	15
Quartered Ham	169	380	100	12	6	—	40	1110	50	3	11	19	6	15	25	15
Supreme	210	460	170	19	9	—	45	1250	52	4	12	22	6	25	25	20
Super Supreme	228	490	190	21	9	—	55	1430	53	4	12	23	8	30	25	20
Chicken Supreme	203	400	110	12	6	—	40	1070	52	3	12	22	6	25	25	15
Meat Lover's®	197	500	200	22	10	—	60	1400	51	3	12	24	6	20	25	20
Veggie Lover's®	203	390	110	12	6	—	30	1030	53	4	12	17	10	25	25	20
Pepperoni Lover's®	195	520	210	24	11	—	65	1370	51	3	12	25	8	10	35	15
Sausage Lover's®	197	510	210	23	10	—	55	1330	51	3	11	23	6	10	25	20

6" Personal Pan Pizza, slice

Cheese Only	63	160	60	7	3	—	15	310	18	<1	4	7	4	0	10	8
Pepperoni	61	170	70	8	3	—	15	340	18	<1	4	7	4	2	8	8
Quartered Ham	62	150	50	6	2	—	15	330	18	<1	4	7	4	6	8	8
Supreme	77	190	80	9	3.5	—	20	420	19	1	4	8	4	6	8	8
Super Supreme	83	200	90	10	4	—	20	480	19	1	4	9	4	10	8	10
Chicken Supreme	73	160	50	6	2.5	—	15	320	19	<1	4	8	4	6	8	8
Meat Lover's®	75	200	90	10	4	—	20	470	18	1	4	9	4	8	8	10
Veggie Lover's®	69	150	50	6	2	—	10	280	19	1	4	6	4	6	8	10
Pepperoni Lover's	72	200	90	10	4.5	—	25	440	18	1	4	9	4	2	10	10
Sausage Lover's®	71	190	90	10	4	—	20	400	18	1	4	8	4	4	8	10

Fit'N Delicious™ 12" Medium

Chicken, Red Onion, & Green Pepper	106	170	40	4.5	2	—	15	460	23	2	6	10	6	30	8	8
Chicken, Mushroom Jalapeno	105	170	45	5	2	—	15	690	22	2	5	10	8	8	8	8
Ham, Red Onion, & Mushroom	101	160	40	4.5	2	—	15	470	22	2	6	8	4	10	8	8

(continues)

TABLE 1
Fast Food Composition (*continued*)

Food	Serving Size (g)	Calories	Calories from Fat	Total Fat (g)	Saturated Fat (g)	Trans Fat (g)	Cholesterol (mg)	Sodium (mg)	Total Carbs (g)	Dietary Fiber (g)	Total Sugar (g)	Protein (g)	Vitamin A, %DV	Vitamin C, %DV	Calcium %DV	Iron %DV
Ham, Pineapple, & Diced Red Tomato	99	160	35	4	2	–	15	470	24	2	7	8	6	20	8	8
Green Pepper, Red Onion, & Tomato	104	150	35	4	1.5	–	10	360	24	2	6	6	8	35	8	8
Tomato, Mushroom, & Jalapeno	104	150	40	4	2	–	10	590	22	2	5	6	10	10	8	8
Appetizers																
Hot Wings (2 pieces)	57	110	60	6	2	–	70	450	1	0	0	11	10	0	0	2
Wing Ranch Dipping Sauce	43	210	200	22	3.5	–	10	340	4	0	2	<1	0	0	0	0
Wing Blue Cheese Dipping Sauce	43	230	210	24	5	–	25	550	2	0	2	2	0	0	2	0
Breadsticks, each	50	150	60	6	1	–	0	220	20	<1	4	4	0	0	0	20
Breadstick Dipping Sauce	99	50	0	0	0	–	–	370	11	2	6	1	8	15	2	2
Desserts																
Cinnamon Sticks (2 pieces)	57	170	45	5	1	–	0	170	27	<1	10	4	0	0	0	20
White Icing Dipping Cup	57	190	0	0	0	–	0	0	46	0	39	0	0	0	0	0
Apple Dessert Pizza (1 slice)	98	260	30	3.5	0.5	–	0	250	53	1	14	4	0	0	2	6
Cherry Dessert Pizza (1 slice)	102	240	30	3.5	0.5	–	0	250	47	1	24	4	2	10	2	6

Glossary

absorption The transfer of nutrients and fluids from the gut lumen across the epithelium into the blood or lymphatic system. The mechanisms involved depend on the chemical nature of the specific nutrient involved.

absorption period (postprandium) The 3- to 4-hour period that follows the last ingestion of a meal during which the most nutrients are absorbed. This period is associated with wide swings in blood glucose and insulin concentrations, even under normal conditions.

Academy of Nutrition and Dietetics The national organization responsible for the credentialing of registered dietitians.

acetic acid (acetate) A simple organic acid with two carbon atoms that results from the metabolism of alcohol, glucose, fatty acids, and other organic molecules.

acetyl coenzyme A (acetyl CoA) The activated form of acetate. Because of the addition of coenzyme A, this molecule can enter the citric acid (Krebs) cycle or other metabolic pathways, including those involved in fatty acid synthesis, ketogenesis, and cholesterol synthesis.

achlorhydria Condition of essentially no production of hydrochloric acid (HCl) by the stomach.

acid–base balance The maintenance of a normal balance with respect to acidity (H^+) and alkalinity (basicity). Human fluids usually maintain a pH of 7.4.

acid group See carboxyl group (carboxylate group, COOH).

acidic food A food that, when metabolized, leaves an acid-ash (mineral) residue. Acidic foods include cereals, meats, nuts, a few vegetables (corn and lentils), and many fruits (cranberries, plums, and prunes). See also alkaline (basic) food.

acidosis A serious disorder of the blood characterized by the pH falling considerably below 7.4, the healthy normal human value, because of increased generation of hydrogen ions (H^+) or insufficient bicarbonate (base) production. May result from excessive production of ketones. See also ketoacidosis.

acquired immunity Specific antibody production in response to an infection by an adaptive mechanism. Immunoglobulins produced in response to an antigen of an infectious agent contain the same structure because they are derived from a unique clonal line of cells (lymphocytes) that are produced as a result of the primary stimulation of antigen; these clones remain in readiness for secondary or additional stimulations because of the "memory" of this specific clone for the specific antigen.

active transport The movement of a molecule across a membrane from a region of lower to higher concentration (i.e., up a concentration gradient), which requires both a carrier (porter) and cellular energy (ATP). Uphill transport applies to water-soluble molecules and ions, including nutrient molecules and ions, that are not soluble in the lipophilic membranes of cells.

acute Short-term effects; the opposite of chronic.

adenosine triphosphate (ATP) The major intracellular energy molecule that is used for the synthesis of many molecules and for active transport of molecules across membranes. It contains three phosphates.

Adequate Intake (AI) A designation under the Dietary Reference Intakes (DRIs) of recommended intakes for several nutrients that do not have an Estimated Average Requirement (EAR). Usually used with nutrients where not enough information is available to set a more exact requirement (RDA).

adipocyte A fat cell. Adipocytes take up fatty acids and glucose to synthesize triglycerides and undergo lipolysis to generate glycerol and free fatty acids that diffuse to blood for distribution to other body tissues.

adipose (fat) tissue Fat storage tissue containing fat cells, or adipocytes, whose function is to store and mobilize fats (triglycerides).

adolescence Period of life beginning at puberty (ending of childhood) and continuing until skeletal development is complete (i.e., approximately 11 to 18 years of age for females and 13 to 20 years for males).

adolescent pregnancy Pregnancy in females younger than 18 years of age. Many teenagers are not fully developed and may not be adequately nourished to support a pregnancy, thus increasing the risk for adverse outcomes.

adrenal cortex The outer portion of the adrenal gland that produces corticosteroid hormones, (e.g., cortisol, a glucocorticoid) and aldosterone (a mineralocorticoid). Part of the hypothalamic-pituitary-adrenal (HPA) axis.

adrenal medulla The inner portion of the adrenal gland that produces epinephrine, a catecholamine.

Adult Treatment Panel (ATP III) Guidelines based on extensive research that have been developed by the National Cholesterol Education Program (NCEP) on the detection, evaluation, and treatment of high blood cholesterol.

adulteration The process, which is forbidden by law, of modifying a food through the addition of a relatively inert filler. Adulterated foods fall under the regulation of the Food and Drug Administration (FDA).

adulthood Period of life beginning after the conclusion of skeletal growth (height) (approximately age 18 to 20 years in females and 20 to 22 years in males). The main divisions are early adulthood from 20 to 30 years of age and later adulthood up to age 60.

aerobic Refers to processes requiring oxygen. The oxidative metabolic pathways, such as the citric acid (Krebs) cycle, are aerobic processes. *See also* anaerobic.

aerobic respiration Cellular respiration that requires the presence of oxygen. *See also* citric acid cycle (Krebs cycle).

aflatoxin Toxic molecule produced by fungi that grow on moist grains, peanuts, and other legumes in storage. These mycotoxins are potentially cancer promoting because they act as mutagens.

age-related macular degeneration (AMD) Condition characterized by cell damage to a small portion of the retina (i.e., the macula), which captures images and relays them via the optic nerve to the brain. Oxidative damage via free radicals to the macula reduces its ability to transmit sharp images to the brain.

aging The decline in biological functions that typically begins after age 50 years and leads to variable decrements in organ functions, reduced cell renewal, and losses of tissue in the lean body mass compartment, especially in muscle mass and bone mass.

AI *See* Adequate Intake (AI).

alanine A nonessential amino acid. Alanine is required for protein synthesis and to carry hydrocarbon backbones from muscle tissue to the liver as part of the alanine–glucose cycle during periods of fasting.

alanine–glucose cycle Cycle whereby alanine moves from muscle via the blood to the liver and as glucose back to the blood. Provides hydrocarbon backbones for hepatic gluconeogenesis, after which glucose is delivered to tissues, especially to the brain and red blood cells, which have an essential requirement for it. *See also* gluconeogenesis.

albumin The most abundant serum (plasma) protein in blood. Albumin has a powerful osmotic effect, which is partly lost after long periods of undernutrition. Responsible for transport in blood of several nutrients, including calcium ions and fatty acids.

alcohol (ethanol) A simple organic molecule that can cause intoxication. It is metabolized by a two-step process in many cells of the body, but especially in the liver. The metabolism of alcohol yields energy and toxic byproducts.

alcohol effects Adverse effects on nutritional status and organ systems resulting from excessive intake of alcohol. Alcoholism is typically associated with poor nutritional status. *See also* fetal alcohol effects (FAE) *and* fetal alcohol syndrome (FAS).

alcohol metabolism The degradation of alcohol by two enzymatic steps, the first being the slow, or rate-limiting, step requiring alcohol dehydrogenase and the second requiring acetaldehyde dehydrogenase. The final product is acetic acid (acetate), which enters the citric acid (Krebs) cycle after combining with coenzyme A for oxidation to carbon dioxide and water, and some ATP and heat generation.

alcoholic beverage A beverage that contains alcohol (ethanol). Includes beer, wine, and distilled liquors or spirits, which have varying amounts of alcohol.

alcoholism Compulsive and uncontrolled consumption of alcoholic beverages, usually to the detriment of the drinker's health, personal relationships, and social standing. It is medically considered a disease, specifically an addictive illness.

aldehyde An organic group that is also known as a carbonyl group (CH=O).

aldosterone A mineralocorticoid (steroid) hormone produced by specific cells of the adrenal cortex. Aldosterone enhances renal reabsorption of sodium and excretion of potassium, and thereby conserves

sodium in the body. It is part of the renin-angiotensin-aldosterone sequence.

alginate Seaweed (kelp) derivative used as a food additive to hold water in foods such as ice creams and other dairy products. Also used to thicken and stabilize foods.

alkaline (basic) food Food that, when metabolized, yields an alkaline (basic) ash (mineral) residue. Examples include most fruits and vegetables, dairy products, a few nuts (almonds), and coconut. *See also* acidic food.

alkalosis A disorder of the blood occurring when the body's pH exceeds 7.4, the healthy normal human value, because of excess generation of carbon dioxide/bicarbonate (base) or too little acid (hydrogen ion) production. *See also* acidosis.

allergen A protein in food or other environmental material that induces an allergic response (i.e., excess production of antibodies and other immune defense molecules); a type of antigen.

allowances *See* Recommended Dietary Allowance (RDA).

alternate dietary pattern Diets that do not contain red meats (the standard American diet) or diets in which the protein is primarily obtained from legumes. Some consumption of eggs and dairy products may be permitted; various types of alternate diets exist, including vegan diets, but they are all assumed to be balanced diets.

amenorrhea Never beginning menstrual cycles (primary amenorrhea) or absence of menstrual cycles for at least three consecutive months (secondary amenorrhea). *See also* oligomenorrhea.

American (U.S.) eating trends Trends since 1980 include decreases in the consumption of animal fats, cholesterol, meats, eggs, and dairy products, especially whole milk, and increases in the consumption of vegetable oils, poultry, fish, vegetables, fruits, low-fat dairy products, and whole grain products.

American Heart Association A nonprofit organization in the United States that fosters appropriate cardiac care in an effort to reduce disability and deaths caused by cardiovascular disease and stroke. Advocates the use of physical activity and diet to reduce the risk of developing cardiovascular disease.

amino acid An organic molecule with one carbon that contains four groups: COOH, NH_2, H, and R. The R-group is unique to each amino acid; amino acids are the structural units of peptides and proteins.

amino acid degradation The breakdown of an amino acid by the removal of the amine group (NH_2) that is either transferred to a keto acid or deaminated and shuttled into the urea cycle in the liver. The hydrocarbon backbone of the amino acid is further metabolized via the citric acid (Krebs) cycle to generate ATP, water, and carbon dioxide.

amino group (NH_2) A side group found in every amino acid that can combine with a carboxyl group to form a peptide bond, be transferred to an organic keto acid to form a new amino acid via transamination, or be removed via deamination in the liver and used to make urea. Also called an amine group.

ammonia (NH_3) A degradation product of amino acid metabolism; its ammonium cation, NH_4^+, is excreted into the urine by the kidneys.

amylase Enzyme that hydrolyzes α-1,4-glycosidic bonds in starch molecules. It is secreted by the salivary glands, where it acts in the mouth and the stomach (until inactivated), and by the pancreatic (exocrine) gland as a proenzyme.

amylopectin Branched-chain starch with branching points (α-1,6-glycosidic bonds) every 6 to 10 glucose units. The main chain consists only of α-1,4-glycosidic bonds; branching points permit more efficient storage of starches.

amylose Straight-chain starch with no branching points and consisting solely of α-1,4-glycosidic bonds between glucose units.

anabolic steroid Commonly used term for synthetic steroid molecules used by bodybuilders and power athletes to improve their muscle mass, muscle definition, or strength. These drugs are illegal for these purposes, but they can be used clinically to improve strength and bone mass of elderly subjects.

anabolism The synthetic (building) pathways within a cell or tissue that convert small molecules into larger, more complex molecules; for example, the synthesis of a fatty acid (palmitic acid) from eight acetyl CoA molecules, of a triglyceride from glycerol and three fatty acids, of cholesterol, of glycogen, and of protein. *See also* catabolism *and* metabolism.

anaerobic A process that does not require oxygen. Fermentation is an anaerobic process. *See also* aerobic.

anaerobic metabolism (respiration) Cellular respiration that does not require oxygen. *See also* glycolysis.

androgens Male sex steroid hormones responsible for male secondary sex characteristics; also present in females at lower concentrations because of its production by the adrenal cortex in both sexes. Act as growth promoters.

android fat distribution Fat distribution pattern where fat has a greater propensity to distribute around the abdomen as measured by the waist-to-hip ratio (WHR). It is the typical fat distribution pattern in adult males. *See also* gynoid fat distribution.

anemia A deficiency of hemoglobin that results in inadequate oxygen-carrying capacity by red cells. Can be caused by a nutrient deficiency (iron or one of several vitamins), increased red blood cell degradation, blood losses, genetic defect, or other reason. Iron deficiency anemia is a classic deficiency disease.

angina pectoris A myocardial condition in which the heart muscle does not get adequate oxygen delivery because of a partial, but not total, occlusion (blockage) of a coronary artery or arteriole.

angular stomatitis A set of epithelial lesions associated with the corners of the mouth that result from one or more B vitamin deficiencies.

animal fat Fat in animal-based foods. Animal fats (triglycerides) are typically high in saturated fatty acids (SFAs) and low in monounsaturated fatty acids (MFAs) and polyunsaturated fatty acids (PFAs). They exist as solids at room temperature.

animal protein foods Dietary protein from animal sources, such as meat, poultry, seafood, and eggs. Animal proteins typically provide greater quantities of specific amino acids, such as arginine, that give rise to hormones that following a meal stimulate insulin and glucagon release. Animal proteins are usually more complete than those obtained from plants. *See also* plant protein foods.

anion A molecule or mineral that carries a negative charge because it takes on one or more extra electrons in solution; for example, chloride ions carry a net negative charge of one (–1), as do most organic acids. *See also* cation.

anorexia A loss of appetite that is often, though not necessarily, associated with severe reduction in body weight for any reason, such as occurs in many cancer patients.

anorexia nervosa A psychological disorder characterized by refusal to eat, extreme weight loss, loss of menstrual cycles, and depressed gonadotropin hormones. *See also* bulimia nervosa.

anorexia of running Loss of appetite and tissue wastage in endurance runners who are running 80 to 100 miles per week. Prevalence and severity are not currently well understood.

antacid A class of drugs used to buffer the acid (H^+) produced by the gastric glands of the stomach. *See also* buffer.

anthropometric assessment The use of physical measurements of the body in determining the fitness of the body with respect to overweight, underweight, excessive fatness, and other parameters of body composition.

anthropometry The science of measurement of body dimensions, such as weight, height, waist circumference, skinfold thicknesses, body fat, body composition, and calculated variables, such as body mass index, waist-to-hip ratio, and others.

antibody An immunoglobulin made in response to antigenic stimulation by specific lymphocytes. Certain antibodies in the circulation exist because of a prior exposure to an antigen from a bacteria or other microorganism (i.e., acquired immunity), whereas others are in the blood at birth (innate). *See also* milk.

anticaking agent A class of additives used to protect against clumping of dry mixes and other dry powders by drawing water from the powder or dry mix and holding the water without affecting the powder or mix.

These anhydrous drying agents include salts of long chain fatty acids, calcium phosphates, and aluminum silicate and other silicate salts.

anticarcinogen A molecule that blocks the action of a carcinogen or reverses the promotion of an initiated cell.

antigen A molecule, typically a protein from a bacteria or virus, that produces an antibody response (i.e., increased synthesis of immunoglobulins by specific lymphocytes and release of them into the circulation).

antioxidant A molecule that prevents the reaction between an oxygen free radical and macromolecules of cells (e.g., unsaturated fatty acids, proteins, and nucleic acids).

antioxidant additive A class of food additives used to protect foods, especially fatty foods, from being oxidized and becoming rancid. Examples of such additives include BHT and BHA, which are used in many snack foods containing fair amounts of fat.

antioxidant nutrient Nutrient that acts as an antioxidant in the body, such as vitamin C, vitamin E, beta-carotene, and selenium.

apolipoprotein (apo) Class of proteins associated with plasma lipoproteins, such as very low density lipoproteins (VLDL), chylomicrons, low-density lipoproteins (LDL), and high-density lipoproteins (HDL).

apoptosis Programmed cell death that occurs when cells senesce and undergo death at a time characteristic of the cell type. Apoptosis may also occur due to toxic effects; the opposite of cell changes that lead to the induction of cancer cells.

appetite The desire to obtain and consume food. The appetite center in the brain, along with a satiety center, controls food intake. It is also influenced by external cues whether true hunger exists or not.

appetite center Part of the brain that acts to increase food gathering and ingestion, whether the person is hungry or not. *See also* satiety center.

apple fat distribution *See* android fat distribution.

arachidonic acid A polyunsaturated omega-6 fatty acid essential for the synthesis of eicosanoids, particularly inflammatory eicosanoids.

arterial wall A thick elastic structure consisting of three layers, the intima, middle (smooth muscle) layer, and the serosa. The intima is the site of initial fatty deposits, but advanced pathologic changes affect the smooth muscle cells that often convert to bone-producing cells.

arteriosclerosis Cardiovascular disease of the arteries with advanced pathology that is preceded by atherosclerosis.

ascorbic acid Another name for vitamin C.

Asian diet Diet characterized by high-carbohydrate foods, such as rice and other grains, low amounts of animal foods, and good amounts of vegetables (greens) and fruits. This type of diet is commonly consumed in Japan, parts of China, Korea, and other Asian nations. It typically contains small amounts of many different food items per meal including fish and other seafood, many vegetables, and heavily salted pork (especially in Japan).

assessment of nutritional status Procedures designed to capture as much information on nutritional intake and health as possible about an individual or population. Techniques include the ABCDs of assessment: anthropometrics, biochemical measurements of blood and other compartments, clinical observation and measurements, and dietary intake measures.

atheroma A fatty deposit (or plaque) on the wall of an artery or arteriole formed as part of the atherosclerotic process; less advanced in development than an atherosclerotic lesion. It is similar to a fatty streak but more defined.

atherosclerosis An early form of arteriosclerosis characterized by plaques or lipid accumulations (atheromas) in the arterial wall; any such lesion can become sufficiently extensive to interfere with or even to block blood flow through the vessel, causing a clot (thrombus) to form at the site of obstruction. Plaques contain cholesterol, triglycerides, other fatty molecules, and tissue debris, including mineralizations.

atmospheric packaging The use of oxygen-free gases such as nitrogen and carbon dioxide to replace oxygen-containing air so that certain foods, such as salads, pastas, and breads, can be stored for longer than normal.

ATP *See* adenosine triphosphate (ATP).

atrophy The loss of tissue mass, typically because of disuse.

Atwater equivalent The energy equivalent per gram of macronutrient or alcohol (ethanol). For example, 1 gram of carbohydrate yields 4 kilocalories of energy, 1 gram of fat yields 9 kilocalories, 1 gram of protein yields 4 kilocalories, and 1 gram of alcohol (pure or 200 proof) yields 7 kilocalories.

B cells (beta cells) Insulin producing cells located within the pancreatic islets of Langerhans.

B vitamins A group of water-soluble vitamins that includes thiamin, riboflavin, niacin, pyridoxin, folic acid, cobalamin, pantothenic acid, and biotin. These vitamins play important roles in the body's metabolic pathways in the synthesis of RNA and DNA. *See also specific vitamins.*

bacteria Microbes, such as *Escherichia coli*, that inhabit the gastrointestinal tract. Most are beneficial, but others are not. Breakdown of the gut barrier may lead to serious infection caused by invasion of gut bacteria or gut flora into body fluid compartments. *See also* gut bacteria.

bactericidal Refers to a substance that kills bacteria.

bacteriostatic Any action by an agent or process that keeps bacteria or their spores at low levels in foods, in blood, or in culture media.

balance (nutrient) Positive, zero, or negative difference between input and output with respect to nutrient or energy intake into the body. Status of balance aids in understanding the health outcome(s) of macronutrient consumption. *See also* calcium, iron balance, *and* protein.

balanced diet A diet balanced with respect to macronutrients, micronutrients, and non-nutrients, providing all the essential nutrients and energy from foods to support the daily activities in a healthy individual. Energy intake is not excessive, maintaining energy balance. Such diets for healthy males and females contain nutrient intakes at approximately RDA levels.

basal metabolic rate (BMR) The minimal expenditure of energy of the body under basal conditions, basically when awake and quietly resting. Approximately equivalent to resting energy expenditure (REE). *See also* resting energy expenditure (REE).

basal metabolism The basic set level of minimal metabolism in active cells of the body (i.e., lean body mass) that is under gene-driven thyroid hormone regulation.

basolateral membrane The membrane of intestinal absorbing epithelial cells or enterocytes at the serosal side that allow exit of nutrients to blood or lymphatic lacteals.

behavior modification (dietary) The use of psychological techniques for changing individual behaviors related to food consumption, including wise selection of foods, meal planning, and food preparation. Involves unlearning old, unhealthy habits and learning new, healthy behaviors.

beriberi A classic deficiency disease resulting from severe deficiency of thiamin; "wet" beriberi results from very low protein intake and the development of edema. May develop in people who eat large amounts of white rice.

beta-carotene A yellow pigment found in many fruits and vegetables, including carrots. Can be split into two vitamin A molecules by an enzyme located in the brush border surface of absorbing epithelial cells of the small intestine. It is a provitamin that has antioxidant properties that are distinctly different from vitamin A.

beta-oxidation The degradation of fatty acids to acetate molecules via a mitochondrial enzyme system.

bicarbonate ion (HCO_3^-) Acts as a base in body fluids and helps to buffer fluids by counteracting hydrogen ions (H^+) in solution. *See also* buffer.

bile A secretion of the liver (and by the gallbladder after storage) containing water, bile salts, cholesterol, and phosphatidylcholine, in addition to fat-soluble waste products. It is secreted into the small intestine, where it is critical to the digestion and absorption of fats.

bile pigment Degradation products of the heme component of hemoglobin (i.e., bilirubin). Icterus, or jaundice, occurs when the liver cannot secrete bile pigment into the gut lumen and it backflows into the blood.

bile salts (acids) Synthesized by liver cells from cholesterol, the primary bile acids, such as cholic acid, aid in fat digestion and absorption by acting as detergents in forming micelles in the small intestine. Bile salts can be modified in the gastrointestinal tract by bacteria to secondary bile acids through the loss of one or more hydroxyl groups. Secondary bile acids are considered to be carcinogenic in the large intestine.

bilirubin A bile pigment resulting from the degradation of the heme component of hemoglobin. If a blockage occurs in a biliary duct or the common bile duct of the liver, bilirubin backs into the blood, giving the body the yellowish hue characteristic of jaundice.

binding protein Blood binding proteins, such as vitamin-D binding protein (DBP), are used to carry water-insoluble molecules in the watery environment of body fluids.

binge-eating disorder (BED) An eating disorder characterized by excessive eating without control. *See also* bulimia *and* bulimia nervosa.

bioavailability The availability of micronutrients from foods within the lumen of the small intestine for absorption. This term especially applies to mineral cations that can be bound by several organic molecules in the lumen and thereby made unavailable for absorption.

biochemical assessment The component of nutritional assessment involving biochemical measurements of molecules and ions in body fluids, such as blood serum/plasma and urine, and in tissues, including skin, hair, exfoliated cells, and blood cells.

bioelectric impedance analysis (BIA) A technique using the body's resistance to electrical current to estimate total body fat.

biotin A B vitamin that is involved in multiple pathways that interconvert nutrients and energy-providing molecules throughout the body.

birth defect Developmental deformities that result in reduced functional capabilities; an example is spina bifida (unclosed spinal cord) at birth.

blanching The heating of fresh vegetables and other foods with steam or boiling water (scalding) in order to inactivate the enzymes that potentially cause food spoilage. In commercial food processing, foods that are blanched are either canned or frozen.

blood The central fluid compartment of the body containing blood cells and serum (or plasma). It is part of the extracellular fluid (ECF) compartment of the body. Serum contains many molecules and ions, including water-soluble and lipid-soluble species; lipid-soluble molecules require special carrier molecules or they must be aggregated as part of lipoproteins.

blood cholesterol (total) The total concentration of cholesterol in either fasting blood serum or plasma; the total blood cholesterol (TC) includes cholesterol in the circulating lipoproteins—VLDL, LDL, and HDL. A high level of total blood cholesterol is a risk factor for heart disease. *See also* cholesterol.

blood circulation The vasculature or vessels carrying blood from the heart to the lungs (i.e., pulmonary circulation) and from the heart to the rest of the body (i.e., systemic or general circulation), including the capillary beds.

blood glucose The concentration of glucose in blood that changes from low fasting values to the higher values of the postprandial period in healthy, normal individuals. High blood glucose levels are indicative of a potential disease state, such as diabetes.

blood pressure Arterial pressure measured at peripheral sites such as in the upper arm (brachial artery). It is the amount of pressure required to push blood throughout the body. Blood pressure depends on both cardiac output (the ability of the heart to pump) and peripheral resistance (the back pressure from the capillary beds of the body).

blood urea nitrogen (BUN) The concentration of urea in blood as determined by measuring the nitrogen (N) in urea. BUN is a measure of the kidney's ability to efficiently excrete waste.

body cell mass The metabolically active cells of the body; equivalent to the lean body mass, exclusive of fat tissue.

body composition Division of the body into two or more compartments, depending on the model used, based on the different chemical properties of those compartments. The two-compartment model consists of the fat tissue (compartment 1) and lean body mass (compartment 2). The three-compartment model consists of the fat compartment, lean body mass, and bone mass.

body mass index (BMI) An estimation of body fatness based on the equation of weight (kg)/height (m)^2 that is used to delineate overweight and obesity. Also referred to as the Quetelet index.

bone A mineralized tissue providing structural support for the body that contains an organic matrix (osteoid) that mineralizes and forms hydroxyapatite crystals.

bone formation The production of an organic bone matrix and mineralization of that matrix in an organized array through the action of osteoblasts.

bone mass (bone mineral content) The mineral phase of the entire skeleton, exclusive of the organic component of the skeleton; it consists primarily of hydroxyapatite. *See also* body composition.

bone mineral density (BMD) A measure of how much calcium and other minerals are in an area of bone.

bone modeling The building of bone from a genetic (DNA) program; osteoblasts that form bone dominate over osteoclasts that degrade bone.

bone remodeling The restructuring or recycling of bone after the cessation of growth and continuing throughout adulthood. The normal sequence is activation of the osteoclasts that degrade bone, which is then followed by the formation of new bone by osteoblasts to replace the bone lost during degradation. In older adults, the amount of bone formed is not enough to replace the amount lost, which results in a net loss of bone mass.

bone resorption The degradation of both the organic matrix (osteoid) and the mineral phases of bone tissue through the action of osteoclasts, which make a uniform resorption cavity on the bone surface.

bone turnover The sequential degrading and rebuilding of bone tissue; the rates of these processes vary at different stages of the life cycle, being higher during the early growth phases and in the early postmenopausal years and lower later in life.

botulism A common type of food poisoning caused by toxins produced by *Clostridium botulinum* bacteria that results in characteristic symptoms and death in a high percentage of those afflicted.

branched-chain amino acids (BCAAs) Essential amino acids with carbon backbones containing a branch point in the R-group. They include leucine, isoleucine, and valine. Primarily used for protein synthesis and also secondarily for energy.

branching point Additional bonds of complex carbohydrates; for example, α-1,6-glycosidic bonds in storage starches, such as amylopectin. Amylose starches contain only α-1-4-glycosidic bonds.

Brassica family Family of plants that includes broccoli, Brussels sprouts, cabbage, cauliflower, collards, horseradish, kale, mustard, radish, turnip, and watercress. Members of the Brassica family contain good quantities of many essential nutrients plus non-nutrient phytochemicals, especially indoles, that may help to prevent cancer.

breast feeding (lactation) The act of giving a baby human breast milk. Pediatricians currently recommend that mothers breast-feed their infants for a minimum of 6 months. Also called *nursing*.

browning reaction Several types of reactions, both nonenzymatic and enzymatic, cause browning and discoloration of foods during cooking or when exposed to ambient temperatures.

brush border The microvilli on the luminal surfaces of absorbing cells. They look like microscopic paint brushes with lengthy, well-organized cytoplasmic extensions. Similar to the villi, these membrane modifications of the epithelial cells of the small intestine greatly increase the surface area available for absorption.

buffer A molecule in solution that can neutralize the effects of both acids (H$^+$) and bases (OH$^-$) and thereby help to maintain acid–base balance within a narrow range. Also a class of food additives used to maintain a specific pH in order to prevent deterioration.

buffering effect of foods Partial neutralization of gastric pH by minerals and other components of food that helps prevent gastric and duodenal ulcers.

bulimia Refers to having a huge appetite for foods.

bulimia nervosa A psychological disorder characterized by bingeing and purging. *See also* anorexia nervosa.

bulk An old term for dietary fiber or indigestible residue of plant foods.

butter A dairy product made by churning fresh or fermented cream or milk. It is generally used as a spread and a condiment, as well as in cooking, such as baking, sauce making, and pan frying. Like many animal-based foods, it is high in saturated fat.

buttermilk A cultured type of skim milk resulting from the removal of butter from cream and the subsequent introduction of a bacterial culture to the remaining liquid.

C-H bond A carbon–hydrogen bond in organic compounds that is converted by metabolic pathways in cells into other useful bonds, such as the energy-rich phosphate bonds in ATP.

C-terminal (protein) The carboxyl (C) end of a peptide chain, as compared to the amino (N) end of a peptide chain (i.e., primary structure).

calcidiol Another name for 25-hydroxycholecalciferol.

calciferol Another name for vitamin D.

calcitriol Another name for 1,25-dihydroxycholecalciferol, the hormonally active form of vitamin D.

calcium A macromineral necessary for the mineralization of the skeleton and for many other functions, including extracellular blood clotting and intracellular regulation.

calcium homeostasis The regulation of blood calcium concentration (total) at about 10 milligrams per deciliter through the integrated actions of parathyroid hormone (PTH), the hormonal form of vitamin D (i.e., 1,25-dihydroxycholecalciferol), and other hormones working on the skeleton, gut, and kidneys.

calcium loading High intakes of supplemental calcium. Research suggests that it may promote arterial calcification, and thus increase the risk of cardiovascular disease.

calcium-to-phosphorus (Ca:P) ratio The ratio of calcium to phosphorus in the diet or in a food.

calciuria The normal presence of calcium in the urine. Calcium excretion in the urine varies from day to day in normal excretors, depending on calcium intake. It can also vary by age, gender, and race.

calorically dense foods Foods that have many calories (or kilocalories) per unit of weight but few micronutrients. Examples of calorically dense foods include many desserts, snack foods, cooking oils, salad dressings, and mayonnaise.

calorie The approximate amount of energy needed to raise the temperature of 1 gram of water by 1 degree Celsius; 1,000 calories is equal to 1 kilocalorie (kcal).

Canada's Guidelines for Healthy Eating Canadian food guidelines that include many of the same recommendations as made in the *Dietary Guidelines for Americans, 2010*.

cancer A disease of uncontrolled cell growth (proliferation). Cancer cells do not conduct the normal functions characteristic of their cell type, but they do keep the general characteristics of their tissue of origin. Cancer cells exist in varying degrees of undifferentiation; they may be contained or some may break away from their point of origin and spread (metastasize) to other tissues of the body. Cancer is the second most common cause of death in the United States.

capillary The smallest of the body's blood vessels.

carrageenan An extract of a common seaweed (Irish moss) that is rich in dietary fiber. It is used as a filler in many processed foods.

carbohydrate One of the macronutrients required by the body. Dietary carbohydrates include sugars, starches, and fibers. Commonly found in grains and root crops.

carbohydrate (glycogen) loading A technique used by endurance athletes to increase muscle glycogen before an event. It involves consuming high-carbohydrate (starch-based) meals several days (typically 6) prior to an event while at the same time decreasing training time.

carbon dioxide (CO$_2$) Exhaled gaseous product of aerobic respiration. Also found in tissues, where it must either be utilized to make urea in the liver or be eliminated via the lungs.

carbon–nitrogen (C-N) bond The chemical linkage between these two atoms in amino acids (also called a peptide bond) and many other molecules.

carbonyl group (CH=O) A functional organic group found in aldehydes, ketones, and keto acids.

carboxyl group (carboxylate group, COOH) Functional group that is added or removed in metabolic reactions; also known as an organic acid.

carboxylation An enzymatic reaction involving addition of a carboxyl group or carbon dioxide via a carboxylase enzyme to one keto acid, such as pyruvate, to form another, such as oxaloacetate, and that requires biotin as a coenzyme.

carcinogen A cancer-causing molecule that may or may not result in a gene mutation. Carcinogens can act by either initiating cancer through mutations or through the promotion of cancer cells that have already been initiated. In general, any molecule that causes cancer.

carcinogenesis The process of cancer cell formation and growth.

cardiac output (CO) The volume of blood pumped per beat (systole) by the left ventricle and the right ventricle; this variable is part of the equation that determines blood pressure.

cardiovascular disease (CVD) A disease that develops from atherosclerosis in the arteries and arterioles of the general circulatory system; includes coronary heart disease, peripheral artery disease, and stroke.

caries Erosion or decay of tooth surfaces in the oral cavity caused, in part, by bacterial plaque formation and acid etching of enamel.

carotene Typically beta-carotene, a yellow pigment found in many fruits and vegetables, including carrots. Beta-carotene can be split into two vitamin A molecules by an enzyme located in the brush border surface of absorbing epithelial cells of the small intestine; it is a provitamin that has antioxidant properties that are distinctly different from those of vitamin A.

carotenoid Family of molecules found in plants; includes beta-carotene. Some have vitamin A activity.

carrier (1) A protein molecule in a membrane that transfers molecules across the membrane, also known as a *transporter* or simply as a *porter*. (2) A molecule in the blood that transfers other molecules from a storage site to the site of use, such as retinol-binding protein (RBP) and vitamin D-binding protein (DBP).

case-control study A retrospective investigation of cases (defined as having a disease of interest) in comparison to control subjects without the disease but with similar backgrounds as the cases; other variables, including diet, are assessed in order to determine any statistical differences between the groups.

catabolism Degradative metabolic pathways within cells and in body fluids in which complex molecules are broken down into simpler ones. *See also* anabolism.

catalyst A molecule that increases the rate of a reaction without being part of the reaction itself. In biological systems, catalysts (known as enzymes) typically are proteins.

cation Mineral ions (or sometimes organic ions) that carry a positive charge because of the loss of one or more electrons when dissolved in fluids; examples include sodium, potassium, and calcium ions. *See also* anion *and* electrolyte.

cataract Clouding of the eye, leading to decreased vision.

CDC *See* Centers for Disease Control and Prevention (CDC).

cell The basic structural, functional, and biological unit of a living organism. The typical cell of a tissue in an organ system contains a plasma membrane, cytosol, nucleus, and organelles (mitochondria, endoplasmic reticulum, Golgi apparatus, and others). An exception is the mature circulating red blood cell, which does not have organelles or a nucleus. The function of a cell depends on the specific tissue and other factors.

cell-mediated immunity Specific circulating cells of the immune system, especially B cells, T cells, and NK cells, that help the body defend against the invasion of foreign organisms.

cellulose A nondigestible polysaccharide that makes up a large fraction of the dietary fiber in plant foods. It is classified as a water-insoluble fiber and is found mainly in the cell walls of plants.

cell organelle Structures within cells that perform specific functions: mitochondria, the nucleus, endoplasmic reticulum (smooth and rough), Golgi complex, and others.

cell renewal The replacement (turnover) of cells in a tissue through normal tissue maintenance; for example, epithelial cells are continuously replaced throughout life at a fairly constant renewal rate, which decreases with age.

Centers for Disease Control and Prevention (CDC) A federal agency within the Public Health Service charged with investigating disease outbreaks, maintaining health statistics, mounting prevention programs, and conducting periodic National Health and Nutrition Examination Surveys (NHANES).

cephalic phase A phase of the eating or pre-eating process involving the brain (mind), such as thinking of food and smelling and tasting food.

cereals and grains One of the basic food groups of the MyPlate food guidance system that consists of breads, baked goods, breakfast cereals, corn products, and rice products; whole grains are rich in dietary fiber.

chemical bond A linkage between atoms in molecules (or their ionic forms). The various types of chemical bonds vary in strength and other characteristics. For example, the C-H bond yields much of its energy for cellular generation of ATP. Disulfide bonds, hydrogen bonds, and other bonds are responsible for the secondary, tertiary, and quaternary structures of proteins.

chemoprevention The use of nutrients (or other molecules) to prevent the development of cancer or to decrease the growth of cancer that has already been initiated.

chief cells Secretory cells in gastric glands or pits that make and secrete pepsin.

childhood The period of life between infancy and adolescence; typically includes the onset of puberty. This period is marked by extensive growth (both general and skeletal) and extends from 1 year of age to 11 to 13 years in girls and 13 to 15 years in boys.

chloride Macromineral required by the body. Exists as an anion (Cl^-) in the body's fluids, balancing cations in solution. Extracellular concentrations are higher than intracellular concentrations.

cholecalciferol A form of vitamin D, also called D_3.

cholecystokinin (CCK) A hormone synthesized and secreted by gut cells (enterocytes) that has several effects following food ingestion, including inhibition of the feeding center of the brain.

cholesterol A lipid consisting of a characteristic four-ringed sterol structure that is used by the body for many functions. It is used either as is or after modification to cholic acid and other bile acids, steroid hormones, vitamin D, and other structures. Cholesterol can be produced by most cells and also obtained in the diet from animal products. Serum levels are routinely monitored because of linkage of high serum cholesterol with heart disease.

cholesterol ester A storage form of cholesterol formed by the addition of a fatty acid to cholesterol by an ester bond.

cholesterol synthesis The generation of new cholesterol molecules, especially in the liver; however, practically all cells of the body can synthesize cholesterol.

cholic acid A primary bile acid made by liver cells and secreted in bile as a salt of cholic acid with the amino acids taurine or cysteine.

choline An organic base used in the synthesis of phosphatidylcholine and other organic molecules. It is a source of methyl groups for the body.

ChooseMyPlate The food guidance system developed by the USDA for the U.S. population. It includes five food groups: grains, proteins, vegetables, fruits, and dairy. It uses an icon that shows a plate and drink to provide a pictorial display of how much of a meal should be represented by each food group. It provides an entire website with menus, a food composition table, and many other dietary tools. Sometimes simply referred to as MyPlate.

chromium An essential trace mineral whose function has not been established. It is possibly involved with insulin regulation as a glucose tolerance factor.

chromosome The highly coiled form of DNA and associated nucleoproteins that exists in the nucleus during mitosis and meiosis;

23 pairs of chromosomes exist in each cell except mature red blood cells (no chromosomes) and gametes (i.e., eggs and sperm, which have 23 unpaired chromosomes).

chronic Refers to long-term effects; the opposite of acute.

chronic disease A disease typically diagnosed in adulthood as a result of suboptimal dietary intake patterns, environmental risk factors, hormonal factors, or heredity. Common chronic diseases include cardiovascular disease, type 2 diabetes, chronic obstructive pulmonary disease (COPD), and cancer.

chronic kidney disease A degenerative disease of the kidneys that leads to reductions in the glomerular filtration of nitrogenous and other waste products, such as creatinine and urea. It is closely linked with hypertension and type 2 diabetes mellitus.

chylomicron A type of lipoprotein made by intestinal absorbing cells after a meal to carry triglycerides around the body. After most of the lipid contents are removed by peripheral tissues, a chylomicron remnant is taken up by the liver for degradation.

chylomicron formation Synthesis of lipoprotein by intestinal absorbing cells of the small intestine following the absorption of fatty acids and other lipids. The chylomicron is released to the lymphatic circulation for distribution of resynthesized triglycerides and other fat-soluble molecules to tissues of the body.

chylomicron remnant The residual and smaller part of the chylomicron left after partial degradation of triglycerides by lipoprotein lipase and release of other lipids in the peripheral capillary beds. The remnant is taken up by the liver and degraded. They are not found in the circulating blood of healthy fasting individuals.

chyme The viscous mixture of partially digested food contents and water in the lower stomach and small intestine. This partially digested material (i.e., digesta) is distinguished from a food bolus, which is essentially undigested.

circulatory system All of the body's blood vessels (arteries, veins, and capillaries) plus the heart. The lymphatic circulation is included as a special subsystem.

citric acid (citrate) An organic acid generated in metabolic pathways that is especially important in the citric acid (Krebs) cycle. It is also used as a food additive.

citric acid cycle (Krebs cycle) The cyclic metabolic pathway in the mitochondria that begins with the combining of oxaloacetate and acetyl CoA and ends with the regeneration of oxaloacetate after the oxidation of two carbon units to carbon dioxide and water, along with the generation of ATP and heat. The citric cycle also generates water (metabolic) and carbon dioxide through the complete oxidation of glucose, fatty acids, amino acids, and alcohol.

clearance The removal of a molecule from the blood; for example, by renal clearance, such as for creatinine, or by degradation of lipoproteins in the liver by hepatocytes.

clinical assessment The assessment of an individual with respect to clinical status. Involves the assessment of characteristic signs and symptoms that a clinician recognizes with the eye, hand, or instruments. Typically, a thorough physical examination can discover any abnormalities of the face, body surface (skin), or hair; fluid accumulation (edema); enlargement of the liver or spleen; or other changes that suggest a disease condition.

clinical sign An objective indicator of health status. Includes vital signs, such as body temperature, pulse rate, and heart rate.

clinical symptom Subjective evidence of disease, usually as described by a patient to a physician or nurse. Assessed during a physical examination as part of a clinical assessment to determine the health status of an individual.

clinical trial Investigation of a treatment using the double-blind, placebo-controlled method. Involves the comparison of a minimum of two experimental groups, one getting a treatment (e.g., a nutrient supplement) and the other a placebo. Subjects are randomly assigned to each group and the investigators and subjects do not know who is in which group (i.e., blinded).

clone (1) A cell line where all cells have the exact same DNA. (2) A selected lymphocyte cell line that has been established in the body as a result of stimulation by a specific antigen. Clones are the offspring cells of a single progenitor cell.

clotting (coagulation) The process whereby specific blood proteins combine with calcium ions in the blood, starting a cascade of reactions that results in a fibrin clot or plug of an artery or arteriole at the site of an atheroma dissection or break or other damage to a vessel.

clotting protein A protein that participates in the clotting of blood and coagulation. These proteins are usually called *factors* followed by a Roman numeral; e.g., factor VIII. Four of these proteins are vitamin K–dependent because they must have carboxyl groups inserted in glutamic acid residues in their polypeptides before they become active; these post-translational modifications require a carboxylase (enzyme) and vitamin K.

cobalamin (vitamin B$_{12}$) A B vitamin with a complex structure containing a cobalt atom. It is found only in animal foods and is produced by a few specific intestinal microorganisms. It requires binding by intrinsic factor (IF) before it can be absorbed and participate in the transfer of methyl groups. Humans have a large storage capacity in the liver for cobalamin. It is essential for cell division and nucleic acid synthesis.

cocarcinogen A molecule that promotes or enhances the development of cancer.

coenzyme An organic molecule, typically a B vitamin or modified B vitamin, that activates an enzyme and enhances the specific reaction catalyzed by the enzyme.

coenzyme A (CoA) A derivative of pantothenic acid that combines with the acid group of many organic acids prior to their degradation in metabolic pathways such as beta-oxidation and the citric acid (Krebs) cycle.

cofactor A molecule that participates with enzymes and coenzymes to increase the rate of a reaction. Cofactors typically are mineral ions such as calcium or magnesium.

collagen A protein molecule found in connective tissues that consists of a triple helix of polypeptide coils. It provides strength to connective tissues in tendons and ligaments. It is part of the organic matrix (osteoid) of skeletal tissues, where collagen fibers are arranged in an orderly array.

coloring agent A food additive, either natural or synthetic, used to improve the attractiveness of foods. Some coloring agents, such as some red dyes, are suspected of contributing to cancer in animal models.

colostrum The first milk produced by a mother during the first 2 to 3 days following birth of an infant. Colostrum is rich in immunoglobulins that provide a short period of acquired immunity for the breastfeeding infant before the infant can adequately synthesize his or her own immunoglobulins.

common bile duct The duct that carries both bile and pancreatic juice into the lumen of the upper duodenum. If blocked, jaundice can result.

complementation (complementarity) of proteins The combining of two or more plant proteins in the same meal to provide adequate amounts of all essential amino acids for the synthesis of proteins; for example, the use of corn and beans or other legumes together in a meal.

complete protein A high-quality protein that contains all the essential amino acids in reasonable quantities. *See also* incomplete protein.

conditionally essential vitamin A vitamin that is essential in the diet because it cannot be synthesized in human tissue. Choline is a conditionally essential vitamin.

connective tissue Body tissue composed of fibers (collagen and others) and other substances. Bones, teeth, tendons, and cartilage are all formed from connective tissue.

control of food intake The regulation of the intake of food by the integrated actions of the feeding center and the satiety center in the hypothalamus. *See also* food intake center *and* satiety center.

control group A group of subjects in an experiment (human, animal, or cell study) that do not get the treatment, but rather are treated with a placebo; that is, they receive a control (inert) material or substance or perhaps nothing at all. *See also* experimental group.

Cori cycle Pathway for removing lactic acid from peripheral tissues, principally exercising skeletal muscle, via the blood circulation to the liver for gluconeogenesis. Lactate derived from anaerobic respiration in peripheral tissues, especially exercising muscle of endurance athletes, is converted by the liver to glucose using the malate shuttle and the gluconeogenic pathway.

coronary artery A blood vessel supplying the heart muscle (myocardium) with oxygen and nutrients. Coronary arteries have a predilection to atherosclerotic lesions and blockage of blood flow.

coronary heart disease (CHD) Narrowing of the small blood vessels that supply blood and oxygen to the heart.

cortical (bone) tissue The compact component of bones, such as found in the shafts of long bones and in the outer surfaces of all bones.

corticosteroid (adrenocorticosteroid) A steroid hormone made by the adrenal cortex, such as cortisol and aldosterone. These hormones function in various metabolic pathways.

cortisol A corticosteroid of the glucocorticoid class. It is synthesized and secreted by the adrenal cortex and is involved in the metabolism of carbohydrates, fats, and proteins.

cow's milk Milk from cows and other dairy products are one of the basic food groups upon which a healthy diet is based. Milk is a good source of nutrients, especially calcium and protein.

creatine phosphate The high-energy molecule in skeletal muscle that serves as a readily available store of energy for muscle contractility and the events associated with movement.

creatinine A waste product produced through the muscle's use of creatine phosphate that can be used as a measure of renal function. It is found in both blood and urine.

crop yield Average production of a specific crop, such as bushels of corn, per acre or hectare.

cruciferous vegetables Vegetables of the Brassica family, such as cauliflower, broccoli, Brussels sprouts, and others. The name is derived from the crucifix pattern of their four-leaved flowers. These vegetables contain good amounts of cancer chemopreventive molecules, both nutrients and non-nutrients.

crypts (of Lieberkuhn) The epithelial cells lining these crypts at the base of the intestinal villi are continuously dividing to generate new cells that migrate up the villi and, after maturation, function as nutrient absorbing cells. Often referred to as an intestinal gland.

cytochrome An enzyme in mitochondria that is part of the electron transport chain that captures energy from the C-H bonds of acetate molecules (and other molecules that convert to acetate) from the citric acid (Krebs) cycle. It enables the oxidation of the two hydrocarbons (C-H) of acetate to carbon dioxide and water (metabolic).

cytokine General name given to signaling proteins (or polypeptides) secreted by white blood cells and other cells involved in host defense. These molecules serve as messengers to other cells to initiate responses to injury and infection. Subclasses include monokines (from white blood cells) and lymphokines (from lymphocytes).

cytoplasm (cytosol) The fluid (water) compartment of cells that contains dissolved molecules and ions. Organelles, especially the nucleus, are not considered part of the cytosol.

dairy group One of the basic food groups of the MyPlate food guidance system. This food group includes milk and foods made from milk, such as cheese, sour cream, and yogurt. Foods in this group are generally good sources of calcium.

dairy product A food derived from milk. Part of the basic MyPlate food groups. Consists of milks of varying fat content, cheeses, yogurts, buttermilk, and other products.

D-binding protein (DBP) A protein synthesized and secreted by the liver that has the capacity to bind all vitamin D molecules and metabolites in the blood. *See also* 1,25-dihydroxyvitamin D, 25-hydroxyvitamin D, *and* vitamin D.

DASH diet *See* Dietary Approaches to Stop Hypertension (DASH) diet.

deadly quartet A clustering of four diet-related chronic diseases, two or more of which are frequently found in the same individual and in a large proportion of Americans, namely, obesity, hypertension, atherosclerosis, and type 2 diabetes mellitus.

deamination The enzymatic removal of an amine group; in the liver these amine groups enter the urea cycle for elimination from the body.

death rate Another term for mortality rate.

decarboxylation Enzymatic reaction involving removal of a carboxyl group or carbon dioxide from an organic molecule. It requires a decarboxylase enzyme.

deficiency disease A disease that results from a severe deficiency of a particular macronutrient or micronutrient.

dehydration (1) Excessive loss of fluids from the body that contributes to water imbalance. (2) Removal of water from food products.

dehydroascorbic acid An oxidized form of vitamin C.

Delaney Clause An addition to the Food Additives Amendment of 1958 that specifically outlaws the use of any additive in human foods that has been shown to be carcinogenic in humans or animals.

dementia Loss of cognitive ability that results in problems with memory, language, and thinking. May be temporary or permanent, depending on the condition or disease causing it. Alzheimer's disease is a type of dementia resulting from plaques that form on the brain.

demography The study of the statistical characteristics of populations, such as births, deaths, fertility, and other health-related data collected by the National Center for Health Statistics.

denaturation Disruption of the three-dimensional structure of a protein resulting from chemical or physical treatment of the molecule; for example, heat will denature the protein of egg white (albumen).

dental caries Erosion or decay of tooth surfaces in the oral cavity caused, in part, by bacterial plaque formation and acid etching of enamel.

dental plaque Plaque formed by bacterial colonies on tooth surfaces.

deoxyribonucleic acid (DNA) A complex molecule that has a double-helix structure. Portions of DNA comprise genes. Long DNA strands are linked to nucleoproteins in chromosomes in the nucleus of cells; these molecules comprise the genetic code, regulating all cellular activities at the most fundamental level through the synthesis of specific functional proteins.

dermatitis Peeling of skin or desquamation. It is characteristic of many nutrient deficiency diseases, such as pellagra, and is especially prominent in kwashiorkor.

desertification The process through which fertile land becomes a desert due to poor agricultural methods, drought, deforestation, or climate change.

determinants of food intake The major factors that drive people to choose the foods that they consume: emotions, social and cultural factors, and food availability.

dextrin Derivative short and long polysaccharides resulting from the partial degradation of food starches, such as cornstarch. Beta-limit dextrins typically contain one α-1,6-glycosidic bond, which cannot be hydrolyzed by pancreatic amylase. Also used as a food additive.

dextrose Another name for glucose used mainly by the food industry. *See also* glucose.

DHA *See* docosahexaenoic acid (DHA).

diabesity Term coined to describe the presence of both diabetes and obesity. Can be defined as a metabolic dysfunction that ranges from mild blood sugar imbalance to full-fledged type 2 diabetes that occurs concomitantly with obesity.

diabetes mellitus A disease characterized by high levels of blood glucose. The two major types are type 1 and type 2. Type 1 diabetes mellitus is an autoimmune disease typically striking early in life. Type 2 diabetes mellitus is a chronic disease typically arising from overweight or obesity in mid-adult life or later.

diastolic blood pressure Component of blood pressure measured while the heart is at rest between beats. In a blood pressure reading, it is the second of the two values reported. For example, the diastolic blood pressure for a reading of 120/80 is 80 mm Hg. *See also* systolic blood pressure.

diet An eating pattern. May reflect a healthy eating pattern or that of a particular culture (e.g., Mediterranean diet). Often used to refer to weight-loss regimens, such as the Atkins Diet (low-carbohydrate) or the Zone Diet.

diet–disease linkage The linkage between a long-term dietary pattern and the development of a chronic disease.

Dietary Approaches to Stop Hypertension (DASH) diet Diet formulated by scientists and physicians to reduce hypertension. This diet is low in saturated fat, cholesterol, and total fat and focuses on fruits, vegetables, and fat-free or low-fat dairy products. Contains less sugar and red meat than the typical American diet. This diet also promotes maintenance of a healthy weight and can help to prevent the development of chronic diseases such as type 2 diabetes and cardiovascular disease.

dietary assessment The elicitation of information on dietary intake through questionnaires, such as a 24-hour dietary recall; a food diary or food record; or a food frequency instrument.

dietary fiber A broad class of indigestible plant polysaccharides and related molecules. Dietary fiber can be divided into water-soluble and water-insoluble fiber. Found in whole unrefined grains and fruits and vegetables, dietary fiber is part of a healthy diet and plays a role in reducing the risk of several chronic diseases.

dietary fiber intake The intake per day of dietary fiber. In the United States, intake averages 10 to 12 grams per day, whereas the recommended intake is 25 to 30 grams per day.

Dietary Goals Goals related to nutrition and health published by the Senate Select Committee on Nutrition and Human Health in 1970. These goals have been replaced by other documents, such as the *Dietary Guidelines for Americans* and the Recommended Dietary Allowances.

Dietary Guidelines for Americans Document prepared by a committee representing both the U.S. Department of Agriculture and the Department of Health and Human Services that provides guidelines that Americans should follow to ensure a healthy diet. The guidelines stress reductions in the consumption of fat, cholesterol, and sodium; increased consumption of complex carbohydrates, dietary fiber, and fruits and vegetables; maintenance of a desirable body weight; and limited alcohol consumption. The guidelines are updated every 5 years.

dietary pattern A typical pattern of eating within a society or culture. For example, in the United States and many Western nations traditional meals have contained one or more servings of red meat plus dairy products, breads, potatoes, beans, or one other vegetable. Alternate dietary patterns, including various forms of vegetarianism, have greatly modified the traditional "meat and potatoes" approach to eating in recent decades.

Dietary Reference Intakes (DRIs) Recommended intakes of nutrients that are presented in a series of books from the Institute of Medicine. Each nutrient either has a Recommended Dietary Allowance (RDA) or an Adequate Intake (AI), depending on the availability of information upon which to make a recommendation.

dietary risk factors for chronic diseases Several major dietary risk factors have been found by epidemiologic investigations to be associated with one or more of the chronic diseases, namely, excessive energy, sodium (salt), saturated fatty acids, and insufficient dietary fiber, fruits, vegetables, whole grains, calcium, potassium, and magnesium.

dietetic food A food that is marketed for individuals with a specific disease who require a modified diet, such as those with diabetes mellitus. Dietetic foods typically contain low amounts of sugar or no sugar, but they may contain artificial sweeteners. Such foods may also be low in fat and in total energy.

diet-induced thermogenesis (DIT) Energy expended and waste heat generated as a result of processes required for macronutrient digestion and absorption. DIT for proteins represents approximately 20% of the energy contained in the protein in the meal; DIT is lower for carbohydrates and lowest for fats (triglycerides). The overall DIT for a mixed meal is approximately 10% of the calories the meal contains.

differentiation The characteristic (normal) changes of cells as they mature from newly formed daughter cells (via cell division) to functional cells in a tissue (or organ). Cancer cells do not undergo normal differentiation.

diffusion Passive transfer of molecules or ions across a membrane from a region of higher concentration to one of lower concentration; net downhill movement of chemical species, especially of nutritionally important fat-soluble molecules.

digestibility The ability of food materials to be degraded to their macronutrient and micronutrient components within the gut lumen. Animal foods are more easily digested than plant foods. Plant foods are often high in fiber, which decreases their digestibility.

digestion The physical and chemical (enzymatic) degradation of foods that results in the release of nutrients, especially macronutrients (i.e., proteins, fats, and carbohydrates), so that the digestion products can be absorbed across the gut mucosa. The major role of digestion in the stomach and small intestine is to create many small absorbable molecules from the large macronutrient molecules.

digestive tract Also known as the gastrointestinal (GI) tract, alimentary tract, or gut. This organ system consists of the tube that runs from the mouth to the anus and the associated organs, such as the salivary glands, pancreas, liver, and glands of the tube itself. Although the fluids in the lumen of the gut are technically part of the external environment, they are significantly modified by secretions of the contents of the various glands to allow for digestion and then absorption of nutrients.

diglyceride A lipid containing two fatty acids linked to glycerol, with one hydroxyl (alcohol) group of glycerol remaining unbound.

1,25-dihydroxyvitamin D (calcitriol) The hormonal form of vitamin D that is made in the kidneys from 25-hydroxyvitamin D. It acts on cells in the small intestine to increase calcium absorption. Also known as 1,25-dihydroxycholecalciferol.

disaccharide A sugar consisting of two monosaccharide units. Examples include sucrose, lactose, and maltose. *See also* monosaccharide *and* polysaccharide.

disease Any abnormality or derangement in tissue anatomy or function that affects the host (i.e., pathologic change). Sometimes referred to as a disorder, condition, or dysfunction. Lay terms include sickness, ailment, and malady.

disease prevention Interventions taken before the onset of a disease. May include drug therapy, behavior modification, dietary changes, lifestyle changes, and public health initiatives.

distribution of macronutrients in U.S. diet The current approximate percentages of the macronutrients are as follows: carbohydrate 50%; fat 35%; protein 15% (alcohol is minimal).

diuretic A class of drugs, typically antihypertensive agents, that increases water (fluid) loss via the kidneys. Typically increase urinary losses of sodium and sometimes potassium in addition to water. Alcohol and a few dietary ingredients also act as diuretics.

DNA *See* deoxyribonucleic acid (DNA).

docosahexaenoic acid (DHA) An essential fatty acid of the omega-3 family (C22:6) that is commonly found in fish oil.

double-blind study A clinical trial in which neither the subjects nor the investigators know which subjects are receiving treatment (e.g., nutrient or drug) or placebo.

double bond A type of carbon-to-carbon atomic bond that involves two bonds (C=C) rather than one (C-C). Represents a point of unsaturation with respect to hydrogen atoms in a hydrocarbon.

down-regulation A decrease in the number of hormone receptors in a cell membrane. For example, the number of insulin receptors decreases when cells contain too much glucose, as in insulin resistance.

DRIs *See* Dietary Reference Intakes (DRI).

drug metabolism The metabolism of foreign molecules, such as drugs and other organic molecules from the environment. Occurs primarily in the liver hepatocytes. The hepatocytes typically oxidize these molecules, thus inactivating them and increasing their solubility in body fluids for excretion in the urine or in bile. Biliary excretion usually is greater for drugs that are conjugated by the liver with other molecules (glucose derivative and others).

drying A traditional method of food preservation to remove moisture and thereby preserve a food. This method is often used to preserve cereal grains and legumes.

dual-energy x-ray absorptiometry (DXA) A scan of bone and soft tissues of the body by a machine that uses two energy sources of x-rays to separate measurements of bone from soft tissues (i.e., adipose tissue). The total body scan permits estimations of mass of bone and fat, which enables the determination of lean body mass (primarily muscle). DXA is used to measure bone mineral content (BMC) and bone mineral density (BMD).

duodenum The first segment of the small intestine, approximately 12 inches in length, where intestinal absorption is typically highly efficient.

DV *See* Percent Daily Value (PDV or %DV).

DXA *See* dual-energy x-ray absorptiometry (DXA).

dyspigmentation (hair) Change in hair color because of loss of production of normal pigment. It often appears as a flag, with stripes of abnormal dyspigmented light bands alternating with normal dark bands. It is a characteristic of kwashiorkor.

EAR *See* Estimated Average Requirement (EAR).

early life programming Theory that common chronic diseases in adult life originate during fetal life, such that low birth weight may be linked to later development of hypertension, diabetes, obesity, and cardiovascular disease. Also called the "Barker hypothesis."

eating disorder An abnormal eating pattern that affects a person's health. Examples include anorexia nervosa and bulimia nervosa.

edema Fluid accumulation outside the blood vascular compartment, especially in extracellular tissues of the ankles, wrists, and abdomen; appears as a swelling of the lower legs and arms.

eicosanoids The general name of hormone molecules derived from specific 20-carbon (eicosa-) polyunsaturated fatty acids. Examples include arachidonic acid (AA, C20:4) found in vegetable oils and eicosapentaenoic acid (EPA, C20:5) found in fish oils.

eicosapentaenoic acid (EPA) An essential fatty acid of the omega-3 family (C20:5) that is an eicosanoid precursor. It is found in good amounts in fish oil.

EIT *See* exercise-induced thermogenesis (EIT).

elderly period The period after adulthood from about 60 years to the end of life. The young-old (early elderly) includes those ages 60 to 80 years; the old-old (late elderly) includes those from 80 to 100 years. Centenarians are those 100 years and older.

electrolyte A charged ion in solution. The three major mineral ions found in serum (and also in cells) are sodium (Na^+), potassium (K^+), and chloride (Cl^-) ions. *See also* anion *and* cation.

electron transport chain Part of cellular respiration that occurs in the mitochondria. It requires enzymes (cytochromes) and water-soluble vitamins, riboflavin (FAD), and niacin (NAD). It is an important generator of ATP.

elevated body temperature A condition that may result from many conditions and diseases; it typically occurs in the hypermetabolic response to infections, especially of bacteria, as a result of increased catabolism, inflammation, and heat production.

embolism The lodging of a clot (thrombus) that has broken away from the site of origin and is caught in the capillaries of the lungs, brain, heart, or other tissues.

embryo An early stage of development of a fertilized egg prior to implantation in the uterus; the human embryo exists *in utero* for approximately 4 weeks, after which the circulation of the placenta supplies the nutrients and oxygen necessary for development as a fetus, the second stage of pregnancy.

emulsification The process of mixing molecules that are not compatible, such as water and oil, through the use of a detergent or a similar complex, such as bile, that has both water-soluble and fat-soluble chemical groups. Used in food processing to make products such as mayonnaise.

emulsifier A food additive or other molecule that enhances the mixing of lipid-soluble and water-soluble components in processed foods. Also acts as a food stabilizer. Examples include monoglycerides, diglycerides, lecithin, and other phospholipids.

emulsion Mixtures of water- and fat-soluble molecules that hold together because of the presence of an emulsifier. Emulsions form in the presence of bile in the small intestine following the physical breakdown of fat globules from foods in the stomach. Emulsions are typically larger than micelles, which also form in the small intestine from emulsions.

enamel The hard outer layer of teeth that contains a highly ordered array of the mineral, hydroxyapatite. Can be strengthened by fluoride.

endemic goiter Increase in the incidence of an enlarged thyroid within the population of a circumscribed geographic area that results from either too little intake of iodine or from the consumption of a goitrogen that interferes with the uptake of iodine by the thyroid gland.

endocrine gland A gland that synthesizes and secretes endocrine hormones. Part of the diffuse endocrine system. Examples include the hypothalamus, anterior pituitary, thyroid, islets of Langerhans, gonads (ovaries and testes), the GI tract, and the kidney.

endoplasmic reticulum (ER) The membrane complex within the cytosol that plays important roles in the synthesis of fatty acids, triglycerides, lipoproteins, and other molecules. Smooth ER (sER) synthesizes molecules for use within the cell, whereas rough ER (rER) synthesizes molecules that have a protein component and that are secreted for export to other parts of the body.

energy (calorie) A physical unit of energy that is derived from food macronutrients and alcohol; 1 kilocalorie is the amount of heat required to raise the temperature of a gram of water 1 °C. Energy can be also expressed in joules, where 1 kilocalorie is equal to 4.2 kilojoules.

energy allowance (RDA) The recommended energy intake for males and females at moderate levels of activity that will sustain good health. Females 19 years and older have an energy RDA of 2,400 kilocalories; the value for males 19 years and older is 3,100 kilocalories.

energy balance The balance between energy intake and energy expenditure. Energy imbalance represents either higher intake than expenditure or the reverse. Positive (+) energy balance results in weight gain. Negative (−) energy balance results in weight loss.

energy consumption The typical pattern of caloric intake from diverse foods containing macronutrients. Energy consumed should equal energy expenditure in activities on a regular basis so that body weight remains reasonably constant.

energy expenditure in activities The energy spent over 24 hours in various activities, including walking, eating, reading, writing, sports, and other tasks. It is the most variable component of total daily energy expenditure.

enrichment A specific type of fortification for cereal flours and products. Traditional fortificants in wheat and corn flours are thiamin, riboflavin, niacin, and iron, and, more recently, folate.

enterocyte The primary columnar absorbing cell type of the gut epithelium. Also used to refer to any cell type, including goblet cells, in the epithelial lining of the gastrointestinal tract.

enterohepatic circulation (EHC) The circulation of bile acids and salts and fat-soluble components of bile fluid from the liver (and gallbladder) into the gastrointestinal tract and then the absorption of a percentage of these molecules in the ileum for return to the liver for reuse.

enterokinase Enzyme located (fixed) on the brush border surface of epithelial cells of the small intestine that cleaves pancreatic proenzymes to active enzymes.

enzyme A protein or protein complex that acts as a biological catalyst that speeds up a chemical reaction. Also a type of food additive used in the processing of foods. *See also* catalyst, digestion, food additive, *and* hydrolytic enzyme.

EPA *See* eicosapentaenoic acid (EPA).

epidemiology The quantitative science that examines the risk factors or determinants that contribute to the prevalence of a disease or the incidence of new cases in populations. *See also* incidence *and* prevalence.

epinephrin(e) A hormone, also known as adrenalin, secreted by the adrenal medulla and sympathetic nerve endings that acts to speed up energy availability for muscular activity, such as hepatic glycogenolysis.

epithelial cell Cells that line tubes and cavities in the body. They have rapid turnover or renewal and are typically susceptible to carcinogens and mutagens. *See also* cancer, enterocyte, epithelial sheet (epithelium), *and* mucus.

epithelial sheet (epithelium) Epithelial tissue that consists of specialized epithelial cells that line the gastrointestinal tract (gut), respiratory tract, and the urogenital tract. These tissues act as barriers and as absorbing surfaces. They also contain cells that secrete mucus that coats the luminal surface and thereby protects the epithelia. *See also* absorption, epithelial cell, host defense mechanisms, *and* mucus.

ergogenic aid Molecules that improve physical performance or exercise; nutritional ergogenic aids typically are substances found in common foods, but that are provided in larger quantities to provide a druglike dose; other types of ergogenic aids also exist.

erythrocyte Mature red blood cells that carry oxygen to all cells bound to hemoglobin. They have a finite life of approximately 120 days. Anemic erythrocytes do not deliver adequate amounts of oxygen; a mature erythrocyte does not contain a nucleus, mitochondria, or other cell organelles.

essential (indispensable) amino acid Amino acid that must be supplied in the human diet because humans do not have enzymes that can synthesize them, as opposed to nonessential amino acids, which can be synthesized by the body. Animal products generally contain greater amounts of the essential amino acids than plants. *See also* nonessential amino acid.

essential fatty acid (EFA) Fatty acids that must be supplied in the diet because humans do not have enzymes that can synthesize them. Includes two categories: those with the first unsaturation at the omega-6 position (n-6 fatty acids) and those with the first unsaturation at the omega-3 position (n-3 fatty acids). Omega-6 fatty acids are found in vegetable oils such as corn oil; omega-3 fatty acids are found in fish oils.

essential nutrients Approximately 50 nutrients that are essential for life and good health.

ester bond A chemical bond formed between an organic acid (COOH) and an organic hydroxyl group (OH) through the removal of a water (H_2O) molecule; binds fatty acids to glycerol in triglycerides.

Estimated Average Requirement (EAR) The amount of intake of a nutrient needed by the average individual to maintain good health. If a nutrient has an EAR, its Recommended Dietary Allowance (RDA) is based on the mean (average) + 2 standard deviations above the mean.

estrogens Female sex hormones. Natural estrogens are responsible for female sexual development and play an essential role in fertility, pregnancy, and lactation.

ethnic foods (diets) Foods prepared and eaten by different ethnic groups. In the United States, ethnic foods are represented by Asian (Chinese, Japanese, and others), Italian, Greek, French, Mexican, and many other specific ethnic diets.

etiology The causation of a disease. Often based on one or more risk factors that contribute to the development of a disease. The etiology of most chronic degenerative diseases involves multiple risk factors.

exercise-induced thermogenesis (EIT) Energy expended as heat by the body because of muscular activities; this energy is over and above the energy expended for basal metabolism (BMR).

experimental group The group of subjects in an experiment (human, animal, or cell study) that receives a treatment (e.g., nutrient or other molecule) as opposed to the control group. *See also* control group *and* placebo.

extracellular fluid The fluid compartment of the body, including blood plasma, extravascular fluids, and cerebrospinal fluid, that bathes all tissues and permits exchanges of nutrients, waste products, oxygen, and carbon dioxide with cells.

facilitated diffusion Transfer of solutes (molecules and ions) across a membrane down a concentration gradient (from high to low) through the use of a carrier molecule (protein), but without the expenditure of energy (ATP). Typical transport mechanism for water-soluble chemical species.

FAD *See* flavin adenine dinucleotide (FAD).

fad diets Popular diets that are designed to yield rapid weight loss but that typically are deficient in one or more essential micronutrients because of the limited numbers of foods allowed. Such diets cannot be followed for long periods of time.

FAE *See* fetal alcohol effects (FAE).

failure-to-thrive Condition in infancy (or later) in which poor growth (height and weight) occurs for unknown reasons, but typically because of reduced food consumption or malnutrition.

famine Situation in which food availability becomes so limited that severe undernutrition and disease follow in a widespread geographic area; typically associated with crop failures, adverse weather conditions, soil erosion, war, or pestilence.

FAS *See* fetal alcohol syndrome (FAS).

fast food Foods obtained quickly from outlets that typically are designed to prepare food rapidly and often for take-out. Many fast foods are high in calories and low in nutrients. There are many fast-food chains in the United States.

fasting The absence of food (but not necessarily water or other fluids) for a period of time. For example, an overnight fast typically lasts 12 hours. Fasting becomes total starvation when no food is consumed for 2 days or longer; physiologic mechanisms respond rapidly to fasting to protect vital bodily resources.

fasting blood glucose Measurement of blood glucose under conditions of overnight fasting (approximately 12 hours) for the purpose of assessing regulation of blood glucose. This measurement is occasionally followed by a glucose tolerance test. *See also* blood glucose.

fasting blood lipids Measurement of blood lipids under conditions of overnight fasting (approximately 12 hours) for the purpose of assessing the concentrations of total cholesterol, triglycerides, and lipoprotein fractions of cholesterol, such as from HDL and LDL. Fasting typically removes all chylomicrons from the blood and allows for a more stable measurement of triglycerides.

fasting hypoglycemia A condition of abnormal low blood sugar.

fat A type of lipid molecule. Another name for triglyceride molecules containing glycerol and three fatty acids. The fatty acid composition determines whether the fat is solid or liquid at room temperature. *See also* adipose (fat) tissue *and* triglyceride.

fat digestion The enzymatic degradation of fats in the gastrointestinal tract after micelle formation in the presence of bile. The products are glycerol and free fatty acids and mono- and diglycerides.

fat distribution Distribution of fat in the body. Fat is typically distributed around the waist or hips and thighs. *See also* android fat distribution *and* gynoid fat distribution.

fat flavor Desirable flavor (and often odor) arising from the organic molecules in fatty foods.

fat mass The body compartment consisting of all fat tissue, including subcutaneous fat, abdominal fat, and other stores of fat tissue. *See also* body composition.

fat-soluble vitamin Vitamins that are soluble in lipids or organic solvents. Includes vitamins A, D, E, and K; beta-carotene is also considered a fat-soluble vitamin. *See also* water-soluble vitamin.

fat substitute Substances used to replace fats in foods in an effort to reduce fat intake. They have not found wide acceptance due to their lack of flavor, relative solubility compared to real fats, and the fact that most cannot be used in baking or frying.

fatty acid Class of lipids that contains a hydrocarbon chain of 10 to 22 carbons and a carboxyl group at one end; these molecules can be fully saturated or unsaturated. Typically they are obtained as part of the diet in triglycerides or phospholipids. *See also* saturation (fatty acid) *and* unsaturated.

fatty acid synthesis A complex enzyme system in the endoplasmic reticulum synthesizes palmitic acid in human tissues, starting with acetyl CoA molecules; newly synthesized fatty acids are incorporated into triglycerides for distribution from the liver via very low density lipoprotein (VLDL) particles to other tissues of the body. Certain other fatty acids may be elongated and unsaturated enzymatically in cells.

fatty liver Accumulation of fat stores in hepatocytes following excessive calorie and/or alcohol consumption that serves as an indicator of abnormal metabolism.

fatty streak An elongated fat deposit in the intimal layer of the walls of arteries and arterioles. It is the beginning of an abnormality that may develop into an atheroma and more severe atherosclerosis. *See also* atheroma *and* atherosclerosis.

FDA *See* Food and Drug Administration (FDA).

federal food programs USDA programs that provide foods or food vouchers for needy individuals or families. These programs include the School Lunch Program, the Supplementary Food Program for Women, Infants, and Children (WIC), and the food stamp program (SNAP).

feeding center (brain) Food intake center of the hypothalamus that regulates food-gathering and ingestive behaviors. Consists of neurons that receive signals via hormones and cytokines or cues from external stimuli (odors, visual figures, or images).

female athlete triad A condition occurring among some female athletes that is characterized by amenorrhea or oligomenorrhea, poor eating habits (but not true anorexia), and osteopenia (and possibly stress fractures).

ferritin Storage form of iron found primarily in the liver but also measurable in blood serum. It is derived through the combining of iron with apoferritin, a protein synthesized in the liver that is capable of storing large quantities of iron. *See also* anemia, iron, *and* iron deficiency.

fetal alcohol effects (FAE) A disorder observed in babies or young children of mothers who consumed excessive amounts of alcohol during pregnancy. Results in reduced intelligence test scores, but the overall effects on child development may be minor.

fetal alcohol syndrome (FAS) A severe disorder in an offspring resulting from heavy alcohol consumption, frequently binge drinking, by the mother during pregnancy. Results in physical abnormalities in the development of the face, limbs, and internal organs, in addition to retarding brain development and severely affecting intelligence.

fetus The developing human in the uterus that receives its oxygen and nutrients from the mother via the placenta. The fetal nutritional supply depends on the mother's eating habits and other lifestyle practices, such as cigarette smoking, alcohol consumption, and maternal weight gain, and health.

firming agents A class of food additives used to keep foods firm and coherent. Includes calcium carbonate, calcium phosphate, and magnesium sulfate.

flavin adenine dinucleotide (FAD) A coenzyme commonly utilized in oxidation-reduction reactions throughout the body, particularly those related to energy production in glycolysis and the citric acid (Krebs) cycle. Formed from the vitamin riboflavin.

flavoprotein A protein that contains riboflavin in the form of flavin adenine dinucleotide (FAD).

flavor of foods Typical flavor of a food detected by the tongue (not nose), such as strawberry, lemon, coffee, and many others. Flavors result from the organic molecules in the foods, especially those in the fat component.

flavoring agents A class of food additives used to provide a specific flavor in a food that normally does not have the flavor; these molecules may be either natural extracts or artificial substances.

fluoridation Addition of fluoride ions to municipal drinking water for the purpose of preventing dental caries. *See also* dental caries.

fluoride Ionic form of the trace mineral fluorine. Helps maintain healthy tooth enamel and surfaces in the oral cavity.

fluorosis Condition of excess fluoride accumulation in the hard tissue of teeth and bones. Teeth become discolored and, in extreme cases, flake off pieces, giving them an etched appearance. In bone, the quality of tissue is diminished and fractures (especially microfractures) are more likely to occur.

foam cell Cells that contain fat and cholesterol that develop from macrophages or monocytes in early atherosclerotic lesions of arteries. Such cells are typical of the pathologic changes in the artery wall.

folic acid (folate, folacin) A B vitamin that is essential for the renewal of tissues that are turned over because of its role in facilitating cell division (mitosis) and nucleic acid synthesis. If not present in adequate amounts during pregnancy, neural tube defects may occur in the fetus.

food additive A chemical added to a food to maintain or preserve its desirable qualities, including color, flavor, appearance, and nutrient content. *See also* GRAS list.

Food and Drug Administration (FDA) The federal agency that regulates the safety of the U.S. food supply and that mandates food labeling. It is also responsible for all drug safety and licensing issues.

food assistance Food provided by countries with food surpluses to countries that are experiencing food shortages. International organizations such as the United Nations are often responsible for identifying areas in need of assistance and in coordinating the delivery of supplies.

food availability The availability of food or foods in a particular geographic region because of production, distribution, or cultivation of the foods for human consumption. It is one of the basic determinants of food intake, particularly in poorer nations. *See also* food habit.

food bolus The partially moistened food cluster that leaves the mouth, passes through the esophagus, and enters the stomach still containing active salivary amylase molecules, where it becomes chyme. A vitamin or mineral pill may also be consumed as a "bolus" dose.

food composition table A table or database that contains data on the nutrient content of foods. Such tables are published by U.S. government agencies, such as the USDA, and in other sources, such as *McCance and Widdowson's The Composition of Foods.*

food diary A record of foods and beverages consumed over a period of time, typically 3 to 7 days, that is used as part of a nutritional assessment.

food disappearance data Data collected by USDA economists to estimate the kinds of foods purchased in the United States. Such data are a crude indicator of total food consumption, but they do not take into consideration food waste in preparation of food for actual consumption.

food fallacies Beliefs about the properties of foods that are not substantiated by scientific data.

food groups Groupings of foods that are used to aid consumers in the wise selection of a variety of foods to meet the body's needs and to maintain health. The USDA's ChooseMyPlate food guidance system currently includes five groups of foods: grains, vegetables, fruits, protein (meat and beans or legumes), and dairy foods. *See also* ChooseMyPlate.

food habit The usual selection of foods by an individual or a defined population on a long-term basis that characterizes a pattern of eating that reflects traditions, culture, and availability.

food insecurity Condition when people do not have adequate access to safe, nutritious foods to meet their dietary needs and to sustain an active, healthy life.

food intake center An area of the brain in the lateral nucleus of the hypothalamus that controls food intake behavior. This feeding center is connected with the satiety center and other neuronal pathways in the lower brain. *See also* satiety center.

food intolerance An adverse effect or reaction that arises from consuming a specific food (e.g., intolerance to milk) but that is not an allergic response to a food protein.

food irradiation The use of penetrating x-rays or gamma rays to kill all microorganisms in a food. It has been used successfully by the military to preserve foods. More recently, it has been approved for use with meats, such as hamburger, to reduce *E. coli.*

food labeling Legally required information that must appear on the label of a food item, such as the manufacturer, ingredients, and nutrient composition. *See also* Nutrition Facts panel.

food laws Federal laws enacted to govern the safety of the food supply through regulation of food additives, food labeling, and other food-related issues.

food myths Old beliefs about foods or the benefits of foods that are totally or partially incorrect.

food preparation Altering foods so that they are edible, such as peeling, cutting, cooking, and other steps.

food preservation Preparing foods for storage through methods such as freezing, canning, irradiating, pasteurizing, drying, or salting. It enables foods to be stored, distributed, processed, and marketed.

food preservative A food additive used to control bacterial growth, thus increasing a food's shelf life, portability, and safety. Two common food preservatives are salt and sugar.

food processing The modification of a food by physical or chemical means. With extensive food processing, it may be difficult to know what the original raw food looked or tasted like. The techniques used by food processsors enable foods to be brought efficiently and economically from fields and barns to our tables.

food pyramid An older food guide established by the USDA for Americans to follow in selecting a balanced diet each day. The base of the pyramid was cereals and grain products, followed by fruits and vegetables, meats and protein foods, and dairy products. It was capped by miscellaneous foods, including nuts and seeds and olive and other vegetable oils. The USDA replaced the food pyramid with ChooseMyPlate. *See also* ChooseMyPlate *and* pyramid.

food questionnaire Tool used to assess usual intakes of foods over a long period of time, usually a month to a year. Questionnaires may be qualitative, asking about the frequency of a targeted variety of specific foods, or semiquantitative, asking about frequency and about serving sizes of a comprehensive set of foods. The resulting data are used to estimate food and nutrient intakes.

food safety Protection of the food supply so that it is safe for human consumption. Many laws and regulations exist to ensure the safety of foods. The Food and Drug Administration (FDA) oversees most food safety regulations, but the U.S. Department of Agriculture (USDA) and a few other federal agencies are also involved in the safety of the U.S. food supply.

food selection Choosing foods from the basic food groups to ensure adequate intake of all the required macronutrients, micronutrients, and phytochemicals to maintain health.

food shortages Shortages in food supplies that are typically local in nature due to crop failures and armed conflicts. These shortages can affect the nutritional status and disease rates of a population. They can be life-threatening for many people, especially the very young and very old who have depressed immune systems.

food spoilage The breakdown of food products that can occur by browning reactions, oxidation reactions, and contamination with microorganisms, such as molds and bacteria.

foodborne illness An illness resulting from the consumption of foods contaminated with pathogenic bacteria or viruses or natural toxins. Most foodborne illnesses are caused by insufficient cooking, poor sanitation, and inadequate storage. Characteristic symptoms include diarrhea and other disturbances, such as vomiting and cramping; elevated body temperature; and fluid losses.

fortificant The specific nutrient added to a food during fortification.

fortification of foods The addition of nutrients to foods for the purpose of improving intakes of nutrients that are not consumed in adequate amounts.

fortified B vitamins The three vitamins added to wheat flour in the early 1940s (along with iron) were thiamin, riboflavin, and niacin because these nutrients were low or deficient in the diets of many U.S. citizens; only in the late 1990s was folate (folic acid) also included in fortification because this vitamin protects against birth defects.

fracture Breaking of bone by external forces. Most occur due to impact from a large force (strain), such as being thrown by a horse, being in an auto accident, or other high-impact collision. May also occur due to weakness of the bone due to osteoporosis.

fragility fracture Fracture occurring as a result of minor trauma, such as falling, coughing, or other activities of daily living, because of osteoporosis or other bone weakness.

Framingham Heart Study A study that was started in 1948 to investigate heart disease. Over time, it has been used to study practically all chronic diseases. Many of the epidemiologic and clinical findings of this study have had broad implications for the entire U.S. population.

free fatty acid A fatty acid that has been released from a triglyceride by lipase enzymes operating in the gut lumen or in adipose tissue. Lipolysis releases free fatty acids from adipocytes that then enter the blood and are taken up by muscle cells.

free radical A highly reactive chemical species (of very short life)—typically oxygen atoms containing a free electron—that combine with a carbon atom of an unsaturated fatty acid (at the double bonds) or of other molecules, including proteins and DNA; the result is an alteration at the point of the unsaturation. Damage to DNA may result in mutations. *See also* antioxidant.

French paradox The French diet is characterized by rich cream sauces, cheeses, fatty foods, fresh vegetables, bread, and wine. However, this diet is considered to be quite healthy because the French have fairly low heart disease rates. This French paradox has yet to be explained, but some think it has to do with protective substances in red wines.

freeze-drying A method of food preservation that freezes foods and removes water in a vacuum chamber.

freezing A method of food preservation whereby the food is stored below water's freezing point, which stops the growth of most microorganisms.

Friedewald equation An equation used to calculate LDL-cholesterol based on known values of triglycerides, HDL-cholesterol, and total cholesterol.

fructose A six-carbon monosaccharide sugar. Also called fruit sugar, it has a very sweet taste. Together with glucose it makes up sucrose, a disaccharide. It is an intermediary molecule in glycolysis. Often used as a sweetener that when consumed in large quantities may have adverse metabolic effects.

fruit group One of the basic food groups of the MyPlate food guidance system. This food group includes the fruits of any plant or 100% fruit juice. In addition to supplying macronutrients, fruits are rich in micronutrients, dietary fiber, and phytochemicals. *See also* ChooseMyPlate.

functional food A food that contains, in addition to normal amounts of nutrients and non-nutrients, other molecules that promote health or prevent disease. Functional foods are often rich in phytochemicals. Examples include blueberries, broccoli, and salmon. They are also referred to as pharmfoods or nutraceuticals.

galactose A monosaccharide similar to glucose. Lactose contains galactose and glucose as its two monosaccharides.

gallbladder A muscular sac that collects and concentrates bile (fluid) released by the liver. During a meal, the gallbladder contracts periodically and releases some of its contents through the common bile duct into the lumen of the gastrointestinal tract to aid in the digestion and absorption of dietary fats. *See also* bile, common bile duct, digestive tract, *and* liver.

gallstone A crystalline deposit that forms in the gallbladder. Can be as large as a golf ball or as small as a grain of sand.

gastric An adjective referring to the stomach.

gastric acid Hydrogen ions (H^+) secreted by gastric glands lower the pH of the stomach food contents during eating so that the digestion of proteins can be initiated and the digestion of cobalamin (vitamin B_{12}) can free up the vitamin from its protein complex for subsequent binding with the intrinsic factor (IF) secreted by the gastric glands.

gastric gland Secretory glands (or pits) within the wall of the stomach that generate hydrogen ions (acid) along with chloride ions; they also synthesize intrinsic factor (IF).

gastroenteritis Gastrointestinal infection typically caused by microorganisms in contaminated foods that results in diarrhea, headaches, chills, nausea, vomiting, and abdominal disturbances and pain.

gene A unit of hereditary information consisting of DNA that usually encodes for a specific protein (i.e., the amino acid sequence). *See also* deoxyribonucleic acid (DNA) *and* genetic code.

Generally Recognized as Safe (GRAS) list *See* GRAS list.

genetic code The code by which sequences of nucleotides in a gene are translated into a sequence of amino acids in a protein. Each three-nucleotide sequence encodes a single amino acid.

genetically modified Development of new varieties of plants or animals that have had changes made to their DNA through genetic engineering methods. Allows for the rapid development of new varieties that have increased resistance to specific crop diseases as well as enhanced nutritional value (e.g., golden rice that has enhanced vitamin A content).

genome The genetic material of an organism that consists of tens of thousands of different genes coding for specific proteins.

gestation Period of fetal development in the uterus from conception to birth; normally 280 days (or approximately 9 months) in humans.

gestational diabetes A form of type 2 diabetes that may develop late in pregnancy. Occurs in 3% to 10% of pregnancies and may result in adverse outcomes for both the baby and mother. Development of gestational diabetes increases a woman's risk of type 2 diabetes after pregnancy.

globesity A term coined by the World Health Organization to refer to global obesity trends.

glucagon Hormone produced by alpha (α) cells of the islets of Langerhans that acts primarily on the liver to stimulate gluconeogenesis and glycogenolysis, especially during periods of fasting, to make glucose available to the body's cells.

glucocorticoid A steroid hormone made by adrenocortical cells that has a role in glucose metabolism and lipolysis in fat cells.

gluconeogenesis Production of glucose in the liver from alanine, lactate, glycerol, and other amino acids in order to keep the blood glucose concentration at a level that will supply the body with glucose, especially the brain and red blood cells. Typically occurs under conditions of extended fasting (i.e., beyond an overnight fast). *See also* alanine–glucose cycle.

glucose A six-carbon monosaccharide sugar used by cells for many purposes, including energy (ATP) production and glycogen synthesis. It is the principal energy source for brain and red blood cells.

glucose polymer Synthetic polysaccharide containing glucose molecules that is used in sports drinks and other beverages as an energy source. Such polymers have a shorter chain length than amylose starch molecules.

glucose porter (carrier) A membrane protein that facilitates the transport of glucose across the plasma membrane.

glucose regulation The control of blood glucose concentration by insulin on one side and by glucagon, cortisol, growth hormone, and other insulin counterregulatory hormones on the other.

glucose tolerance The state of responding appropriately to a glucose challenge (oral load) by lowering the blood glucose concentration in a normal fashion. Glucose intolerance refers to not being able to appropriately lower the blood glucose concentration after a challenge.

glucose tolerance factor A suggested, but still not established, molecule containing chromium that enhances the interaction of insulin with its membrane receptor on extrahepatic cells, such as muscle and fat cells.

glycation A nonenzymatic chemical reaction in which glucose binds to proteins in blood or tissue, reducing the proteins' ability to function.

glycemic index (GI) Refers to the rise in serum glucose concentration from baseline (fasting) following the ingestion of a single carbohydrate-rich food item (experimental food) in comparison with the glucose rise following the consumption of the same amount of glucose itself, which is arbitrarily assigned a GI value of 100%. High GI foods cause a rapid increase in blood glucose concentration after ingestion.

glycemic load Represents the total amount of carbohydrate in a meal; that is, the sum of all glucose sources, especially foods with high glycemic indexes. A meal with a high glycemic load would be one that contains one or more foods with a high glycemic index.

glyceride Any molecule that contains glycerol and one or more fatty acids, including monoglycerides, diglycerides, and triglycerides.

glycerol A three-carbon carbohydrate molecule with three hydroxyl groups. It is the backbone of triglycerides and phospholipids.

glycogen A storage form of starch (a polysaccharide) found in almost all human tissues, especially the liver. It serves to keep the blood glucose concentration near normal between meals.

glycogenesis The synthesis of glycogen in the liver and in most other cells of the body.

glycogenolysis The degradation of glycogen in the liver and in other cells of the body to glucose.

glycolysis An anaerobic respiration pathway in the cell cytosol that begins with glucose and ends with pyruvate or lactate and the generation of two ATP molecules. *See also* anaerobic metabolism (respiration).

glycoprotein A complex molecule containing protein and carbohydrate.

glycosidic bonds Bonds between the rings of disaccharide or polysaccharide molecules.

glycosuria The presence of sugar (glucose) in the urine, which is not the normal condition. It is a warning sign of type 2 diabetes mellitus.

goiter (simple) A classic deficiency disease of iodine that results in simple enlargement of the thyroid gland. Endemic goiter refers to the prevalence of many individuals in a population with goiter because of iodine deficiency or consumption of goitrogens in the usual diet. Other types of goiter (i.e., metabolic) are not simple goiter.

goitrogen Molecules in foods that can interfere with iodine uptake by cells of the thyroid gland, leading to the enlargement (hypertrophy) of the gland in an attempt to trap as much iodine as possible to synthesize thyroid hormones.

Golgi complex An organelle within cells that is connected to the endoplasmic reticulum. It serves as the final stop for the addition of components (e.g., carbohydrates) to newly synthesized molecules just prior to secretion into the blood or lumen.

gradual weight loss Weight loss of 1 pound or so per week, based on decreasing daily intake by 500 kilocalories per day for 7 days, or 3,500 kilocalories.

grain group One of the basic food groups of the MyPlate food guidance system. This food group includes any food made from wheat, rice, oats, cornmeal, barley, or other cereal grains. Grains can be divided into whole grains and refined grains. Grains are an important source of macronutrients as well as dietary fiber and B vitamins. *See also* ChooseMyPlate.

GRAS list The food additives on the FDA's Generally Recognized As Safe (GRAS) list have stood the test of time and scientific evaluation and have been determined by scientists and health experts to be safe for human consumption.

Green Revolution A large increase in crop production in developing countries achieved by the use of fertilizers, pesticides, and high-yield crop varieties.

growth (general) The increase in tissue mass, especially soft tissues and hard (skeletal) tissues, through the formation of new cells (hyperplasia) and the enlargement of these cells (hypertrophy).

growth hormone Hormone secreted by the anterior pituitary that stimulates growth early in life and helps maintain and renew adult tissues. It exerts metabolic effects on fats cells by increasing lipolysis via hormone-sensitive lipase.

growth pattern The continuous growth from birth to late adolescence, as measured by weight and height (or length up to 3 years) along grids that indicate specific growth paths according to percentile; going up or down on the percentile tracks may indicate growth problems or even more commonly excessive growth characteristic of overweight or obesity.

growth plate The growing hyperplastic tissue at the ends of long bones that appears as a horizontal plate when a section of a long bone is dissected lengthwise. The plate consists of cartilage-like cells (chondrocytes) that actively undergo mitoses and migrate in two different (vertical) directions during the growth period that lasts to the end of adolescence.

gum A type of water-soluble dietary fiber classified as a type of mucilage. It is a relatively small polysaccharide that is partially degraded by gut bacteria. *See also* mucilage.

gums (swollen) A lesion resulting from a deficiency of ascorbic acid. Gums may also bleed on minimal abrasion, such as when brushing teeth. May also result from infection of the gingiva due to poor dental hygiene.

gut bacteria The flora that normally exist only in the lower small intestine and the large intestine. The number of bacteria is much larger in the large intestine than in the ileum.

gynoid fat distribution Fat distribution pattern where fat has a greater propensity to distribute around the hips and thighs as measured by the waist-to-hip ratio (WHR). It is the typical fat distribution pattern in adult females. *See also* android fat distribution.

H-P-A axis *See* hypothalamic-pituitary-adrenal cortex (H-P-A) axis.

H-P-O axis *See* hypothalamic-pituitary-ovarian (H-P-O) axis.

half-life The amount of time it takes for half of a particular molecule to disappear from the blood. For example, the half-life of insulin is 5 to 10 minutes. *See also* clearance.

Harris-Benedict equations Equations used to estimate resting energy expenditure (REE), where W = weight in kilograms, H = height in centimeters, and A = age in years. *Females:* REE = 655 + 9.6W + 1.9H − 4.7A. *Males:* REE = 66 + 13.8W + 5H − 6.8A.

HDL *See* high-density lipoproteins (HDL).

health claim A statement of an established beneficial association between a nutrient or food ingredient and a disease or health condition. The claim must be reviewed and approved by the FDA and must establish a definite linkage (e.g., calcium may help to prevent osteoporosis).

Healthy People 2020 Health objectives set by the U.S. Public Health Service for the year 2020 to promote longer lives free of preventable diseases, to achieve health equity, to create environments that promote good health, and to promote healthy behaviors across all life stages.

health promotion Encouragement of behaviors that enhance health, such as healthy eating, physical activity, and refraining from smoking or using tobacco. May be part of a formal health improvement program.

heat treatment A traditional food preservation method where a food is heated to a high enough temperature to kill microorganisms, including most pathogens.

hematocrit Packed cell volume of blood after centrifugation that is expressed as a percentage of cells to the total volume in the capillary tube. *See also* hemoglobin.

heme The iron-containing portion of the hemoglobin molecule. Also called porphyrin.

heme iron Iron that is combined with the heme metalloprotein (e.g., hemoglobin, myoglobin). *See also* iron *and* nonheme iron.

hemicellulose A type of dietary fiber that contains both soluble and insoluble polysaccharides, depending on their length (i.e., molecular weight).

hemochromatosis Iron storage disease that results from increased intestinal absorption and excessive accumulation or overload of iron in the major storage organs (i.e., liver, spleen, bone marrow, and the heart). Complications resulting from this disorder have a severe negative impact on long-term health.

hemoglobin The oxygen-carrying molecule in red blood cells that utilizes iron in the heme portion to hold oxygen atoms being delivered from the lungs to other tissues.

hemoglobin A1c concentration A marker of glucose binding (glycation) to the protein in hemoglobin that serves, when elevated, as a warning of poor glucose control and prediabetes or even full diabetes; this marker takes weeks to months to increase (or reduce) so that it represents long-term glucose control, i.e., eating pattern.

hepatic An adjective referring to the liver.

hepatic portal vein Large vein that runs from the intestines to the liver. It collects water-soluble nutrients absorbed across the gastrointestinal tract and carries them to the liver for initial processing and utilization.

hepatocyte The major cell type in the liver. The hepatocytes are responsible for most of the liver's synthetic and storage functions.

HFCS *See* high-fructose corn syrup (HFCS).

high-density lipoproteins (HDL) A type of lipoprotein that is protective against heart disease and stroke because it brings cholesterol back from the body tissues to the liver. Often referred to as the so-called good cholesterol. *See also* lipoproteins *and* low-density lipoproteins (LDL).

high-fructose corn syrup (HFCS) A sweetener made from corn starch through several enzymatic reactions and purification steps that has about the same concentration of fructose and sweetness as sucrose. A rather controversial product partially blamed for the increased intake of sweetened beverages and the rise in childhood obesity.

high-protein, low-carbohydrate diet A hypocaloric diet that is high in proteins and low in carbohydrates in an effort to promote weight loss. Examples include the Atkins Diet and the South Beach Diet. These diets minimize intakes of certain nutrients and therefore can be detrimental if followed for a long period of time. *See also* hypocaloric weight-loss diet.

homeostasis Regulatory systems or mechanisms that attempt to maintain constancy in the internal environment of the body, such as with blood pH, blood calcium concentration, body temperature, and oxygen uptake and carbon dioxide removal.

homocysteine An intermediary molecule in cells that builds up when folate or vitamin B_{12} is deficient. Linked with high blood pressure; high levels are also a risk factor for cardiovascular disease risk.

hormonal response to fasting The secretion of hormones during fasting or temporary starvation that are counterregulatory to insulin. These hormones degrade extrahepatic proteins so that the liver can generate glucose via gluconeogenesis. Other tissues can then use the generated glucose to meet cellular energy needs.

hormone A messenger molecule (protein/peptide, steroid, or other) that is produced by an endocrine gland or other organ (e.g., kidney) and is secreted into the blood for distribution to tissues in other parts of the body where the hormone acts; typically act as part of homeostatic mechanisms.

host defense mechanisms A broad class of protective components of the body that defend against foreign microorganisms and viruses and cancer cells. Includes nonspecific responses of epithelial barriers, macrophages, and other tissue cells and the specific responses of immune cells (white cells or leukocytes) and their products, including immunoglobulins (antibodies) and other proteins (factors or cytokines). *See also* acquired immunity, immune response, *and* immune system.

humectants A class of food additives that prevent a food from drying out. They attract and hold water (hygroscopic). Examples include glycerol and sorbitol.

hunger Basic physiologic drive for finding and consuming food that is under the control of the feeding center of the brain; various internal stimuli and external cues may influence the feeding center. *See also* feeding center *and* satiety center.

hydrocarbon chain The carbon backbone of organic molecules that typically contains only hydrogen (H) atoms attached to each carbon in the chain; the hydrocarbon portion of fatty acids and amino acids is hydrophobic.

hydrogen ion (H⁺) Ion formed by removal of the electron from atomic *hydrogen*. Found in all aqueous solutions of acids. It can be formed by the dissociation of the carboxylic acid group in organic acids or from other sources, such as inorganic acids. *See also* acidosis, alkalosis, *and* pH.

hydrogenation The addition of hydrogen (H) atoms to double bonds, or points of unsaturation, in a hydrocarbon. This industrial process is usually done by passing hydrogen gas through liquid vegetable oils. *See also* trans fatty acids (trFA).

hydrolysis The chemical process whereby an ester bond is split with addition of water. The hydrogen ion is added to the carboxylic group and the hydroxyl group is added to the other (hydrocarbon) portion of the ester, resulting in two new molecules, an organic acid and an alcohol. Peptide bonds are also split by hydrolysis with the aid of specific enzymes.

hydrolytic enzyme An enzyme that hydrolyzes ester bonds in organic molecules.

hydrophilic An adjective that means "love of water." Refers to the portion of an organic molecule that is attracted to water, such as the organic acid (COOH) portion of fatty acids and amino acids. *See also* hydrophobic, lipophilic, *and* lipophobic.

hydrophobic An adjective that means "fear of water." Refers to the portion of an organic molecule that is repelled by water, such as the hydrocarbon chain of fatty acids and amino acids. *See also* hydrophilic, lipophilic, *and* lipophobic.

hydroxyapatite The mineralized crystal typical of mature bone tissue that contains calcium, phosphate, and hydroxyl ions in an organized lattice structure.

hydroxyl group An OH group (i.e., alcohol group) found in many organic molecules, including ethanol, glycerol, and glucose. Exists in ionic form in bone mineral (i.e., hydroxyapatite).

hydroxylation The addition of a hydroxyl group (OH) to an organic molecule. Hydroxylation increases the water solubility of lipid molecules.

25-hydroxyvitamin D (calcidiol) A vitamin D metabolite made in the liver via a hydroxylation at the 25-carbon position. This is the major circulating and storage form of vitamin D. *See also* vitamin D.

hypercalcemia Significantly elevated blood concentration of calcium beyond the normal range.

hypercalciuria Excess calcium in the urine.

hyperglycemia Significantly elevated fasting blood concentration of glucose (i.e., beyond the range of normality of the laboratory measurement used). Often an indicator of diabetes mellitus or prediabetes.

hyperinsulinemia An abnormally and excessively elevated serum insulin concentration either after a meal or during fasting (overnight); characteristic of type 2 diabetes mellitus and obesity.

hypermetabolism The state of a critically ill individual who has a marked increase in basal metabolic rate (BMR). Patients in this state also have negative nitrogen balance, alterations in blood hormonal concentrations, metabolism of macronutrients in body tissues, and poor blood hemodynamics (flow rates).

hyperplasia An increase in production of new cells by mitosis (cell division). Common in growing and developing tissues in children and adolescents as well as in the adipose tissue of people with obesity. *See also* hypoplasia.

hypertension Also called high blood pressure. Abnormally elevated blood pressure resulting from either an increase in cardiac output, peripheral resistance, or both; a risk factor for cardiovascular disease.

hypertrophy Cells that are larger in size than normal. A characteristic of adipose cells of people with overweight and obesity. *See also* hypotrophy.

hypervitaminoses Toxicities of vitamins A and D.

hypocalcemia Abnormally low levels of calcium in the blood. Typically found in individuals who have had thyroid or parathyroid surgery. *See also* hypercalcemia.

hypocaloric weight-loss diet A diet low in calories (usually 1,200 to 1,600 kilocalories) that is followed for the purpose of weight reduction.

hypochlorhydria Condition of too little production of hydrochloric acid (HCl) by the stomach. *See also* achlorhydria.

hypochromic The partial loss of color of red blood cells because of a reduction in hemoglobin. Characteristic of iron deficiency.

hypoglycemia The state when plasma glucose concentration is depressed below normal fasting concentration (70 to 110 mg/dL). *See also* hyperglycemia.

hypometabolism A state of lowered metabolism. *See also* hypermetabolism.

hypoplasia The loss of cells due to cell death with no replacement or renewal. This state is typical of elderly individuals who begin to lose lean tissue (LBM) because they are unable to replace it. *See also* hyperplasia.

hypothalamic-pituitary-adrenal (H-P-A) axis The interactions among the hypothalamus, pituitary, and adrenal glands in the stress response and regulation of many body processes, including digestion, the immune system, mood, and emotions. Considered to be overactive in the female athlete triad.

hypothalamic-pituitary-ovarian (H-P-O) axis The complex interactions among the hypothalamus, the pituitary, and the ovary that regulate the female reproductive cycle.

hypothalamus The part of the brain that regulates food intake, satiety, water consumption, thirst, and other basic functions of life. It is where the feeding center and satiety center are located. *See also* feeding center *and* satiety center.

hypotrophy Cell or tissue shrinkage, typically from disuse. *See also* atrophy *and* hypertrophy.

ileum The final segment of the small intestine that joins the colon. It is responsible for the absorption of significant amounts of macronutrients, micronutrients, and bile acids. Large numbers of bacteria (gut flora) live within its lumen. The intrinsic factor (IF)–vitamin B_{12} complex combines with a receptor in the lower ileum prior to absorption.

immune cells Class of white blood cells or leukocytes named *lymphocytes* that are responsible for specific immune effects. Consist primarily of two types: B cells and T cells. Other cells involved in immune defense secrete cytokines that enhance the activities of lymphocytes.

immune response The body's response to foreign agents, especially microorganisms (bacteria, viruses) and parasites, through the actions of lymphocytes and other cells, the production of immunoglobulins and cytokines, as well as the activation of diverse cells (lymphocytes and others) by antigens or foreign cells. The immune response is greatly blunted if nutrients are inadequate.

immune system The network of cells, tissues, and organs that work together to defend the body against attacks by foreign invaders, such as bacteria, parasites, and fungi that can cause infections.

immunity Innate and acquired immunity refers to antibodies (immunoglobulins) circulating in the blood either through natural production (innate) of nonspecific antibodies or through the stimulation by infecting organisms of the production of specific antibodies (acquired). Also includes temporary immunity or passive acquired immunity against infection obtained by giving preformed antibodies by injection, such as used in the prophylactic control of flu epidemics.

immunoglobulins The class of large glycoproteins that are produced by plasma cells and lymphocytes and function as antibodies in the immune system. The classes of immunoglobulins are abbreviated IgA, IgD, IgE, IgG, and IgM.

immunologic Adjective referring to the immune system.

incidence The number of new cases of a disease in a given time frame, such as a year, for a given population. *See also* prevalence rate.

incomplete protein A protein that is deficient or lacking in one or more essential amino acids. Examples include corn protein and collagen. *See also* complete protein.

indirect calorimetry (gas exchange) The estimation of heat production by the body under basal conditions or during different activities by measuring oxygen uptake and carbon dioxide production during a timed period.

infancy Period of life from birth to 1 year of age. Typically a period of rapid growth, with almost a doubling of birth weight and a significant enlargement of the head (and brain) relative to the rest of the body.

infant formulas Milk substitutes that contain nutrients in approximately the same concentrations as human breast milk. These formulas are typically modified cow's milk or soy milks. They are very important for infant growth for mothers who cannot produce their own milk or who choose not to breast feed. *See also* milk.

infection The entry of a foreign organism into the body that initiates the body's defense mechanisms, including a local inflammatory response and the immune response involving white cells and lymphocytes and other cells, such as macrophages. *See also* immune response.

inflammatory response A physiologic response to environmental and physical insults, such as infection, injury, burn, arthritis, surgery, and smoking; involves a rise in body temperature, changes in blood variables, and an enhanced immune response.

ingestion The act of consuming (eating) food by mouth; intake or input of food.

ingredients list A list of all ingredients in a food item in order from high to low in mass units of each component or nutrient. It is required on all food labels in the United States.

inhibition (of cancer) Blockage of further cancer progression through chemical or physical agents; dietary antioxidant molecules may operate in this way.

initiation (of cancer) The first stage of a cancer that is characterized by damage to DNA; generally irreversible. *See also* cancer.

inorganic Refers to the chemistry of molecules that are not organic (not carbon based). *See also* organic.

insensible water loss Loss of body fluids through the skin and from the lungs that is not sensed by the individual. Such losses may lead to dehydration.

insoluble fiber The components of dietary fiber that are not soluble in water and do not, therefore, exert an osmotic force. *See also* dietary fiber *and* soluble fiber.

insulin Hormone produced by beta (β) cells of the islets of Langerhans in the pancreas that primarily acts on cells of the body, especially liver, muscle, and fat cells, to permit glucose entry into cells from blood and extracellular fluids, especially during the postprandial (meal) period. *See also* blood glucose, diabetes mellitus, *and* glucose regulation.

insulin counterregulatory hormones Several hormones that work in opposition to insulin to increase blood glucose concentration during periods of fasting and starvation. They include glucagon, epinephrin(e), growth hormone, and cortisol.

insulin resistance The resistance of peripheral tissues (e.g., muscle and adipose) to the action of insulin to take up glucose. This condition precedes the development of type 2 diabetes mellitus.

intercurrent infection Repeated persistent infections that come and go in terms of severity causing some undernourished children to have severe growth retardation because of depressed appetite and poor immune defense. It is the leading cause of deaths of infants in developing nations. *See also* malnutrition–infection cycle.

intimal damage of arteries Damage typically caused by fatty deposits (atheromas) in the intimal layer of arteries. It is often the initial step in the development of cardiovascular disease.

intimal layer The endothelial layer of cells on the inner or luminal surface of an artery or arteriole.

intracellular fluid compartment The water compartment of cells derived primarily from the cytosol but also in a limited amount from the fluids within the cell organelles. *See also* extracellular fluid.

intrinsic factor (IF) A glycoprotein secreted by the stomach that binds vitamin B_{12} in the upper small intestine prior to absorption of the vitamin in the lower ileum of the small intestine.

iodine An essential trace mineral that exists as iodide (I^-) in solution. Iodide is taken up by the thyroid gland so that the thyroid cells can synthesize the thyroid hormones thyroxin (T_4) and triiodothyronine (T_3). *See also* thyroid hormones.

ion Anions and cations that have an electrical charge when in solution.

iron A micronutrient that serves as a component of hemoglobin, myoglobin, cytochromes, and enzymes. It seldom exists in the free state. Present in foods in heme and nonheme forms. *See also* heme iron *and* nonheme iron.

iron balance The difference between iron taken into the body and iron lost from the body. Positive iron balance occurs with adequate dietary iron intake from all food sources and it signifies normal hemoglobin and hematocrit values plus sufficient blood concentration of serum ferritin, a marker of the storage form equivalent of ferritin. Negative balance results in low measurements of all of these blood variables and may result in anemia.

iron deficiency A form of deficiency of iron resulting from inadequate consumption of iron-rich foods characterized by low hematocrit and blood hemoglobin content; typically also characterized by low, but not exhausted, iron stores (ferritin).

iron deficiency anemia A severe form of iron deficiency characterized by low hemoglobin and depressed values of virtually all biochemical indices of iron status. Symptoms include tiredness and lack of energy. *See also* microcytic anemia.

islets of Langerhans The endocrine portion of the pancreas that contains specific cell types that secrete insulin (beta or B cells), glucagon (alpha or A cells), and other hormones.

jaundice Yellowish color, especially of mucosal tissues and the whites of the eye, because of abnormal accumulation of bilirubin and other bile pigments in the blood. Typically results from a blockage of the common bile duct and backflow into the liver and blood.

jejunum The segment of the small intestine between the duodenum and the ileum. It is approximately 8 feet in length. *See also* duodenum *and* ileum.

joule (kilojoule) Metric unit of energy (as opposed to calories and kilocalories) used for calculating energy content of foods and energy consumption; 1 calorie = 4.18 joules. *See also* calorie *and* kilocalorie (kcal).

keratin A skin protein made by cells of the skin and eyes (keratinocytes) that provides strength to these thin surfaces (i.e., skin, conjunctivae, and corneas).

keto acid An organic molecule with a keto group and a carboxylic group (e.g., pyruvic acid). Essential reactant (molecule) in transamination, as well as being a product molecule of this reaction.

ketoacidosis Acidosis of the blood (i.e., low pH), because of an excess of circulating acidic ketones. *See also* acidosis.

ketogenic Refers to a type of diet or specific molecules that generate ketones. Fatty acids and a few amino acids contribute to the metabolic generation of ketones.

ketogenesis The pathway through which ketones are formed in the mitochondria of the liver due to insufficient amounts of oxaloacetate or excessive generation of acetate from fatty acid oxidation or alcohol degradation.

ketone Molecule produced from the accumulation of excess acetic acid molecules. The three most common ketones are acetone (a true ketone) and the organic acids acetoacetic acid and hydroxybutyric acid. Ketones are typically elevated in uncontrolled diabetes mellitus (type 1) and, to a lesser extent, during conditions of fasting or starvation. *See also* ketoacidosis, ketogenesis, *and* ketonemia.

ketonemia (ketosis) The state of metabolism in which ketone production is high, blood pH is lowered, and acetone is exhaled from the lungs and excreted in the urine. Excessive ketones circulating in the blood result in both ketotic breath and urine. *See also* ketoacidosis.

kidney Organ that helps maintain homeostasis of the blood and other body fluids. Reabsorbs much of the filtered load of blood of sodium, calcium, glucose, and other important nutrient molecules and ions, keeping these substances in the body. Removes and eliminates waste products such as urea, uric acid, and creatinine.

kilocalorie (kcal) A unit of energy (calories) used to estimate both energy consumption from foods and energy expenditure in activities; 1 kcal is the amount of energy required to raise the temperature of 1 kilogram of water 1 degree Celsius (1 °C); 1 kcal is often written as1 Cal (capital C as opposed to lowercase c). *See also* joule (kilojoule).

knowledge of nutrient content of foods An established determinant of food habits that has resulted from increased knowledge of food composition and an understanding of the use of ChooseMyPlate for selecting foods each day.

kwashiorkor A severe form of undernutrition characterized by extremely low protein intake as well as inadequate energy intake. Changes to the skin and hair and edema are characteristic of this protein–energy deficiency disease. *See also* malnutrition, protein–energy malnutrition (PEM), *and* undernutrition.

lactase An enzyme of the small intestine that metabolizes lactose, the milk sugar, to glucose and galactose. In infants, this enzyme is present in adequate amounts during the breastfeeding period, and thereafter it declines. *See also* lactose *and* lactose intolerance.

lactation (breastfeeding) The production and release of milk by the mammary glands for nourishing the infant. Pediatricians currently recommend that mothers breast-feed their infants for a minimum of 6 months.

lactational amenorrhea Temporary postnatal infertility that occurs when a woman is amenorrheic (not menstruating) and fully breast-feeding.

lacteal (vessel) A lymphatic vessel that collects lymph within the villi of the small intestine.

lactic acid (lactate) A derivative (reduced form) of pyruvate formed by the addition of two hydrogen atoms in the liver and other cells after glycolysis. In exercising skeletal muscle tissue deprived of oxygen, such as following physical exertion, lactate is released by the muscles to the blood circulation for return to the liver and use in the gluconeogenic pathway. *See also* Cori cycle, gluconeogenesis, *and* pyruvic acid (pyruvate).

lacto-ovo-vegetarian A type of vegetarian who avoids meats, fish, and poultry but does consume eggs and dairy products. *See also* vegetarian eating pattern.

lacto-vegetarian A vegetarian who consumes dairy products but avoids eggs, fish, and meats. *See also* vegetarian eating pattern.

lactose A disaccharide composed of glucose and galactose found in milk and milk products. The intestinal enzyme lactase metabolizes lactose to its monosaccharides. *See also* lactose intolerance.

lactose-free milk products Milks and other dairy foods that have been treated with lactase to degrade most of the lactose in the food. Lactose causes adverse effects in people who have low lactase enzyme production in their small intestine (i.e., lactose intolerance). These products enable people with lactose intolerance to consume dairy products.

lactose intolerance The inability to digest milk sugar (lactose) after the consumption of milk or other lactose-containing products. Consumption of products containing lactose can cause adverse effects in people who do not produce enough lactase, the enzyme required to break down lactose in the small intestine. *See also* lactase *and* lactose.

lard Pork fat that has been rendered.

latency period Delay in appearance or presentation of specific events related to disease pathology; time between initiation of carcinogenesis and detection of a cancer. For chronic diseases such as cancer, the latency period may be 20 years or longer.

laxative Food components, such as dietary fiber, or over-the-counter formulations that enhance the flow of the contents of the large bowel (colon) toward elimination.

LBM *See* lean body mass (LBM).

LDL *See* low-density lipoproteins (LDL).

lean body mass (LBM) The compartment of the body that includes skeletal muscle and other tissues but excludes fat tissue and generally bone. *See also* body composition.

legume A special subset of vegetables that includes a variety of beans, peas, and soybeans. The macronutrient composition of legumes differs from other vegetables, especially their protein and fat content. Because of their high protein content, they are often grouped with other protein-rich foods, such as meats.

leptin A hormone produced by fat cells and released into the blood that inhibits the feeding center of the hypothalamus in the brain and thereby helps regulate body weight.

life cycle The human life cycle from prenatal life to old age and death.

life expectancy The average lifetime age expected at birth. In the United States, life expectancy is approximately 81 years for females and 76 years for males.

life span The oldest possible age achievable for the human species. Estimates range from 110 to 130 years; however, few people live the full life span. The number of centenarians in the United States, nevertheless, is steadily increasing.

lifestyle risk factors A collection of behaviors that can adversely or favorably impact health; for example, cigarette smoking and excessive alcohol consumption (more than two drinks a day on a regular basis) are deleterious risk factors, whereas regular physical activity, a nutritious, balanced diet, and adequate sleep are beneficial risk factors for health.

lignin A nondigestible fiber found in the cell walls of plants.

limiting amino acid One or more amino acids deficient in a food that limits the ability of cells to synthesize a protein containing all the required amino acids. *See also* essential (indispensable) amino acid.

linoleic acid (C18:2) An essential double-unsaturated fatty acid (PFA) of 18 carbon atoms of the omega-6 series. It is commonly found in vegetable oils and other plants; it is not synthesized by animals or humans.

linolenic acid An essential, triple-unsaturated fatty acid (PFA) of 18 carbon atoms of the omega-3 series; i.e., the first double bond is three carbons from the beginning of the hydrocarbon chain. It is commonly found combined with glycerol in linseed oil and other vegetable oils; it is not synthesized by animals or humans.

lipase Class of enzymes that are located in a variety of tissues (e.g., liver and adipose), as well as in gut lumen (e.g., pancreatic lipase) and in the capillary beds of the general circulation (e.g., lipoprotein lipase). Hormone-sensitive lipase is responsible for lipolysis in fat cells. *See also* adipose (fat) tissue, capillary, digestion, lipolysis, lipoprotein degradation, lipoprotein lipase, *and* liver.

lipid A broad class of water-insoluble molecules that includes triglycerides, phospholipids, cholesterol, steroids, eicosanoids, waxes, fat-soluble vitamins, and many phytomolecules. *See also* cholesterol phospholipid, steroid hormone, *and* triglyceride.

lipid soluble A substance that dissolves in fats, oils, lipids, and nonpolar substances, but not water. Also known as being fat soluble. *See also* water soluble.

lipogenesis The synthesis of a new fatty acid in the liver through the combining of two acetyl CoA molecules and the successive addition of acetyl CoA molecules. The fatty acids produced by the liver are fully saturated. The acid or carboxyl end of each fatty acid can be linked to glycerol phosphate to produce a triglyceride or phospholipid.

lipolysis Fat (triglycerides) degradation in adipose tissue via hormone-sensitive lipase. Results in the release of free fatty acids and glycerol that then diffuse into the blood for distribution to other body tissues. *See also* lipase.

lipophilic Adjective that means "lover of fats." Used to refer to fat- or lipid-soluble molecules. *See also* hydrophilic, hydrophobic, *and* lipophobic.

lipophobic Adjective that means "fear of fats." Used to refer to water-soluble molecules. *See also* hydrophilic, hydrophobic, *and* lipophilic.

lipoprotein degradation Enzymatic degradation of lipid components of lipoproteins by lipoprotein lipase and other enzymes located in peripheral capillaries following lipoprotein uptake (clearance) by liver cells and subsequent enzymatic degradation within the hepatocytes.

lipoprotein lipase Enzyme found in the capillary beds that degrades triglycerides in lipoproteins during their passage through the circulation.

lipoproteins Complex aggregates or particles that contain specific proteins, triglycerides, cholesterol esters, and phospholipids. They transport lipids in the blood and carry triglycerides and cholesterol esters to and from the peripheral tissues. The modified lipoproteins are taken up (cleared) by liver cells. *See also* lipogenesis, lipoprotein degradation, *and* lipoprotein lipase.

liver A large organ that has many functions relating to energy and protein metabolism. It plays important roles in the urea cycle, the ketogenic pathway, bile acid synthesis, bile (fluid) production, and lipoprotein production (except for chylomicrons) and degradation. It is also responsible for the metabolism of alcohol, drugs, toxic chemicals, and vitamin D. Alcoholic liver has characteristic pathologic changes, including excess fatty deposits and cirrhosis. *See also* alcohol effects *and* liver cirrhosis.

liver cirrhosis A disease of the liver typically caused by alcoholism in which most of the normal hepatic cells are replaced by scar tissue so that liver function is severely suppressed.

long-chain fatty acid A fatty acid containing 12 or more carbon atoms. Long-chain polyunsaturated fatty acids (PFA) typically fill essential biological roles, whereas long-chain saturated fatty acids (SFA) do not.

longevity The typical length of life of males and females in a society. *See also* life expectancy *and* life span.

low-birth-weight (small-for-term) baby A baby born at or near full term that is less than 5.5 pounds (2,500 grams) in weight.

Low-birth-weight infants are at higher risk for poor nutrition and disease outcomes.

low-density lipoproteins (LDL) A type of lipoprotein derived from very low density lipoproteins (VLDL) in the capillary beds through the action of lipoprotein lipase and other enzymes. This lipoprotein has the highest concentration of cholesterol (as ester) and the longest half-life. High circulating concentrations of LDL-cholesterol is a risk factor for cardiovascular disease. *See also* high-density lipoproteins (HDL) *and* very low density lipoproteins (VLDL).

lower esophageal sphincter (LES) The muscular segment between the esophagus and the stomach that, when closed, prevents acid reflux from the stomach into the esophagus. Heartburn occurs when the LES does not close adequately and stomach acid enters the sensitive esophagus.

lumen The inner open space or cavity of a tubular organ, such as the GI tract or blood vessels.

lymph The fluid of the lymphatic system. It is collected from the interstitial spaces between the cells and contains low levels of proteins and electrolytes. The lymph also collects chylomicrons from the GI tract for transport to the circulatory system.

lymphatic circulation The collection of lymph, or fluids basically devoid of cells, from the tissues and the return of albumin-rich and chylomicron-rich (only after meals) fluid from the body cavities to the blood vascular circulation.

lymphocytes A type of white blood cell whose roles are related to immune defense. B-lymphocytes undergo changes into plasma cells that synthesize immunoglobulins (antibodies). T-lymphocytes become involved in other aspects of immune defense against bacteria, viruses, and other microorganisms.

macrocytic, megaloblastic anemia A type of anemia characterized by large immature red blood cells that typically results from a deficiency of either folic acid or cobalamin. Oxygen insufficiency results because of an inadequate number of red blood cells with too little hemoglobin within them. *See also* anemia, microcytic anemia, *and* pernicious anemia.

macromineral Mineral elements needed in large amounts in the diet each day. Calcium, phosphorus, magnesium, sodium, potassium, and chloride are the macrominerals needed by the body each day. *See also* micromineral (trace element).

macronutrient Class of nutrients that generate energy (carbohydrates, fats, proteins) and provide nitrogen (N) and amino acids (protein). Sometimes other molecules, such as dietary fiber and water, are included in this class because they are consumed in large amounts. *See also* micronutrient *and* phytonutrient.

macrophage Type of cell of the body's host defense mechanism that engulfs and breaks down foreign organisms (e.g., bacteria). Macrophages also enter the extensive fatty deposits or plaques of atheromas in arteries and arterioles. When they engulf a certain amount of fat material (debris), they then become foam cells.

magnesium An essential intracellular divalent cation (Mg^{2+}) that is abundant in the body, particularly the skeleton. Functions mainly within cells where it acts as an enzyme cofactor or enzyme activator. Most magnesium-requiring enzymes are involved in ATP synthesis or degradation.

malate shuttle The shuttle that carries malate from the mitochondria to the cytosol so that it can begin the cytosolic pathway of gluconeogenesis.

malic acid (malate) A key intermediary molecule in the citric acid (Krebs) cycle that normally feeds into oxaloacetate. However, the reverse reaction (oxaloacetate to malate) also can occur in hepatic gluconeogenesis. The malate shuttle then carries this glucose precursor from the mitochondrion to the cytosol.

malignancy A cancer that may remain localized or spread to distant sites, such as the liver, lungs, and skeleton. *See also* metastasis.

malnutrition "Bad" nutrition that can be either over- or undernutrition. For example, obesity results from chronic malnutrition on the high side, whereas marasmus (starvation) results from chronic malnutrition on the low side. *See also* overnutrition *and* undernutrition.

malnutrition–infection cycle The circular sequence starting with poor nutrition, especially among infants and young children, that leads to an infectious disease that, in turn, enhances malnutrition. This cycle may possibly even lead to death.

maltase Enzyme complex at the luminal surface of epithelial cells of the small intestine that degrades maltose (disaccharide) and dextrins (short chains containing 3 to 10 glucose units) derived from starches (polysaccharides) into glucose.

maltose A disaccharide containing two glucose units that is derived from starch.

maltotriose A three-unit saccharide containing glucose that is derived from a starch molecule.

manganese Essential micromineral that serves as an enzyme cofactor. Plays an important role in the body's energy-deriving pathways and in protein metabolism.

marasmus A form of undernutrition characterized by emaciation, tissue wasting, and other signs. The body literally consumes itself, with all body compartments losing mass. *See also* malnutrition *and* undernutrition.

margarine (oleomargarine) Imitation spread developed as a replacement for butter that is composed of modified fats, often hydrogenated vegetable oils. Recent modifications have greatly reduced the amount of trans fats in margarines.

Maslow's hierarchy of food needs The diverse needs of foods, such as physiological needs for survival and security of health, and social and psychological needs for higher levels of uses of the individual or family in society.

maternal nutrition (pregnancy and lactation) Nutrition during the critical periods of pregnancy and lactation, and even in the prenatal period. Good maternal nutrition is critical in ensuring a healthy outcome of pregnancy (i.e., a healthy baby and a healthy mother).

meal planning The preplanning of meals for a week or an extended period so that nutritious balanced meals are consumed. Meal planning may be repeated on 1- or 2-week cycles, but with some variation. Use of ChooseMyPlate is critical in order to obtain the recommended numbers of servings of all the basic food groups.

Mediterranean diet A food guidance system inspired by the traditional dietary patterns of Greece and Italy. It recommends proportionally high consumption of olive oil, legumes, unrefined cereals, fruits, and vegetables, moderate to high consumption of fish, moderate consumption of dairy products (mostly as cheese and yogurt), moderate wine consumption, and low consumption of meat and meat products. Some studies have found that this diet may reduce the risk of coronary heart disease, possible because of the high amounts of monounsaturated fats this diet provides.

medium-chain fatty acid A fatty acid that has 6 to 10 carbon atoms. It is available in very limited amounts in the typical diet. A triglyceride containing medium-chain fatty acids is called a medium-chain triglyceride (MCT).

megadose Excessive consumption of a particular nutrient, typically as a supplement in pill form. For water-soluble vitamins, a megadose is greater than 5 times the RDA; for fat-soluble vitamins, it is greater than 10 times the RDA. For the more toxic minerals, the ratios of megadose intakes to the RDAs are much lower. *See also* nutrient toxicity.

melanin Pigment that gives skin (and other skin derivatives, such as hair) dark coloration. Responsible for the brown skin coloration of dark-skinned people.

memory loss Unusual forgetfulness. Occurs in some people as part of the normal aging process or it may signal the onset of dementia caused by a disease process such as Alzheimer's disease.

menarche The physiological/hormonal events surrounding the first menstruation (menses), which marks the pubertal transition of girls from late childhood (prepuberty) into adolescence. *See also* puberty.

menopause The cessation of menstruation and ovarian production of estrogens and progestins and the physiological changes in organ systems such that a woman can no longer become pregnant. Usually occurs in women ages 45 to 55.

Metabolic Equivalent of Task (MET) Metabolic energy unit that reflects energy expended in physical activities or sports. One MET is proportional to the basal metabolic rate (BMR), so that an activity with an expenditure of 1.5 METs would require 1.5 times the amount of energy used to support basal metabolism.

metabolic pathway A named pathway through which a molecule enters and is changed to one or more products. Examples include anaerobic metabolism and the citric acid (Krebs) cycle.

metabolic syndrome A complex of conditions that results from overweight or obesity and insulin resistance; contributes to several chronic diseases (the "deadly quartet"). Characterized by a large waist, low HDL-cholesterol, high fasting triglycerides, high fasting glucose, and high blood pressure. *See also* deadly quartet.

metabolic water The water generated by the citric acid (Krebs) cycle steps along with carbon dioxide (CO_2).

metabolism The synthetic (anabolic) and degradative (catabolic) biochemical pathways that occur both within and outside of cells. *See also* anabolism *and* catabolism.

metastasis The spread of malignant cancer cells from the original site of production via lymphatics and blood vessels to distant tissues (e.g., lung, liver, or bone), where secondary growth occurs; characterized by invasiveness. *See also* cancer.

Metropolitan Life tables Tables of weight and height by age and gender of reasonably healthy Americans who have applied for health insurance. Data are taken from a sample of mostly white adults and are not broken down by race or ethnicity.

MFA *See* monounsaturated fatty acids (MFA).

micelle A small complex of fat and bile formed in the lumen of the small intestine after the breakdown of large fat emulsions. The smaller micelles permit greater access of lipase enzymes to triglycerides and phospholipids for enzymatic degradation. They also serve to ferry the digestion products of lipid molecules to the brush-border surfaces for absorption.

microcytic anemia Anemia resulting from severe iron deficiency. Red blood cells are not only small but also hypochromic. *See also* iron deficiency anemia.

micromineral (trace element) An essential mineral needed in small quantities in the diet. At present, RDAs or AIs have been set for the following trace elements: iron, zinc, iodine, selenium, manganese, copper, chromium, and fluoride. *See also* macromineral.

micronutrient Class of nutrients that includes vitamins and minerals; nutrients consumed in small amounts each day. *See also* macronutrient, mineral, phytonutrient, and vitamin.

microorganisms Bacteria, viruses, protozoa, and other microscopic organisms, some of which are infectious (i.e., cause disease).

microvilli Projections on the luminal surfaces of absorbing cells. They look like microscopic paint brushes with lengthy, well-organized cytoplasmic extensions. Similar to the villi, these membrane modifications of the epithelial cells of the small intestine greatly increase the surface area available for absorption.

milk Secretion from the mammary glands of mammals. The composition of human breast milk differs considerably from cow's milk, especially in total energy, protein, and micromineral content. *See also* buttermilk, dairy products, *and* infant formulas.

milk proteins The two major proteins found in milk are casein and lactalbumin (whey).

mineral Elements in the earth's surface that are used by the body, such as calcium and iron. *See also* macromineral, micromineral, *and* micronutrient.

mineralization The process whereby calcium salts precipitate on an organic matrix. In skeletal and dental tissues, mineralization (i.e., calcification) occurs in an organized regular structure. In soft tissues, it is irregular and serves no function.

mineralocorticoid A steroid hormone made by the adrenal cortex for the purpose of enhancing renal sodium reabsorption and thereby conserving sodium, while at the same time secreting and losing potassium in the urine.

misbranding The inaccurate and fraudulent labeling of foods, such as horsemeat for beef. This unlawful practice is regulated by the FDA.

miscellaneous food group One of the basic food groups of the older Pyramid Food Guide that consists of many foods that are high in energy but low in nutrients (e.g., sugary foods and lard). Frequent consumption from this group typically provides excessive energy intake.

mitochondrion A cell organelle with many unique functions, including production of most of the energy (ATP) needed by the cell.

mitosis Cell reproduction and division. In adulthood, some tissues, such as nerve and muscle, typically undergo no turnover and mitosis. In contrast, epithelial cells, such as enterocytes, have high mitotic rates.

molybdenum An essential micronutrient that exists as a cation (Mo^{6+}) in the body. Is required only as a component of the xanthine oxidase system.

monoglyceride A glyceride containing only one fatty acid. Often used as an additive to stabilize foods.

monosaccharide Simple sugars. Glucose, galactose, and fructose are naturally occurring monosaccharides. The preferred molecular arrangement of these simple sugars in foods and in our bodies is a ring structure. *See also* disaccharide *and* polysaccharide.

monosodium glutamate (MSG) A flavor enhancer used in foods, especially Chinese foods. It is a source of sodium for those concerned about high blood pressure. Some people are allergic to it.

monounsaturated fatty acids (MFA) Fatty acids with one point of unsaturation (double bond), usually at omega-9 position. Olive oil is a good source of MFA. *See also* polyunsaturated fatty acids (PFA).

morbidity Existence of a specific disease in a defined population in a given time frame, such as a year; it can refer to incidence (only new cases) or to prevalence (all cases). *See also* incidence *and* prevalence.

morbid obesity (severe obesity) Obesity characterized by having a BMI greater than 40. Usually associated with severe complications of several organ systems and premature mortality. Is a very high risk factor for type 2 diabetes. People with morbid obesity are candidates for gastric bypass surgery. *See also* obesity *and* overweight.

mortality (death) rate The annual number of deaths in a population (i.e., deaths per year). Often adjusted for specific factors.

mottling Changes to the surface of the tooth enamel, such as discoloration and etching. Commonly seen with fluorosis.

mucilage A type of dietary fiber that is soluble in water.

mucosa The epithelial layer that contains the columnar absorbing cells, such as those in the small intestine. This layer extends into the lumen of the small intestine, and it serves as the barrier to nutrients entering the blood. The absorbing cells of this layer have mechanisms for transporting nutrients from the lumen to the blood.

mucus A proteinaceous fluid secreted by mucous cells in the body's epithelial tracts. Mucus helps to lubricate and protect these surfaces.

multifactorial Adjective referring to diseases that have many determinants or risk factors involved in their etiology.

muscle wasting A characteristic of marasmus (starvation) caused by the proteolytic degradation of muscle tissue for glucose generation. Also a common characteristic of wasting diseases such as cachexia of cancer, tuberculosis, and HIV.

mutagen An agent, chemical or physical, that initiates a mutation to DNA within a gene by direct damage to nuclear DNA; the result often is a gene that is dysfunctional. May lead to cancer in some instances.

mutation A change in the DNA within a gene that changes the gene's genetic role; the change could be beneficial, but it usually is not. A mutation can contribute to the development of cancer. *See also* carcinogen *and* mutagen.

mycotoxin Toxin produced by molds that may exert adverse effects if consumed in sufficient amounts with contaminated foods, especially grains and peanuts. A common example is aflatoxin in poorly dried corn and peanuts. *See also* aflatoxin.

myocardial infarction (MI) Also called a heart attack. Death of myocardial tissue in an area of the heart because of total occlusion of a coronary artery or arteriole by a blood clot. Tissue death occurs because the heart muscle does not get any blood supply and thereby delivery of oxygen and nutrients. Preceded by atherosclerosis, which causes a narrowing of the artery or arteriole. Often leads to death.

myoglobin An iron-rich protein in skeletal muscles that binds small amounts of oxygen for use in muscle contractility.

MyPlate (ChooseMyPlate) The food guidance system developed by the USDA for the U.S. population. It includes five food groups: grains, proteins, vegetables, fruits, and dairy. It uses an icon that shows a plate and drink to provide a pictorial display of how much of a meal should be represented by each food group. It provides an entire website with menus, a food composition table, and many other dietary tools.

N-terminal (protein) The amino (N) end of a peptide chain, as compared to the C-terminal or carboxyl end of the chain (i.e., primary structure).

National Center for Health Statistics (NCHS) The branch of the Centers for Disease Control and Prevention (CDC) that is responsible for the NHANES and for assessing the disease rates and health status of the U.S. population.

National Cholesterol Education Program (NCEP) The National Heart, Lung, and Blood Institute (NHLBI) launched the NCEP in November 1985. The goal of the NCEP is to contribute to reducing illness and death from coronary heart disease (CHD) in the United States by reducing the percentage of Americans with high blood cholesterol.

National Health and Nutrition Examination Survey (NHANES) Continuous surveys conducted by the National Center for Health Statistics (NCHS) that are conducted for the purpose of assessing the health status of Americans through various clinical tests, blood and urine analyses, anthropometrics, and clinical and nutritional assessments.

National Institutes of Health (NIH) The research arm of the U.S. Public Health Service that has a primary function to investigate the causation of human diseases and to explore new therapies for the treatment and control of diseases.

natural foods Foods that contain no preservatives or other additives and otherwise appear in their natural form with little or no processing. *See also* organic food.

neural tube defect (NTD) Birth defect resulting from incomplete closure of the neural tube during fetal development. Results, in part, from insufficient folate intake during prepregnancy and early gestation (first 2 months). Defects may be severe, resulting in spina bifida. *See also* folic acid (folate, folacin) *and* spina bifida.

neuropathy A complication of diabetes caused by damage to the nerve fibers by high blood sugar. Most often damages nerves in the legs or feet, resulting in pain or numbness of the extremities.

neutral foods (neutral-ash foods) Foods that when metabolized yield neutral-ash residue (mineral) with respect to body fluids at a pH of approximately 7.4. Examples include butter, margarine, vegetable oils, cornstarch, sugar, maple syrup, tapioca, and plain (clear) candies. *See also* acidic food *and* alkaline (basic) food.

niacin An essential B vitamin found in meats, whole grains, and legumes. Its deficiency disease is pellagra. It is converted into two key cofactors—NAD and NADP—that are used in many energy pathways.

nicotinic acid A form of niacin used as a drug in the treatment of patients with high total blood cholesterol and low high-density lipoprotein concentrations.

night-blindness An early condition of vitamin A deficiency resulting from insufficient retinal. Rhodopsin (opsin–retinal combination) is needed to detect black-and-white patterns of light.

nitrate (NO$_3$) A nitrogen-containing food additive used in the curing of meats, hot dogs, and luncheon meats that inhibits bacterial growth. It combines with the amines of meat proteins to form nitrosamines, which are potential carcinogens.

nitrite (NO$_2$) A food additive used to cure meats and meat products, especially ham, bacon, frankfurters, and related products. It combines with the amines of meat proteins to form nitrosamines, which are potential carcinogens.

nitrogen (N) An element that is a component of amino acids, nucleic acids, and numerous other organic molecules. Nitrogen typically exists in the form of an amino group (NH$_2$) in these molecules. Two nitrogen atoms are used to synthesize urea.

nitrogen balance The state when nitrogen intake from protein equals nitrogen losses in excreta, sweat, and exfoliated cells (i.e., input = output and the balance is zero). Positive nitrogen balance would be an excess of input, and negative nitrogen balance would be an excess of output.

nitrosamines Molecules resulting from the combination of a nitrate or nitrite with a protein in foods or tissues. In meats, the combination of nitrite with the secondary amine groups of myoglobin or other muscle proteins results in potentially carcinogenic nitrosamines.

nonessential amino acid An amino acid whose structure can be synthesized by usual pathways in the body and, therefore, does not need to be consumed in the diet. *See also* essential (indispensable) amino acid.

nonessential nutrients Approximately 10 amino acids are considered nonessential because cells can make them. Apart from the essential fatty acids, the other fatty acids are nonessential as well. For example, phosphatidylcholine, a nonessential phospholipid, can be synthesized by cells from smaller molecules.

nonheme iron Iron that is consumed in foods as ionic iron rather than as a component of heme (porphyrin plus iron); nonheme iron is absorbed less efficiently than heme iron. *See also* heme iron *and* iron.

non-nutrient Food molecules that are not considered nutrients because they are not essential for cellular or tissue needs but that may be important for other aspects of human health. For example, dietary fibers and many phytomolecules may protect against cancer and other chronic diseases.

nucleic acids Deoxyribonucleic acid (DNA) and ribonucleic acid (RNA). These molecules, which consist of nucleotides in long polymer chains, govern protein synthesis. *See also* deoxyribonucleic acid (DNA) *and* ribonucleic acid (RNA).

nucleotide A complex molecule consisting of a base (adenine, guanine, thymine [or uracil], or cytosine), a five-carbon sugar (ribose or deoxyribose), and a phosphate group linked together. Three nucleotides together in a sequence of DNA and RNA serve as the genetic code for an amino acid that is to be part of a specific protein. Other nucleotides become part of ATP and other essential cellular molecules. *See also* deoxyribonucleic acid (DNA), genetic code, *and* ribonucleic acid (RNA).

nucleus The central organelle of cells (except for mature red blood cells) that controls all activities through diverse genes in the 23 pairs of chromosomes in humans. *See also* deoxyribonucleic acid (DNA), gene, *and* ribonucleic acid (RNA).

nutrient Essential or nonessential molecules or minerals derived from foods that are used by cells of the body to carry out diverse functions.

nutrient additive A food additive used in the enrichment, fortification, or restoration of foods. For example, iron, thiamin, riboflavin, niacin, and folate are nutrient additives used to enrich wheat and corn flours and cereals. Vitamins A and D are added back to milk products following processing. Calcium, iron, and vitamin C are also added to many food items. *See also* enrichment, fortification of food, *and* restoration (nutrients).

nutrient density The amounts (in units) of nutrients per 1,000 kilocalories of a food. It is a good index of the nutritional value of a food.

nutrient–drug interaction Typically negative effects of a nutrient on a drug or of a drug on a nutrient, either in the GI tract and affecting intestinal absorption or within organs such as the liver, resulting in increased nutrient degradation.

nutrient–nutrient interaction One nutrient may interfere with the absorption or utilization of another nutrient, thereby reducing the effectiveness of one or both nutrients.

nutrient supplement A product that provides nutrients in pill, tablet, or powder form for the purpose of improving nutritional status.

Many micronutrients are available in pill form. Protein and energy may also be obtained through specific macronutrient supplements.

nutrient toxicity Adverse effects resulting from megadoses of nutrient supplements. Does not usually occur from high intakes of nutrients in foods consumed in excess. Most commonly observed with vitamins A and D. *See also* megadose.

nutrition The branch of science dealing with foods, nutrient composition, eating habits, nutritional status, and health and diseases of individuals and populations.

nutrition education The provision of information about the nutrient quality of foods, healthy eating patterns, and disease prevention. Such education is given to those who wish to lose weight or who are otherwise seeking to improve their diets and health.

Nutrition Facts panel A label on packaged food that provides information about the serving size, calories, nutrients, and ingredients contained in the food product. Most provide information on saturated fats, trans fats, calories, sodium, and beneficial nutrients such as calcium, iron, and fiber. *See also* food labeling.

nutrition–population dilemma The global problem of producing and distributing food to the world's poor in order to improve their nutritional status and reduce undernutrition.

nutrition transition Global phenomenon whereby the emerging middle classes in many developing countries are attaining the purchasing power to consume more than adequate amounts of food and achieving the means to limit much of the physical activity previously required for everyday living, resulting in an increasing prevalence of overweight and obesity.

nutritional assessment A complete nutritional assessment of an individual includes the ABCDs: anthropometric measurements, biochemical measurements, clinical evaluation for physical signs and other changes from normal, and dietary assessment (dietary questionnaires).

nutritional deficiency A deficit in the intake of a specific nutrient(s), such as iron, calcium, or vitamin C.

nutritional status The health of an individual with respect to nutrient intake. Also known as nutritional state.

nutritionist A trained professional who has expertise in the functional uses of nutrients, developing nutritional programs and services, or other nutrition-related activities. *See also* registered dietitian (RD).

nuts and seeds Plant foods that fall under the protein food group of ChooseMyPlate.

obesity Excess accumulation of body fat mass. By definition, an individual is obese when his or her BMI is 30 or greater. *See also* body mass index (BMI).

obesity prevention diet A diet that is low in fats, animal proteins, sugars, and alcohol and high in complex carbohydrates and dietary fibers, with a focus on fruits and vegetables. This diet is also protective against the development of diabetes, dental caries, hypertension, coronary artery disease, and possibly cancer.

observational study A type of study in which individuals are observed or certain outcomes are measured. No attempt is made to affect the outcome.

Okinawa diet A Japanese diet consumed mainly by those living on the island of Okinawa, one of the Japanese prefectures, where the consumption of fish and other seafood plus fruits and vegetables represents the main food items; meats and other animal foods are eaten only in small amounts. Residents of Okinawa are known for their longevity.

oleic acid A monounsaturated fatty acid (C18:1) found in olive oil and other vegetable oils.

oligomenorrhea Having fewer menstrual cycles than normal; for example, fewer than nine menses per year. *See also* amenorrhea.

omega-3 (n-3) fatty acids Subclass of essential polyunsaturated fatty acids (PFA) whose first double bond begins at the third carbon from the end (omega-3) in the hydrocarbon chain. *See also* essential fatty acids (EFA).

omega-6 (n-6) fatty acids Subclass of essential polyunsaturated fatty acids (PFA) whose first double bond begins at the sixth carbon

from the end (omega-6) in the hydrocarbon chain. *See also* essential fatty acids (EFA).

omnivorous eating pattern Dietary pattern where an individual eats food from both plants and animals. *See also* vegetarian eating pattern.

oral feeding Administration of nutrients by mouth (i.e., the normal way of feeding). Also includes tube feeding of ill patients by the mouth.

oral glucose tolerance test (OGTT) A test of glucose tolerance involving an overnight fast and fasting glucose measurement, followed by an oral challenge (load) of glucose (75 grams) or a meal and serial measurements of blood glucose at several times following the time of the load. *See also* glucose tolerance.

organ systems (of the body) The 10 organ systems are as follows: circulatory (blood), digestive, endocrine, immune, integumentary (skin), musculoskeletal, nervous, reproductive, respiratory, and urinary (renal).

organic Molecules that are based on carbon atoms. *See also* inorganic.

organic food An additive-free food that has been grown on soil that has not been treated with chemicals and that has been fertilized with natural fertilizers. The USDA's Certified Organic label carries specific requirements, including that the organism has not been genetically modified. *See also* natural foods.

organic matrix of bone The proteins of bone tissue, namely, collagen and matrix proteins, that must first be in place before mineralization can occur.

osmotic effect Applies to sufficient proteins, especially albumin, in circulating blood, so that this fluid can retain sufficient water and, hence, blood volume. Following long-term undernutrition, protein levels decrease and this effect declines, causing edema to occur in locations most affected by gravity, such as the ankles, wrists, and abdomen. *See also* edema.

osmotic pressure The pressure exerted in a membrane-bound fluid compartment (e.g., blood circulation) by dissolved proteins and other molecules and ions that have osmotic forces (i.e., draw water to them). The normal physiological osmotic pressure is 300 mOsm per liter of fluid. This iso-osmotic or isotonic value compares to low (hypo) and high (hyper) values that may exist at different times. Hypo-osmotic values of blood occur in children or adults with kwashiorkor, who develop edema as a result. *See also* edema *and* kwashiorkor.

osteoblast Type of bone cell that makes new bone, first by synthesizing collagen and other matrix proteins and then by enhancing mineralization on the organic matrix.

osteocalcin A vitamin K–dependent matrix protein in bone that may be involved in the mineralization process. It serves as a marker of bone turnover.

osteoclast Type of bone cell that degrades old bone as part of the remodeling process and in order to maintain calcium homeostasis. Both the mineral phase and the organic matrix are removed through the acid medium and the degradative enzymes created by the osteoclasts.

osteomalacia An adult form of rickets resulting from deficiency of both vitamin D and calcium. This classic deficiency disease is characterized by widened osteoid seams that fail to mineralize; however, there is no distortion of the skeleton as in rickets. *See also* rickets.

osteopenia Low bone mass; a precursor to osteoporosis. Defined by the World Health Organization (WHO) as a bone mineral density (BMD) 1.0 to 2.5 standard deviations (SDs) below that of healthy 20 to 29 year olds.

osteoporosis A disease of the skeleton characterized by too little bone mass and deterioration of bone tissue. The thinning of bone trabeculae increases fragility and likelihood of fracture of cancellous-rich (trabecular-rich) bone sites. Defined by the World Health Organization (WHO) as a bone density (BMD) that is 2.5 standard deviations (SDs) below the mean for young, healthy adults plus poor bone quality at the microscopic level.

ovary Reproductive organ that produces eggs and estrogen hormones and progestins; part of the H-P-O axis.

overnutrition A form of malnutrition characterized by excessive energy and nutrient consumption. *See also* malnutrition *and* undernutrition.

overweight Body weight that exceeds the normal weight range (i.e., BMI between 25 and 30). This definition does not consider whether the excess weight is fat or lean tissue. *See also* obesity.

ovo-vegetarian A vegetarian who consumes eggs but not dairy products. *See also* vegetarian eating pattern.

oxalic acid (oxalate) A short organic acid found in some plant foods, such as rhubarb, that binds calcium ions and to a lesser extent other divalent cations in the gut lumen, thereby reducing the intestinal absorption of calcium and other minerals. Also involved in renal tubular formation of oxalate stones (kidney stones).

oxaloacetic acid (oxaloacetate) A key intermediary molecule in the citric acid (Krebs) cycle that must be available for combination with acetyl-CoA to make citrate and start the cycle. *See also* citric acid cycle (Krebs cycle).

oxidation The complete degradation of an organic molecule in the presence of oxygen to carbon dioxide, metabolic water, and heat. The loss of electrons or hydrogens is another form of oxidation, such as occurs when ascorbic acid is oxidized to dehydroascorbic acid.

oxidation-reduction (redox) A system in which a molecule, such as ascorbic acid, is oxidized to dehydroascorbic acid by donating two hydrogen ions and two electrons to another species, such as ferric ions, to reduce the ferric ions (Fe^{3+}) to ferrous ions (Fe^{2+}). Ascorbic acid can be regenerated from dehydroascorbic acid by the addition of the hydrogen ions and electrons. *See also* oxidation *and* reduction.

oxidative phosphorylation The linking of two processes in the electron transport chain of mitochondria with the end result being the oxidation of nutrients to produce adenosine triphosphate (ATP). Although this process is quite efficient, some of the energy generated is lost as heat. *See also* adenosine triphosphate (ATP).

oxidize To combine with oxygen or to lose an electron.

oxidizing agent Molecule or ion that accepts an electron or donates an oxygen to another molecule or ion.

palmitic acid (palmitate) The saturated fatty acid produced in abundance in hepatic cells and most other cells in the body from eight acetyl CoA molecules via the fatty acid synthase system. Also found in palm oil, beef, and dairy products.

pancreas (exocrine and endocrine) A large gland associated with the digestive system that produces enzyme precursors, such as trypsinogen, and fluids (pancreatic juice) that are secreted into the gastrointestinal tract, where the enzymes are then activated. The pancreas also has the islets of Langerhans, which produce insulin. *See also* islets of Langerhans.

pancreatic duct The duct that carries the secretory products of the exocrine pancreas to the common bile duct. The pancreatic fluid is then secreted into the intestinal lumen.

pantothenic acid (pantothenate) A B vitamin that is essential for human function. It contributes to the structure of coenzyme A (CoA). It is widely available in foods.

paracellular transfer The movement of solutes *between* the cells of the small intestine rather than *through* them in the absorptive step. The molecules or ions must be small to be able to penetrate the tight junctions of the epithelium. *See also* transcellular transfer (absorption).

parathyroid glands The structures that are in the neck, often embedded in the thyroid gland but more frequently separate, that make and secrete parathyroid hormone.

parathyroid hormone (PTH) Hormone produced by the parathyroid glands that has a major role in regulating blood calcium concentration through its direct actions on bone and the kidneys and indirect actions on the small intestine via the hormonal form of vitamin D (1,25-dihydroxyvitamin D).

parenteral nutrition The delivery of nutrition to patients who cannot use their guts, typically by a venous catheter; also known as intravenous feeding or nutrition.

parturition The act of giving birth to a baby that ends a pregnancy. Also referred to as delivery.

passive diffusion Intestinal absorption through or between epithelial cells that requires no energy (ATP) because of movement of nutrients from high concentration to low concentration.

pasta Carbohydrate-rich food of Italian origin. It is made from wheat flour and comes in a variety of diverse shapes and sizes (e.g., spaghetti, macaroni, vermicelli).

pasteurization Heating of milk or other beverages at high temperature (161°F) for 20 seconds in order to kill pathogenic bacteria. *See also* ultrapasteurization.

pathogenic Adjective referring to a disease-producing effect, as from the activities of microorganisms in the body or in foods and from the effects of adverse risk factors, such as those for chronic, noninfectious diseases.

pathogenic bacteria Bacteria, such as most forms of *E. coli*, that reside in the lumen of the lower small bowel and the colon that can enter body tissues following a perforation or break in the intestinal wall and distribute all over the body; if the load or titer of bacteria is high, bacteremia may result, in which condition antibiotic drugs are needed because natural defense mechanisms become rapidly overwhelmed.

pathophysiology The loss or decline of function of tissues caused by disease.

PDV *See* Percent Daily Value (PDV or %DV).

peak bone mass (PBM) The point at which greatest bone mass is attained. Typically occurs by 30 years of age or the decade thereafter.

pectin A type of water-soluble dietary fiber that is used in the making of fruit jelly.

pellagra A classic deficiency disease resulting from chronically low intakes of niacin that manifests as a skin disorder. Alcoholic pellagra results from the combination of low dietary niacin and excessive alcohol consumption. *See also* niacin.

pepsin An active enzyme that degrades peptide bonds of food proteins within the lumen of the stomach to smaller peptides and, to a lesser extent, to free amino acids. It is made and secreted as pepsinogen by the chief cells of the gastric glands.

pepsinogen The inactive precursor (proenzyme) of pepsin whose short peptide segment at the C-terminus must be cleaved within the lumen of the stomach to generate the active enzyme, pepsin.

peptidase A type of enzyme that attacks peptide bonds in proteins, starting at either the N-terminus (i.e., aminopeptidase) or the C-terminus (i.e., carboxypeptidase).

peptide A short version of a protein containing approximately 2 to 10 amino acids. *See also* polypeptide *and* protein.

peptide absorption The entry step of absorption from the lumen into the cell that occurs via dipeptides and free amino acids. Tripeptides have also been reported to be absorbed by this entry step; these peptides probably require peptide hydrolase (enzyme) degradation in the columnar absorbing cells after absorption before the amino acids can be transferred to the blood via the exit step.

peptide bond An organic bond formed between two amino acids, the organic acid group of one and the amine group of the other; formation of the peptide bond involves the removal of a water (H_2O) molecule. *See also* amino acid.

Percent Daily Value (PDV or %DV) The percentage value of selected nutrients of a food in a 2,000-kilocalorie diet. Federal law requires that these be listed on food labels. *See also* Nutrition Facts panel.

percentage (%) energy contributions of macronutrients The percentage of energy contributed by each of the three macronutrients based on total energy consumption. Americans consume approximately 49% of kilocalories from carbohydrates, 35% from fats, and 16% from proteins, with no calories estimated from alcohol consumption.

periodontal disease Dysfunction of the gums and underlying tissues. Often related to poor diet.

peripheral resistance (PR) to blood flow Resistance to blood flow generated by capillary beds throughout the body; both PR and cardiac output (CO) affect blood pressure.

peripheral insulin resistance The resistance of peripheral tissues (e.g., muscle and adipose) to the action of insulin to take up glucose. This condition precedes the development of type 2 diabetes mellitus.

pernicious anemia A classic form of macrocytic anemia resulting from a deficiency of intrinsic factor (IF) or some defect in its linkage with cobalamin or in the IF–cobalamin receptor in the lower ileum, but not from a deficiency of cobalamin in the diet. *See also* macrocytic, megaloblastic anemia.

pesco-vegetarian A partial vegetarian who consumes fish, fish products, and seafood. Also called a pescotarian. *See also* vegetarian eating pattern.

petechia Small, reddish spider-like hemorrhages in the skin, commonly found with scurvy.

PFA *See* polyunsaturated fatty acids (PFA).

pH Hydrogen ion concentration in body fluid and other solutions in logarithmic units. A pH of 7.0 is neutral. Solutions with a pH less than 7.0 are acidic, and those with a pH greater than 7.0 are basic (or alkaline).

phosphate bond High-energy bond found in ATP and other molecules. ATP has three phosphate bonds.

phosphate ion Inorganic phosphate ions (i.e., PO_4^{2-}) are present in the body's intracellular fluids, blood, other extracellular fluids, and secretions into the gut lumen. Phosphate is essential for the formation of hydroxyapatite in bone and teeth. Its most important role is in the formation of high-energy molecules, such as ATP and creatine phosphate. It also is a critical component of RNA and DNA.

phosphatide Type of phospholipid that contains phosphorus (as a phosphate group), glycerol, two fatty acids, and a base, such as choline. Examples include phosphatidylcholine, phosphatidylinositol, phosphatidylserine, and similar molecules. *See also* phospholipid.

phosphatidylcholine (PC, or lecithin) A phosphatide found in membranes that has a role in signaling information from hormones and other molecules that influence membrane receptors.

phospholipid Molecule that contains a phosphate group and a fat component. *See also* phosphatide.

phosphorus additive Phosphate salts are added to many foods during processing, including meats, baked goods, and others, but food labels only need to state in the Ingredients list what P salts are added so that no information of the actual amounts of P present is given on food labels.

physical examination As part of a clinical assessment, an individual can be assessed from head to toe by proper clinical technique. *See also* clinical assessment.

physical signs Objective indications of disease found during a physical examination by a trained professional.

phytic acid (phytate) Plant molecule found associated with fiber, especially in cereal grains, that binds divalent and monovalent cations. When degraded in the gut, the minerals are freed and available for absorption.

phytochemical (phytomolecule) Non-nutrient molecules made by plants and found in diverse fruits, vegetables, grains, nuts, and seeds. Many of these molecules are considered to protect against cancer development, especially as antioxidants. *See also* non-nutrient *and* nutrient.

phytonutrient Nutrients provided by plants that have the same activities as nutrients derived from animal foods. Nutrients differ from phytochemicals, which are not classified as nutrients. *See also* phytochemical (phytomolecule).

phytosterol A type of sterol made by plants that is in the same chemical family as cholesterol. However, unlike cholesterol, phytosterols do not elevate serum cholesterol concentrations when consumed.

pica Abnormal eating behavior characterized by eating clay, ice, or starch. May occur during pregnancy; often associated with iron deficiency.

pituitary gland The anterior portion of this gland functions as an endocrine gland with five specific cell types responsible for the production of follicle-stimulating hormone (FSH), luteinizing hormone (LH), prolactin, growth hormone, adrenocorticotropic hormone (ACTH), and prolactin. The cells of the anterior pituitary receive signals from other cells in the hypothalamus that govern the synthesis and secretion of these hormones.

placebo An inert substance that has no active ingredient and that is used as a comparator or control for an active substance in a clinical trial. *See also* control group.

placebo effect A beneficial effect observed on human subjects treated with a placebo. Such an effect has been explained to occur as a result of the intervention alone or the involvement of the subject in the study.

placenta The organ formed within the uterus following the fertilization of an egg and implantation of the embryo that permits transfer of nutrients and oxygen from the mother to the growing fetus; some waste products from the fetus cross the placenta to the maternal circulation.

plant protein foods Proteins obtained from plant sources, including cereal grains, vegetables, nuts, and seeds. Protein quality typically is lower for plant proteins than for animal proteins, with legumes having the highest quality plant proteins. *See also* animal protein foods *and* protein quality.

plaque (atheroma) A fatty deposit on the wall of an artery or arteriole formed as part of the atherosclerotic process; less advanced in development than an atherosclerotic lesion. It is similar to a fatty streak but more defined.

plasma The fraction of blood consisting of fluid and any dissolved molecules after centrifugation. Differs from serum because an anticlotting agent is added to the blood prior to centrifugation. *See also* blood *and* serum.

plasma membrane The membrane ipid-bilayer enveloping cells and often connecting to other intracellular membranes, such as of the endoplasmic reticulum and Golgi complex. The lipophilic membranes must be crossed by hydrophilic molecules and ions, almost always via carriers or transporters. Fat-soluble molecules move across these membranes within the lipid component either as free molecules or as part of micelles (gut) or lipoproteins (gut and liver).

platelets A type of very small white blood cell. They are easily damaged in the circulation and can initiate the formation of a thrombus (clot) that can plug the artery and stop blood flow.

polypeptide A polymer of many amino acids (i.e., 20 or so different types in human proteins) that includes numerous peptide bonds. *See also* peptide, peptide bond, *and* protein.

polyphenol Group of molecules with a chemical structure of several hydroxyl groups on aromatic rings. They are derived from the amino acid phenylalanine and are metabolized to thousands of different chemical structures in plants. Many of these molecules act as antioxidants. *See also* antioxidant.

polysaccharide Long carbohydrate molecules consisting of monosaccharide units joined together by glycosidic bonds. Examples include starch and cellulose. *See also* disaccharide *and* monosaccharide.

polyunsaturated fatty acids (PFA) A class of fatty acids containing two or more double bonds (points of unsaturation). Two types exist in plants and animals: omega-6 and omega-3. *See also* monounsaturated fatty acids (MFA) *and* saturated fatty acids (SFA).

population growth Increases in population over time. Population growth can be problematic for poor developing nations, which often lack the resources to feed more people.

portal circulation of the liver The hepatic portal vein carries water-soluble nutrients from the gut to the liver. They then travel to the rest of the body via the inferior vena cava to the heart.

portal vein The large vein that collects absorbed nutrients from the small veins draining the small intestinal villi after a meal and then carries the blood to the liver for first use prior to entering the general circulation for use by other organs.

porter A protein molecule in a membrane that transfers molecules across the membrane, also known as a *transporter* or simply as a *carrier*.

postprandium (absorption period) The 3- to 4-hour period that follows the last ingestion of a meal during which the most nutrients are absorbed. This period is associated with wide swings in blood glucose and insulin concentrations, even under normal conditions.

post-translational insertion A modification of a protein immediately after its synthesis. Carboxyl groups are added to gamma-carbons in glutamic acid residues in the polypeptides after the clotting proteins and osteocalcin are synthesized (translation) through carboxylase activity and vitamin K as a coenzyme.

potassium A major intracellular cation (K$^+$) that is essential for the function of neurons and muscle cells and for growth of muscle tissue. Also serves as an enzyme activator in several reactions involving energy production. The body's total potassium content is directly related to lean body mass (LBM), especially muscle mass.

poverty–disease cycle People living in poverty are often unable to purchase adequate amounts of food, which may eventually lead to malnutrition and disease. Poor people who suffer from disease and malnutrition are often unable to work, thus making it even more difficult for them to escape poverty.

Poverty Index Ratio (PIR) The ratio of a USDA-calculated income needed by a family of four to cover all basic living expenses, including 25% of that income earmarked for food and beverages, compared with the actual intake of a family of four. If income is greater than the calculated amount, then the family is above the PIR and does not qualify for federal food programs, such as SNAP (food stamps).

prandium (meal or eating period) The period of eating a meal, typically lasting from 15 minutes to an hour. The eating period follows the cephalic phase of the premeal period; it is followed by the absorption (postprandial) period. *See also* absorption period (postprandium) *and* cephalic phase.

prebiotic Dietary fiber components that serve as food or fodder for the bacteria in the gut and influence the intestinal absorption, especially lowering cholesterol absorption and adverse effects of bile acids on the colonic mucosa that may contribute to colon cancer.

preeclampsia A condition in pregnancy that includes high blood pressure, edema, and protein in the urine (proteinuria). It can cause further eclampsia and may result in fetal death.

pregnancy The period of gestation (280 days) that consists of three terms (trimesters). Normally leads to a healthy baby and mother. *See also* gestation *and* pregnancy outcome.

pregnancy outcome Ideally, the birth of a healthy, well-developed, full-term baby of weight greater than 5.5 pounds or 2,500 grams and of good length accompanied by good health of the mother.

prematurity Preterm delivery of a baby, usually defined as occurring before 8 months of gestation or 250 days.

prenatal development Growth of the fetus from the fertilized egg and embryo up until parturition (delivery) of a baby, even if premature. Full-term development implies the delivery of a baby greater than 5.5 pounds (2,500 grams) at approximately 280 days of gestation.

prepregnancy (preconception) The phase of life of a potentially child-bearing woman when good nutrition serves to promote optimal health of the woman and fetus once conception occurs; folate (folic acid) is only one critical nutrient that optimizes chances for a healthy baby as the outcome of an uneventful pregnancy when the woman is also healthy.

preservative A food additive that increases the shelf-life of a food; for example, sulfur dioxide is used to preserve lettuce on salad bars of restaurants and salt is used to inhibit the growth of microorganisms in meats and vegetables. *See also* food additive.

prevalence The total number of cases of a specific disease existing at any one time; for example, the prevalence rate of coronary heart disease would include all individuals with this disease in the United States at a specific time, including both old cases from previous years and any new (incident) cases from the current year. *See also* incidence.

prevention Procedures, including diet and physical activities, that prevent chronic diseases so common in Western nations, such as cardiovascular diseases, obesity, type 2 diabetes, and several others; the term also has broader usage in the prevention of infectious diseases, accidents, and other ways in which health may be compromised making illness or death more likely.

primary osteoporosis of Type I and Type II Classes of osteoporosis related to low gonadal hormones (Type I) and late life (Type II). *See also* osteoporosis.

primary structure (protein) The chain of amino acids linked by peptide bonds in a specific order; sometimes referred to as the backbone of a protein. *See also* secondary structure (protein).

probiotic Bacteria or other microorganisms that can be added in the gut by foods that contain live cultures, such as yogurt; the probiotics aid in digestion and may have other health benefits such as reducing cholesterol absorption and general health of colonic function.

procarcinogen A cancer-inactive molecule that becomes an active carcinogen once it is metabolized. *See also* carcinogen.

processed food The result of conversion of raw food by various steps, such as removal of the bran and other components of wheat grains plus the addition of other chemicals, including nutrient fortificants and chemical additives that enhance the appearance and keeping quality of foods.

proenzyme An inactive precursor of an enzyme.

prolactin Female hormone synthesized by the anterior pituitary that stimulates milk production near the time of delivery.

progestins Progesterone and related progestational agents that help to maintain the uterine lining after ovulation and following fertilization of an egg and pregnancy.

progression (of cancer) The final stage in the development of a cancer. Changes in a tumor, such as increased rates of cell division, abnormal microscopic appearance of cells, and malignant or invasive characteristics. *See also* cancer, initiation, (of cancer), *and* promotion (of cancer).

proliferation An increase in the number of cells as a result of cell growth and cell division. Cancer is a disease characterized by uncontrolled cell proliferation.

promoter (of cancer) A dietary or environmental molecule or endogenous hormone/factor that promotes cancer development, including its progression and promotion. *See also* cancer, inhibition (of cancer), progression (of cancer), *and* promotion (of cancer).

promotion (of cancer) The second stage of a cancer that is characterized by development of a population of abnormal cells through the support of a cocarcinogen or promoter (e.g., dietary factors). *See also* cancer, initiation (of cancer), *and* progression (of cancer).

prostaglandin A class of eicosanoids derived from specific polyunsaturated fatty acids (PFA) having 20 carbon atoms. Prostaglandins exist in essentially all human tissues, and they act as local factors to induce a variety of activities.

prostate (gland) Male reproductive organ that secretes seminal fluid components into the urethra. Benign prostatic hypertrophy and then cancer development are common in older men.

protein Macronutrient composed of a polymer of amino acids; also contributes nitrogen (N) for synthesis of biological molecules.

protein balance Balance of nitrogen (protein) intake and output of nitrogen from waste products being equal over a period of time; negative balance refers to a net loss of nitrogen, and positive balance to a net gain over time.

protein deficiency Represents negative protein balance. If sufficiently low and prolonged, it can lead to kwashiorkor. *See also* kwashiorkor.

protein–energy malnutrition (PEM) Balanced or unbalanced undernutrition with respect to calorie and protein intake. Can be a severe life-threatening nutritional disorder that requires medical attention. PEM is often coupled with infection as part of a malnutrition–infection cycle. *See also* kwashiorkor, marasmus, *and* undernutrition.

protein group One of the basic food groups of the MyPlate food guidance system. This food group includes foods that share one feature—they are very rich sources of protein. Includes both animal and plant sources of proteins. *See also* ChooseMyPlate.

protein-induced hypercalciuria The increase in urinary calcium following a high-protein meal (mainly animal proteins) and during the regular pattern of high-protein meals from animal sources. The mechanism for this increased loss of calcium may be related to increased stimulation of insulin or insulin and glucagon by the hormone-stimulating amino acids found in animal proteins.

protein powder Powder containing extracted protein from milk (whey) or other source that is used to increase protein intake, especially by endurance athletes, wishfully to enhance muscle growth and strength and improve performance; evidence that protein powder helps is not clear.

protein quality An index of the amount of all essential amino acids in a single food protein; protein quality of animal and plant foods varies considerably, with animal proteins generally having higher values; milk and egg proteins have the highest quality for humans. *See also* essential (indispensable) amino acid *and* nonessential amino acid.

protein-sparing modified fast A severe dietary approach to weight loss involving low-energy, high-protein intake. *See also* hypocaloric weight-loss diet *and* very low calorie diet.

protein synthesis A complex system that involves the ribosome, enzymes, and messenger RNA derived from nuclear DNA (genetic information) to assemble amino acids into proteins. *See also* amino acid *and* protein.

protein-to-energy ratio Ratio of protein content relative to energy (kilocalories). A good source of protein has about 4 grams of protein per 100 kilocalories of food energy.

protein turnover The dynamic synthesis and breakdown of proteins by the body.

proteinuria Abnormal finding of high levels of protein in the urine. Occasionally occurs after heavy exercise and occasionally in late pregnancy as a consequence of preeclampsia. It is also a sign of kidney failure.

proteolysis The degradation (catabolism) of protein molecules to their constituent amino acids by proteolytic enzymes (peptidases) that hydrolyze peptide bonds. Occurs both within the GI tract and within cells.

provitamin A precursor molecule of a vitamin. For example, carotenoids such as beta-carotene are provitamins of vitamin A and can be converted into vitamin A (retinol) in the GI tract. *See also* beta-carotene *and* vitamin A.

prudent diet A diet plan prepared by the American Heart Association (AHA) for the prevention of cardiovascular diseases and hypertension; several editions of the prudent diet have been published since the 1960s.

PTH *See* parathyroid hormone (PTH).

puberty The transitional period between late childhood and early adolescence that is marked by sexual development, including hormonal changes and increased physical development of the skeleton. In boys, it is also characterized by added muscle mass.

pull date Date that must be placed on packaged food products after which the product is no longer assured to be safe based on the product's estimated shelf-life.

pulmonary Adjective referring to the lung.

purchasing power (money) The economic capability of a family (or individual) to purchase items for a family unit. A major determinant of food habits.

pyloric sphincter Thick muscular portion of the lower stomach that contracts and occasionally relaxes during gastric digestion. The closing permits gastric grinding and digestion of food molecules until small quantities of chyme are released into the duodenum.

pyramid A food guidance tool used to help consumers choose foods wisely so that they meet their nutrient needs every day but do not consume too many calories, salt, and other less healthy constituents of foods; examples include the Mediterranean pyramid and the vegetarian pyramid. *See also* food pyramid.

pyridoxin(e) (vitamin B$_6$) An essential B vitamin that plays a role in amino acid metabolism by transferring amino groups to other keto acids or to intermediate molecules in the urea cycle.

pyruvic acid (pyruvate) A three-carbon keto acid that allows entry of degraded carbohydrates and selected amino acids to the citric acid (Krebs) cycle for oxidative metabolism. *See also* citric acid cycle (Krebs cycle) *and* glycolysis.

quackery In the context of this book, marketing or promoting healthful benefits of a concoction that has no proven health benefit; products typically designed for economic gain but without consideration of potentially adverse health consequences, such as Lydia Pinkham's concoction with alcohol or a plant extract like ephedrine that has recently been withdrawn from the market by the FDA.

R The residual or remainder of a molecule (e.g., of an amino acid, triglyceride, or other molecule).

rancidity The oxidation and spoilage of unsaturated fats in foods through the action of oxygen and often the presence of metallic ions, such as copper, manganese, or iron. Typically, these reactions occur under conditions of elevated temperature, and they result in molecules whose odor and taste are not acceptable. *See also* food safety.

randomized clinical trial (RCT) The investigation of a treatment using the double-blind placebo-controlled method. Involves the comparison of a minimum of two experimental groups, one getting a treatment (e.g., a nutrient supplement) and the other a placebo. Subjects are randomly assigned to each group and the investigators and subjects do not know who is in which group (blinded). *See also* control group, placebo, *and* treatment group.

RBP *See* retinol-binding protein (RBP).

RCT *See* randomized clinical trial (RCT).

RDA *See* Recommended Dietary Allowance (RDA).

ready-to-eat cereal A processed grain product, such as wheat, oats, rice, and corn, that contain nutrient fortificants and chemical additives before being packaged and sealed in plastic bags.

receptor A molecule on the outer plasma membrane or in the nuclear DNA of a cell that accepts a hormone (or similar type of molecule or factor); this interaction of hormone and receptor leads to other complex actions in the cell and subsequently to a response (i.e., effect). *See also* hormone.

Recommended Dietary Allowance (RDA) Recommended intakes of specific nutrients; generally the Estimated Average Requirement (EAR) plus an additional safety factor specific for each nutrient. Age-gender groups are considered for different RDAs, as are women who are pregnant or lactating.

red blood cells (erythrocytes) The most common type of the cell in the blood. They contain hemoglobin but do not have a nucleus or other cell organelles. They are responsible for carrying oxygen to cells of the body and returning carbon dioxide to the lungs via the circulation. Comprise almost the entire amount of the packed cell volume or hematocrit after centrifugation of blood.

redox agent Molecule that can either be oxidized or reduced by donating or accepting one or more electrons and one or more hydrogen ions. An example is ascorbic acid.

reducing agent Molecule or ion that donates an electron or receives an oxygen from another molecule or ion.

reduction The addition of one or more electrons to an atom, ion, or molecule; it is the opposite of oxidation. An example is the conversion of ferric (Fe^{3+}) to ferrous (Fe^{2+}) iron. In organic reactions, the gain of a hydrogen atom (with its electron) is another form of reduction. *See also* oxidation.

refrigeration (cooling) A traditional method of food preservation in which foods are stored at cool temperatures in order to slow the metabolic activity of fruits and vegetables and to inhibit the enzymatic activities of microorganisms.

registered dietitian (RD) Professional who is credentialed to work with foods and menus and to counsel patients or community members about their diets. Has received training under the guidance of criteria established by the Academy of Nutrition and Dietetics. *See also* Academy of Nutrition and Dietetics *and* nutritionist.

religious food practices Practices or customs, often written in religious law, that proscribe certain foods, such as specific meats or seafood, caffeine-containing sources, or other foods, possibly as a result of historical problems of food poisonings or other adverse effects of the banned foods.

renal An adjective referring to the kidney.

required nutrient Nutrient that must be provided by foods or by supplements. The required amounts of the different nutrients vary according to gender and other variables. *See also* essential nutrients.

respiratory quotient (RQ) The ratio of carbon dioxide produced to oxygen consumed by a human subject. This ratio can be used to determine the proportion of metabolic fuels (carbohydrates or fats) being metabolized. The RQ of carbohydrate is near 1.0, whereas the RQ for fat is near 0.7.

resting energy expenditure (REE) The amount of energy expended in cellular metabolic activities while the body is at rest. *See also* basal metabolic rate *and* basal metabolism.

restoration (nutrients) A type of fortification that applies to the replacement (addition) only of vitamins A and D to milk after removal of these vitamins with the cream. *See also* fortification *and* nutrient additive.

retinal The aldehyde form of vitamin A.

retinoic acid The acid (organic) form of vitamin A.

retinoid Considered to be a type of vitamin A molecule; its biochemical actions in the body are essentially the same as those for vitamin A.

retinol The hydroxyl (alcohol) form of vitamin A.

retinol-binding protein (RBP) A serum protein made by the liver that circulates in the blood with transthyretin. Transports retinol from liver stores to extrahepatic tissues. RBP has a short half-life in the blood circulation. *See also* transthyretin.

retinopathy A complication of diabetes that affects the eyes. It is caused by damage to the blood vessels of the light-sensitive tissue at the back of the eye (retina).

rhodopsin A color pigment in the rods of the retina (eye) that participates in the black-and-white visual cycle. The pigment requires retinal. *See also* retinal *and* retinol.

riboflavin An essential B vitamin that is a component of flavonoid proteins, flavin adenine dinucleotide (FAD), and other coenzymes that play key roles in the body's energy pathways. Good sources include liver, dairy products, and fortified cereal products.

ribonucleic acid (RNA) Nucleic acid polymer that controls protein synthesis in ribosomes by transferring the genetic code for a specific protein from the DNA to the ribosome; also the genetic material of many viruses. *See also* deoxyribonucleic acid (DNA) *and* protein.

ribose Five-carbon sugar and its closely related pentoses, especially deoxyribose, that are required for a number of structures, including nucleic acids and nucleotides.

ribosome The molecular complex in cells that serves as the assembly line for protein synthesis. Free ribosomes (cytosolic) synthesize proteins for use in the cell; fixed ribosomes (on microsomal membranes) synthesize proteins for export from the cell. *See also* protein synthesis *and* ribonucleic acid (RNA).

rickets A classic deficiency disease that results from vitamin D and calcium deficiency in infants and children. Characterized by misshapen bones, especially of the tibia (bowed) and pectoral (chest) region (pigeon-breasted). *See also* osteomalacia.

ring structure The arrangement of atoms in the form of a loop or ring, also known as a cyclic structure; many organic molecules important in human metabolism contain ring structures; some of these molecules are provided by the diet, such as phytic acid and polyphenols, and many others are made by cells for specific uses, such as cholesterol, vitamin D, steroid hormones, bile acids (salts), and others.

risk factor A contributor to disease, such as genetic predisposition, lifestyle, or an environmental factor. Also called a determinant.

RNA *See* ribonucleic acid (RNA).

runner's anemia (athletic anemia) Anemia of unknown origin often found in distance runners. *See also* anemia.

saccharin A sugar substitute often used to decrease calories but to maintain sweetness in beverages, desserts, and other foods.

saliva The fluid secreted by the salivary glands into the mouth to facilitate chewing and swallowing. Saliva is responsible for the initial digestion of complex carbohydrates (i.e., starches).

salivary glands Secretory glands located in the oral cavity that provide saliva that mixes food with water, mineral ions, and amylase enzymes. Also bathes the teeth with caries-preventing water and mineral ions.

Salmonella A bacterial genus responsible for food poisoning.

salt Sodium chloride has been used as a food preservative for thousands of years. Salt also enhances the taste of food. However, it is a source of concern for hypertension.

salt preservation Classic method of food preservation that was heavily used before refrigeration became widespread for the preservation of foods such as meats and vegetables. *See also* food preservation.

salt sensitivity Condition, possibly hereditary, whereby individuals have a strong desire for salty foods or discretionary salt use.

salt taste The taste for salt or salty foods on the tongue. One of the four basic chemical tastes. It can be developed or it can be partially depressed through learned behaviors.

sarcopenia Age-related loss of muscle mass. It usually begins around age 45, when muscle mass begins to decline at a rate of about 1% per year.

satiety The feeling of fullness or satisfaction after eating.

satiety center The portion of the hypothalamus that inhibits food intake behavior by sending signals to inhibit activity of the feeding center of the brain.

saturated fatty acids (SFA) A fatty acid with no double bonds (and no points of unsaturation). Common in meat and dairy products; excess consumption has been found to be a dietary risk factor for heart disease. *See also* monounsaturated fatty acids (MFA) *and* unsaturated fatty acids (UFA).

saturation (fatty acid) The presence of the maximum number of hydrogen atoms in a hydrocarbon chain of a fatty acid (no double bonds). *See also* unsaturated.

School Lunch Program A federal program that reimburses schools for serving low-cost and free lunches to qualifying students. The program uses surplus and low-cost foods to the benefit of the U.S. agricultural market. Standards recently have been raised to improve the nutritional quality of the meals provided. Many of these students also qualify for the Summer Food Service Program. *See also* federal food programs.

scurvy A classic deficiency disease of ascorbic acid (vitamin C) characterized by bleeding gums, skin hemorrhages, and developmental defects in infants and children. *See also* deficiency disease.

seafood A staple food in many coastal areas that is a source of high-quality protein plus minerals and many vitamins.

seaweed (kelp) A major source of dietary fiber used in the food supply, often as an additive, such as alginates, or a filler, such as carrageenan. *See also* food additive.

secondary structure (protein) The structure that results from hydrogen bonds between amino acid residues along the peptide backbone of the protein; these bonds form automatically and help stabilize the structure of the protein.

secretions The fluid products of many glands and organs of the body, including those of the GI glands, the endocrine glands, and organs such as the liver and kidney.

sedentary lifestyle Lifestyle characterized by low levels of physical activity. Believed to be a key factor in the development of obesity.

selenium An essential micromineral that exists as a divalent anion (Se^{2-}). It activates the enzyme glutathione peroxidase, which protects fatty acids and other molecules against oxidative damage.

semistarvation The deliberate consumption of less than the recommended number of calories for a period of time. A diet that has roughly 30% fewer calories than the normal diet.

Senate Select Committee on Nutrition and Human Needs The committee under the leadership of Senator George McGovern that formulated the Dietary Goals in 1970. *See also* Dietary Goals.

sequelae Various pathological consequences in tissues following the development of a disease.

sequestrants A class of food additives that bind metal ions and keep them from affecting taste or other properties of foods. *See also* food additive.

serosa The outer layer of the gastrointestinal tract that is in contact with the venous and lymphatic collection vessels. It surrounds the middle muscular layer, which, in turn, surrounds the mucosal layer of the gastrointestinal tract. *See also* mucosa.

serotonin Neurotransmitter that inhibits the feeding center and hence reduces food ingestion. It is derived from the amino acid tryptophan.

serum The liquid fraction of blood remaining after clotting. *See also* blood *and* plasma.

serum albumin A stable protein in blood that is largely responsible for maintaining the osmotic pressure of blood. Levels decline slowly during periods of protein deficiency, so it is not a good short-term marker of protein deficiency. However, with chronic deficiency it does serve as a good indicator of protein insufficiency.

serum (plasma) proteins Albumin, globulins (immunoglobulins), fibrinogen, and many other proteins in the liquid portion of blood.

Seven Countries Study (Ancel Keys) A study that found links between coronary heart disease (CHD) and blood cholesterol levels in five European countries, the United States, and Japan that helped establish the lipid hypothesis for the etiology of CHD and an early understanding of the benefits of the Mediterranean diet against heart disease. *See also* Mediterranean diet.

SFA *See* saturated fatty acids (SFA).

shelf-life The maximum time a processed food product is allowed to be on the shelf of a food market.

short-chain fatty acids Fatty acids with eight or fewer carbon atoms that are produced when dietary fiber is fermented in the colon. *See also* long-chain fatty acid *and* medium-chain fatty acid.

side group Atoms in a special group added to a core molecular structure that may modify the molecule's function; many organic molecules have side groups attached to the hydrocarbon backbone, such as amino groups, carboxyl groups, sulfur groups, phosphate groups, and others.

skeletal growth The increase in size of the skeleton in both length (height) and width through osteoblastic activity and bone modeling. Growth in height in childhood is typically concluded by late adolescence; continuing accumulation of bone mass (mineral content) occurs during early adulthood (bone consolidation).

skeletal muscle The striated muscle found in motor-controlled muscle groups of the body. These muscles comprise the largest fraction of lean body mass and represent 60–70% of body weight. Men have greater muscle mass than women.

skeleton The structural framework of the body that supports and protects the internal organs. It also serves as a reservoir of calcium, inorganic phosphate, and other minerals. During growth and development, the bones of the skeleton undergo modeling to achieve adult height and size (dimensions). During adulthood, the bones of the skeleton undergo remodeling.

small intestine The segment of the gastrointestinal tract between the stomach and large intestine that functions primarily in digestion and absorption. It consists of three segments: duodenum, jejunum, and ileum.

small-for-gestational-age (SGA) baby A baby who is low birth weight (i.e., less than 5.5 pounds or 2,500 grams) at term or a premature baby whose birth weight is lower than it should be for its gestational age.

smooth muscle Nonstriated muscle that exists in the middle layers of arterial walls, the intestinal tube, and other epithelial tissues of the body.

social and cultural value Values applied to foods by a group, culture, or society; in the United States, societal food values exist, but they have been greatly affected by the marketing of a tremendous array of processed foods. A major determinant of food habits. *See also* Maslow's hierarchy of food needs.

sodium A monovalent mineral cation (Na^+) found predominantly in blood and extracellular fluids. Excess sodium consumption can lead to hypertension.

sodium-induced hypercalciuria Excess dietary sodium enhances urinary calcium losses. The kidney tubules reabsorb much more of the sodium ions, which tends to reduce the reabsorption of calcium ions by the cotransport mechanism. *See also* hypercalciuria.

sodium–potassium (Na^+-K^+) pump The pump that transfers sodium out of and potassium into cells in order to maintain the electrical charge differential across cell membranes. The energy (ATP) required by the Na^+-K^+ pump is a major portion of the basal metabolic rate.

soil exhaustion Condition that occurs when the same crops are grown multiple times in the same location, leading to depletion of soil nutrients and eventual loss of the ability of the soil to support crops or other plant life. Can be prevented by crop rotation and application of fertilizer.

soluble fiber The components of dietary fiber that are soluble in water and that exert an osmotic force in body fluids, such as in the gut. A significant fraction of soluble fiber can be degraded (fermented) by gut bacteria, thereby improving a number of diverse bodily functions. *See also* insoluble fiber.

soybeans Plant food containing high-quality proteins and phytomolecules (e.g., isoflavones). Processed and used in many food products.

spina bifida A severe neural tube defect resulting, in part, from insufficient folate intake during prepregnancy and early gestation (first 2 months of pregnancy). *See also* folic acid (folate, folacin) *and* neural tube defect.

sports drink Electrolyte-enriched fluid that is formulated to replace electrolytes lost during a sporting event or physical activity.

stabilizer A food additive or other molecule that enhances the mixing of lipid-soluble and water-soluble components. Examples include monoglycerides, diglycerides, lecithin, and other phospholipids.

staple foods A food that is eaten routinely and in large quantities such that it constitutes the large portion of the diet of a population. In much of the world, rice, cassava, wheat, and corn are staples. Many staple foods, such as rice, are high in carbohydrates and energy but low in many other nutrients.

starch A complex carbohydrate (polysaccharide) consisting of amylose, amylopectin, or glycogen molecules.

starvation Also called marasmus; a form of undernutrition characterized by emaciation, tissue wasting, and other signs. The body literally consumes itself, with all body compartments losing mass. *See also* malnutrition *and* undernutrition.

statins Class of cholesterol-lowering drugs that have proven to be highly effective in reducing total cholesterol and LDL-C.

stearic acid A saturated fatty acid found most commonly in meats.

stem cell An undifferentiated cell that has the potential to develop into one of many different kinds of cells, such as a skin cell or red blood cell.

steroid hormone A hormone that is derived from cholesterol and has a similar chemical ring structure; examples include estrogens and androgens.

sterol The complex four-ring structure of many steroids; cholesterol is the precursor molecule in animal tissues, but plant tissues have several sterols that differ from cholesterol. *See also* cholesterol.

stomach An organ of the GI tract that has several functions, including temporary storage, digestion, and secretion, but not absorption (except for alcohol and fluoride). The gastric glands secrete acid (H^+), intrinsic factor (IF), and pepsinogen in addition to fluids (water).

stress fracture A small bone fracture, especially in the femur and feet, that may occur in athletes, especially runners, due to the strain of forces at specific sites; such fractures are often difficult to find on x-rays because they are so small.

stroke A blockage of an artery of the brain (ischemic stroke) or a bursting of a vessel in the brain (hemorrhagic stroke).

subclinical condition Medical condition that is not noticeable upon clinical examination; usually not severe or debilitating. An example is iron deficiency (subclinical) compared to iron deficiency anemia (clinical).

sucralose A sweetener used in foods that is poorly absorbed so that almost no kilocalories are generated. Structure is that of sucrose with three chloride substitutions for hydroxyl groups.

sucrase An enzyme of the small intestine that degrades sucrose.

sucrose A disaccharide containing fructose and glucose. It is most well known as common table sugar.

sugar A monosaccharide or disaccharide that is characterized by a sweet taste; naturally occurring sugars include sucrose, fructose, and lactose; refined and processed sugars include high-fructose corn syrup (HFCS).

sugar alcohol A type of alcohol derived from sugar. Sugar alcohols are used widely in the food industry as thickeners and sweeteners. They are absorbed more slowly that sugar and do not contribute to the formation of dental caries.

sulfite Sulfur-containing additive originally used to preserve lettuce and other foods; it may provoke an allergic response in some individuals.

Supplemental Nutrition Assistance Program (SNAP) A federal food aid program, more commonly referred to as food stamps, that provides food assistance to low-income individuals and families. It is funded through the U.S. Department of Agriculture and administered through the states. *See also* federal food programs.

Supplementary Food Program for Women, Infants, and Children (WIC) A federal food-assistance program that provides nutrition education for medically qualified mothers and certain high-quality foods free for enrolled mothers and their children. Is considered the most cost-effective of the U.S. Department of Agriculture's food programs due to the strong gains in birth weights and growth of infants and children.

supplementation Usually purified micronutrients in pill form; nutrients consumed through the ingestion of pills or tablets for the purpose of improving nutritional status; protein and energy may also be increased by specific macronutrient supplements; supplements are distinguished from nutrient fortificants, i.e., nutrients added to foods.

sweat Salty fluid produced by the sweat glands that helps the body to dissipate heat through evaporation.

sweetener Food additive used to add sweetness to a food. May be nutrient (sugar) or non-nutrient molecules, such as aspartame, saccharin, sucralose, and others.

sweetness scale A scale based on perceptions of sweetness, with sucrose arbitrarily given a value of 1.0. Fructose has a value of about 1.75; glucose has a value greater than 0.75; saccharin and other artificial sweeteners have very high values.

symptom Subjective indication of ill health that may be a precursor of disease (e.g., pain in the lower abdomen that could be related to the appendix, cancer of the colon, or nonspecific change in condition).

systolic blood pressure Arterial pressure when the heart is pumping; first number of the reported blood pressure. For example, for a blood pressure of 120/80 mm Hg, the systolic pressure is 120 mm Hg. *See also* diastolic blood pressure *and* hypertension.

tallow Beef fat obtained from the fat of beef carcasses and rendered by liquefying and solidifying. *See also* lard.

taste preferences Sweet and salty are the primary taste preferences desired in foods, but acid and sour are also desired by some. Taste is an extremely important quality in the selection of foods.

teeth Hard, mineralized tissue in the oral cavity that helps in the initial mechanical breakdown of food.

teratogen Molecule or other agent that causes developmental abnormalities either of the embryo or fetus.

thermogenesis Generation of heat by the body's metabolic activities. *See also* diet-induced thermogenesis (DIT) *and* exercise-induced thermogenesis (EIT).

thiamin A B vitamin found in pork and whole grains and fortified cereals. Plays a critical role in the body's energy-producing pathways. The deficiency disease is beriberi. It was the first vitamin discovered. *See also* beriberi.

thrombosis The formation of a clot within an artery or arteriole, which leads to total blockage of blood flow at that specific site. Can lead to a myocardial infarction or stroke. *See also* myocardial infarction and stroke.

thrombus (clot) The plug that is formed in the arteries due to thrombosis.

thyroglobulin A protein found in the thyroid gland that is used to produce the hormones thyroxine (T_4) and triiodothyronine (T_3).

thyroid hormones Thyroxin(e) (T_4) and triiodothyronine (T_3), which contain four and three iodine atoms, respectively.

thyroxin(e) (T_4) A hormone produced by the thyroid gland that contains four atoms of iodine.

tight junction A microanatomic structure between adjacent cells of the epithelial tract. These structures tend to prevent the entry of large molecules into the blood from the lumen of the small intestine.

tocopherol A form of vitamin E.

tocotrienol A form of vitamin E.

Tolerable Upper Limit of Safety (UL) The safe upper limit of intake of a nutrient from foods and supplements; determined when establishing the Dietary Reference Intake (DRI) of a nutrient.

total blood cholesterol (TC) The total concentration of cholesterol in either fasting blood serum or plasma; includes cholesterol in the circulating lipoproteins—VLDL, LDL, and HDL. A high level is a risk factor for heart disease. *See also* cholesterol.

toxin A molecule that produces an adverse effect, sometimes lethal. Sometimes produced by a microorganism (e.g., fungus or mold) that has adverse effects, including severe toxicity, in individuals consuming the contaminated food.

trabecular tissue The sponge-like cancellous tissue consisting of plates and spicules (trabeculae) found at the ends of the long bones and in the vertebrae.

trace element Another term for micromineral. An essential mineral needed in small quantities in the diet. At present, RDAs or AIs have been set for the following trace elements: iron, zinc, iodine, selenium, manganese, copper, chromium, and fluoride. *See also* macromineral.

transamination The transfer of an amine group from an amino acid to an organic keto acid to form a new amino acid.

transcellular transfer (absorption) Transfer of nutrients across membranes and through the cells of the small intestine from the gut lumen to the serosa.

transcription Transfer of information from the DNA genetic code to RNA, specifically to messenger RNA (mRNA). *See also* deoxyribonucleic acid (DNA), ribonucleic acid (RNA), *and* translation.

trans fatty acid (trFA) Unsaturated fatty acid that results from partial hydrogenation of vegetable oils for the purpose of preparing fats of varying hardness for commercial use. The three-dimensional configuration of the remaining double bonds (one or more) in the fats takes on the *trans* form rather than remaining in the natural *cis* configuration. Trans fatty acids are metabolized much more like saturated fatty acids than monounsaturated or polyunsaturated fatty acids. They have been found to increase the risk of heart disease.

transferrin A liver protein secreted into the blood to carry iron from the liver to tissues, especially the red bone marrow, where red blood cells are forming. A marker for acute disease because synthesis increases when the body is under stress.

transferrin saturation (%) The percentage of the molecule that is carrying iron compared to its total iron-binding capacity; normally the % saturation is approximately 30%, but in iron deficiency it can decrease. In iron deficiency anemia, it is typically near 10–15%.

transient ischemic attack (TIA) A mini-stroke that may result in only a brief blockage of an artery in the brain. May cause a blackout or temporary loss of function of the brain. A risk factor for stroke. *See also* stroke.

translation The conversion of genetic information from RNA into a protein via protein synthesis. *See also* ribonucleic acid (RNA) *and* transcription.

transthyretin Travels in blood with retinal-binding protein in a complex with retinol. Also transports T_3 and T_4 hormones. *See also* retinol-binding protein (RBP).

treatment group A group of subjects given an experimental treatment in an experiment; for example, the group that receives a nutrient supplement or a drug. The control group receives a placebo. *See also* control group *and* randomized clinical trial (RCT).

trends in calorie consumption (U.S.) The direction of changes in mean total energy intake; this intake has actually decreased over the last five or six decades in spite of the increase in mean body weight during this post-WWII period; the reduction in exercise and routine activities because of cars and other labor-saving devices has resulted in a slight lowering of the quantities of food intake.

trends in macronutrient intake (U.S.) The direction of changes in macronutrient intake; trends for this intake over the last 5 or 6 decades includes more carbohydrate, especially sugars and processed grains, about the same or slightly less fat but more saturated fats, and slightly more protein, especially animal protein; fewer plant sources of the macronutrients are consumed, but more processed foods and snacks are eaten.

triacylglycerol Another term for triglyceride.

triglyceride A triacylglycerol or fat that contains glycerol linked to three fatty acids by ester bonds.

triglyceride synthesis The synthesis of a triglyceride in the cytosolic endoplasmic reticulum that requires activated glycerol plus three fatty acids.

triiodothyronine (T$_3$) A hormone produced by the thyroid gland that contains three atoms of iodine.

trimester A term in the course of pregnancy. A normal full-term pregnancy contains three trimesters over approximately 9 months (280 days).

trypsin An enzyme that hydrolyzes (splits with the addition of water) peptide bonds in dietary proteins in the small intestine.

trypsinogen A proenzyme secreted by the pancreas that must be partially cleaved within the small intestinal lumen to yield the active enzyme trypsin, which degrades peptide bonds.

tumor An abnormal growth that may be benign (relatively harmless) or malignant (cancer). *See also* cancer.

UL *See* Tolerable Upper Limit of Safety (UL).

ultrapasteurization Heating of milk or other beverages at high temperature (600 °F) for a second or so to kill all bacteria and other microorganisms. *See also* pasteurization.

ultraviolet (UV) light The light wavelength that is essential for the biosynthesis of vitamin D by the skin. Excess UV light may cause sunburn and skin cancer.

undernutrition A form of malnutrition characterized by insufficient energy and nutrient consumption. *See also* malnutrition *and* undernutrition.

undernutrition–infection cycle A cycle whereby inadequate nutrition depresses the immune system, thus reducing the body's ability to respond to invading organisms. During sickness, the body responds by decreasing appetite, digestion of ingested nutrients, and utilization of absorbed nutrients and increasing mobilization and wasting of the body's stored nutrients, which further decreases the body's immune response, further driving the cycle.

underwater weighing A method used for estimating body fat by submerging the body in water and measuring the amount of water that is displaced.

underweight Body weight that is 10% or more below the lower range of normal weight (Metropolitan or NHANES); also, a BMI of less than 18.5.

unsaturated A point in a hydrocarbon chain from which two hydrogen atoms have been lost from adjacent carbons; a carbon-to-carbon double bond. *See also* saturation (fatty acid).

unsaturated fatty acids (UFA) Mono- or polyunsaturated fatty acids. The double bonds in these molecules represent points of unsaturated carbon atoms with respect to hydrogen atoms. The double bonds of monounsaturated and polyunsaturated fatty acids are subject to oxidative attack by free radicals. *See also* monounsaturated fatty acids (MFA) *and* polyunsaturated fatty acids (PFA).

upregulation Increase in the number of receptors or porters inserted in a cell membrane; for example, glucose receptors or porters are upregulated when cells need glucose, as in fasting or in the downregulated state.

urbanization An increase in the number of people living in urban areas. In many poor and developing countries, the rural poor migrate to urban areas in search of employment opportunities. Urbanization often results in the development of so-called shanty towns that are characterized by substandard nutrition and sanitation.

urea The major waste product of nitrogen metabolism.

urea cycle The hepatic cycle that synthesizes urea from two amine groups and one carbon dioxide molecule.

uremia Elevation of blood urea (BUN) and other nitrogenous waste products that have toxic effects at very high levels; typically results from failing kidneys.

uric acid A degradation product of nucleic acids that must be removed from the blood or else it will accumulate in joints and cause joint irritations and dysfunction (gout).

urinary hydroxyproline A general marker of the breakdown of bone collagen, and to a lesser extent the degradation of other connective tissue collagens in the body.

urine The fluid made by the kidneys that contains nitrogenous waste products (urea, creatinine, ammonia, uric acid, and hydroxyproline), various chromes (colored products), water-soluble metabolites of vitamins, and minerals, such as potassium, calcium, sodium, and many others. Does not usually contain sugar (glucose) or proteins.

U.S. Census Bureau Federal agency responsible for conducting the U.S. Census every 10 years and for projecting population trends in the United States.

U.S. Department of Agriculture The federal agency responsible for developing and executing policy on farming, agriculture, forestry, and food.

U.S. Department of Health and Human Services (USDHHS) Includes the Public Health Service, Centers for Disease Control and Prevention, and the National Institutes of Health.

U.S. RDAs U.S. Daily Recommended Allowances. These differ from the RDAs but are derived from them. They were used on food labels until the mid-1990s, when they were replaced by Percent Daily Values.

USDA *See* U.S. Department of Agriculture.

USDHHS *See* U.S. Department of Health and Human Services.

vacuum dehydration A modern type of food preservation that removes most of the water from a powdered foodstuff (i.e., it dehydrates it), thereby allowing it to be packaged in a sealed pouch. It can later be reconstituted with water and eaten. Examples includes dried soups and complete dinners.

valves (heart) The heart has four valves that open to let blood flow through or out of the heart and then shut to keep blood from flowing backward.

vascular depression A form of depression resulting from damage to the major arteries of the brain. May have a strong linkage with diets that promote arterial plaque formation, which generally occurs much earlier in life than when the depression is clinically identified.

vegan A strict vegetarian who consumes no animal products, excluding all meat, poultry, seafood, dairy products, and eggs. *See also* vegetarian eating pattern.

vegetable group One of the basic food groups of the MyPlate food guidance system. This food group includes any vegetable or 100% vegetables juice. Can be divided into five subgroups based on nutrient content: dark green, leafy vegetables, starchy vegetables, beans and peas (legumes), red and orange vegetables, and other. In addition to supplying macronutrients, vegetables are rich in micronutrients and dietary fiber. *See also* ChooseMyPlate.

vegetable oils Triglycerides extracted from plants. They are typically high in poly- and monounsaturated fatty acids, but lower in saturated fats than animal fats. They are typically liquid at room temperature. Examples include corn, soy, olive, and sunflower oils.

vegetarian diet In general, a diet that does not include meat or meat products. The strictest type of vegetarian diet, the vegan diet, does not include any animal products. Other types of vegetarian eating patterns allow consumption of dairy products and eggs.

vegetarian eating pattern A diet in which no meats are consumed. The strictest type of vegetarian diet, the vegan diet, does not include any animal products. Other types of vegetarian eating patterns allow consumption of dairy products and eggs. *See also* lacto-ovo-vegetarian, lacto-vegetarian, ovo-vegetarian, pesco-vegetarian, *and* vegan.

very low calorie diet (VLCD) Any diet that provides approximately 400 to 600 kilocalories per day for the purpose of weight loss (e.g., protein-sparing modified fast). *See also* hypocaloric weight-loss diet.

very low density lipoproteins (VLDL) The class of lipoproteins made by the liver for export to extrahepatic tissues. They contain triglycerides, cholesterol, and phospholipids in addition to protein. They are converted in the capillary beds to low-density lipoproteins (LDL) through the action of lipoprotein lipase and other enzymes. *See also* lipoprotein lipase *and* low-density lipoproteins (LDL).

villi (villus) Finger-like projections of the small intestinal mucosa into the gut lumen; they increase the surface area for absorption of nutrients.

visual cycle The biochemical cycle in the eye that permits vision; both the black-and-white cycle in the rods and the color cycle in the cones utilize the vitamin A molecules retinol and retinal.

vitamin An essential organic micronutrient needed in the diet in small amounts; consists of both water-soluble and fat-soluble vitamins. *See also* fat-soluble vitamin *and* water-soluble vitamin.

vitamin A An essential fat-soluble vitamin with three distinct forms: retinol (an alcohol), retinal (an aldehyde), and retinoic acid (an organic acid). Retinol is a storage form found in the liver; it is carried by retinol-binding protein (RBP) to the eye and other tissues for use. Retinal participates in the visual cycle; retinoic acid functions like a steroid hormone in cells and is responsible for growth and epithelial integrity. *See also* retinol-binding protein (RBP) *and* visual cycle.

vitamin B$_{12}$ Also called cobalamin. A B vitamin with a complex structure containing a cobalt atom. It is found only in animal foods and is produced by a few specific intestinal microorganisms. It requires binding by intrinsic factor (IF) before it can be absorbed and participate in the transfer of methyl groups. Humans have a large storage capacity in the liver for cobalamin. It is essential for cell division and nucleic acid synthesis.

vitamin C (ascorbic acid) An essential water-soluble vitamin that functions as an oxidation-reduction system in tissues and in the gut. It is also responsible for the hydroxylation of collagen and is a powerful antioxidant. If intake is inadequate, the deficiency disease scurvy will develop.

vitamin D Fat-soluble vitamin made in the skin under the influence of ultraviolet light. Dietary sources include dairy products and other fortified foods. Vitamin D plays a critical role in calcium absorption and homeostasis. The deficiency disease in children is rickets.

vitamin E A fat-soluble antioxidant vitamin that operates in the highly lipophilic portion of cell membranes to protect polyunsaturated fatty acids and monounsaturated fatty acids from oxidation.

vitamin K A fat-soluble vitamin essential for blood clotting and formation of bone matrix proteins, including osteocalcin. Gut bacteria synthesize some vitamin K that is then absorbed by the GI tract.

VLDL *See* very low density lipoproteins (VLDL).

waist circumference A measure of abdominal girth that is a fairly good surrogate measurement for BMI.

waist-to-hip ratio (WHR) A ratio of two measurements that serves as a prognostic index of health; a high WHR, a pattern typical in men, is associated with more metabolically active fat tissue in the abdominal cavity, which favors development of the chronic diseases. A low WHR represents more fat in the hips and buttocks, a pattern typical in women, which has less of an influence on the development of the chronic diseases. *See also* android fat distribution *and* gynoid fat distribution.

water A molecule consisting of two hydrogens and one oxygen (H_2O) that normally exists as a liquid at room temperature. The human body requires water to function.

water activity (A_W) The amount of water that is available to support the growth of bacteria, yeast, or mold. It is based on a scale of 0 to 1.0, with water having a value of 1.0. Products that have lower water content have lower water activity. Foods with low water activity are more resistant to spoilage by bacteria.

water balance The maintenance of the body's water compartments, both extra- and intracellular, through the consumption of water and the generation of metabolic water to equal the losses in urine, feces, sweat, and evaporation via the lungs and skin. *See also* metabolic water.

water-insoluble fiber molecules Dietary fibers that are not soluble in water. Because they are not soluble in the watery fluids of the GI tract, they are not subject to digestion by gut bacteria in the lower small intestine and large intestine. Include the celluloses, lignans, and most of the hemicelluloses. *See also* dietary fiber *and* water-soluble fiber molecules.

water loss The loss of water from the body by any route; water is lost in all excretions, sweat, and exhaled air throughout the day and, if not replaced by liquid fluids, dehydration may occur; maintaining water balance requires conscious effort because the thirst mechanism is not as sensitive as needed for adequate water replacement.

water quality A measure of the condition of water in an area and its ability to be used by people. In many parts of the world, water may be contaminated by chemicals or sewage, making it unsuitable for human use.

water soluble A substance that dissolves in water. Organic molecules with hydroxyl (OH), aldehyde (CHO), keto (=O), or carboxylic acid (COOH) groups tend to be water soluble. *See also* lipid soluble.

water-soluble fiber molecules Dietary fibers that are soluble in water. Because they are soluble in the watery fluids of the GI tract, they can be digested by gut bacteria in the lower small intestine and especially in the large intestine. Include the gums, mucilages, pectins, algal polysaccharides, and some hemicelluloses of low molecular weight. *See also* dietary fiber *and* water-insoluble fiber molecules.

water-soluble vitamin Vitamins that are soluble in water. Includes the B complex vitamins and vitamin C. *See also* fat-soluble vitamin.

weight cycling Repetitive weight loss and then regain of the lost weight. This pattern is typical of overweight or obese individuals who temporarily go on hypocaloric diets. Also called yo-yo dieting.

Western diet A dietary habit chosen by many people in some developed countries, and increasingly in developing countries. It is characterized by high intakes of red meat, sugary desserts, high-fat foods, and refined grains. It also typically contains high-fat dairy products, high-sugar drinks, and higher intakes of processed meat. This diet has been found to be correlated with obesity, heart disease, and cancer.

white blood cells (leukocytes) A class of cells or formed elements found in blood that include multinucleated white cells that stain differently. Include eosinophils, basophils, neutrophils, and lymphocytes. When blood is centrifuged with an anticlotting agent, the white cells form a narrow band, the buffy coat, on top of the red blood cells and beneath the plasma.

whole grain Cereal grain that has little or no processing prior to use (e.g., whole wheat and brown rice).

Women, Infants and Children (WIC) food program A federal food-assistance program that provides nutrition education for medically qualified mothers and certain high-quality foods free for enrolled mothers and their children. Is considered the most cost-effective of the U.S. Department of Agriculture's food programs due to the strong gains in birth weights and growth of infants and children.

xerophthalmia An eye disease resulting from a dietary deficiency of vitamin A.

xerosis Dryness or dry patches of the skin or whites (conjunctivae) of the eyes. Thought to be associated with vitamin A deficiency.

zen macrobiotic vegetarianism An extreme form of vegetarianism where the diet consists only of cereal grains. This is not a safe diet. *See also* vegetarian eating pattern.

zinc An essential micromineral that exists in the body as a divalent cation (Zn^{2+}). Plays a role in more than 100 enzyme reactions and is a component of many other tissue proteins.

Index

undernutrition (*cont.*)
  infection cycle, 283*f*, 370, 381, 381*f*
  and infectious diseases, 380–383
  and risk of infectious diseases, 282–283
underweight, 303
unidirectional flow of nutrients, 66, 67*f*
United States
  common cancers in, 357*t*
  diet-related cancers rates, 354–355
unsaturated fatty acid (UFA), 133
urbanization, 376–377
urine, 209
U.S. Department of Agriculture (USDA), 59–60, 60*f*
uterus shrinks, 266

V
valves (heart), 151
vascular depression, 361, 361*f*
vegan diets, 335
vegetable group, 38–39
  subgroups and frequently consumed, 39*t*
vegetarian diet, 36, 36*f*
vegetarian eating pattern, 12–13, 13*t*
vegetarians
  nutritional needs during lactation, 266–267
  proteins need for, 172–173, 172*f*
  special needs for pregnant women, 256
very low calorie diets (VLCDs), 313
very low density lipoproteins (VLDLs), 141, 143
villi, 65–66, 66*f*, 69
Vipeholm study of sugar-related dental caries, 285
visceral fat, 306
vitamin A, 193
  deficiency, 199
  excessive intake of, 258
  functions of, 195–196, 196*t*
vitamin B$_6$. *See* pyridoxin(e)
vitamin B$_{12}$. *See* cobalamin
vitamin C, 38, 180
  food content, 181*t*
  functions of, 185
vitamin D, 43, 193
  biosynthesis of, 197*f*
  deficiency, 199–200
  excessive intake of, 258
  functions of, 197
  interactions between calcium and, 226
  metabolic conversions of, 198*f*
  vitamin D$_2$, 193, 198*f*
  vitamin D$_2$, 193, 198*f*
vitamin E, 193
  deficiency, 200
  functions of, 197–198
vitamin K, 193
  deficiency, 200
  functions of, 198–199
vitamins, 3
  fat-soluble. *See* fat-soluble vitamins
  water-soluble. *See* water-soluble vitamins
VLCDs. *See* very low calorie diets (VLCDs)
VLDLs. *See* very low density lipoproteins (VLDLs)

W
waist circumference, 305
warfarin, 199
waste heat, 90, 92, 92*f*
water, 208–210
  content of body, 208, 208*f*
  digestion and absorption of, 80–81
  -soluble nutritents *vs.* fat-soluble nutrients, absorption of, 75
water activity (A$_w$), 5
water balance, 208
water-insoluble fiber molecule, 109
water quality, 377
water-soluble fiber molecule, 109
water-soluble vitamins, 81, 179–180
  deficiencies, 188–190
  essential for human health, 180*t*
  food sources, 180–183
  foods rich in, 182*f*
  fortified foods, 183, 183*f*
  functions of, 185–187
  RDAs, 190–191
  supplements of, 183–185, 184*f*, 184*t*
  toxicities, 190
weight cycling, 314
weight gain, recommendations during pregnancy, 250–253, 253*t*
weight loss, 313–314
weight management
  behavior modification techniques, 317–318
  dietary recommendations, 314–316
  gastric surgery, 318–319
  pharmacologic therapy, 318
  physical activity, 317
  and type 2 diabetes, 317
Western diets, 49
WHO. *See* World Health Organization (WHO)
whole grain
  foods, 39, 41, 41*t*
  oats, 48
Women, Infants and Children (WIC) Food Program, 60
World Health Organization (WHO), 386

X
xanthine oxidase, 239
xerophthalmia, 199

Y
yo-yo dieting. *See* weight cycling

Z
zinc (Zn^{2+}), 42, 235
  absorption, 236
  content of foods, 236*t*
  deficiency, 236*t*, 372
  excretion, 236
  food sources, 235
  toxicity, 236

Tolerable Upper Intake Levels (ULs[1])

Life stage group	Vitamin A[2] (µg/d)	Vitamin D (µg/d)	Vitamin E[3,4] (mg/d)	Niacin[4] (mg/d)	Vitamin B$_6$ (mg/d)	Folate[4] (µg/d)	Vitamin C (mg/d)	Choline (g/d)	Calcium (g/d)	Phosphorus (g/d)	Magnesium[5] (mg/d)	Sodium (g/d)
Infants												
0-6 mo	600	25	ND[7]	ND	ND	ND	ND	ND	ND	ND	ND	ND
7-12 mo	600	25	ND	ND	ND	ND	ND	ND	ND	ND	ND	ND
Children												
1-3 y	600	50	200	10	30	300	400	1.0	2.5	3	65	1.5
4-8 y	900	50	300	15	40	400	650	1.0	2.5	3	110	1.9
Males, females												
9-13 y	1,700	50	600	20	60	600	1,200	2.0	2.5	4	350	2.2
14-18 y	2,800	50	800	30	80	800	1,800	3.0	2.5	4	350	2.3
19-70 y	3,000	50	1,000	35	100	1,000	2,000	3.5	2.5	4	350	2.3
>70 y	3,000	50	1,000	35	100	1,000	2,000	3.5	2.5	3	350	2.3
Pregnancy												
≤18 y	2,800	50	800	30	80	800	1,800	3.0	2.5	3.5	350	2.3
19-50 y	3,000	50	1,000	35	100	1,000	2,000	3.5	2.5	3.5	350	2.3
Lactation												
≤18 y	2,800	50	800	30	80	800	1,800	3.0	2.5	4	350	2.3
19-50 y	3,000	50	1,000	35	100	1,000	2,000	3.5	2.5	4	350	2.3

Life stage group	Iron (mg/d)	Zinc (mg/d)	Selenium (µg/d)	Iodine (µg/d)	Copper (µg/d)	Manganese (mg/d)	Fluoride (mg/d)	Molybdenum (µg/d)	Boron (mg/d)	Nickel (mg/d)	Vanadium[6] (mg/d)	Chloride (g/d)
Infants												
0-6 mo	40	4	45	ND	ND	ND	0.7	ND	ND	ND	ND	ND
7-12 mo	40	5	60	ND	ND	ND	0.9	ND	ND	ND	ND	ND
Children												
1-3 y	40	7	90	200	1,000	2	1.3	300	3	0.2	ND	2.3
4-8 y	40	12	150	300	3,000	3	2.2	600	6	0.3	ND	2.9
Males, females												
9-13 y	40	23	280	600	5,000	6	10	1,100	11	0.6	ND	3.4
14-18 y	45	34	400	900	8,000	9	10	1,700	17	1.0	ND	3.6
19-70 y	45	40	400	1,100	10,000	11	10	2,000	20	1.0	1.8	3.6
>70 y	45	40	400	1,100	10,000	11	10	2,000	20	1.0	1.8	3.6
Pregnancy												
≤18 y	45	34	400	900	8,000	9	10	1,700	17	1.0	ND	3.6
19-50 y	45	40	400	1,100	10,000	11	10	2,000	20	1.0	ND	3.6
Lactation												
≤18 y	45	34	400	900	8,000	9	10	1,700	17	1.0	ND	3.6
19-50 y	45	40	400	1,100	10,000	11	10	2,000	20	1.0	ND	3.6

[1] UL = The maximum level of daily nutrient intake that is likely to pose no risk of adverse effects. Unless otherwise specified, the UL represents total intake from food, water, and supplements. Due to lack of suitable data, ULs could not be established for vitamin K, thiamin, riboflavin, vitamin B$_{12}$, pantothenic acid, biotin, or carotenoids. In the absence of ULs, extra caution may be warranted in consuming levels above recommended intakes.

[2] As preformed vitamin A (retinol) only.

[3] As α-tocopherol; applies to any form of supplemental α-tocopherol.

[4] The ULs for vitamin E, niacin, and folate apply to synthetic forms obtained from supplements, fortified foods, or a combination of the two.

[5] The ULs for magnesium represent intake from a pharmacological agent only and do not include intake from food and water.

[6] Although vanadium in food has not been shown to cause adverse effects in humans, there is no justification for adding vanadium to food and vanadium supplements should be used with caution. The UL is based on adverse effects in laboratory animals and these data could be used to set a UL for adults but not children or adolescents.

[7] ND = Not determinable due to lack of data on adverse effects in this age group and concern with regard to lack of ability to handle excess amounts. Source of intake should be from food only to prevent high levels of intake.

Sources: Data compiled from *Dietary Reference Intakes for Calcium, Phosphorus, Magnesium, Vitamin D, and Fluoride*. Washington, DC: National Academies Press; 1997. *Dietary Reference Intakes for Thiamin, Riboflavin, Niacin, Vitamin B$_6$, Folate, Vitamin B$_{12}$, Pantothenic Acid, Biotin, and Choline*. Washington, DC: National Academies Press; 1998. *Dietary Reference Intakes for Vitamin C, Vitamin E, Selenium, and Carotenoids*. Washington, DC: National Academies Press; 2000. Institute of Medicine, Food and Nutrition Board. *Dietary Reference Intakes for Vitamin A, Vitamin K, Arsenic, Boron, Chromium, Copper, Iron, Manganese, Molybdenum, Nickel, Silicon, Vanadium, and Zinc*. Washington, DC: National Academies Press; 2000. *Dietary Reference Intakes for Water, Potassium, Sodium, Chloride, and Sulfate*. Washington, DC: National Academies Press; 2005. These reports may be accessed via http://nap.edu.